DIAGNOSIS, SCREENING AND TREATMENT OF ABDOMINAL, THORACOABDOMINAL AND THORACIC AORTIC ANEURYSMS

Edited by **Reinhart T. Grundmann**

Diagnosis, Screening and Treatment of Abdominal, Thoracoabdominal and Thoracic Aortic Aneurysms
Edited by Reinhart T. Grundmann

Published by InTech

Janeza Trdine 9, 51000 Rijeka, Croatia

Publishing Process Manager Mirna Cvijic

Technical Editor Teodora Smiljanic

Cover Designer InTech Design Team

Additional hard copies can be obtained from orders@intechopen.com

Diagnosis, Screening and Treatment of Abdominal,
Thoracoabdominal and Thoracic Aortic Aneurysms, Edited by Reinhart T. Grundmann
p. cm.
978-953-307-466-5

For EU product safety concerns:
IN TECH d.o.o., Prolaz Marije Krucifikse Kozulić 3, 51000 Rijeka, Croatia,
info@intechopen.com or visit our website at intechopen.com.

Meet the editor

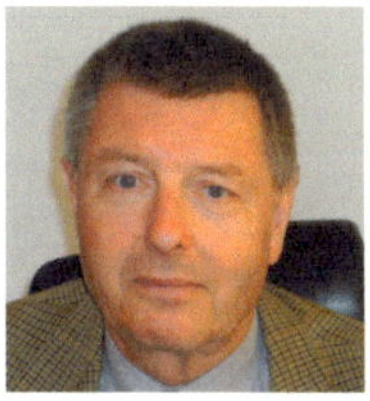

Dr. Reinhart T. Grundmann works currently as an independent medical expert. He is a professor of surgery at the University of Cologne and he has the qualification of general and vascular surgery. He is the former medical director of the B.Braun company, one of the leading providers of healthcare solutions. In the last eight years he has been working as the medical director of the Clinics Altotting-Burghausen, Germany. Dr. Grundmann was from 1992 until 2008 the managing director of the Zentralblatt fur Chirurgie and he is currently a member of the Editorial Board of World Journal of Gastrointestinal Surgery. He edited from 2001 to 2005 the Jahrbuch der Chirurgie- the book which provides an information on the latest developments in surgery. Dr. Grundmann already published more than 260 scientific publications, including books and the book chapters. His recent research interests lie in the field of efficiency and efectiveness in surgery. In this frame, he published a workflows on liver surgery, gastric cancer, obesity surgery and surgery for abdominal and carotide artery stenosis treatment.

Contents

Preface

This book considers mainly diagnosis, screening, surveillance and treatment of abdominal, thoracoabdominal and thoracic aortic aneurysms. It addresses vascular and cardiothoracic surgeons and interventional radiologists, but also anyone engaged in vascular medicine. The high mortality of ruptured aneurysms certainly favors the recommendation of prophylactic repair of asymptomatic aortic aneurysms (AA) and therewith a generous screening. However, the comorbidities of these patients and their age have to be kept in mind if the efficacy and cost effectiveness of screening and prophylactic surgery should not be overestimated. The treatment recommendations, which will be outlined here, have to regard on the one hand the natural course of the disease, the risk of rupture, and the life expectancy of the patient, and on the other hand the morbidity and mortality of the prophylactic surgical intervention. The book describes perioperative mortality after endovascular and open repair of AA, long-term outcome after repair, and the cost-effectiveness of treatment.

Prof. Dr. Reinhart T. Grundmann
Medical Expert
Burghausen, Germany

1

The Abdominal Aortic Aneurysm – Prognosis, Treatment, Screening and Cost-Effectiveness

Reinhart T. Grundmann
Formerly Kreiskliniken Altötting-Burghausen
Germany

1. Introduction

Mass screening is claimed for finding a disease in which symptoms are not yet occurred. The indication for such an examination is given if the early detection of the disease allows treatment with lower morbidity and mortality than treatment at an advanced stage. In addition, the long-term prognosis of the patients must be considered. Screening makes only sense if the overall mortality of a specific population can be diminished by the diagnostic and therapeutic measures. In assessing the screening for an asymptomatic abdominal aortic aneurysm (AAA) that has to be treated surgically to avoid the rupture of the AAA with its associated high fatality rate, the expected extension of life should be weighed against the risk of surgery. It must be ensured that the untreated disease would progress to rupture of the AAA with fatal outcome. The benefits of screening and subsequent prophylactic operation must be contrasted its risk and cost. It is the objective of the following remarks to outline the value of screening for AAA on the basis of studies on the prevalence of AAA, risk of rupture, and the results of surgical treatment. Meanwhile, two different approaches are available for the treatment of AAA, open repair and endovascular aneurysm repair (EVAR). The considerations for prophylactic repair of AAA must therefore also include morbidity and mortality of the two interventions and the evaluation of cost-benefit ratio. This will be shown in the following.

2. Prevalence of abdominal aortic aneurysm and mortality rate

Generally, an AAA is considered to be present when the minimum anterioposterior diameter of the aorta reaches 3.0 cm (Hirsch et al., 2006). The prevalence of AAA depends on various risk factors, as advancing age, family history, male gender, and tobacco use. According to the ACC/AHA guidelines (Hirsch et al., 2006) the prevalence of AAA 2.9 to 4.9 cm in diameter ranges from 1.3 % for men aged 45 to 54 years up to 12.5 % for men 75 to 84 years of age. Comparable prevalence figures for women are 0% and 5.2 %, respectively. Scott et al., 1995 reported in men and women aged 65-80 years a prevalence rate of 4 % overall and 7.6 % of men. Vardulaki et al., 1999 observed in two different areas the prevalence of AAA ranging between 5.3 % and 8% and between 6.18% and 9.88 %, respectively, in men aged between 65 and 79 years. In the Multicentre Aneurysm Screening Study (MASS) the prevalence in men aged 65-74 years was 4.9% (Ashton et al., 2002). In these studies the AAA was defined as an aortic diameter ≥ 3cm. If clinically important aneurysms are only taken into account (AAA measuring ≥ 4 cm in diameter) the indicated prevalence would be lower. Van Walraven et al., 2010 identified the prevalence of incidental AAA during imaging for other reasons. In 79,121 abdominal images 812 incidental AAA with a mean diameter of 4.0 cm (1% of all studies) were detected in patients with a mean age of 74 years. Lederle et al., 1997 reported the results of ultrasonography screening for AAA in 73,451 US veterans who were 50 to 79 years of age and had no history of AAA. The infrarenal aortic diameter was at least 4 cm in 1031 patients (1.4%), 368 patients (0.5%) had an AAA of 5 cm or larger. Smoking was the factor most closely associated with AAA in this study. In men who never smoked the prevalence of AAA 4 cm or larger was 0 % (patient age 50 to 59 years) and 0.8% (patient age > 75 years), respectively. The corresponding figures for men who smoked were 0.9 % and 2.7 %, respectively. A second cohort study of the Department of Veterans Affairs medical centers (Lederle et al., 2000) including 52,745 subjects aged 50 to 79 years confirmed the findings previously reported and supported the hypothesis that AAA is primarily a smoking-related disease. In this study AAA of 4.0 cm or larger were detected in 613 participants (1.2%). The excess prevalence associated with smoking accounted for approximately 75% of all AAA of 4.0 cm or larger. Smoking as a very strong risk factor for AAA was also proven by the Tromsø study (Forsdahl et al., 2009). When subjects who reported to have never been a daily smoker were compared with those who currently were smoking 20 cigarettes or more, the latter group had a > 13 times increased risk of an incident AAA during follow-up. In the women`s health initiative, an observational study involving 161,808 postmenopausal women, too, a strong positive association between smoking and clinically important AAA was found (Lederle et al., 2008). The prevalence defines the number of AAA present in a specific population during a particular point in time. This does not mean that these subjects will die of a ruptured aneurysm. Vardulaki et al., 1999 estimated the prevalence of AAA reaching around 10 % of the population at an age of 74 years, nevertheless in the year 1997 ruptured AAA caused not more than approximately 2.1 % of all deaths in men and 0.75 % of all deaths in women over the age of 65 in England and Wales. These data have not changed in the last 10 years; on the contrary, the mortality rate might be even decreasing. In the year 2009, 2415 men, 72.4 % of them being ≥ 75 years old, and 1239 women, 71.8 % of them being ≥ 80 years old, died of ruptured AAA in England and Wales (Office for National Statistics, 2011). In addition, 402 men and 184 women died of AAA without mention of rupture. With reference to 238,062 deaths in men and 253,286 in women, in 2009 therefore merely 1% of all deaths in men and 0.49 % in women were caused by ruptured AAA in England and Wales. Including the insufficiently defined cases, AAA caused 1.18% of all deaths in men and 0.56 % in women. In men 65 years of age or older, ruptured AAA caused 1.24 % of deaths and 1.45%, respectively, including the insufficiently defined cases. For the USA, 2,423,712 deaths are reported in the year 2007, including 12,986 deaths caused by all kinds of aortic aneurysms and dissections, not only AAA. 58.7 % of these patients were 75 years of age or older. These were 0.53% of all deaths, and 0.58% of the deaths in men and women over the age of 64 years, respectively (Xu et al., 2010). The small percentage of deaths due to AAA and the relatively old age of the population dying of ruptured AAA demonstrate the impossibility to increase significantly the median life expectancy of the total population by an untargeted mass screening for AAA (Dimick & Upchurch, 2003) and call for more sophisticated strategies, also for financial reasons.

3. Risk of rupture

The statements about the natural course of the disease and the risk of rupture are mainly based on the results of the randomized studies that compared immediate repair with surveillance for small AAA (Lederle et al., 2002; UK Small Aneurysm Trial Participants, 1998, 2002). The evidence report prepared for the Agency for Healthcare Research and Quality (AHRQ) analyzed these and further observational studies (Wilt et al., 2006). They came to the conclusion that the annual risk of rupture is 1% or lower for AAA less than 5.5 cm. The 1-year risk of rupture increases with aneurysm size and may exceed 10% in individuals with AAA > 6cm. For AAA that attain a size of > 8 cm, the risk may exceed 25 % at 6 months. Female sex, higher mean arterial blood pressure, current smoking, and poor lung function increase the risk of aneurysm rupture in addition to the size of initial AAA diameter (UK Small Aneurysm Trial Participants, 1999, 2002). A systematic review of the literature concluded that the rupture rate of small AAA with a diameter range 3.0-5.5 cm amounts to 0 to 1.61 ruptures per 100 person-years (Powell et al., 2011). These authors criticized that most studies have been poorly reported and did not have clear ascertainment and diagnostic criteria for aneurysm rupture. The inaccurate assessments of the risk of rupture might be due in part to the bimodal growth pattern of AAA observed by A.R. Thompson et al., 2010. They found nearly 50% of all aneurysms never progressing to surgery and rupture. Conversely, adjusted annual growth rates of at least 2 mm significantly predicted AAA-related events. In addition, medical treatment may influence the growth rate of AAA. Schlösser et al., 2008 reported for small AAA (initial AAA diameter between 3.0 and 5.5 cm) a rupture rate of 0.9 % per patient-year corresponding to the data mentioned above. The mean expansion rate of AAA was 2.5 mm / year in this study. Patients using lipid-lowering drugs had a 1.2 mm/ year lower AAA growth rate compared to non-users.

4. Treatment recommendations

In the absence of symptoms related to an aneurysm, the threat that the aneurysm will rupture is the major consideration. The treatment recommendations have to regard on the one hand the natural course of the disease, the risk of rupture, and the life expectancy of the patient, and on the other hand the morbidity and mortality of the prophylactic surgical intervention. The ACC/AHA guidelines give the following treatment recommendations (Hirsch et al., 2006): - Patients with AAA measuring 4.0 to 5.4 cm in diameter should be monitored by ultrasound or CT scans. - Patients with AAA measuring 5.5 cm or larger should undergo repair to eliminate the risk of rupture. - Intervention is not recommended for asymptomatic AAA measuring less than 5.0 cm in men or less than 4.5 cm in women. - Repair can be beneficial in patients with AAA measuring 5.0 to 5.4 cm in diameter. This latter recommendation is not based on the results of the trials that were cited (Lederle et al., 2002; UK Small Aneurysm Trial Participants, 2002). Both trials reported no benefit from repair of AAA less than 5.5 cm in diameter or in any subgroup of patients defined by aneurysm diameter at entry, a finding that directly refutes the ACC-AHA recommendation, for which no alternative justification is presented (Lederle et al., 2006). Survival was not improved by elective repair of AAA smaller than 5.5 cm compared with surveillance, even when operative mortality was low (Lederle et al., 2002; UK Small Aneurysm Trial Participants, 1998, 2002). In the UK Small Aneurysm Trial, even after 12 years of follow-up mortality in the surgery and surveillance groups actually did not differ (63.9% and 67.3 %, respectively) (Powell et al., 2007). A Cochrane review also found no overall benefit for early surgery of small AAA (4.0 to 5.5 cm) (Ballard et al., 2008). Here are the indications for endovascular aneurysm repair (EVAR) currently the same as for open repair. Under the hypothesis that the perioperative risk might be lower with EVAR compared to open repair, the PIVOTAL study has sought to determine whether EVAR for AAA measuring 4 to 5 cm in diameter compared to surveillance might be of benefit (Ouriel et al., 2010). Among patients randomized to treatment, 89% underwent aneurysm repair. Among patients randomized to surveillance, 31 % underwent aneurysm repair during the course of the study. Significant differences with respect to aneurysm rupture or aneurysm-related death could not be detected between both groups after a mean follow-up of 20 ± 12 months. EVAR and rigorous surveillance appeared to be equally safe alternatives for patients with small aneurysms, at least in the short-term run.

5. Perioperative mortality after endovascular and open repair of AAA

The evidence report prepared for the AHRQ (Wilt et al., 2006) compared EVAR with open repair in patients who were medically fit for open repair. The pooled 30-day mortality was 1.6 % for EVAR vs. 4.7 % for open repair of AAA. This may lead to the conclusion that endovascular repair is preferable to open repair with respect to the 30-day operative mortality. The conclusion is based mainly on the results of the EVAR 1 trial (Greenhalgh et al., 2004) and the DREAM study (Prinssen et al., 2004), which found a perioperative mortality for EVAR vs. open repair of 1.6% vs. 4.6%, and 1.2% vs. 4.6%, respectively. Later on, an additional 170 patients were enrolled in the EVAR 1 trial, with mortality at 30 days after surgery of 1.8% in the endovascular repair group and 4.3 % in the open repair group (United Kingdom EVAR Trial Investigators, 2010a). Also in the Veterans Affairs Cooperative Study, EVAR resulted in fewer perioperative deaths than open repair (0.5 % vs. 3.0%) (Lederle et al., 2009). In patients 67 years of age or older, a study with 22,830 matched patients in each cohort described a perioperative mortality after EVAR of 1.2 % vs. 4.8 % after open repair. The reduction in mortality with EVAR increased with patient age (2.1% difference for patients 67 to 69 years old to 8.5% for those 85 years of age or older) (Schermerhorn et al., 2008). Additional information provides a systematic review and meta-analysis of the literature including 28,862 patients. In this review, the pooled estimate for operative mortality with EVAR was 3.3% (95% confidence interval 2.9 to 3.6%) (Franks et al., 2007). In reverse, a meta-analysis considering 115,273 elective open AAA repairs mentioned a mean mortality rate of 5.56 %, with a significant relationship between higher surgeon caseload and lower mortality (E.L.Young et al., 2007). After all, the German national registry comprising 10,163 elective open repairs of AAA performed in 131 hospitals reported an overall perioperative mortality rate of 3.2% (Eckstein et al., 2007).

5.1 Long-term outcome after endovascular and open repair of AAA

Long-term outcome after aneurysm repair depends on the patient`s age, his risk factors and comorbidities. In the UK Small Aneurysm Trial, the death rate in these patients was about twice that in the general population matched for age and sex (Powell et al., 2007). Others found the long-term survival after elective AAA open repair similar to that in the general population, with a survival rate of 50.7 % and 31.5 % at 10 and 15 years after surgery. The main cause of death was cardiovascular disease (18.2%), followed by cancer (14.5%) (Vega de Céniga et al., 2010). In the Swedish Vascular Registry, crude long-term survival at 10 years after elective AAA repair was 33.8% for women and 40.4 % for men (Mani et al., 2009). Excluding AAA repair-related mortality, defined as death within 90 days after surgery, relative survival at 10 years after repair was 53.6 % for women and 72.2 % for men. Two randomized trials compared the long-term outcome after endovascular vs. open repair of AAA. In the UK EVAR 1 trial, after a median follow-up of 6.0 years 260/626 (41.5 %) patients had died in the EVAR group compared with 264/626 (42.2%) in the open repair group (United Kingdom EVAR Trial Investigators, 2010a). 76 of these 524 deaths were aneurysm related, 5.8% in the EVAR and 6.4% in the open repair group. This means that the early benefit of lower operative mortality in the EVAR group was completely lost in the longer term, with substantially higher aneurysm-related mortality in the EVAR group than in the open repair group during follow-up. In the DREAM study, too, no differences were seen between both procedures in total mortality or aneurysm-related mortality in the long-term run. Six years after randomization, the cumulative overall survival rates were 69.9% for open repair and 68.9 % for endovascular repair (De Bruin et al., 2010). In patients considered to be physically ineligible for open repair of AAA the survival rates are distinctly lower. In the EVAR 2 trial those patients were randomly assigned to undergo EVAR or to have no intervention (United Kingdom EVAR Trial Investigators, 2010b).The mean age of the patients was 76.8 ± 6.5 years, the mean aneurysm diameter was 6.7± 1.0 cm. After a median follow-up of 3.1 years, death from any cause was seen in 145/197 (73.6%) patients of the EVAR group and in 160/207 (77.3%) of the no repair group. Thus, EVAR as compared with no intervention did not lead to an improvement in overall survival, although the aneurysm-related mortality was significantly reduced by the intervention. (The overall aneurysm-related deaths were 25/197 (12.7%) in the EVAR group and 53/207 (25.6%) in the no repair group).

5.2 Reinterventions and readmissions after endovascular and open repair of AAA

Graft-related complications and reinterventions constitute an argument against endovascular repair. In the EVAR1 trial, the overall rates of graft-related complications and reinterventions were higher by a factor of three to four in the EVAR group than in the open repair group (United Kingdom EVAR Trial Investigators, 2010a). The rate of complications for all patients was 12.6 per 100 person-years in the endovascular repair group and 2.5 per 100 person-years in the open repair group. The DREAM study (De Bruin et al., 2010) reported six years after randomization cumulative rates of freedom from secondary interventions of 81.9% for open repair and 70.4 % for EVAR. After open repair, the most frequent reintervention was correction of an abdominal incision hernia, whereas EVAR reinterventions were most often performed because of endograft-related complications, such as endoleak and endograft migration. The French ACE trial compared EVAR and open repair in patients with AAA anatomically suitable for EVAR and at low-risk or intermediate-risk for open surgery (Becquemin et al., 2011). At 3 years of follow-up, there was no difference in in-hospital mortality or survival, however, the crude percentage of reinterventions was higher in the EVAR group than after open surgery (16% vs. 2.4%) with a trend toward a higher aneurysm-related mortality (4% vs. 0.7%). In this study, open repair of AAA proved to be as safe as EVAR in patients with low to intermediate risk factors, but remained a more durable option. In the two cohorts of Medicare beneficiaries described by Schermerhorn et al., 2008 late survival was similar after open repair as compared with EVAR, but late reinterventions related to AAA were more common after EVAR vs. open repair (9.0% vs. 1.7%). This higher reintervention rate was balanced by an increase in laparotomy-related reinterventions and hospitalizations after open repair (overall, at 4 years these interventions occurred in 4.1% of patients in the EVAR group and 9.7 % in the open repair group). This research team reported subsequently long-term results without any change in the conclusion (Giles et al., 2011). Through 6 years of follow-up, overall reinterventions or readmissions were slightly more common after EVAR vs. open repair (7.6 vs. 7.0/100 person-years). Reinterventions or readmissions accounted for 9.6% of all EVAR deaths and 7.6% of all open repair deaths in the follow-up period. The difference likely contributed to the erosion of the perioperative survival benefit of EVAR over time.

5.3 Cost-effectiveness of endovascular and open repair of AAA

A detailed cost analysis of EVAR and open repair was provided in the EVAR 1 trial (United Kingdom EVAR Trial Investigators, 2010a). The mean cost of the primary aneurysm repair was £13,019 in the EVAR group and £11,842 in the open repair group. During 8 years of follow-up, the mean cost of aneurysm-related readmissions was £2,283 in the EVAR group and £442 in the open repair group. The total average cost of aneurysm-related procedures in the EVAR group was £3,019 more than in the open repair group. A Health Technology Assessment (HTA) report analyzed the cost-effectiveness of endovascular repair of AAA in patients at varying levels of risk on the basis of six published decision models (Chambers et al., 2009). Both models considered relevant for the decision in the UK concluded that EVAR was not cost-effective on average compared with open repair at a threshold of £20,000 per quality adjusted life-year (QALY). Based on the results of this assessment of clinical effectiveness and cost-effectiveness, open repair should be the treatment of choice for patients with AAA who have good or moderate fitness. In subgroup analysis, EVAR was likely to be cost-effective in patients with a poor risk of operative mortality. In patients considered of very poor fitness or unfit of open repair, EVAR may be cost-effective at a threshold of £20,000 per QALY up to 77 years in patients with an 8 cm aneurysm, up to 74 years in patients with a 6 cm aneurysm, and up to 71.5 years in patients with a 5 cm aneurysm. Increasing the threshold to £30,000 per QALY increases the age at which EVAR is cost-effective by about 2 years. The HTA report (Chambers et al., 2009) besides concluded that EVAR cannot currently be recommended for the treatment of ruptured aneurysms. Hayes et al., 2010 came to the opposed argumentation. In their health economic model EVAR dominated open repair in the base case analysis, with a mean cumulative cost/patient of £17,422 for EVAR and £18,930 for open repair of acute (ruptured or symptomatic) AAA. In the emergency setting, EVAR was cost-effective compared with open repair at a threshold value of £20,000 to 30,000 per QALY.

5.3.1 Cost-effectiveness of surgery vs. surveillance in small aneurysms

Cost was analyzed in the UK Small Aneurysm Trial (Powell et al., 2007). After 12 years of follow-up, three-quarters of the surveillance group eventually had aneurysm repair. Estimates suggested that the cost of treatment was 17% higher in the early surgery group compared with the surveillance group, with a mean difference of £1326. In this trial, most of the patients underwent open aneurysm repair. Whether EVAR would be more cost effective in small aneurysms compared with surveillance was analyzed by K.C. Young et al., 2010 in a Markov model. The model demonstrated that early EVAR for 4.0 cm-5.4 cm AAA led to fewer QALYs at greater costs when compared with observational management and elective repair at 5.5 cm. From this data it must be concluded that in patients with small aneurysms surveillance is more cost effective than early surgery independently of the kind of surgical procedure.

6. Mortality of ruptured AAA (rAAA)

Heikkinen et al., 2002 assessed the mortality of rAAA in a defined geographic area. The mean annual incidence of rAAA was 6.3/100,000 inhabitants. Out of 221 patients presenting with rAAA, 82 (37%) died before arriving at hospital. 79.8 % of the admitted patients underwent emergency surgery. The overall hospital mortality was 63.3 %, including the nonadmitted cases the cumulative mortality of rAAA was 76.9 %. Similar ratios were observed by Qureshi et al., 2007. In this study, 48% (225/468) of patients with rAAA died before surgical repair (including the patients dying in the community). The 30-day perioperative mortality of rAAA was 43 % (105/243 patients), while overall mortality was 70% (330/468), including the deaths in the community. Filipovic et al., 2007 analyzed treatment and outcome after emergency hospital admission for rAAA in England. A total of 2463 women and 7615 men were admitted with a primary diagnosis of rAAA (mean age 79.8 and 74.9 years, respectively). Only 60% of patients underwent surgical repair (39.6 % of women and 66.4% of men). Overall, 75.6 % of women and 61.7 % of men died within 30 days of admission. McPhee et al., 2007 used the Nationwide Inpatient Sample of the USA to identify 37,016 patients presenting with rAAA between the years 2001 and 2004. In this analysis, too, women were less likely to undergo surgical intervention compared to men (59% vs. 70%). For those that underwent repair, women had higher in-hospital mortality rates than men (43% vs. 36%). A metaanalysis of 116 studies published between 1991 and 2006 and comprising 60,822 patients suggested that overall mortality of open repair for rAAA was 48.5 % and did not change significantly over the years (Hoornweg et al., 2008).

6.1 Endovascular vs. open repair of ruptured AAA

The question arises whether EVAR might be superior to open surgery for treatment of rAAA. No randomized trials could be identified so far by a Cochrane review to answer this issue (Dillon et al., 2007). There was no high quality evidence to support the use of emergency EVAR in the treatment of rAAA. Nevertheless, these authors assumed that in selected cases EVAR may be associated with a trend towards reduction in blood loss, duration of intensive care treatment, and mortality. This assumption is confirmed by a series of 104 consecutive patients with rAAA, of whom 25 underwent endovascular repair, and 79 open surgery (Ten Bosch et al., 2010). In this study the intraoperative, 30-day, and 6-month mortality was 4%, 20%, and 28% after EVAR compared with 6.1%, 45.5%, and 54.5% after open surgery. Davenport et al., 2010 examined the National Surgical Quality Improvement Program database from the years 2005 to 2007 to compare 30-day multicenter outcomes for endovascular vs. open repair of rAAA. After adjustment for preoperative mortality risk factors, the mortality risk was higher for open repair vs. EVAR but did not reach significance. However, composite 30-day morbidity risk was significantly lower after EVAR vs. open repair of rAAA. Open repair was associated with increased transfusion requirements. Veith et al., 2009 argued that EVAR has a lower procedural mortality at 30 days than open repair at least in selected cases and that EVAR is better than open repair for treating patients with rAAA provided they have favorable anatomy. In this collected experience with use of endovascular repair in 1037 patients with rAAA overall 30-day mortality after EVAR was 21.2%. Centers performing EVAR for rAAA whenever possible, did so in 28% to 79% of their patients, and had a 30-day mortality of 19.7% for 680 EVAR patients and 36.3 % for 763 open repair patients. In addition, outcome following endovascular and open repair of rAAA was evaluated by Giles et al., 2009 interrogating the

Nationwide Inpatient Sample database to identify all repairs between 2000 and 2005 for rAAA. In the study period, 2323 patients (1794 men; median age 75 years) with rAAA had endovascular repair, while 26,106 patients (20,311 men; median age 73 years) had an open procedure. Overall mortality after rAAA repair was 40.8%, 32.6% for endovascular and 41.5% for open repair. Mortality after EVAR was significantly lower than after open surgery for patients ≥70 years (36% vs. 47%), but not for those <70 years (24% vs. 30%). McPhee et al., 2009 used the same database for the years 2001- 2006. They as well demonstrated lower overall in-hospital mortality for EVAR than open repair of rAAA (31.7% vs. 40.7%). The survival benefit of EVAR over open repair was amplified by institutional volume. Higher elective open repair as well as rAAA volume increased the mortality advantage for EVAR.

6.2 Long-term outcome after repair of ruptured AAA

In the Swedish Vascular Registry (Mani et al., 2009) the 10-year crude survival after rAAA repair was 13.2 % in women and 24.9 % in men; the relative survival, excluding AAA repair-related mortality, was 46% and 68.4%, respectively. Schlösser et al., 2010 have quantified the age-and gender-specific mortality risks for 1,463 patients hospitalized for rAAA. Mean age was 79 years in women and 72 years in men. Mortality risks at 28-day, 1-year, and 5-year increased significantly with age (28-day: from 36 to 91 % in men, and 59 to 92% in women; 5-year: from 51 to 97% in men and 79 to 96 % in women). In patients aged <80 years, mortality risks were significantly higher in women than in men. Cerebrovascular disease and previous hospitalization for congestive heart failure were significant predictors of short- and long-term mortality. It must remain an open question whether a prophylactic aneurysm repair before rupture would have had a major influence on the life expectancy of these patients.

7. Screening for AAA

The essential findings regarding screening are subsumed in a Cochrane review on the basis of four completed randomized controlled studies (Cosford & Leng, 2007). These were conducted in Chichester, UK (Scott et al., 1995), in the UK (Multicentre Aneurysm Screening Study) (MASS) (Ashton et al., 2002), in Perth, Western Australia (Norman et al., 2004), and in Viborg, Denmark (Lindholt et al., 2005). In these trials, 15,775 men and women aged 65 to 80 years (Chichester), 67,800 men aged 65 to 74 years (MASS), 41,000 men aged 65 to 83 years (Western Australia), and 12,639 men aged 64 to 73 (Viborg) were randomly allocated to ultrasound screening for AAA or no intervention. The Cochrane review concluded that, in summary of the results, there was a significant reduction in mortality from AAA in men aged 65 to 79 years who undergo ultrasound screening (odds ratio (OR) 0.60; 95% Confidence Interval (CI) 0.47 to 0.78). There was insufficient evidence to demonstrate benefit in women (Cosford & Leng, 2007). All-cause mortality was not significantly different between screened and unscreened groups three to five years after screening (men, OR 0.95; 95% CI 0.85 to 1.07); women, OR 1.06; 95% CI 0.93 to 1.21). This had been expected given the relative infrequency of AAA as a cause of death. Meanwhile the final results of the Chichester study have been reported (Ashton et al., 2007) with respect to 6040 men randomized to ultrasound screening or to the control group. Screening detected an AAA in 170 patients. In the group of men invited for screening, AAA-related mortality was reduced over a median 15-year follow-up period from 1.8 to 1.6 %, although the results were not significant for this population size. A mortality benefit from screening men aged 65 to 74 years for AAA was seen in MASS over 10 years of follow-up (S.G. Thompson et al., 2009). In this trial 33,883 men were invited to screening and 27,204 (80%) attended. 1334 aneurysms ≥ 3.0 cm were detected at initial scan. Patients were referred to a hospital for possible elective surgery when the aneurysm reached 5.5 cm, the aneurysm had expanded by 1cm or more in one year, or symptoms attributable to the AAA were reported. Surveillance involved rescanning: annually for those with AAA diameters of 3.0 - 4.4 cm and every three months for those with diameters of 4.5 to 5.4 cm. Over the 10 years of the trial 552 elective operations took place in the invited group and 226 in the control group. Overall, 155 deaths related to AAA (absolute risk 0.46 %) occurred in the invited group and 296 (0.87%) in the control group. Total mortality, however, did not differ significantly between both groups (30.3 % in the invited group and 30.9% in the control group, respectively), because deaths from AAA comprised only about 2% of all deaths. A comparable long-term benefit was observed in the Viborg trial. The relative risk reduction of the screening program in AAA-related mortality was 66%, but the risk reduction in all-cause mortality amounted merely 2% (Lindholt et al., 2010). The number needed to screen to save one life was 352 (Lindholt et al., 2005). Pooled mid-term and long-term effects of screening on AAA-related and total mortality were examined by Lindholt & Norman, 2008 in a meta-analysis including new data not considered in the Cochrane review (Cosford & Leng, 2007). Screening offered a significant mid-term reduction in AAA-related mortality. In addition, all-cause mortality was reduced after 3 to 5 years, but not significantly. The long-term results showed a significant reduction in AAA-related mortality and overall mortality. A significantly greater number of elective operations, and significantly fewer emergency operations were also noticed in the invited group compared to the controls. An updated meta-analysis of randomized controlled trials of AAA screening in men aged ≥ 65 years revealed also a strong trend toward a significant benefit provided by screening. Screening for AAA showed a reduction in all-cause long-term mortality by 5 per 1000 compared with controls (number needed to screen to save one life was 217) (Takagi et al., 2010a). The recommendations of the U.S. Preventive Services Task Force (USPSTF) are consistent with the results of the studies mentioned. One-time screening for AAA by ultrasonography in men aged 65 to 75 years who have ever smoked is recommended (grade B recommendation). No recommendation is made for or against screening for AAA in men age 65 to 75 years who have never smoked (grade C recommendation). The USPSTF recommends against routine screening for AAA in women (grade D recommendation) (U.S. Preventive Services Task Force, 2005). The Society for Vascular Surgery (SVS) greatly expanded these recommendations (Chaikof et al., 2009) in contrast to the USPSTF. The SVS recommends one time ultrasound screening for AAA for all men at or older than age 65, or as early as age 55 years for those with a family history of AAA (Level of recommendation: strong. Quality of evidence: high). One-time ultrasound screening for AAA is recommended for all women at or older than 65 years with a family history of AAA or who have smoked (Level of recommendation: strong. Quality of evidence: moderate). As a direct consequence of these recommendations the Screen Abdominal Aortic Aneurysms Very Efficiently (SAAAVE) Act is effective in the USA since January 2007. Medicare beneficiaries have access to a free, one-time ultrasound screening to check for AAA. The screening will be available for men who have smoked at least 100 cigarettes during their life, and men and women with a family history of AAA. On this basis, a total of 2918 veteran males 65 to 75 years of age (average age, 71 +/- 6 years) were screened for AAA over a 1-year period (Lee et al., 2009). An AAA was diagnosed in 5.1% (148/2918) of patients. The majority of aneurysms (83%)

were small (3.0 - 4.4 cm). A clear-cut indication for prophylactic repair (aneurysm diameter > 5.5 cm) was given in 4.1 % (6/148) of aneurysms and 0.2 % of patients, respectively. The NHS in the UK also announced an AAA screening program being introduced gradually across England from spring 2009. Once fully implemented, the program will invite all men for screening during the year that they turn 65. Depending on the results from the scan surveillance imaging (follow-up scan) will be offered in a year for patients with an AAA of 3 to 4.4 cm, and in three months for patients with an aortic diameter of 4.5 to 5.4 cm. Men with a large aneurysm of over 5.5 cm are referred to a consultant vascular surgeon to discuss treatment (NHS Abdominal Aortic Aneurysm Screening Programme, 2011).

7.1 Aneurysm surveillance/ rescreening

The optimal frequency of aneurysm surveillance has not been defined by randomized clinical studies. The SVS (Chaikof et al., 2009) recommends the following procedure. Re-screening patients for AAA is not recommended if an initial ultrasound scan performed on patients 65 years of age or older demonstrates an aortic diameter of < 2.6 cm (Level of recommendation: strong. Quality of evidence: moderate). Follow-up imaging at 5-year intervals is recommended for patients with a maximum aortic diameter between 2.6 and 2.9 cm (Level of recommendation: weak. Quality of evidence: low). Follow-up imaging at 3 years is recommended for patients with an AAA between 3.0 and 3.4 cm (Level of recommendation: strong. Quality of evidence: low). Surveillance imaging at 12-month intervals is recommended for patients with an AAA of 3.5 to 4.4 cm (Level of recommendation: strong. Quality of evidence: low). Surveillance imaging at 6-month intervals is recommended for patients with an AAA of 4.5 to 5.4 cm (Level of recommendation: strong. Quality of evidence: low).

7.2 Cost effectiveness of screening for AAA

The high mortality of rAAA, particularly when the patients who die before surgical repair are considered and not exclusively the procedure related mortality, certainly favors the recommendation of prophylactic repair of asymptomatic AAA and therewith a generous screening. However, the comorbidities of these patients and their age have to be kept in mind if the efficacy and cost effectiveness of screening and prophylactic surgery should not be overestimated.The cost effectiveness of ultrasound screening for AAA has been assessed in several studies. In MASS, the adjusted mean additional cost per patient screened was £ 63.4 at 4 years follow-up (Multicentre Aneurysm Screening Study Group, 2002). 47 fewer deaths related to AAA were observed in the screening group than in the control group at total additional costs of £ 2.2m. Over 4 years the estimated mean incremental cost effectiveness ratio for screening was £ 28,400 per life year gained. Because the main costs of the program (initial screening and elective surgery for those with aneurysm diameter > 5.5 cm) occur early on, whereas the benefit in terms of life years increases over time, the cost per life year gained was estimated to fall around £ 8000 after 10 years. This estimation was confirmed later on. The extent of reduction in number of deaths related to AAA in the invited group led to an estimated incremental cost effectiveness ratio of £ 7600 per life year gained over the 10 years of the trial (S.G. Thompson et al., 2009). The cost effectiveness of screening for AAA was also estimated in the Viborg trial. The costs per life year saved were Euro 9057 after 5 years (Lindholt et al., 2006). In the long-term run screening was found to be even more cost effective, at a probability above 0.97 for a willingness to pay threshold of

Euro 5000 (Lindholt et al., 2010). In contrast, the cost effectiveness of screening Danish men aged 65 for AAA was rejected by Ehlers et al., 2009a. They developed a decision tree and Markov model to simulate the short-term and long-term effects of screening for AAA. In this analysis, the incremental cost effectiveness ratio varied from £32,640 to £ 66,001 per QALY with a mean cost of £43 485. At a willingness to pay threshold of £30,000 the probability of screening being cost effective was less than 30%. Their study contradicted the widespread conception that screening for AAA is cheap. A possible reason for the discrepancy between this study and that by S.G. Thompson et al., 2009 might be that the MASS results (S.G. Thompson et al., 2009) reflect a sample group screened at age 65-74. Ehlers et al., 2009a, however, have directly modeled the effects of the current policy of inviting men aged 65 to participate in a screening program, what is fundamentally different from a one-time screening of all elderly men (Buxton, 2009; Ehlers et al. 2009b). This latter approach will benefit from a higher prevalence of AAA and thus show a better cost effectiveness (Ehlers et al. 2009b). Ehlers et al., 2009a emphasized that ultrasonography may be cheap on a per person basis, but screening is not just a test but a program. If screening is to be effective then overall administration of the program, operational planning, a communication strategy, a quality assurance system, and more are needed. Hoffmann et al., 2009 assessed routine screening for asymptomatic AAA in high-risk patients in an emergency department. The sonographers were able to completely visualize and correctly measure the abdominal aortas of only 71% of patients. AAA ultrasonography performance varied markedly among sonographers, depending on training and experience (Hoffmann et al., 2010). Even in a special aortic screening program, out of 2918 patients 9.9 % were inappropriately screened (Lee et al., 2009). How the quality of ultrasonography influences the cost effectiveness of screening programs has to be carefully monitored. In all published decision analytic models of AAA screening, patients with an AAA ≥ 5.5 cm were assumed to face a constant probability of rupture no matter how many years they have had a large AAA (Ehlers et al., 2008). If all men are screened in the year that they turn 65 the calculated number of gained life years due to screening could be overestimated as the age of males dying of ruptured AAA is well over 65 years (72.4 % of men who died in 2009 of ruptured AAA in England and Wales were ≥ 75 years old, see above). In MASS, the mean age of the men who died at 10-year follow-up was 74.7 years in both, invited group and control group, respectively. These findings did not suggest any major general differences in health care between the groups as a result of screening (S.G. Thompson et al., 2009). In addition, economic evaluations did not incorporate evidence that the lives of tobacco smokers are generally shorter than those of the general population (> 90% of patients with AAA have a history of smoking) (Ehlers et al., 2008). MASS found an association between AAA death and participation in the AAA screening program, but life-style issues were not controlled. The gained life years could be due to other things than surgery such as smoking cessation and further life-style changes (Ehlers et al., 2009b). In this context it should be noted that statin therapy was not analyzed in the cost effectiveness studies. The use of statins seems to slow the growth of small aneurysms and to improve freedom from aneurysm repair and rupture (Schouten et al., 2006; Mosorin et al., 2008; Takagi et al., 2010b). If these results should be confirmed in randomized studies, the recommendations for small aneurysm repair would have to be modified and the cost effectiveness of screening would be diminished. Moreover, the introduction of EVAR could have a negative impact on cost effectiveness of screening what must be evaluated in the future. Provided that screening and/or repair are employed on a much wider scale than occurred in the trials, the ratio of benefit to harm would be reduced or even reversed. EVAR is assumed to be a moderately risky procedure, if screening leads to a large increase in elective EVAR in patients whose AAA would never have ruptured, the expected benefit of screening on AAA-related mortality may never be realized (Lederle, 2008). Instead screening all men during the year that they turn 65, a selective screening might be more cost effective. Mani et al., 2010 evaluated the long-term outcome and the cost effectiveness of selective AAA screening among patients referred to the vascular laboratory for arterial examination. An AAA was detected in 181 of 5924 (3%) patients (mean age 72.8 years), of whom 21.5% underwent elective repair (perioperative mortality 5.1%) after 7.5 years of follow-up. In this analysis, screening was cost effective (11,084 Euro/life year gained) which suggests that screening patients with atherosclerotic disease, rather than the whole population, might be more cost effective (Greenhalgh, 2004).

8. Conclusion

The available data have proven the benefit of screening with respect to a reduction of AAA-related mortality. One-time screening for AAA by ultrasonography in men aged 65 to 75 years who have ever smoked is therefore recommended (U.S. Preventive Services Task Force, 2005). Whether these recommendations should be further extended as suggested by the Society for Vascular Surgery (Chaikof et al., 2009) is debatable. So far, the risk reduction in all-cause mortality by screening is small. Changes in the management of ruptured and non-ruptured aneurysms such as EVAR might have a significant impact on efficiency and cost effectiveness of screening programs that is not elucidated. Some doubts remain with respect to the NHS screening program (Johnson, 2008) inviting all men for screening during the year that they turn 65. At least for smaller aneurysms the risk of rupture is difficult to estimate. Statins and other new treatments are expected to decelerate the growth of small aneurysms found by screening. The mortality of prophylactic AAA repair can be greater than the likelihood of rupture. Operative results of hospitals are central to whether screening saves or looses lives (Greenhalgh & Powell, 2007). Operative mortality may be lower with EVAR compared with open repair; however, EVAR comprises frequent follow-up examinations. In addition, reinterventions which impair patient's quality of life are more common after EVAR than after open repair. People who have been screened and found to have an aorta that is dilated less than 5.5 cm, will be condemned to six monthly or annual ultrasound examinations to estimate the size of the aneurysm. These people have felt comfortable as long as they were not informed about the diagnosis; the impact of the knowledge of the diagnosis on quality of life is scarcely investigated. The demand for national screening programs concerns not only patients with a possible indication for operation but also the much greater group of persons in whom the size of the aneurysm is small and constitutes no indication for treatment (and will never be so). Johnson, 2008 claims rightly, that persons taking the test will need intensive counseling about the possible consequences that screening might have for their future lives and psychological wellbeing. The psychological consequences of screening were described by Lindholt et al., 2000. Quality of life was lower among men with a small AAA compared to the controls and declined further below control values during the period of conservative treatment. Diagnosis of an AAA impaired quality of life permanently and progressively in conservatively treated patients, anything but surprising, since a cohort of patients find it intolerable to have what they often describe as a "time bomb inside" them (Johnson, 2008). As far as cost effectiveness of screening for AAA is concerned, the society in question has to decide whether £ 7600 up to more than £ 44,000 per life year gained is adequate. In the case of limited resources it is justified to ask whether the funds should be used for search of an asymptomatic disease or whether it would be better to invest in prophylactic measures like smoking cessation. The lack of attention that smoking cessation receives in some primary and specialist settings is a concern; > 90% of patients with AAA have a history of smoking. Nicotine replacement therapy and brief counseling by physicians costs around US $ 2000 to 6000 per life year saved compared with no treatment (Lancet, 2009). These caveats emphasize that costs and outcomes of screening for AAA need to be carefully monitored.

9. References

Ashton HA, Buxton MJ, Day NE, Kim LG, Marteau TM, Scott RA, Thompson SG & Walker NM; Multicentre Aneurysm Screening Study Group. (2002). The Multicentre Aneurysm Screening Study (MASS) into the effect of abdominal aortic aneurysm screening on mortality in men: a randomised controlled trial. *Lancet* 360(9345):1531-1539

Ashton HA, Gao L, Kim LG, Druce PS, Thompson SG & Scott RA. (2007). Fifteen-year follow-up of a randomized clinical trial of ultrasonographic screening for abdominal aortic aneurysms. *Br J Surg* 94(6): 696-701

Ballard DJ, Filardo G, Fowkes G & Powell JT. (2008). Surgery for small asymptomatic abdominal aortic aneurysms. *Cochrane Database Syst Rev* 8; (4): CD001835

Becquemin JP, Pillet JC, Lescalie F, Sapoval M, Goueffic Y, Lermusiaux P, Steinmetz E & Marzelle J; ACE trialists.(2011). A randomized controlled trial of endovascular aneurysm repair versus open surgery for abdominal aortic aneurysms in low- to moderate-risk patients. *J Vasc Surg* 53(5): 1167-1173

Buxton MJ. (2009). Screening for abdominal aortic aneurysm. *BMJ* 338:b2185

Chaikof EL, Brewster DC, Dalman RL, Makaroun MS, Illig KA, Sicard GA, Timaran CH, Upchurch GR Jr & Veith FJ; Society for Vascular Surgery.(2009). The care of patients with an abdominal aortic aneurysm: the Society for Vascular Surgery practice guidelines. J Vasc Surg 50 (4 Suppl): S2-49

Chambers D, Epstein D, Walker S, Fayter D, Paton F, Wright K, Michaels J, Thomas S, Sculpher M & Woolacott N. (2009). Endovascular stents for abdominal aortic aneurysms: a systematic review and economic model. *Health Technol Assess* 13(48): 1-189, 215-318, iii

Cosford PA & Leng GC. (2007). Screening for abdominal aortic aneurysm. *Cochrane Database Syst Rev* (2): CD002945

Davenport DL, O'Keeffe SD, Minion DJ, Sorial EE, Endean ED & Xenos ES. (2010). Thirty-day NSQIP database outcomes of open versus endoluminal repair of ruptured abdominal aortic aneurysms. *J Vasc Surg* 51(2): 305-309.e1

De Bruin JL, Baas AF, Buth J, Prinssen M, Verhoeven EL, Cuypers PW, van Sambeek MR, Balm R, Grobbee DE & Blankensteijn JD; DREAM Study Group.(2010). Long-term outcome of open or endovascular repair of abdominal aortic aneurysm. *N Engl J Med* 362(20): 1881-1889

Dillon M, Cardwell C, Blair PH, Ellis P, Kee F & Harkin DW. (2007). Endovascular treatment for ruptured abdominal aortic aneurysm. *Cochrane Database Syst Rev* (1): CD005261

Dimick JB, Upchurch GR Jr. (2003). The quality of care for patients with abdominal aortic aneurysms. *Cardiovasc Surg* 11(5): 331-336

Eckstein HH, Bruckner T, Heider P, Wolf O, Hanke M, Niedermeier HP, Noppeney T, Umscheid T & Wenk H. (2007). The relationship between volume and outcome following elective open repair of abdominal aortic aneurysms (AAA) in 131 German hospitals. *Eur J Vasc Endovasc Surg* 34(3): 260-266

Ehlers L, Sørensen J, Jensen LG, Bech M & Kjølby M. (2008). Is population screening for abdominal aortic aneurysm cost-effective? *BMC Cardiovasc Disord* 8: 32

Ehlers L, Overvad K, Sørensen J, Christensen S, Bech M & Kjølby M. (2009a). Analysis of cost effectiveness of screening Danish men aged 65 for abdominal aortic aneurysm. *BMJ* 338: b2243

Ehlers L, Kjølby M, Christensen S, Bech M, Overvad K & Sørensen J. (2009b). The Danish health economic modelling study on AAA screening is not flawed. Rapid response to: Analysis of cost effectiveness of screening Danish men aged 65 for abdominal aortic aneurysm. *BMJ* 338: b2243

Filipovic M, Seagroatt V & Goldacre MJ. (2007). Differences between women and men in surgical treatment and case fatality rates for ruptured aortic abdominal aneurysm in England. *Br J Surg* 94(9): 1096-1099

Forsdahl SH, Singh K, Solberg S & Jacobsen BK. (2009). Risk factors for abdominal aortic aneurysms: a 7-year prospective study: the Tromsø Study, 1994-2001. *Circulation* 119(16): 2202-2208

Franks SC, Sutton AJ, Bown MJ & Sayers RD. (2007). Systematic review and meta-analysis of 12 years of endovascular abdominal aortic aneurysm repair. *Eur J Vasc Endovasc Surg* 33(2): 154-171

Giles KA, Hamdan AD, Pomposelli FB, Wyers MC, Dahlberg SE & Schermerhorn ML. (2009). Population-based outcomes following endovascular and open repair of ruptured abdominal aortic aneurysms. *J Endovasc Ther* 16(5): 554-564

Giles KA, Landon BE, Cotterill P, O'Malley AJ, Pomposelli FB & Schermerhorn ML. (2011). Thirty-day mortality and late survival with reinterventions and readmissions after open and endovascular aortic aneurysm repair in Medicare beneficiaries. *J Vasc Surg* 53(1): 6-12,13.e1

Greenhalgh RM. (2004). National screening programme for aortic aneurysm. *BMJ* 328(7448): 1087-1088

Greenhalgh RM, Brown LC, Kwong GP, Powell JT & Thompson SG; EVAR trial participants. (2004). Comparison of endovascular aneurysm repair with open repair in patients with abdominal aortic aneurysm (EVAR trial 1), 30-day operative mortality results: randomised controlled trial. *Lancet* 364(9437): 843-848

Greenhalgh R, Powell J. (2007). Screening for abdominal aortic aneurysm. *BMJ* 335(7623): 732-733

Hayes PD, Sadat U, Walsh SR, Noorani A, Tang TY, Bowden DJ, Gillard JH & Boyle JR. (2010). Cost-effectiveness analysis of endovascular versus open surgical repair of acute abdominal aortic aneurysms based on worldwide experience. *J Endovasc Ther* 17(2): 174-182

Heikkinen M, Salenius JP & Auvinen O.(2002). Ruptured abdominal aortic aneurysm in a well-defined geographic area. *J Vasc Surg* 36(2): 291-296

Hirsch AT, Haskal ZJ, Hertzer NR, Bakal CW, Creager MA, Halperin JL, Hiratzka LF, Murphy WR, Olin JW, Puschett JB, Rosenfield KA, Sacks D, Stanley JC, Taylor LM Jr, White CJ, White J, White RA, Antman EM, Smith SC Jr, Adams CD, Anderson JL, Faxon DP, Fuster V, Gibbons RJ, Halperin JL, Hiratzka LF, Hunt SA, Jacobs AK,

Nishimura R, Ornato JP, Page RL & Riegel B. (2006). ACC/AHA 2005 guidelines for the management of patients with peripheral arterial disease (lower extremity, renal, mesenteric, and abdominal aortic): executive summary a collaborative report from the American Association for Vascular Surgery/Society for Vascular Surgery, Society for Cardiovascular Angiography and Interventions, Society for Vascular Medicine and Biology, Society of Interventional Radiology, and the ACC/AHA Task Force on Practice Guidelines (Writing Committee to Develop Guidelines for the Management of Patients With Peripheral Arterial Disease) endorsed by the American Association of Cardiovascular and Pulmonary Rehabilitation; National Heart, Lung, and Blood Institute; Society for Vascular Nursing; TransAtlantic Inter-Society Consensus; and Vascular Disease Foundation. *J Am Coll Cardiol* 47(6): 1239-1312

Hoffmann B, Um P, Bessman ES, Ding R, Kelen GD & McCarthy ML. (2009). Routine screening for asymptomatic abdominal aortic aneurysm in high-risk patients is not recommended in emergency departments that are frequently crowded. *Acad Emerg Med* 16(11): 1242-1250

Hoffmann B, Bessman ES, Um P, Ding R & McCarthy ML. (2011). Successful sonographic visualisation of the abdominal aorta differs significantly among a diverse group of credentialed emergency department providers. *Emerg Med J* 28(6): 472 - 476

Hoornweg LL, Storm-Versloot MN, Ubbink DT, Koelemay MJ, Legemate DA & Balm R.(2008). Meta analysis on mortality of ruptured abdominal aortic aneurysms. *Eur J Vasc Endovasc Surg* 35(5): 558-570

Johnson JN.(2008). Should we screen for aortic aneurysm? No. *BMJ* 336(7649): 863

Lancet. (2009). Editorial: Cardiologists should be less passive about smoking cessation *Lancet* 373(9667): 867

Lederle FA, Johnson GR, Wilson SE, Chute EP, Littooy FN, Bandyk D, Krupski WC, Barone GW, Acher CW & Ballard DJ. (1997). Prevalence and associations of abdominal aortic aneurysm detected through screening. Aneurysm Detection and Management (ADAM) Veterans Affairs Cooperative Study Group. *Ann Intern Med* 126(6): 441-449

Lederle FA, Johnson GR, Wilson SE, Chute EP, Hye RJ, Makaroun MS, Barone GW, Bandyk D, Moneta GL & Makhoul RG. (2000). The aneurysm detection and management study screening program: validation cohort and final results. Aneurysm Detection and Management Veterans Affairs Cooperative Study Investigators. *Arch Intern Med* 160(10): 1425-1430

Lederle FA, Wilson SE, Johnson GR, Reinke DB, Littooy FN, Acher CW, Ballard DJ, Messina LM, Gordon IL, Chute EP, Krupski WC, Busuttil SJ, Barone GW, Sparks S, Graham LM, Rapp JH, Makaroun MS, Moneta GL, Cambria RA, Makhoul RG, Eton D, Ansel HJ, Freischlag JA & Bandyk D; Aneurysm Detection and Management Veterans Affairs Cooperative Study Group. (2002). Immediate repair compared with surveillance of small abdominal aortic aneurysms. *N Engl J Med* 346(19): 1437-1444

Lederle FA, Powell JT & Greenhalgh RM. (2006). Repair of small abdominal aortic aneurysms. *N Engl J Med* 354(14): 1537-1538

Lederle FA. (2008). Screening for AAA in the USA. *Scand J Surg* 97(2): 139-141

Lederle FA, Larson JC, Margolis KL, Allison MA, Freiberg MS, Cochrane BB, Graettinger WF & Curb JD; Women's Health Initiative Cohort Study. (2008). Abdominal aortic aneurysm events in the women's health initiative: cohort study. *BMJ* 337: a1724

Lederle FA, Freischlag JA, Kyriakides TC, Padberg FT Jr, Matsumura JS, Kohler TR, Lin PH, Jean-Claude JM, Cikrit DF, Swanson KM & Peduzzi PN; Open Versus Endovascular Repair (OVER) Veterans Affairs Cooperative Study Group. (2009). Outcomes following endovascular vs open repair of abdominal aortic aneurysm: a randomized trial. *JAMA* 302(14): 1535-1542

Lee ES, Pickett E, Hedayati N, Dawson DL & Pevec WC. (2009). Implementation of an aortic screening program in clinical practice: implications for the Screen For Abdominal Aortic Aneurysms Very Efficiently (SAAAVE) Act. *J Vasc Surg* 49(5): 1107-1111

Lindholt JS, Vammen S, Fasting H, Henneberg EW. (2000). Psychological consequences of screening for abdominal aortic aneurysm and conservative treatment of small abdominal aortic aneurysms. *Eur J Vasc Endovasc Surg* 20(1): 79-83

Lindholt JS, Juul S, Fasting H & Henneberg EW. (2005). Screening for abdominal aortic aneurysms: single centre randomised controlled trial. *BMJ* 330(7494): 750

Lindholt JS, Juul S, Fasting H & Henneberg EW. (2006). Cost-effectiveness analysis of screening for abdominal aortic aneurysms based on five year results from a randomised hospital based mass screening trial. *Eur J Vasc Endovasc Surg* 32(1): 9-15

Lindholt JS & Norman P. (2008). Screening for abdominal aortic aneurysm reduces overall mortality in men. A meta-analysis of the mid- and long-term effects of screening for abdominal aortic aneurysms. *Eur J Vasc Endovasc Surg* 36(2): 167-171

Lindholt JS, Sørensen J, Søgaard R & Henneberg EW. (2010). Long-term benefit and cost-effectiveness analysis of screening for abdominal aortic aneurysms from a randomized controlled trial. *Br J Surg* 97(6): 826-834

Mani K, Björck M, Lundkvist J & Wanhainen A. (2009). Improved long-term survival after abdominal aortic aneurysm repair. *Circulation* 120(3): 201-211

Mani K, Alund M, Björck M, Lundkvist J, Wanhainen A. (2010). Screening for abdominal aortic aneurysm among patients referred to the vascular laboratory is cost-effective. *Eur J Vasc Endovasc Surg* 39(2): 208-216

McPhee JT, Hill JS & Eslami MH. (2007). The impact of gender on presentation, therapy, and mortality of abdominal aortic aneurysm in the United States, 2001-2004. *J Vasc Surg* 45(5): 891-899

McPhee J, Eslami MH, Arous EJ, Messina LM & Schanzer A. (2009). Endovascular treatment of ruptured abdominal aortic aneurysms in the United States (2001-2006): a significant survival benefit over open repair is independently associated with increased institutional volume. *J Vasc Surg* 49(4): 817-826

Mosorin M, Niemelä E, Heikkinen J, Lahtinen J, Tiozzo V, Satta J, Juvonen T & Biancari F. (2008). The use of statins and fate of small abdominal aortic aneurysms. *Interact Cardiovasc Thorac Surg* 7(4): 578-581

Multicentre Aneurysm Screening Study Group. (2002). Multicentre aneurysm screening study (MASS): cost effectiveness analysis of screening for abdominal aortic aneurysms based on four year results from randomised controlled trial. *BMJ* 325(7373): 1135

NHS Abdominal Aortic Aneurysm Screening Programme. February 2011. Available from http://aaa.screening.nhs.uk/cms.php?folder=2436

Norman PE, Jamrozik K, Lawrence-Brown MM, Le MT, Spencer CA, Tuohy RJ, Parsons RW & Dickinson JA. (2004). Population based randomised controlled trial on impact of screening on mortality from abdominal aortic aneurysm. *BMJ* 329(7477): 1259

Office for National Statistics. Mortality statistics. Review of the national statistician on deaths in England and Wales, 2009. February 2011. Available from www.statistics.gov.uk/downloads/theme_health/dr2009/dr-09.pdf

Ouriel K, Clair DG, Kent KC & Zarins CK; Positive Impact of Endovascular Options for treating Aneurysms Early (PIVOTAL) Investigators. (2010). Endovascular repair compared with surveillance for patients with small abdominal aortic aneurysms. *J Vasc Surg* 51(5): 1081-1087

Powell JT, Brown LC, Forbes JF, Fowkes FG, Greenhalgh RM, Ruckley CV & Thompson SG. (2007). Final 12-year follow-up of surgery versus surveillance in the UK Small Aneurysm Trial. *Br J Surg* 94(6): 702-708

Powell JT, Gotensparre SM, Sweeting MJ, Brown LC, Fowkes FG & Thompson SG.(2011). Rupture rates of small abdominal aortic aneurysms: a systematic review of the literature. *Eur J Vasc Endovasc Surg* 41(1): 2-10

Prinssen M, Verhoeven EL, Buth J, Cuypers PW, van Sambeek MR, Balm R, Buskens E, Grobbee DE & Blankensteijn JD; Dutch Randomized Endovascular Aneurysm Management (DREAM)Trial Group. (2004). A randomized trial comparing conventional and endovascular repair of abdominal aortic aneurysms. *N Engl J Med* 351(16): 1607-1618

Qureshi NA, Rehman A, Slater N, Moss E, Shiralkar S, Patel RT, Grimley RP & Jayatunga AP. (2007). Abdominal aortic aneurysm surgery in a district general hospital: a 15-years experience. *Ann Vasc Surg* 21(6): 749-753

Schermerhorn ML, O'Malley AJ, Jhaveri A, Cotterill P, Pomposelli F& Landon BE. (2008). Endovascular vs. open repair of abdominal aortic aneurysms in the Medicare population. *N Engl J Med* 358(5):464-474

Schlösser FJ, Tangelder MJ, Verhagen HJ, van der Heijden GJ, Muhs BE, van der Graaf Y & Moll FL; SMART study group. (2008). Growth predictors and prognosis of small abdominal aortic aneurysms. *J Vasc Surg* 47 (6): 1127-1133

Schlösser FJ, Vaartjes I, van der Heijden GJ, Moll FL, Verhagen HJ, Muhs BE, de Borst GJ, Tiel Groenestege AT, Kardaun JW, Reitsma JB, van der Graaf Y & Bots ML. (2010). Mortality after hospital admission for ruptured abdominal aortic aneurysm. *Ann Vasc Surg* 24(8): 1125-1132

Schouten O, van Laanen JH, Boersma E, Vidakovic R, Feringa HH, Dunkelgrün M, Bax JJ, Koning J, van Urk H & Poldermans D. (2006). Statins are associated with a reduced infrarenal abdominal aortic aneurysm growth. *Eur J Vasc Endovasc Surg* 32(1): 21-26

Scott RA, Wilson NM, Ashton HA & Kay DN. (1995). Influence of screening on the incidence of ruptured abdominal aortic aneurysm: 5-year results of a randomized controlled study. *Br J Surg* 82(8): 1066-1070

Takagi H, Goto SN, Matsui M, Manabe H & Umemoto T. (2010a). A further meta-analysis of population-based screening for abdominal aortic aneurysm. *J Vasc Surg* 52(4): 1103-1108

Takagi H, Matsui M & Umemoto T. (2010b). A meta-analysis of clinical studies of statins for prevention of abdominal aortic aneurysm expansion. *J Vasc Surg* 52(6): 1675-1681

Ten Bosch JA, Teijink JA, Willigendael EM & Prins MH. (2010). Endovascular aneurysm repair is superior to open surgery for ruptured abdominal aortic aneurysms in EVAR-suitable patients. *J Vasc Surg* 52(1): 13-18

Thompson AR, Cooper JA, Ashton HA & Hafez H .(2010). Growth rates of small abdominal aortic aneurysms correlate with clinical events. *Br J Surg* 97(1): 37-44

Thompson SG, Ashton HA, Gao L & Scott RA; Multicentre Aneurysm Screening Study Group. (2009). Screening men for abdominal aortic aneurysm: 10 year mortality and cost effectiveness results from the randomised Multicentre Aneurysm Screening Study. *BMJ* 338: b2307

United Kingdom EVAR Trial Investigators, Greenhalgh RM, Brown LC, Powell JT, Thompson SG, Epstein D & Sculpher MJ. (2010a). Endovascular versus open repair of abdominal aortic aneurysm. *N Engl J Med* 362(20): 1863-1871

United Kingdom EVAR Trial Investigators, Greenhalgh RM, Brown LC, Powell JT, Thompson SG & Epstein D. (2010b). Endovascular repair of aortic aneurysm in patients physically ineligible for open repair. *N Engl J Med* 362(20): 1872-1880

UK Small Aneurysm Trial Participants. (1998). Mortality results for randomised controlled trial of early elective surgery or ultrasonographic surveillance for small abdominal aortic aneurysms. *Lancet* 352 (9141): 1649-1655

U.K. Small Aneurysm Trial Participants. (1999). Risk factors for aneurysm rupture in patients kept under ultrasound surveillance. *Ann Surg* 230(3): 289-297

UK Small Aneurysm Trial Participants. (2002). Long-term outcomes of immediate repair compared with surveillance of small abdominal aortic aneurysms. *N Engl J Med* 346(19): 1445-1452

U.S. Preventive Services Task Force. (2005). Screening for abdominal aortic aneurysm: recommendation statement. *Ann Intern Med* 142(3): 198-202

van Walraven C, Wong J, Morant K, Jennings A, Jetty P & Forster AJ. (2010). Incidence, follow-up, and outcomes of incidental abdominal aortic aneurysms. *J Vasc Surg* 52(2): 282-289

Vardulaki KA, Prevost TC, Walker NM, Day NE, Wilmink AB, Quick CR, Ashton HA & Scott RA. (1999). Incidence among men of asymptomatic abdominal aortic aneurysms: estimates from 500 screen detected cases. *J Med Screen* 6(1): 50-54

Vega de Céniga M, Estallo L, Barba A, de la Fuente N, Viviens B & Gómez R. (2010). Long-term cardiovascular outcome after elective abdominal aortic aneurysm open repair. *Ann Vasc Surg* 24(5): 655-662

Veith FJ, Lachat M, Mayer D, Malina M, Holst J, Mehta M, Verhoeven EL, Larzon T, Gennai S, Coppi G, Lipsitz EC, Gargiulo NJ, van der Vliet JA, Blankensteijn J, Buth J, Lee WA, Biasi G, Deleo G, Kasirajan K, Moore R, Soong CV, Cayne NS, Farber MA, Raithel D, Greenberg RK, van Sambeek MR, Brunkwall JS, Rockman CB & Hinchliffe RJ; RAAA Investigators. (2009). Collected world and single center experience with endovascular treatment of ruptured abdominal aortic aneurysms. *Ann Surg* 250(5): 818-824

Wilt TJ, Lederle FA, Macdonald R, Jonk YC, Rector TS & Kane RL. (2006). Comparison of endovascular and open surgical repairs for abdominal aortic aneurysm. *Evid Rep Technol Assess (Full Rep)* 144: 1-113. Rockville (MD): Agency for Healthcare Research and Quality (US)

Xu J, Kochanek KD, Murphy SL & Tejada-Vera B. (2010). Deaths: Final Data for 2007. *National Vital Statistics Reports* 58, Number 19. Available from www.cdc.gov/NCHS/data/nvsr/nvsr58/nvsr58_19.pdf

Young EL, Holt PJ, Poloniecki JD, Loftus IM & Thompson MM. (2007). Meta-analysis and systematic review of the relationship between surgeon annual caseload and mortality for elective open abdominal aortic aneurysm repairs. *J Vasc Surg* 46(6): 1287-1294

Young KC, Awad NA, Johansson M, Gillespie D, Singh MJ & Illig KA. (2010). Cost-effectiveness of abdominal aortic aneurysm repair based on aneurysm size. *J Vasc Surg* 51(1): 27-32

2

Pathophysiology of Abdominal Aortic Aneurysm – Genetic Factors and Homocysteine Metabolism

Christopher L Delaney, Hafees A Saleem, Yew-Toh Wong and J Ian Spark
Department of Vascular Surgery, Flinders Medical Centre and Flinders University, Bedford Park, Australia

1. Introduction

Homocysteine (Hcy) is a non-protein amino acid resulting from the demethylation of the essential amino acid methionine. This is an important step in the metabolism of nucleic acids, fats and high-energy bonds and for this reason, the transmethylation reaction of Hcy back to methionine requiring Vitamin B12 and folic acid, is equally important. This pathway is dependent on a form of folate produced by methylenetetrahydrofolate reductase (MTHFR). Hcy can also be metabolised to cystathionine, an intermediate of the non-essential amino acid cysteine. Vitamin B6 is necessary for this transulphuration reaction to occur (Figure 1) (Warsi et al, 2004; Guilliams, 2004; Moroz et al, 2007; Castro et al, 2006)
Excess levels of Hcy are excreted to the plasma where the liver and kidney are the organs achieving catabolism and excretion of Hcy. Despite this, mild hyperHcy is present in 5-7% of the general population, due to either inherited or acquired dietary deficiencies of vitamin B6, B12 and folic acid. Other causes include renal failure, malignancy, hypothyroidism and use of folate and vitamin B6 antagonists (Halazun et al, 2007).

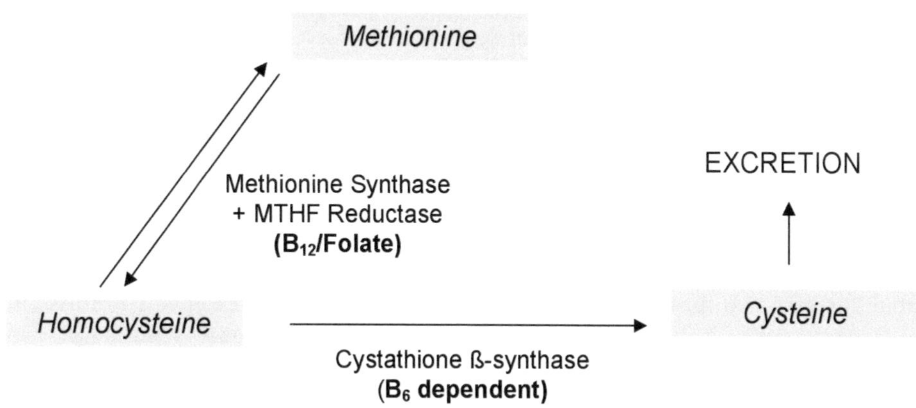

Fig. 1. Brief summary of homocysteine metabolism

2. Historical perspective

HyperHcy has been linked to vascular disease since the early 1960's when children with mental retardation, accelerated growth and propensity to arterial and venous thrombosis were found to have homocysteinuria. An emerging pattern of atherosclerosis was detected in these patients and it was concluded that genetic defects in homocysteine metabolism and associated homocysteinuria was responsible for these vascular lesions (Guilliams, 2004).

Endothelial vascular injury and atherosclerosis was subsequently demonstrated through intravenous infusion of Hcy in an animal model (Warsi et al, 2004).

Several studies followed this, reporting the association between Hcy concentrations and vascular disease and more recent large scale meta-analyses have supported these findings (Castro et al, 2006). A causal relationship between homocysteine and cardiovascular disease is felt to be highly likely and hyperHcy is now an established modifiable risk factor for cardiovascular disease. Raised Hcy levels are present in significant numbers of patients with peripheral, cerebrovascular and coronary heart disease (CHD). High values have also been proven to predict the failure of vascular intervention and more rapid progression of CHD and peripheral vascular disease (Halazun et al, 2007).

3. Evidence for homocysteine in aneurysmal disease

While the importance of homocysteine in atherosclerotic disease has been established, there is also evidence to suggest that raised Hcy levels could play a role in the pathogenesis of abdominal aortic aneurysm (AAA).

A number of recent studies have demonstrated the prevalence of raised Hcy levels in AAA to be as high as 50% and one study has demonstrated a link between Hcy levels and the rate of expansion of AAA (Halazun et al, 2007). Despite this, data is still relatively limited. Confounding has not been excluded with male sex, smoking, hypertension and raised low-density lipoprotein levels all shown to be independently associated with AAA (Naydeck et al, 1999), while the possibility of reverse causality needs consideration. Current large scale genotypic studies are attempting to deal with this and will be discussed later in the chapter.

4. How does homocysteine contribute to aneurysmal disease

Their is no doubt that the pathogenesis of AAA is multi-factorial, in brief, the degradation of key structural proteins such as elastin and collagen results in weakening of the aortic wall and subsequent dilatation and aneurysm formation. HyperHcy has been shown to enhance this process through several mechanisms.

4.1 Oxidative damage and thrombogenicity

Homocysteine has been shown to cause endothelial dysfunction through mechanisms felt to be attributable to oxidative stress. This is an important event preceding manifestation of vascular disease and its involvement is strengthened by the fact that administration of antioxidant vitamins can prevent the impairment of endothelial vasodilator function induced by experimental hyperHcy (Stuhlinger et al, 2003).

One such mechanism is the impaired production of nitric oxide (NO) as an effect of hyperHcy. This is possibly through increasing levels of asymmetric dimethylarginine (ADMA), a strong inhibitor of endothelial nitric oxide synthase (Guilliams, 2004; Stuhlinger

et al, 2003). NO contributes to vessel homeostasis by inhibiting vascular smooth muscle contraction and growth, platelet aggregation, and leukocyte adhesion to the endothelium. The resultant over-production of oxidative free radicals has been shown to induce intimal injury, activate elastase and increase calcium deposition (Brunelli et al, 2000).
The toxic effects of hyperHcy on the endothelium extend to the prothrombotic environment that is created at several levels. These include increased platelet aggregation, activation of clotting factors V, X and XII, along with depressed activation of protein C and cell surface thrombomodulin and modulation of tissue plasminogen activator binding to its cell surface receptor, annexin II (Perna et al, 2003).

4.2 Elastolysis and proteolysis

While the above mechanisms are undoubtedly contributors to aneurysm formation, there is strong evidence to suggest that hyperHcy can enhance proteolysis and this maybe particularly relevant to the pathogenesis of AAA. In the normal aorta, arterial wall structures elastin, collagen and smooth muscle bear the vast majority of wall stress and act as a strong almost indistensible safety net to limit expansion. Histological features of aneurysmal aortic wall show failure of this safety net by way of elastin fragmentation and degeneration, collagen degradation, a medial attenuation and a reduction in tensile strength (Arapoglou et al, 2009).

4.2.1 Serine elastase

Serine elastase is a member of a large family of protein-cleaving enzymes (proteases) that play an essential role in processes like blood coagulation, apoptosis and inflammation. Regulation of proteolysis induced by these serine proteases is essential to prevent self-induced damage.
Vascular smooth muscle cells (VSMC's) are felt to contribute to the homeostasis of the vessel wall by synthesising elastin and elastinolytic enzymes. HyperHcy has been demonstrated to induce the synthesis of serine elastase in vascular smooth muscle cells. While the mechanism for this is currently unclear, through the activation of serine elastase, Hcy increases the rate of elastoylsis and subsequent degradation of the extra-cellular matrix. The associated release of elastin peptides are chemotactic for VSMC's which then proliferate and migrate into the sub-endothelium, resulting in neointimal formation and progressive vascular occlusion. This suggests a possible mechanism to explain the proposed link between aneurysmal and atherosclerotic disease. Such a mechanism is supported by studies demonstrating that inhibition of serine elastase limits the fragmentation of elastic laminae in the aortic wall while also preventing the VSMC alterations and the associated progressive vascular disease (Jourdheuil-Rahmani et al, 1997).

4.2.2 Matrix metalloproteinases

Abdominal aortic aneurysm (AAA) development and expansion are multifactorial in pathogenesis (Ailawadi et al, 2003). Inflammatory response plays a significant role in the pathogenesis of development and expansion of aneurysm. Normal aorta undergo a constant remodelling pocess involving various proteases that degrade elastin and collagen, and the production of new elastin and collagen by the smooth muscle cells of the aortic wall. Disturbance of the normal balance in this process results in AAA initiation and expansion (Davies, 1998; Grange et al, 1997). Three proteolytic systems seem to be involved in the degradation of aorta (Lindholt et al, 2003).

- The serine-dependent proteases are elastases that degrade elastin in the aorta
- The cysteine-dependent proteases are lysosomal proteases such as cathepsin K, L, S that plays a role in apoptosis of the smooth muscles cells of aorta
- The metalloproteinases (MMP) are elastases and collagenases that degrade aortic elastin and collagen. Elastin degradation is associated with aneurysm initiation and expansion and collagen destruction is responsible for eventual AAA rupture.

MMPs are the most widely studied proteolytic system in the pathogenesis of AAA. Many MMPs have been implicated in the pathogenesis of AAA including MMP-1, MMP-2, MMP-3, MMP-8, MMP-9, MMP-12, MMP-13 and MMP-14(Wilson et al, 2005a; Longo et al, 2005; Wilson et al, 2005b; Tromp et al, 2004). MMP-9 is an elastase most frequently implicated in the aneurysm initiation, expansion and rupture. MMP-9 knockout mice do not form aneurysm and their ability to form aneurysm is restored after wild type bone marrow transplantation (Pyo et al, 2000). MMP-9 has also been implicated in asymmetrical regional wall expansion in the anterior wall of aorta (Sinha et al, 2006). Its level in ruptured AAA has been found to be significantly higher than large AAA (Petersen et al, 2000). MMP-2 and MMP-12 (macrophage elastase) are elastases that are also found in increased concentration in aneurysmal aortic tissue. High concentration of MMP-2 is found in small AAA suggesting its role in early AAA formation (Crowther et al, 2000). MMP-12 is highly expressed in tissue along the leading edge of AAA suggesting a role in AAA initiation (Warsi et al, 2004). MMP-1, MMP-3, MMP-8, MMP-13 are collagenases involved in degradation of extracellular matrix during aortic wall remodelling (Tromp et al, 2004; Pyo et al, 2000; Sinha et al, 2006; Petersen et al, 2000; Crowther et al, 2000; Abdul-Hussien et al, 2007). MMP-14 is a membrane type MMP expressed at cell surface and is responsible for activation of MMP-2 (Apte et al, 1997). The exact mechanism of MMPs interactions with other inflammatory cytokines, inflammatory cells, microbes and aortic wall tissue is unknown. MMPs can be activated by a range of stimuli including other MMPs, cytokines released by the inflammatory cells, elastin degradation products, microbes such as chlamydiae pneumoniae, reactive oxygen species, and mechanical alteration in the aortic wall stress (Warsi et al, 2004).

Several genetic polymorphisms are associated with MMP and some have been linked with increased frequency in AAA (Thompson et al, 2008; Sandford et al, 2007). Genetic polymorphism is a difference in DNA sequence among the population that gives rise to different forms such as in the case of human blood groups. Its occurrence cannot be accounted for by just recurrent mutation and is present in greater than 1% of the population. MMP-9 polymorphism has been implicated in AAA. A cytosine to thymidine substitution in position 1562 of the promoter region (MMP-9 -1562C>T) produces a 1.5 fold increase in promoter activity (Zhang et al, 1999). Jones et al. reported increased frequency of TT and CT genotypes in people with AAA compared to normal population (Jones et al, 2003). However, other studies on MMP-9 had not demonstrated similar genetic predisposition (Yoon et al, 1999; Higashikata et al, 2004). Platelet activating factor (PAF) can induce MMP-1, MMP-2, and MMP-9 transcription. The activity of PAF is regulated by PAF acetylhydrolase (PAF-AH). A guanine to thymidine substitution in position 994 of the exon 9 (PAF-AH +994 G>T) results in lower enzymatic activity of PAF-AH with increased PAF level. GT and TT genotype are associated with AAA with an odd ratio of 2.48 (CI 1.36-4.65) (Thompson et al, 2008). In general there is a lack of clear evidence that upregulation of MMPs in AAA has a genetic basis (Sandford et al, 2007).

Dampening the overactivity of MMPs in AAA can potentially slow the progression of AAA. Recent review in the area suggest that statins, non steriodal antiinflammatory drugs (NSAIDS) and antibiotics hold the most promise (Bergqvist et al, 2011). Statin has been shown in metaanalysis to be beneficial in slowing the expansion of AAA (Takagi et al, 2010). The median expansion rate decreased by about 1.2mm per year. Aortic tissue obtained at the time of surgery has shown a reduction in the level of MMP-3 and MMP-9 for patients who are taking statin (Wilson et al, 2005a). The evidence for antibiotics and NSAIDS is less convincing. Roxythromycin and doxycycline have been shown to modulate MMP concentrations and were associated clinically with decreased aneurysm expansion rate in some studies but not others (Hogh et al, 2009; Karlsson et al, 2009; Morosin et al, 2001; Vammen et al, 2001). NSAID's reduce the release of cytokines (IL-1β and IL-6) and in turn reduce the production of elastases in rat aortic tissue (Parodi et al, 2006). A case control study shows that it potentially can reduce AAA expansion rate (Lindholt et al, 2008).

4.2.3 Tissue Inhibitors of MMP's and plasminogen activator Inhibitors

Regulation of the MMP system is provided by Tissue Inhibitors of Metalloproteinases (TIMP's) and Plasminogen Activator Inhibitors (PAI's), which inhibit the action of plasmin (an MMP activator). Platelet Activating Factor (PAF) has been shown to induce MMP formation.

An imbalance of MMP's and their inhibitors/activators leads to an excess of MMP's resulting in the degradation of the structural proteins elastin and collagen and subsequent aneurysm formation (Thompson et al, 2008; Sandford et al, 2007).

Polymorphisms have been identified in the genes encoding each of these protein systems. A relative decrease in TIMP expression has been found in aneurysmal aortas. Although this study concluded that this deficiency was not a result of a primary gene mutation (Tilson et al, 1993), more recent studies have identified both a TIMP-1 and TIMP-2 polymorphism to be expressed in higher frequencies in patients with AAA (Ogata et al, 2005; Wang et al 1999). Despite this, the observed single base pair change does not change translation and is therefore unlikely to be involved in the pathogenesis of AAA. It does however, raise the possibility that other polymorphisms identified within the TIMP gene (G418C and C177T), maybe linked to AAA formation (Sandford et al, 2007), although this has not been investigated to date.

Polymorphisms of both PAF and PAI genes have also been linked to AAA. A 5G allele in position 675 of the PAI-1 gene is associated with reduced transcription and is expressed more frequently in patients with a family history of AAA (Rossaak et al, 2000). Those patients with homozygosity for the 5G allele were found to have more rapid rates of aneurysmal expansion (Jones et al, 2002).

PAF acetylhydrolase controls the activity of PAF. A common polymorphism (G994T) in this gene reduces enzyme activity and results in increased levels of PAF. A significant association with the T-allele and AAA has been demonstrated (Thompson et al, 2008).

4.2.4 Fibrillin

In addition to the mechanisms described above, in a process known as homocysteinylation, Hcy can damage elastin and other matrix proteins through non-enzymatic chemical reactions resulting in protein inactivation (Moroz et al, 2007).

Firbrillin is a glycoprotein essential for the formation of elastic fibres found in connective tissue. It is secreted into the extracellular matrix by fibroblasts and becomes incorporated into the insoluble microfibrils which appear to provide a scaffold for the deposition of elastin (Kielty et al, 2002).

Fibrillin appears to be particularly susceptible to the process of homocysteinylation. This involves a post-biosynthetic acylation of free amino groups in proteins and is mediated by Hcy thiolactone, an intermediate of Hcy metabolism. It is felt that the epidermal growth factor (EGF)-like domains found in fibrillin are preferential sites of homocysteinylation (Krumdieck & Prince, 2000).

The effect of homocysteinylation is protein damge with an altered electrophoretic mobility and loss of enzymatic activity through protein denaturation. This essentially renders the protein useless and may result in elastolysis and damage to other matrix proteins.

When we consider that Marfans syndrome is due to a mutation in the fibrillin 1 (FBN1) gene and the clinical manifestations include aortic aneurysmal disease, it strengthens the evidence that the toxic effects of hyperHcy and associated homocysteinylation of fibrillin, are directly implicated with AAA formation.

5. Genetic polymorphisms and homocysteine

There is increasing evidence supporting an inheritable component to AAA. Although several factors, including age, vitamins and hormones can influence plasma Hcy levels, candidate gene analysis has recently demonstrated that mutations in genes coding for enzymes involved in Hcy metabolism may also play a role in HyperHcy and subsequently the pathogenesis of AAA.

5.1 MTHFR gene

As mentioned previously, the metabolism of Hcy requires several enzymes, nutrient co-factors and a methyl donor. Genetic control of all of these pathways is essential, however, as with any gene their are inherited or acquired errors that effect the efficiency by which Hcy can be metabolised.

The most common of these errors are felt to occur in the gene encoding for the enzyme MTHFR. This enzyme catalyses the conversion of 5,10-methylenetetrahydrofolate to 5-methyltetrahydrofolate, a cosubstrate for Hcy remethylation to methionine.

Currently, 33 MTHFR gene mutations have been reported as causing severe hyperHcy. Perhaps more clinically relevant to aneurysmal disease is a polymorphism in the MTHFR gene at the 677 locus which involves substitution of a cytosine nucleotide for a thymine (Strauss et al, 2003; Jones et al, 2005; Khandanpour et al, 2009; Sunder-Plassman & Fodinger, 2003; Klerk et al, 2002). It is subsequently referred to as the T-allele. This polymorphism leads to an alanine to valine change in the enzyme, resulting in 55-65% loss of enzyme activity. Individuals who are homozygous for the T-allele (TT homozygous) are most likely to manifest this level of enzyme inactivity, while those who are CT heterozygous will experience only 25% loss of activity compared to a CC homozygous individual (Guilliams, 2004).

The frequency of the T allele exhibits marked geographic variability. In those of African descent the frequency is <1%, ranging to >20% in the Hispanic population. The frequency of TT homozygotes shows similar variability (Castro et al, 2006).

The homozygous and heterozygous genotypes (CT) and (TT) have been shown to be associated with raised Hcy levels and lower MTHFR enzyme concentrations. In one study

there was a 36% difference in mean Hcy levels between wildtype and TT genotypes (Khandanpour et al, 2009), while a 47% difference was demonstrated in another study (Rassoul et al, 2000). Further to this, a strong association has been demonstrated between the TT genotype, hyperHcy and coronary, cerebro and peripheral atherosclerotic disease (Khandanpour et al, 2009; Klerk et al, 2002; Moat et al, 2004). Significantly, the association of the MTHFR genotype with Hcy levels is only observed when concomitant inadequate folate concentrations are present (Guilliams, 2004; Castro et al, 2006), although low folate levels independent of MTHFR have not been shown to cause hyperHcy (Spark et al, 2003).
Several studies have investigated the link between MTHFR gene polymorphisms and AAA (Brunelli et al, 2000; Jones et al, 2002; Strauss et al, 2003; Ferrara et al, 2006). All but one of these demonstrated a link between the T allele polymorphism and AAA, a meta-analysis of these studies confirmed a significant effect in favour of the T-allele variant increasing the risk of AAA (Thompson et al, 2008). Interestingly, the study that did not provide evidence to suggest a link between the T-allele and AAA, did suggest that it may be a contributory factor in AAA severity as indicated by aneurysm size (Strauss et al, 2003). This is consistent with results suggesting that hyperHcy patients have faster expansion rates of AAA when compared to patients with normal Hcy (Halazun et al, 2007).
Two further known polymorphisms exist in the MTHFR gene. The T1317C polymorphism has been found to show no association with vascular disease. A1298C alone influences neither folate status or Hcy levels. However, compound heterozygosity for the C677T and A1298C alleles can be associated with decreased folate concentrations and raised levels of Hcy (Sunder-Plassman & Fodinger, 2003). To date there has been no link demonstrated between the A1298C allele and AAA.

5.2 Other genes effecting homocysteine metabolism

In addition to genetic errors effecting folate metabolism and causing subsequent hyperHcy, it is worth mentioning that hyperHcy can also result from genetic mutations in the genes encoding cystathione beta-synthase (the enzyme responsible for the trans-sulphuration of Hcy to cysteine) and enzymes responsible for B12 metabolism or absorption (the co-factor required for remethylation of Hcy to methionine) (Guilliams, 2004).
These mutations occur at a significantly lower frequency than those in the MTHFR gene and are classically associated with severe hyperHcy, leading to clinical features including marfanoid features, mental retardation and early onset of vascular disease (Lievers et al, 2003).

6. Genetics and AAA

The burden of evidence for genetic influence on the aetio-pathogenesis of aneurysmal disease is small. Genetic links have been shown in the initiation and formation of abdominal aortic aneurysms (AAA). There have also been studies showing genetic evidence of familial clustering of AAA (Johansen & Koepsell, 1986).
It is estimated that about 15% of patients with AAA without any recognizable connective tissue disorders, such as Ehlers-Danlos syndrome or Marfan syndrome, have a positive family history for AAA (Frydman et al, 2003; Rizzo et al, 1989). A few studies favoured a genetic model in explaining the familial aggregation of AAA and suggested the presence of a major gene effect. However, these studies do not agree on whether the gene inheritance is recessive or dominant.

Finding a familial susceptibility gene could lead to easy identification of individuals prone to AAA's due to the fact that AAA's are largely asymptomatic prior to their rupture. The study of gene pathways may also provide potential new targets for pharmacological intervention.

It is difficult to independently assess familial tendency by gene analysis due to the presence of confounding overlap by other risk factors that have been described to have a genetic predisposition such as hypertension and atherosclerosis.

6.1 Candidate genes and AAA

If sibling risk results from genetic susceptibility, it may be inferred that this would be attributable to a few gene polymorphisms. Candidate genes for AAA that have been investigated in population studies include those encoding type III collagen, matrix metallo-proteinases and protease inhibitors, angiotensin converting enzyme, nitric oxide synthase and HLA loci. Mutations in any of these candidate genes may explain the hereditary background of AAA (Thompson et al, 2008; Sandford et al, 2007).

There are several plausible candidate genes implicated in the pathogenesis of AAA. *IL15* (interleukin 15; a plausible candidate gene with respect to inflammation in AAA), *GAB1* (GRB2-associated binding protein 1; an important mediator of branching tubulogenesis and a central protein in cellular growth response, transformation, and apoptosis), and *EDNRA* (endothelin receptor type A; an endothelin-1 receptor expressed in many human tissues with the highest level in the aorta) around 140 cM on chromosome 4, as well as *LRP3* (LDL receptor–related protein 3), *HPN* (transmembrane protease, serine 1; a serine-type peptidase involved in cell growth and maintenance), *PDCD5* (programmed cell death 5; a protein expressed in tumor cells during apoptosis independent of the apoptosis-inducing stimuli), and *PEPD* (peptidase D; an Xaa-Pro dipeptidase important in collagen catabolism) on chromosome 19.

Candidate gene studies have certainly shown causal pathways predisposing to developing AAA. Isolated mutations of one of several candidate genes are seen in some patients with AAA. But those did not always translate to similar mutations in first-degree relatives who were found to have AAA.

6.1.1 ACE gene

The renin-angiotensin-aldosterone (RAS) system plays a major role in cardiovascular homeostasis at many levels. The angiotensin converting enzyme (ACE) converts angiotensin I into the active angiotensin II. In an animal model, infusion of angiotensin II produces large AAA (Daugherty et al, 2000), while ACE has been shown to be highly expressed in human aneurysmal aorta (Nishimoto et al, 2002). This suggests a role for increased local levels of angiotensin II in the pathogenesis of AAA and may explain the protective effect to the medial layers of the infra-renal aorta provided by treatment with captopril-hydrochlorothiazide. This was shown to reduce MMP activity, both directly and by inhibiting the release of the MMP activator Angiotensin II from smooth muscle cells (Moroz et al, 2007). This suggests a role for ACE-inhibitors in the treatment and prevention of AAA.

There is a polymorphic site in the ACE gene which consists of the presence or absence of 287 base pairs. It has been termed 'I' for insertion of the fragment or 'D' for its deletion. The polymorphism accounts for three genotypes (DD and II homozygotes and ID heterozygotes. Because the alleles are co-dominant with an additive effect on plasma levels, DD homozygotes have the highest plasma levels of ACE, while II homozygotes have the lowest (Thompson et al, 2008; Sandford et al, 2007; Fatini et al, 2005). Patients in whom the polymorphism is present have been found to have a 50% reduction in ACE levels with subsequent reduction of angiotensin II levels (Fatini et al, 2005). Given the physiological processes undertaken by these enzymes, it fits therefore that the D allele has been associated with hypertension and IHD.

More recently, an association with AAA has been demonstrated by several studies who have found a significantly increased D allele frequency in AAA patients compared to controls (Fatini et al, 2005a). Furthermore, it has been shown that this polymorphism affects AAA development independently of any association with blood pressure (Pola et al, 2001). Interestingly, aldosterone does not mediate angiotensin induced increases in AAA diameter. This suggests that increased ACE levels found in aneurysmal wall may be independent of the physiological RAS system (Cassis et al, 2005).

6.1.2 Nitric oxide synthase gene

Nitric oxide (NO) contributes to vessel homeostasis by inhibiting vascular smooth muscle contraction and growth, platelet aggregation, and leukocyte adhesion to the endothelium. Humans with atherosclerosis, diabetes, or hypertension often show impaired NO pathways (Dessy & Ferron, 2004).

Endothelial Nitric Oxide Synthase (eNOS) is responsible for the production of NO. Several polymorphisms have been identified in the gene coding for eNOS and these may affect the function of the enzyme.

One polymorphism consists of a 27 base pair repeat, present in intron 4 of the eNOS gene. Commonly, 5 repeats are identified at this polymorphic site, however, when analysing patients with AAA, it was found that 4 repeats at this site may be associated with rapid progression of AAA (Kotani et al, 2000).

A further polymorphism is the G894T, in which the rarer T allele has been found to be more frequent in AAA patients compared with age/sex-matched controls (Fatini et al, 2005b). The reduction in NO tissue levels resulting from the T-allele has been suggested to contribute to AAA formation (Thompson et al, 2008).

6.1.3 Chemokine receptor genes

Chemokines are a family of small secreted proteins that selectively recruit monocytes, neutrophils, and lymphocytes to sites of vascular injury, inflammation, and developing atherosclerosis.

Recently, a polymorphism of the chemokine receptor gene 5 (CCR5) has been identified. This is a 32 base pair deletion in the promoter region of the gene, resulting in reduced receptor expression, inhibition of leukocyte recruitment and reduction of inflammatory infiltrate (Smith et al, 1997). This deletion polymorphism has been investigated in vasculopaths with a higher incidence detected among AAA patients compared with patients exhibiting peripheral arterial or carotid disease and healthy controls (Ghilardi et al, 2004).

6.1.4 Interleukin genes

Adventitial and medial inflammatory responses have been implicated as playing a key role in AAA pathogenesis (Arapoglou et al, 2009). Interleukins are associated with this inflammatory process and studies have investigated a link between interleukin gene polymorphisms and AAA. Only the gene encoding the anti-inflammatory cytokine IL-10 was found to have a polymorphism expressed more frequently in AAA patients than controls. It is felt the reduced production of IL-10 as a result of this polymorphism impairs the ability to regulate inflammatory processes, leading to AAA formation (Bown et al, 2003).

6.1.5 Human leukocyte antigen genes

The Human Leukocyte Antigen (HLA) system is a genetically determined series of antigens that are expressed on leukocytes and tissues. They control a variety of cell-cell interactions and certain subtypes have been associated with chronic inflammatory conditions such as rheumatoid arthritis (Sandford et al, 2007).

An autoimmune component to the pathogenesis of AAA has been proposed, implicating HLA subtypes. In a Japanese population, an increased frequency of the HLA-DR2(15) allele has been demonstrated in aneurysm patients. Other studies have shown HLA-DR B1*02 and B1*04 subtypes as well as HLA-A2 and HLA-B61 antigens to be more common in AAA patients (Rasmussen et al, 2002; Monux et al, 2003; Hirose et al, 1998). Despite this, a more recent study of 241 AAA patients failed to demonstrate a risk association between AAA and these alleles suggesting that the role of these particular genes and the autoimmune component in AAA etiology does not appear to be as crucial as previously proposed (Badger et al, 2007).

Several additional candidate gene association studies have been performed in AAA patients in genes encoding proteins ranging from collagen to heme-oxygenase. No statistically significant difference has been observed in such studies, however, the evolution of genetic analysis is likely to uncover several new potential genetic links to AAA in years to come.

Inevitably, whole human genome studies in the future will identify a combination of polymorphisms contributing to the pathogenesis of AAA and it is unlikely that a single gene will underpin this process.

6.2 Collagen and AAA

Collagen (type I and III) is the principle component of the aortic adventitia. The tensile characteristics are attributed to type III collagen and the load-bearing characteristics to type I collagen. The tensile strength of the aortic wall can be influenced by synthesis of structurally abnormal type III collagen that constitutes the basis for the aneurysm formation (Rizzo et al, 1989). A mutation of the Type III collagen gene could result in inherited propensity to develop AAA (Kontusaari et al, 1990).

Abdominal aortic aneurysms, dissections and ruptures are common disorders in different syndromes that are caused by collagen defects. Phenotypic overlap of heritable disorders of connective tissue might be a possible explanation of familial aneurysms. Ehlers Danlos Syndrome (EDS) IV is caused by genetically determined type III collagen (COL3A1) defect or a deficiency. There were some initial studies that correlated levels of Type III collagen and AAA, suggesting even that some of the familial AAA patients could be a manifestation of a subclinical EDS IV. Subsequent studies measuring Type III collagen levels in family members of patients with AAA were inconclusive to suggest a causal relationship between familial clustering and type III collagen.

6.3 Aneurysmal disease in twins

The sibling risk for developing AAA has led to research into associations of AAA in twins. The most significant study is from the Swedish Twin Registry. The investigators provide robust epidemiologic evidence that heritability contributes to aneurysm formation. Concordances and correlations were significantly higher in MZ (monozygotic, identical) compared with DZ (dizygotic, non-identical) compared with DZ twins, indicating genetic effects. There was a 24% probability that the MZ twin of a person with an AAA will have the disease. The twin of an MZ twin with an AAA had a risk of an AAA that was 71 times that of the MZ twin of a person without an AAA. When looking at twins over the age of 55 with an AAA, then possibly excluding genetic connective tissue disorders such as Ehlers-Danlos and Marfan syndrome, the odds ratio was still significantly higher for MZ twins compared to DZ twins. They noted that in other regions the proportions of type of effects could differ because of environmental factors. Also in the cases of aneurysmal disease with several genetic and environmental factors, the liability model assumes that the disease will occur when there are enough contributory factors to push the individual's liability above the threshold (Wahlgren et al, 2010).

The familial clustering of AAA is unlikely to be due to chance alone; the odds ratios for sibling risk in case-control studies are too high. But almost 20 years of work has yielded little persuasive evidence for specific genes underlying this phenomenon. Large, collaborative research proposals are needed to address the reasons for familial clustering of AAA.

7. Therapeutic interventions on homocysteine

The detection of elevated levels of Hcy in patients with large, symptomatic AAA is unlikely to change the treatment because such patients need repair of their AAA. It is in the management of small (30-50mm) AAA's that Hcy levels may have a role. Although surgery is not indicated for these AAA's, a proportion will expand until they are large enough to warrant elective intervention before rupture occurs. Current practice is to monitor the diameter of AAA's with periodic ultrasound or CT scanning, but our understanding of the natural history of these aneurysms remains incomplete.

The identification of risk factors such as Hcy that are associated with greater rates of expansion, may help in the planning of AAA surveillance, the identification of high risk patients who may benefit from early intervention and the development of strategies to prevent expansion (Halazun et al, 2007).

To briefly review the metabolism of Hcy, we know that B12 and folic acid are required for transmethlyation to methionine and that B6 is required for trans-sulphuration to cystathionine. Deficiencies of these vitamins have been implicated with hyperHcy, while normal levels of folate, even in the presence of the MTHFR polymorphism seem to be sufficient to regulate Hcy levels. In fact, it has been proposed that the single most important determinant of Hcy levels in the general population is folate status (Castro et al, 2006).

It seems logical therefore that supplementation with folic acid and vitamins B6 and B12 could act as Hcy lowering therapies, potentially preventing the progression/onset of aneurysmal disease (a risk factor reduction technique).

7.1 Folate, B6 and B12 supplementation

Dietary supplementation with folate has been shown to reduce Hcy levels on average by 25% in individuals with cardiovascular disease. Further reduction in levels has been demonstrated with the addition of B6 and B12, suggesting a synergistic effect. Such a reduction in Hcy has previously been linked to an 11% lower risk of coronary heart disease and 19% lower risk of stroke. Despite this, collective evidence recently published in a large-scale meta-analysis suggests that treating hyperHcy with folate and other B-vitamins had no significant effects within 5 years on cardiovascular morbidity and mortality (Clarke et al, 2010).

Interestingly, these results are associated with patients who already have established cardiovascular disease and may be explained by the potential detrimental effects of B vitamin supplementation. In patients with established atherosclerotic disease it is suggested that B vitamins have the potential to enhance inflammation and proliferation in atherosclerotic lesions (Smulders & Blom, 2011). In contrast to this, several animal studies have suggested that B vitamins delay initial development of atherosclerosis. This is supported by a study in which healthy siblings of patients with premature atherosclerotic disease received dietary folate and B6 supplementation for 2 years, a reduced frequency of abnormal exercise stress tests was detected, which is associated with a reduced risk of ischaemic coronary events. This suggests that Hcy lowering therapy as prophylaxis for at risk patient groups may be beneficial. One such group are patients with small AAA's, in who hyperHcy has been linked with more rapid rate of expansion (Halazun et al, 2007), or indeed patients with familial AAA disease who are at high risk of AAA.

7.2 Trimethylglycine (Betaine)

Trimethylglycine (TMG) is a small trimethylated amino acid that can react with the enzyme betaine methyl-transferase, donating a methyl group to remethylate Hcy to methionine (Steenge et al, 2003).

Moderate Hcy lowering effects have been demonstrated, however, this requires high dose (>6gm/day) TMG and it is not as effective as folate supplementation. To date, TMG administration has not been shown to lower the risk of cardiovascular disease, however, studies are continuing (Steenge et al, 2003).

7.3 N-Acetyl Cysteine (NAC)

NAC is a pharmaceutical drug and nutritional supplement used primarily as a mucolytic agent for the treatment of paracetamol overdose. Recently it has been shown to increase plasma free Hcy, the form removed by the kidney, by breaking the disulfide links of the bound form.

One recent study randomised patients with confirmed hyperHcy and coronary artery disease to 5mg folic acid, 600mg NAC or placebo daily for 8 weeks. Both folic acid and NAC had a similar Hcy lowering effect and improved endothelial function compared to placebo (Yilmaz et al, 2007). A further study found that plasma Hcy levels were reduced during treatment with NAC by 45% (Wiklund et al, 1996).

NAC might therefore be a highly efficient nutritional supplement for reducing plasma Hcy and further research large scale randomised trials are required to identify a potential benefit in lowering risk of aneurysmal and cardiovascular disease.

7.4 Omega-3 Polyunsaturated Fatty Acids (PUFA's)

A growing body of research on marine lipids has revealed that omega-3 rich fish oil supplementation can reduce elevated Hcy levels.

An animal model study examined the effect of fish oil rich in omega-3 PUFA's on Hcy metabolism, treating rats with olive oil, tuna oil or salmon oil for 8 weeks. The plasma Hcy level was significantly reduced in the group fed tuna oil, rich in omega-3 PUFA's (Huang et al, 2011). Similarly, a human trial randomised patients with type 2 diabetes mellitus to either 3g of omega-3 PUFA's or placebo daily for two months. Hcy levels were found to decrease significantly in the treatment group compared with those receiving placebo (Pooya et al, 2010).

7.5 Taurine

Taurine is an organic acid and a major constituent of bile. It is a derivative of the sulphur containing amino acid cysteine and is one of the few known naturally occurring sulfonic acids. Recent studies have shown that taurine can block methionine absorption from the diet, thereby reducing available substrate for Hcy synthesis. One animal study found that taurine normalised hyperHcy and reduced atherosclerosis by 64% over control animals (Zulli, 2011). While in a study of healthy, middle-aged women, plasma Hcy levels exhibited a significant decline after taurine supplementation (Ahn, 2009). The investigators concluded that sufficient taurine supplementation might effectively prevent cardiovascular disease.

8. Conclusion

The pathogenesis of abdominal aortic aneurysm is complex and multi-factorial. The true mechanism underlying the disease process is likely to be underpinned by an interaction between a genetic predisposition and environmental risk factors including smoking and hypertension.

HyperHcy and polymorphisms in the MTHFR gene have been implicated as risk factors for cardiovascular disease and there is some evidence that raised levels of Hcy are associated with an increased risk of having an AAA. Despite this, on the current evidence available, we can not confidently state that hyperHcy is a causative factor in the pathogenesis of AAA, although it may help to explain the variation in expansion rates.

In addition to studies of the MTHFR gene, recent candidate gene analysis has provided us with an improved understanding of the genetic predisposition to AAA development. It is unlikely however, that a single gene polymorphism will hold the key to aneurysm formation and such analysis is susceptible to confounding influences of genetic stratification, in particular genetic overlap with risk factors such as hypertension.

Unanswered questions will remain until large scale genome wide association studies are undertaken to enable a complete understanding of the genetic influence on the pathogenesis of AAA.

With regard to the medical management of AAA, the current available evidence would suggest that pharmacotherapy with statin and ACE-Inhibitor should be implemented to attenuate aneurysmal expansion. Macrolides and NSAID's may play a similar role and are currently being investigated.

There is insufficient evidence to support the routine use of B6, B12 and folate supplementation, though multicentre, prospective randomised trials are urgently recommended. This also applies to the use of PUFA's, NAC and taurine.

Ultimately, as these studies progress and our understanding of the pathophysiology of AAA evolves, it is likely that additional pharmacological and dietary supplements will be identified to form an armamentarium aimed at the prevention of AAA rupture.

9. References

Abdul-Hussien H, Soekhoe RG, Weber E, von der Thusen JH, Kleemann R, Mulder A, van Bockel JH, Hanemaaijer R & Lindeman JH. Collagen degradation in the abdominal aneurysm: a conspiracy of matrix metalloproteinase and cysteine collagenases. *The American journal of pathology* 2007;170(3): 809-817.

Ahn CS. Effect of taurine supplementation on plasma homocysteine levels of the middle-aged Korean women. *Adv Exp Med Biol* 2009;643:415-422.

Ailawadi G, Eliason JL & Upchurch GR, Jr. Current concepts in the pathogenesis of abdominal aortic aneurysm. *J Vasc Surg* 2003;38(3): 584-588.

Apte SS, Fukai N, Beier DR & Olsen BR. The matrix metalloproteinase-14 (MMP-14) gene is structurally distinct from other MMP genes and is co-expressed with the TIMP-2 gene during mouse embryogenesis. *The Journal of biological chemistry* 1997;272(41): 25511-25517.

Arapoglou V, Kondi-Pafiti A, Rizos D, Kotsis T, Kalkandis C & Katsenis K. The Influence of Total Plasma Homocysteine and Traditional Atherosclerotic Risk Factors on Degree of Abdominal Aortic Aneurysm Tissue Inflammation. *J Vasc Endovasc Surg* 2009;43(5):473-479

Badger SA, Soong CV, O'Donnell ME & Middleton D. The role of human leukocyte antigen genes in the formation of abdominal aortic aneurysms. *J Vasc Surg* 2007;45(3):475-480

Baird PA, Sadovnick AD, Yee IML, Cole CW & Cole L. Sibling risks of abdominal aortic aneurysm. *Lancet* 1995;346:601e604.

Bergqvist D. Pharmacological Interventions to Attenuate the Expansion of Abdominal Aortic Aneurysm (AAA) - A Systematic Review. *Eur J Vasc Endovasc Surg.*

Bown MJ, Burton PR, Horsburgh T, Nicholson ML, Bell PRF & Sayers RD. The role of cytokine gene polymorphisms in the pathogenesis of abdominal aortic aneurysms: a case-control study. *J Vasc Surg* 2003;37:999-1005

Brunelli T, Prisco D, Fedi S, Rogolino A, Farsi A et al. High prevalence of mild hyperhomocysteinemia in patients with abdominal aortic aneurysm. *J Vasc Surg* 2000;32:531-536

Cassis LA, Helton MJ, Howatt DA, King VL & Daugherty A. Aldosterone does not mediate angiotensin II-induced atherosclerosis and abdominal aortic aneurysms. *Br J Pharmacol* 2005;144(3):443-448

Castro R, Rivera I, Blom HJ & Jakobs C. Homocysteine metabolism, hyperhomocysteinaemia and vascular disease: An overview. *J Inherit Metab Dis* 2006;29:3-20

Clarke R, Halsey J, Lewington S, Lonn E, Armitage J, Manson JE et al. Effects of Lowering Homocysteine Levels With B Vitamins on Cardiovascular Disease, Cancer, and Cause-Specific Mortality. *Arch Intern Med* 2010;170(18):1622-1631

Crowther M, Goodall S, Jones JL, Bell PR & Thompson MM. Localization of matrix metalloproteinase 2 within the aneurysmal and normal aortic wall. *The British journal of surgery* 2000;87(10): 1391-1400.

Daugherty A, Manning MW & Cassis LA. Angiotensin II promotes atherosclerotic lesions and aneurysms in apolipoprotein E-mice. *J Clin Invest* 2000;105:1605-1612

Davies MJ. Aortic aneurysm formation: lessons from human studies and experimental models. *Circulation* 1998;98(3): 193-195.

Dessy C & Ferron O. Pathophysiological Roles of Nitric Oxide: In the Heart and the Coronary Vasculature. *Current Medical Chemistry – Anti-Inflammatory & Anti-Allergy Agents in Medicinal Chemistry* 2004;3(3):207–216.

Fatini C, Pratesi G, Sofi F, Sticchi E, Lari B et al. ACE DD Genotype: A Predisposing Factor for Abdominal Aortic Aneurysm. *Eur J Vasc Endovasc Surg* 2005;29:227-232

Fatini C, Sofi F, Sticchi E, Bolli P, Sestini I, Falciani M et al. eNOS G894T polymorphism as a mild predisposing factor for abdominal aortic aneurysm. *J Vasc Surg* 2005;42(3):415-419.

Ferrara F, Novo S, Grimaudo S, Raimondi F, Meli F, Amato C et al. Methylenetetrahydrofolate reductase mutation in subjects with abdominal aortic aneurysm subdivided for age. *Clinical Hemorheology & Microcirculation* 2006;34(3):421-426

Frydman G, Walker PJ, Summers K, West M, Xu D & Lightfoot T. The value of screening in siblings of patients with abdominal aortic aneurysm. *Eur J Vasc Endovasc Surg* 2003;26(4):396e400.

Ghilardi G, Biondi ML, Battaglioli L, Zambon A, Guagnellini E & Scorza R. Genetic risk factor characterizes abdominal aortic aneurysm from arterial occlusive disease in human beings: CCR5 Δ32 deletion. *J Vasc Surg* 2004;40(5):995-1000

Grange JJ, Davis V & Baxter BT. Pathogenesis of abdominal aortic aneurysm: an update and look toward the future. *Cardiovascular surgery (London, England)* 1997;5(3): 256-265.

Guilliams TG. Homocysteine - A Risk Factor for Vascular Diseases: Guidelines for the Clinical Practice. *JANA* 2004;7(1):11-24

Halazun KJ, Bofkin KA, Asthana S, Evans C, Henderson M & Spark JI. Hyperhomocysteinaemia is Associated with the Rate of Abdominal Aortic Aneurysm Expansion. *Eur J Vasc Endovasc Surg* 2007;33:391-394

Higashikata T, Yamagishi M, Sasaki H, Minatoya K, Ogino H, Ishibashi-Ueda H et al. Application of real-time RT-PCR to quantifying gene expression of matrix metalloproteinases and tissue inhibitors of metalloproteinases in human abdominal aortic aneurysm. *Atherosclerosis* 2004;177(2): 353-360.

Hirose H, Takagi M, Miyagawa N, Hashiyada H, Noguchi M, Tada S et al. Genetic risk factor for abdominal aortic aneurysm: HLA-DR2(15), a Japanese study. *J Vasc Surg* 1998;27(3):500-503

Hogh A, Vammen S, Ostergaard L, Joensen JB, Henneberg EW & Lindholt JS. Intermittent roxithromycin for preventing progression of small abdominal aortic aneurysms: long-term results of a small clinical trial. *Vascular and endovascular surgery* 2009;43(5): 452-456.

Huang T, Zheng J, Chen Y, Yang B, Wahlqvist ML et al. High consumption of omega-3 polyunsaturated fatty acids decrease plasma homocysteine: A meta-analysis of randomised, placebo-controlled trials. *Nutrition* 2011 [Epub ahead of print].

Johansen K & Koepsell T. Familial tendency for abdominal aortic aneurysms. *JAMA* 1986;256:1934-1936

Jones GT, Phillips VL, Harris EL, Rossaak JI & van Rij AM. Functional matrix metalloproteinase-9 polymorphism (C-1562T) associated with abdominal aortic aneurysm. *J Vasc Surg* 2003;38(6): 1363-1367.

Jones GT, Harris EL, Phillips LV & van Rij AM. The Methylenetetrahydrofolate Reductase C677T Polymorphism Does Not Associate with Susceptibility to Abdominal Aortic aneurysm. *Eur J Vasc Endovasc Surg* 2005;30:137-142

Jones K, Powell J, Brown L, Greenhalgh R, Jormsjo S & Eriksson P. The influence of 4G/5G polymorphism in the Plasminogen Activator Inhibitor-1 gene promoter on incidence, growth and operative risk of abdominal aortic aneurysm. *Eur J Vasc Endovasc Surg* 2002;23:421-425

Jourdheuil-Rahmani D, Rolland PH, Rosset E, Branchereau A & Garcon D. Homocysteine induces synthesis of a serine elastase in arterial smooth muscle cells from multi-organ donors. *Cardiovascular Research* 1997;34:597-602

Karlsson L, Gnarpe J, Bergqvist D, Lindback J & Parsson H. The effect of azithromycin and Chlamydophilia pneumonia infection on expansion of small abdominal aortic aneurysms--a prospective randomized double-blind trial. *J Vasc Surg* 2009;50(1): 23-29.

Khandanpour N, Willis G, Meyer FJ, Armon MP, Loke YK, Wright AJA et al. Peripheral arterial disease and methylenetetrahydrofolate recutase (MTHFR) C677T mutations: A case-control study and meta-analysis. *J Vasc Surg* 2009;49:711-718

Kielty CM, Baldock C, Lee D, Rock MJ, Ashworth JL & Shuttleworth CA. Fibrillin: from microfibril assembly to biomechanical function. *Philos Trans R Soc Lond B Biol Sci* 2002;357(1418):207-217

Klerk M, Verhoef P, Clarke R, Blom HJ, Kok FJ, Schouten EG et al. MTHFR 677C→T Polymorphism and Risk of Coronary Heart Disease: A Meta-analysis. *JAMA* 2002;288:2023-2031

Kontusaari A, Tromp G, Kuivaniemi H, Romanic AM & Prockop DJ. A mutation in the gene for type III procollagen (COL3A1) in a family with aortic aneurysms. *J Clin Invest.* 1990; 86(5): 1465–1473

Kotani K, Shimomura T, Murakami F, Ikawa S, Kanaoka Y, Oghi S et al. Allele frequency of human endothelial nitric oxide synthase gene polymorphism in abdominal aortic aneurysm. *Intern Med* 2000;39(7):537-539

Krumdieck CL & Prince CW. Mechanisms of Homocysteine Toxicity on Connective Tissues: Implications for the Morbidity of Aging. *J Nutr* 2000;130:365S-368S

Lievers KJA, Kluijtman LAJ & Blom HJ. Genetics of hyperhomocysteinaemia in cardiovascular disease. *Ann Clin Biochem* 2003;40:46-59

Lindholt JS, Sorensen HT, Michel JB, Thomsen HF & Henneberg EW. Low-dose aspirin may prevent growth and later surgical repair of medium-sized abdominal aortic aneurysms. *Vascular and endovascular surgery* 2008;42(4): 329-334.

Lindholt JS, Jorgensen B, Shi GP & Henneberg EW. Relationships between activators and inhibitors of plasminogen, and the progression of small abdominal aortic aneurysms. *Eur J Vasc Endovasc Surg* 2003;25(6): 546-551.

Longo GM, Buda SJ, Fiotta N, Xiong W, Griener T, Shapiro S et al. MMP-12 has a role in abdominal aortic aneurysms in mice. *Surgery* 2005;137(4): 457-462.

Moat S, Lang D, McDowell I, Clarke ZL, Madhavan AK, Lewis MJ et al. Folate, homocysteine, endothelial function and cardiovascular disease. *J Nutr Biochem* 2004;15:64-79

Monux G, Serrano FJ, Vigil P & De La Concha EG. Role of HLA-DR in the pathogenesis of abdominal aortic aneurysm. *Eur J Vasc Endovasc Surg* 2003;26:211-214

Moroz P, Le MTQ & Norman PE. Homocysteine and Abdominal Aortic Aneurysms. *ANZ J Surg* 2007;77:329-332

Mosorin M, Juvonen J, Biancari F, Satta J, Surcel HM, Leinonen M, Saikku P et al. Use of doxycycline to decrease the growth rate of abdominal aortic aneurysms: a randomized, double-blind, placebo-controlled pilot study. *J Vasc Surg* 2001;34(4): 606-610.

Naydeck BL, Sutton-Tyrell K, Schiller KD & Newman AB. Prevalence and Risk Factors for Abdominal Aortic Aneurysms in Older Adults With and Without Isolated Systolic Hypertension. *Am J Cardiol* 1999;83:759-764

Nishimoto M, Takai S, Fukumoto H, Tsunemi K, Yuda A, Sawada Y et al. Increased local angiotensin II formation in aneurismal aorta. *Life Sci* 2002;71:2195-2205

Ogata T, Shibamura H, Tromp G, Sinha M, Goddard K, Sakalihasan N et al. Genetic analysis of polymorphisms in biologically relevant candidate genes in patients with abdominal aortic aneurysms. *J Vasc Surg* 2005;41:1036-1042

Parodi FE, Mao D, Ennis TL, Pagano MB & Thompson RW. Oral administration of diferuloylmethane (curcumin) suppresses proinflammatory cytokines and destructive connective tissue remodeling in experimental abdominal aortic aneurysms. *Annals of vascular surgery* 2006;20(3): 360-368.

Perna AF, Ingrosso D, Lombardi C, Acanfora F, Satta E et al. Possible mechanisms of homocysteine toxicity. *Kidney International* 2003;63(84):S137-S140

Petersen E, Gineitis A, Wagberg F & Angquist KA. Activity of matrix metalloproteinase-2 and -9 in abdominal aortic aneurysms. Relation to size and rupture. *Eur J Vasc Endovasc Surg* 2000;20(5): 457-461.

Pola R, Gaetani E, Santoliquido A, Gerardino L, Cattani P, Serricchio M et al. Abdominal aortic aneurysm in normotensive patients: association with angiotensin-converting enzyme gene polymorphism. *Eur J Vasc Endovasc Surg* 2001;21(5):445-449

Pooya SH, Jalali MD, Jazayery AD, Saedisomeolia A, Eshraghian MR et al. The efficacy of omega-3 fatty acid supplementation on plasma homocysteine and malondialdehyde levels of type-2 diabetic patients. *Nutr Metab Cardiovasc Dis* 2010;20(5):326-331.

Pyo R, Lee JK, Shipley JM, Curci JA, Mao D, Ziporin SJ et al. Targeted gene disruption of matrix metalloproteinase-9 (gelatinase B) suppresses development of experimental abdominal aortic aneurysms. *The Journal of clinical investigation* 2000;105(11): 1641-1649.

Rasmussen TE, Hallett JW, Schukte S, Harmsen S, O'Fallon WM & Weyand CM. Genetic similarity in inflammatory and degenerative abdominal aortic aneurysms: a study of human leukocyte antigen class II disease risk genes. *J Vasc Surg* 2002;35(5):988-993

Rassoul F, Richter V, Kuntze T, Mohr F, Geisel J & Herrmann W. Genetic polymorphism of methylenetetrahydrofolate reductase (MTHFR) and coronary artery disease. *International Journal of Angiology* 2000;9(4):205-207

Rizzo RJ, McCarthy WJ, Dixit SN, Lilly MP, Shively VP, Flinn WR et al. Collagen types and matrix protein content in human abdominal aortic aneurysms. *J Vasc Surg*. 1989 Oct;10(4):365-73.

Rossaak JI, Van Rij AM, Jones GT & Harris EL. Association of the 4G/5G polymorphism in the promoter region of plasminogen activator inhibitor-1 with abdominal aortic aneurysms. *J Vasc Surg* 2000;31:1026-1032

Sandford RM, Bown MJ, London NJ & Sayers RD. The Genetic Basis of Abdominal Aortic Aneurysms: A Review. *Eur J Vasc Endovasc Surg* 2007;33:381-390.

Sinha I, Bethi S, Cronin P, Williams DM, Roelofs K, Ailawadi G et al. A biologic basis for asymmetric growth in descending thoracic aortic aneurysms: a role for matrix metalloproteinase 9 and 2. *J Vasc Surg* 2006;43(2): 342-348.

Smith MW, Dean M, Carrington M, Winkler C, Huttley GA, Lomb DA et al. Contrasting genetic influence of CCR2 and CCR5 variants on HIV-1 infection and disease progression. Hemophilia Growth and Development Study (HGDS), Multicenter AIDS Cohort Study (MACS), Multicenter Hemophilia Cohort Study (MHCS), San Francisco City Cohort (SFCC), ALIVE Study. *Science* 1997;277(5328):959-965

Smulders YM & Blom HJ. The homocysteine controversy. *J Inherit Metab Dis* 2011;34:93-99

Spark JI, Laws P & Fitridge R. The Incidence of Hyperhomocysteinemia in Vascular Patients. *Eur J Vasc Endovasc Surg* 2003;26:558-561

Steenge GR, Verhoef P & Katan MB. Betaine Supplementation Lowers Plasma Homocysteine in Healthy Men and Women. *J Nutr* 2003;133:1291-1295

Strauss E, Waliszewski K, Gabriel M, Zapalski S & Pawlak AL. Increased risk of the abdominal aortic aneurysm in carriers of the MTHFR 677T allele. *J Appl Genet* 2003;44(1):85-93

Stuhlinger MC, Oka RK, Graf EF, Schmolzer I, Upson BM et al. Endothelial Dysfunction Induced by Hyperhomocysteinemia: Role of Asymmetric Dimethylarginine. *Circulation* 2003;108:933-938

Sunder-Plassman G & Fodinger M. Genetic determinants of the homocysteine level. *Kidney International* 2003;63(84) S141-S144

Takagi H, Matsui M & Umemoto T. A meta-analysis of clinical studies of statins for prevention of abdominal aortic aneurysm expansion. *J Vasc Surg*;52(6): 1675-1681.

Thompson AR, Drenos F, Hafez H & Humphries SE. Candidate Gene Association Studies in Abdominal Aortic Aneurysm Disease: A Review and Meta-Analysis. *Eur J Vasc Endovasc Surg* 2008;35:19-30

Tilson MD, Reilly JM, Brophy CM, Webster EL & Barnett TR. Expression and sequence of the gene for tissue inhibitor of metalloproteinases in patients with abdominal aortic aneurysms. *J Vasc Surg* 1993;18(2):266-270

Tromp G, Gatalica Z, Skunca M, Berguer R, Siegel T, Kline RA & Kuivaniemi H. Elevated expression of matrix metalloproteinase-13 in abdominal aortic aneurysms. *Annals of vascular surgery* 2004;18(4): 414-420.

Vammen S, Lindholt JS, Ostergaard L, Fasting H & Henneberg EW. Randomized double-blind controlled trial of roxithromycin for prevention of abdominal aortic aneurysm expansion. *The British journal of surgery* 2001;88(8): 1066-1072.

Wahlgren CM, Larsson E, Magnusson PKE, Hultgren R & Swedenborg J. Genetic and environmental contributions to abdominal aortic aneurysm development in a twin population. *J Vasc Surg* 2010;51:3-7

Wang X, Tromp G, Cole CW, Verloes A, Sakalihasan N, Yoon S et al. Analysis of coding sequences for tissue inhibitor of metalloproteinases 1 (TIMP1) and 2 (TIMP2) in patients with aneurysms. *Matrix Biol* 1999;18(2):12-14

Warsi AA, Davies B, Morris-Stiff G, Hullin D & Lewis MH. Abdominal Aortic Aneurysm and its Correlation to Plasma Homocysteine and Vitamins. *Eur J Vasc Endovasc Surg* 2004;27:75-79

Wiklund O, Fager G, Andersson A, Lundstam U, Masson P et al. N-acetylcysteine treatment lowers plasma homocysteine but not serum lipoprotein(a) levels. *Atherosclerosis* 1996;119(1):99-106.

Wilson WR, Evans J, Bell PR & Thompson MM. HMG-CoA reductase inhibitors (statins) decrease MMP-3 and MMP-9 concentrations in abdominal aortic aneurysms. *Eur J Vasc Endovasc Surg* 2005;30(3): 259-262.

Wilson WR, Schwalbe EC, Jones JL, Bell PR & Thompson MM. Matrix metalloproteinase 8 (neutrophil collagenase) in the pathogenesis of abdominal aortic aneurysm. *The British journal of surgery* 2005;92(7): 828-833.

Yilmaz H, Sahin S, Sayar N, Tangurek B, Yilmaz M et al. Effects of folic acid and N-acetylcysteine on plasma homocysteine levels and endothelial function in patients with coronary artery disease. *Acta Cardiol* 2007;62(6):579-585

Yoon S, Tromp G, Vongpunsawad S, Ronkainen A, Juvonen T & Kuivaniemi H. Genetic analysis of MMP3, MMP9, and PAI-1 in Finnish patients with abdominal aortic or intracranial aneurysms. *Biochemical and biophysical research communications* 1999;265(2): 563-568.

Zhang B, Ye S, Herrmann SM, Eriksson P, de Maat M, Evans A et al. Functional polymorphism in the regulatory region of gelatinase B gene in relation to severity of coronary atherosclerosis. *Circulation* 1999;99(14): 1788-1794.

Zulli A. Taurine in cardiovascular disease. *Curr Opin Clin Nutr Metab Care* 2011;14(1):57-60.

3

The Pathohistology of Abdominal Aortic Aneurysm

Gregory T Jones
Vascular Research Group, Dunedin School of Medicine, University of Otago New Zealand

1. Introduction

Atherosclerosis is a chronic condition characterised by the formation of lipid-rich plaques within the walls of medium and large arteries (Ross, 1993; Lusis, 2000) and underlies many forms of vascular disease, including abdominal aortic aneurysm (AAA). The development of all vascular disease phenotypes is dependent on multiple genetic and environmental determinants (Lusis, 2000) though the relative contribution of each of these risk factors may vary with different vascular disease phenotypes. This is certainly true for AAA, which appears to have particularly strong associations with male gender, tobacco smoking (Singh et al., 2001) and a family history of AAA (Verloes et al., 1995; Ogata et al., 2005). Interestingly, diabetes, a well-established occlusive atherosclerotic disease risk factor is not associated, and may even be protective for AAA (Shantikumar et al., 2010).

Abdominal aortic aneurysm is a common condition being responsible for 1.3% of all deaths in 65-85 year old white males (Sakalihasan et al., 2005). The reported prevalence rates vary depending on factors such as the threshold aortic diameter used to define an aneurysm and age strata (relevant when reviewing rates from screening studies). If the most widely accepted value of 30mm is applied, 1% of women and 4.2% of men between the ages of 50 to 79 years are affected in a predominantly white (north American) population (Lederle et al., 2000). In British males, over the age of 65 years, this rate has been reported to be a high as 7.6% (Scott et al., 1995), although there are indications that incidence may be falling internationally (Sandiford et al., 2011). An abdominal aortic aneurysm is typically defined as being localised in the infrarenal abdominal aorta and may either extend up to involve the renal ostia, or down to involve the aortic bifurcation and into common iliac arteries (Sakalihasan et al., 2005).

These epidemiologic and anatomical features are important when considering the pathobiology of AAA. While the initial pathobiology is atherosclerotic, at some stage it diverts to a distinctive dilating, rather than aortic occlusive, phenotype. A schema outlining the key pathogenic components was proposed by Thompson and colleagues in 1995 (Holmes et al., 1995), a modified interpretation of which is shown in Figure 1. This chapter will briefly describe each of the pathohistological features.

2. Histology of the abdominal aorta

2.1 Histological features in the aging arteries

The abdominal aorta is a transitional elastic artery. In the prenatal abdominal aorta the intima consists of an endothelial monolayer and a scant pad of sub-endothelial fibrous connective tissue upon an intact internal elastic lamina (IEL). The only openings between the intima and underlying media are fenestrations in the IEL, which are spanned by elastic tissue trabeculae. The media is composed of approximately 28-30 concentric lamellar subunits (Wolinsky & Glagov, 1969), one lamellar unit consisting of an elastic lamina and the smooth muscle and extracellular matrix contents of the adjacent interlamellar zone (Fig. 2). The medial elastic laminae are approximately two thirds the thickness of the internal elastic lamina and are interconnected by a network of finer elastic fibres. Collagen and elastin fibres are uniformly dispersed around the circumferentially orientated smooth muscle cells (Keech, 1960; Karrer, 1961; Wolinsky & Glagov, 1964).

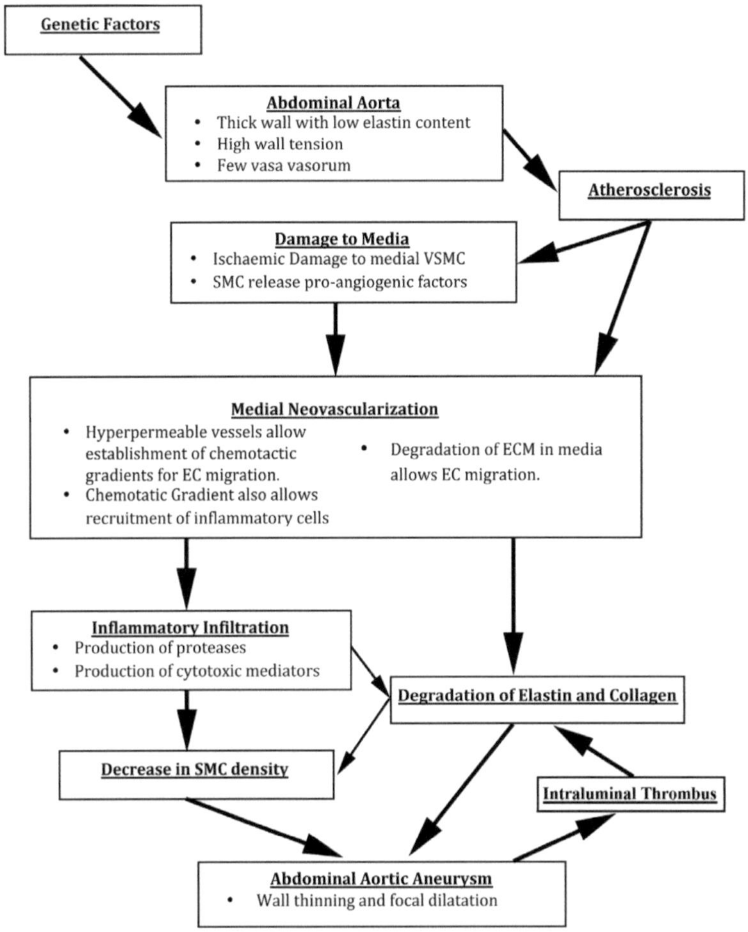

Fig. 1. The Pathogenesis of Abdominal Aortic Aneurysm. This schema is a modification of that proposed by Thompson and colleagues (Holmes et al., 1995). Originally to highlight the central role of medial neovascularisation it shows the progressive steps of aneurysm histopathology outlined in this chapter. Atherosclerosis superimposed on a structurally vulnerable infrarenal abdominal aorta leads to medial degeneration which in-turn stimulates a neovascularisation and inflammatory response from the adventitia. These processes result in a pernicious cycle leading to wall thinning, vessel expansion and eventually aneurysm rupture.

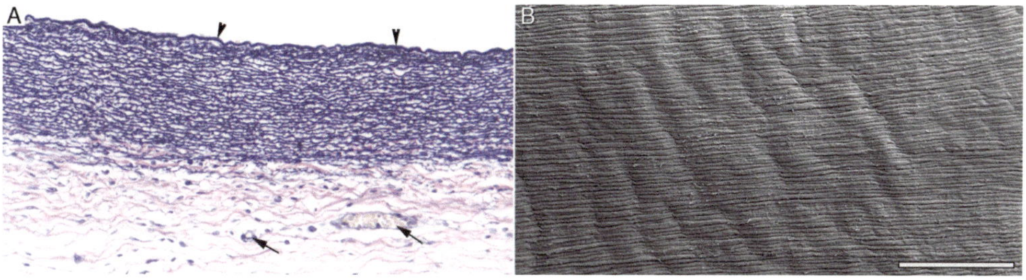

Fig. 2. Infrarenal abdominal aorta, 21 weeks-gestation. A. The intima consists of a monolayer of endothelial cells in close apposition to a thick continuous internal elastic lamina (arrowheads). The aortic media consists of vascular smooth muscle interspaced between approximately 30 elastic laminae (stained black). A network of vasa vasorum (arrows) is found throughout the adventitia but very rare penetrates even the most external layers of the media. Original magnification x50. Verhoeff's elastic stain and van Gieson's counterstain (elastin black, collagen red). B. *An en face* (endothelium removed) scanning electron preparation of the IEL from the same subject. The IEL forms an intact corrugated layer punctuated by small fenestrations (not visible at this magnification. Scale bar 500μm

Within the aortic adventitia a network of vasa vasorum is present that originates from adjacent intercostal, lumbar and mesenteric arteries (Heistad & Marcus, 1979). The vasa vasorum has been shown to only penetrate the media of vessels with greater than 29-30 lamellae (Wolinsky & Glagov, 1969) and consequently the media of the human infrarenal aorta is vastly avascular, despite the presence of the adventitial vasa vasorum (Fig. 3). However, if the luminal diffusion is insufficient to supply nutrients to the intima, vasa vasorum becomes an important alternative nutrient supply (Heistad & Marcus, 1979). Consequently, as the intima thickens, the vasa vasorum extends channels into the outer medial lamellae (Fig. 3B). Significantly however, unlike vasa vasorum in larger vessels such as the thoracic aorta, which are well integrated into the lamellar structure of the wall during its vasculogenesis, these new vessels appear to disrupt the medial structure during their invasion of the wall, as described below in section 2.4.

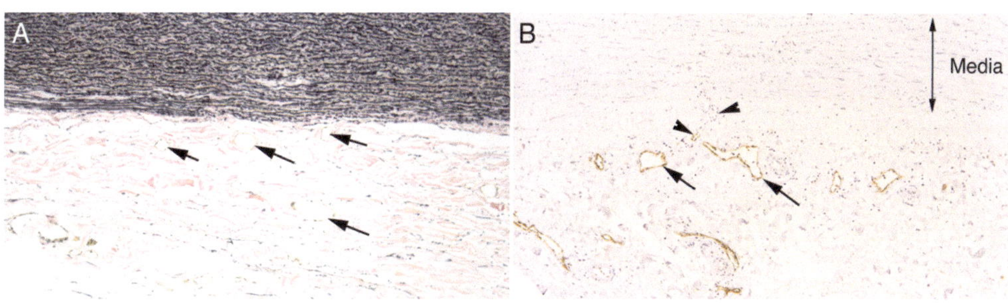

Fig. 3. Vasa vasorum at the medial-adventitial boundary. (A) numerous channels (arrows) within the infrarenal aortic adventitia of a 9-year old female (Verhoeff's elastic stain and van Gieson's counterstain). (B) anti-von-Willebrand factor immunostaining (DAB (3,3-diaminobenzidine) staining resulting in a brown reaction product) showing an extensive network of vessels in the adventitia (arrows), including some small vessels extending into the medial layer (arrowheads) in the infrarenal aorta of a 35-year old male. Original magnification (A) x33, (B) x25

Compared to the thoracic segment and other mammalian aortas of the same thickness, human abdominal aortic media contains less lamellar units, and therefore medial elastic laminae. Consequently, the vessel appears to be stiffer, due to a higher collagen-to-elastin ratio. The flow on effect of this is that the mean tension per lamellar unit is higher in the human abdominal aorta (Wolinsky & Glagov, 1969; Wolinsky, 1970). As will be described below, loss of load bearing elastin, along with the avascular nature of the abdominal aortic media, are key pathologic features of AAA. Therefore the vessels initial lower elastin content and lack of medial vasa vasorum may make it structurally vulnerable to degenerative alteration and the subsequent development of aneurysmal disease later in life (Dobrin, 1989; He & Roach, 1994).

2.2 Early life elastic lamina degeneration, the nidus of atherosclerosis?

After birth one of the first changes in aortic structure consists of disruption of the IEL (Fig. 4). These spontaneous, transversely orientated, elastic lamina defects have been reported within the arteries of newborn and adolescent humans, particularly those vessels known to be prone to the subsequent development of atherosclerosis, such as the aorta (Meyer & Lind, 1972), coronary (Levene, 1956; Moon, 1957; Sims, 1985; Ikari et al., 1999) and carotid (Meyer et al., 1980)] arteries. Critically, Meyer and colleagues demonstrated that elastic lamina defects occur in very young humans, at sites prone to the eventual development of atherosclerosis (Meyer & Lind, 1972; Meyer et al., 1980).

The intima also undergoes early cellular alteration, with the formation of a smooth muscle cell layer between the endothelium and IEL. The origins of these smooth muscle cells has been considered controversial, with some authors suggesting that they are an expansion of a resident intimal cell population (Stary, 2000), while others have argued that they originate from the media and migrate into the intima (Schwartz, 1997; Willis et al., 2004). The most significant contributor to intimal smooth muscle thickening is likely to be a medial origin, as evidenced by the fact that the intima is thicker above regions of IEL disruption in children (Fig. 4). This is further supported by the ApoE deficient mouse model of atherosclerosis, which clearly shows that early intimal smooth muscle cell accumulation is due to medial smooth muscle cell migration through defects in the IEL (Jones et al., 2005). The thickening intima typically forms two distinct layers, a deep musculoelastic layer and a less compact superficial subendothelial layer (Figs 5 & 6C).

The literature also reports the internal elastic lamina beneath the thickened intima and subsequent atherosclerotic plaques as becoming 'frayed', 'reduplicated' or undergoing laminated elastosis. All of these terms refer to intimal elastic tissue deposition and as such should be considered as a distinct, though often co-localised, processes to the disruption of the original IEL. The key cells in producing intimal elastic tissue are smooth muscle cells (Kojimahara, 1988) with a possible contribution by the endothelial monolayer (Jones & Stehbens, 1995) and macrophages (Krettek et al., 2003).

Intimal elastic tissues appear to have an increased affinity for lipoproteins compared with the 'original' elastic laminae (Adams & Tuqan, 1961; Urry, 1975; Meyer et al., 1980). The lipophillic features of intimal elastic tissue (Fig. 5) appears to be a key early contributor to intimal lipid retention (Williams & Tabas, 1995).

Calcification has been shown to be localised to the elastin adjacent to the break edges of spontaneous IEL defects in the arteries of children (Meyer & Lind, 1972; Meyer et al., 1980). While calcium containing matrix vesicles have been shown to preferentially accumulate in microfractures within elastic laminae adjacent to abrupt, haemodynamically induced, elastic tissue defects in experimental animals (Jones & Stehbens, 1995). As such failure of the elastic laminae may facilitate accumulation of granulovesicular debris, including calcospherites, and thereby contribute to vascular connective tissue calcification.

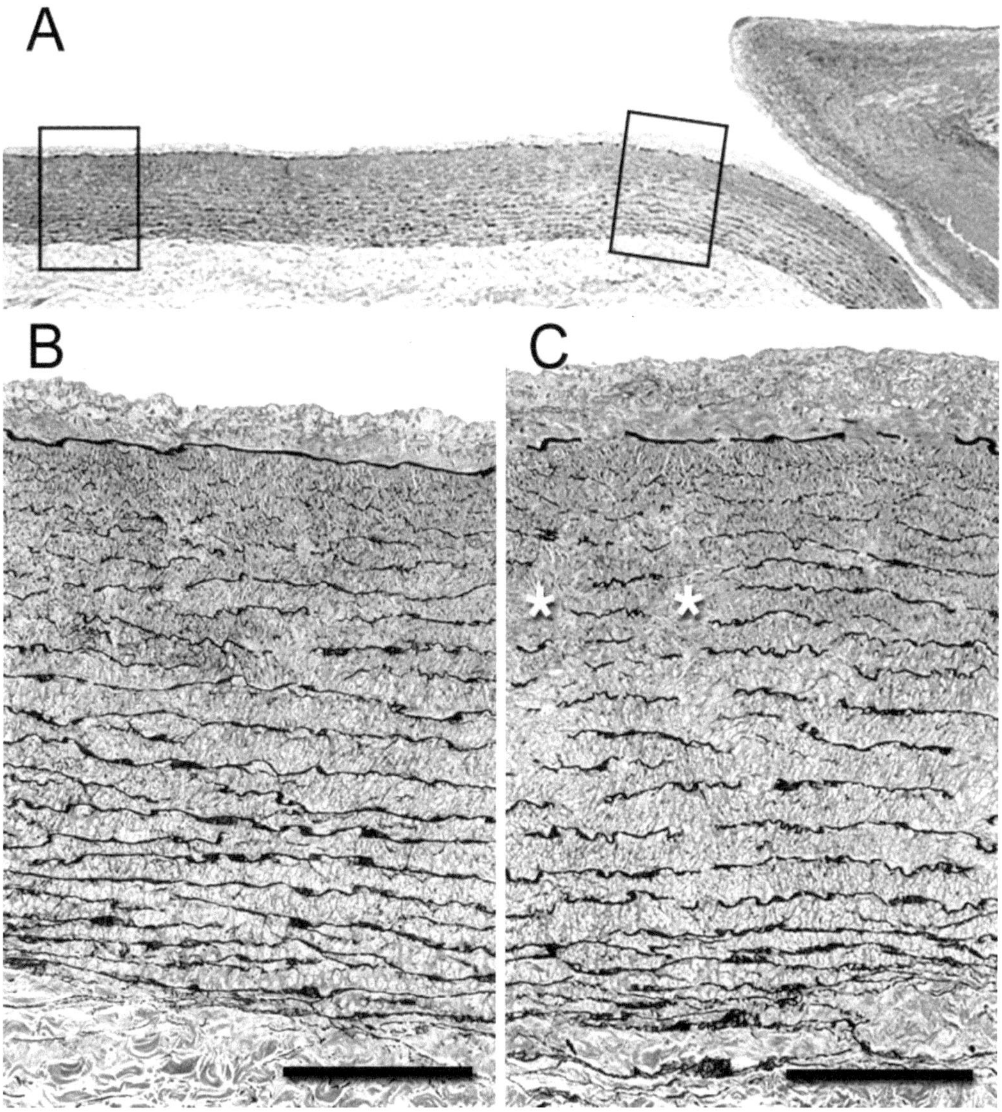

Fig. 4. Longitudinal sections of the anterior infrarenal abdominal aortic wall from a 9 year old female. (A) The two regions indicated represent a proximal segment of the infrarenal aorta (B) and the lateral angle of the inferior mesenteric artery ostium (C). (B) In this young subject IEL defects were not observed in abdominal aortic segments away from branch ostia. (C) In contrast the segment within the lateral branch angle has a fragmented IEL, a more thickened intima, and disrupted medial lamellae (asterisks). Verhoeff's elastic stain. Scale bars 200μm.

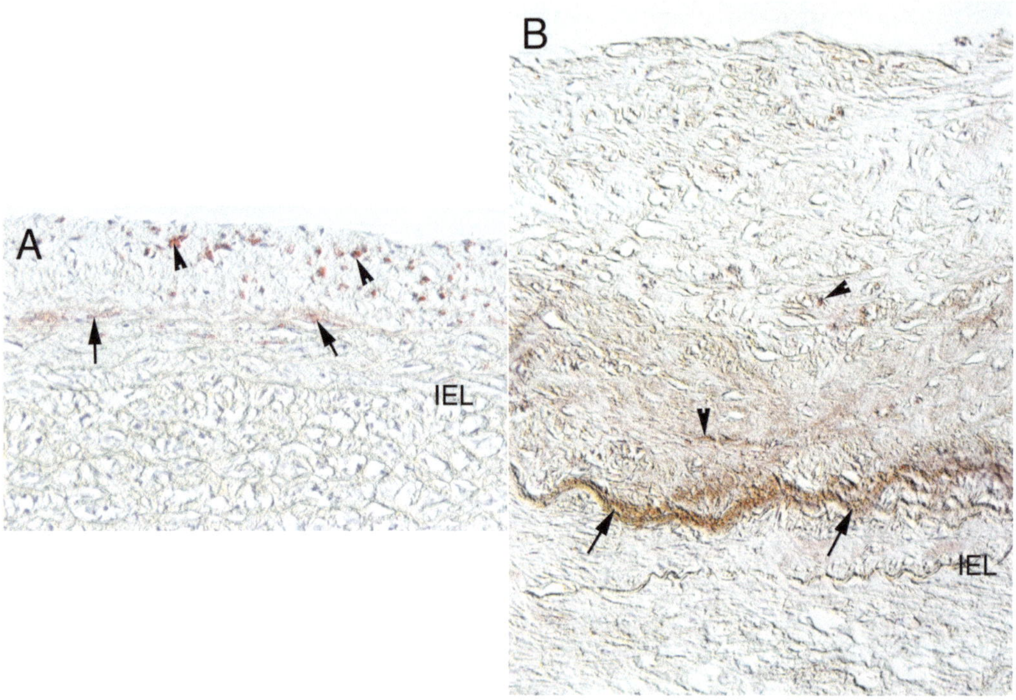

Fig. 5. Intimal lipid disposition. Oil-red-O staining of the distal abdominal aorta in a (A) 37-year old male and an (B) 84-year old female showing diffuse lipid deposits within (subendothelial) macrophages (arrowheads) and bound to extracellular matrix, particularly intimal pseudo-elastic laminae (arrows). The intima is demarcated by the internal elastic lamina (IEL). As the intima thickens with age (B) note the localisation of lipid in the deep (fibroelastic layer) intima as a precursor to the formation of a lipid core. Original magnification both x33. Photographed using differential interference contrast (DIC) microscopy.

The localisation of atherogenic lipids and granulovesicular debris within elastic laminae break edges and the intimal elastic tissue may act as chemotaxic targets for migrating smooth muscle cells and macrophages effectively 'lighting up' these intimal / medial gateways.

When assessing the histopathology of early atherosclerotic lesions, care should therefore be taken to differentiate between intimal elastic tissue and the original IEL. Such a distinction is clearly significant given the possible differences in cell permeability and affinity for lipophilic debris of these two forms of elastic tissue. Certain stains, such as phosphotungstic acid haematoxylin (PTAH), differentially stain these two forms of elastic connective tissue (Gillman et al., 1955), though common elastic tissue stains, such Verhoeff's elastic stain, do not.

Of relevance to the study of abdominal aortic aneurysm histopathology the distal abdominal aorta and common iliac arteries appear to be particularly vulnerable to both IEL degeneration and intimal elastosis (Figs. 4-6).

Even at its earliest stages of development, atherosclerosis displays preferential localisation about the segmental branch ostia of the posterior abdominal aortic wall (Miller et al., 1993; Stehbens, 1995). While systemic factors, such as serum LDL levels, smoking, hypertension and diabetes (Grundy, 1995; Schaefer et al., 1995; Strong & Group, 1995; Jousilahti et al., 1999), have been implicated in the progression of atherosclerosis they fail to fully account for the

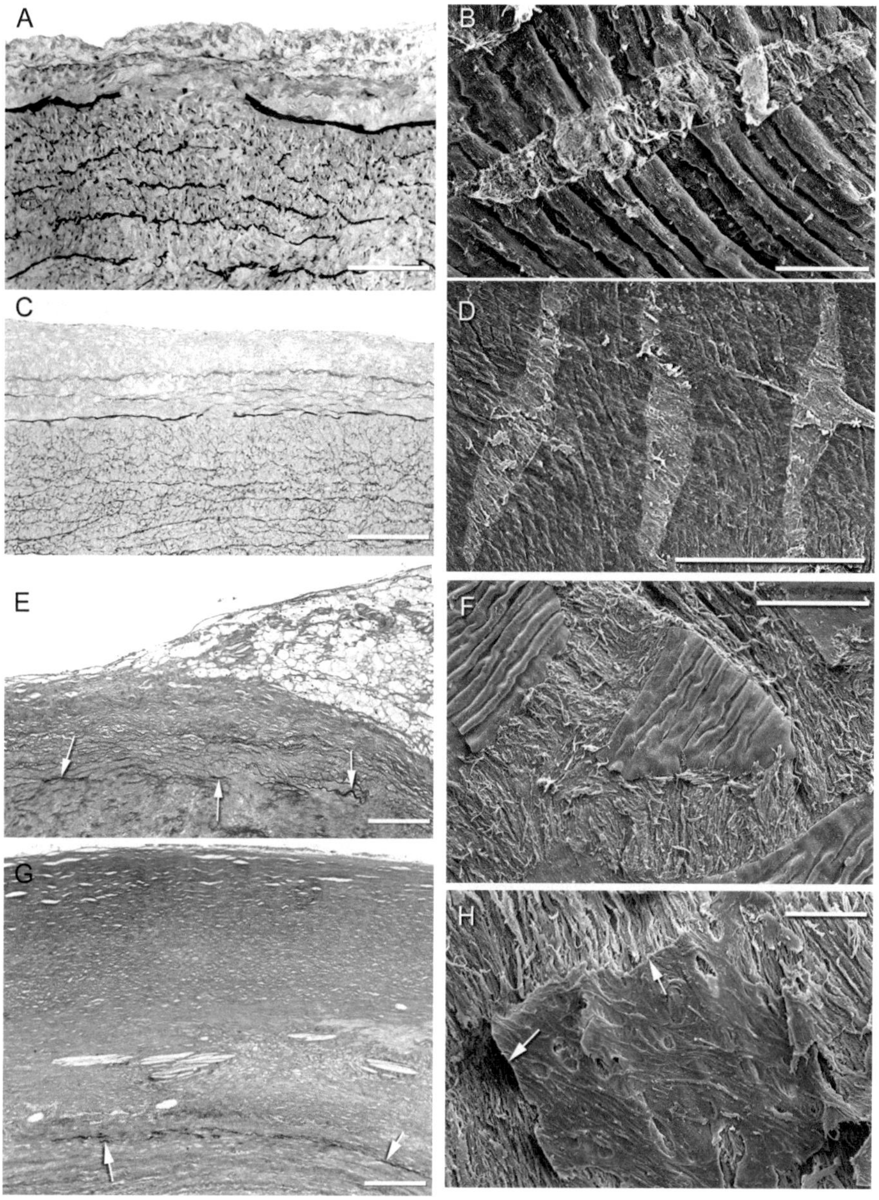

Fig. 6. Histological and en face appearance of abdominal aortic IEL defects. Abdominal aortic specimens from subjects aged (A&B) 9-years, (C&D) 35-years (E&F) 61-years with atherosclerosis, (G&H) 63-year old with abdominal aortic aneurysm. The primary lesions were transversely orientated (B&D), and become interconnected longitudinally in older subjects (F&H). Remnants of the IEL are indicated (E& G arrows). The asterisk in D indicates adherent intimal tissue not fully removed during sample preparation. Note the formation of elastic tissue, within the intimal fibroelastic layer, above the disrupted IEL in early intimal thickenings. In the AAA specimen the small IEL fragment has abrupt break edges (arrows). Scale bars (A&B) 100μm, (C, E-F) 200μm, (D) 500μm, (G) 400μm (H) 50μm.

localised nature of the disease. Haemodynamic stresses, including pulse reflection and summation, may predispose various anatomical sites to the development of vascular disease (Stehbens, 1995) as may local intrinsic wall abnormalities. Early atherosclerotic alterations appear to involve the development of intimal thickenings, which are partly derived from medial smooth muscle cells (Fig. 6). Normally the intact internal elastic lamina (Meyer et al., 1980; Ikari et al., 1999) restricts intimal medial cell migration. In latter stages of atherosclerosis the structural and molecular modification of elastic tissues is believed to reduce arterial compliance leading to increased pulse pressure and pressure wave velocities in aging individuals (Urry, 1975; Robert et al., 1995).

This raises the possibility that early-life structural and functional modification of the aortic wall may directly contribute to the progression of atherosclerosis (Stehbens, 1997) rather than simply being normal physiological remodeling. As shown in figure 6, it is somewhat remarkably that the elastic lamina defect edges remain so abrupt, even in elderly aneurysmal aortae, given the considerable elastolytic activity reported in atherosclerotic tissues, and in particularly AAA (Thompson & Parks, 1996). This is undoubtedly a testament to the stability and low turnover rate of elastin, which is estimated at approximately 70 years in humans (Shapiro et al., 1991).

Nevertheless, given the proteolytic activity that occurs within developing atherosclerotic lesions (Knox et al., 1997) and aneurysms (Vine & Powell, 1991; Gargiulo et al., 1993; McMillan et al., 1995; Thompson et al., 1995), the lack of change to the elastic lamina defect edges, apparently over many decades, is noteworthy in that it may provide a stable cumulative index of connective tissue degeneration, without the confounding effect of connective tissue remodelling (as is the case with the fibrillar collagens).

Though elastolytic activity undoubtedly occurs, the histo-morphological features indicate that the elastin within condensed laminae is remarkably resistant to enzymatic degradation. This is not to say that proteolysis is not a significant pathophysiological process in the loss of elastin, for example proteolytic activity may play an indirect role by degrading structural fibrillar collagens. The effect of this would be to shift mechanical stress from these high tensile strength connective tissue components to the relatively weaker elastic tissues, resulting in their accelerated structural fatigue.

2.3 Early atherosclerotic lesions

The earliest lesion generally considered to be atherosclerotic consists focal accumulations of intracellular lipoproteins in the intima and formation of fatty streaks (Fig. 5A). Fatty streaks may be present in the aorta from early childhood and may even start to develop during the foetal life, especially in foetuses of mothers with hypercholesterolaemia (Napoli et al., 1997). The major cellular constituents of fatty streaks are monocyte-derived macrophages recruited into wall via endothelial cell mediated diapedesis. Within the intima, these macrophages may engulf the blood-derived low density lipoprotein (LDL) and become lipid-filled foam cells. By the age of puberty (12-15 years), almost all children will develop lesions containing macrophages and foam cells in the intima of the aorta. This initial accumulation of lipoprotein and formation of fatty streaks does not protrude into the lumen and are thus asymptomatic (Stary, 2000).

The initial accumulation of lipids within the intima is then followed by progressive accumulation of both intra- and extra-cellular lipids. The origin of these lipoproteins can be classified as either blood-derived or that released from the death of resident macrophage/foam cells (Guyton, 2001). Intimal smooth muscle cells also contain lipid droplets (Stary, 2000), but, not having the oxidised LDL scavenger receptor, never develop

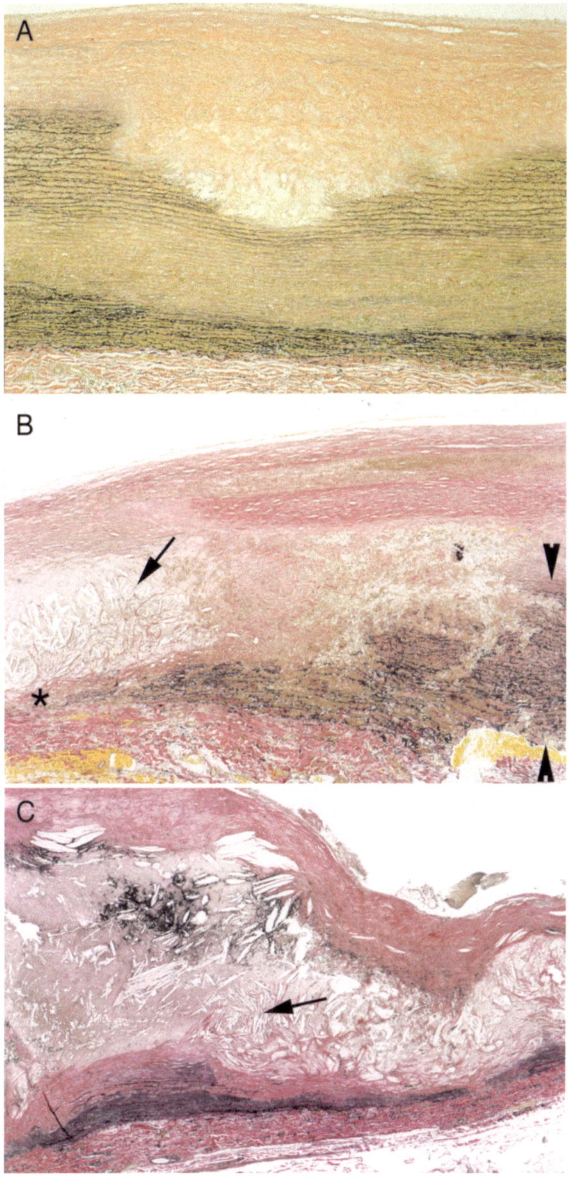

Fig. 7. Infra-renal aortic medial degeneration. A. Mild atherosclerosis (male 84 years). The atherosclerotic intimal lipid core has eroded the medial elastic laminae. (B) Proximal neck of an AAA from a 83-year old female. The region beneath the lipid core (*) has undergone almost complete medial degeneration, while the media on the right hand side still has numerous, at least partially intact, elastic laminae and layers of smooth muscle (between arrow heads). (C) Mid-sac region of an AAA, showing extensive, but heterogenous, medial atrophy (male 69-years). Note accumulation of cholesterol crystals (arrows) and extracellular calicification (black stained region overlying the lipid core in C) in the more advanced lesions. Verhoeff's elastic stain and van Gieson's counterstain (elastin black, collagen red), magnification A x13, B&C x10.

the foam cell appearance observed in tissue macrophages. The process of intimal lipid sequestration is pernicious and eventually results in the formation of a so-called lipid-core within the deep intima. As the size of this region increases it becomes filled with cholesterol ester crystals (Tangirala et al., 1994) and calcium deposits (Fig. 7). Beginning as regions of vesicular debris, termed matrix vesicles (Tanimura et al., 1983; Bobryshev et al., 2008), these small (approximately 20nm in diameter) calcium phosphate rich membrane bound vesicles appear to act as a nidus for subsequent vascular calcification (Fig. 7C). The lipid core is covered by a 'fibrous cap' composed of proteoglycan-rich extracellular matrix, smooth muscle and inflammatory cells (Stary, 2000).

As the disease progresses the atherosclerotic intima becomes more fibrotic, due to the production of extracellular matrix by smooth muscle cells (Davies & Hagen, 1994; Kaiura et al., 2000).

The increased intimal thickness results in decreased luminal diffusion to the deep intima and inner media, producing a hypoxic zone (Pugh & Ratcliffe, 2003). This is generally considered to occur when the intima reaches 500μm in thickness (Moreno et al., 2006).

2.4 Medial atrophy

There are two histopathological features associated with the formation of a hypoxic intimal-medial zone. Firstly the lipid-laden foam cell rich lipid core appears to erode the underlying media (Fig. 7). While, in children and young adults, the initial failure of the internal and medial elastic laminae appears to be driven by biomechanical fatigue, there is little doubt that a strong proteolytic component drives the medial erosion observed in more advanced plaques. The matrix metalloproteinases (MMP), in particular MMP-9 (Fig. 8), have been strongly implicated in the pathogenesis of both atherosclerosis and AAA progression (Thompson & Parks, 1996). It is this outward remodeling of the media, and eventually the adventitia, that preserves luminal patency during the early-mid phases of atherogenesis (Ge et al., 1993; Hermiller et al., 1993).

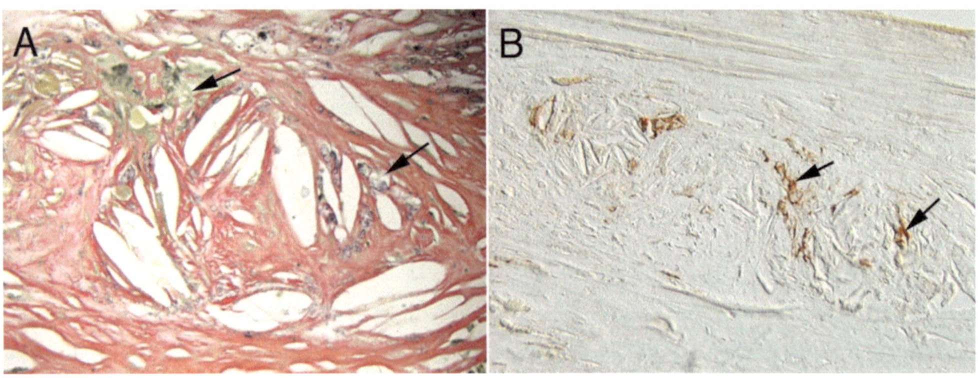

Fig. 8. Proteolytic activity within the developing aneurysm wall (female 70-years). (A) Macrophages (arrows) surrounded by cholesterol ester crystals clefts (Verhoeff's elastic tissue stain). (B) In a matching section, these same macrophages (arrows) are matrix metalloproteinase-9 positive (DAB (brown) reaction product, with DIC microscopy). Magnification A x132, B x66.

Secondly, as a result of the deep intima hypoxia, the adventitial vasa vasorum network begins to penetrate the media (Moreno et al., 2006). In addition, the process of elastic tissue degradation produces small elastin-derived peptides, which have also been shown to stimulate angiogenesis (Nackman et al., 1997; Robinet et al., 2005). The neovascularisation process disrupts the lamellar structure of the media, with heavily vascularised regions of the media having significantly reduced elastic tissue and smooth muscle cell content (Fig. 9). Paralleling the process of medial neovasculisation, the adventitia typically undergoes progressive thickening due to the expansion and proliferation of the vasa vasorum network (Table 1).

Vessel density (channels/0.1mm^2)	**Control n=11**	**AAA n=28**	**p-value**
Media	0.1 (0-1.5)	1.6 (0.4-2.9)	<0.002
Adventitia	3.2 (1.3-5.2)	6.1 (2.8-9.3	<0.003

Table 1. Vasa vasorum (von Willebrand factor positive) channel density in the media and adventitia of the infrarenal aortic wall. Data presented as median and interquartile range. Aneurysmal aortae had significantly increased medial and adventitial vasa vasorum densities compared with controls. Unlike wall cellularity measures (Fig 11), there was no difference in vessel density between different sized aneurysms. *(Data courtesy of Dr Jun Li).*

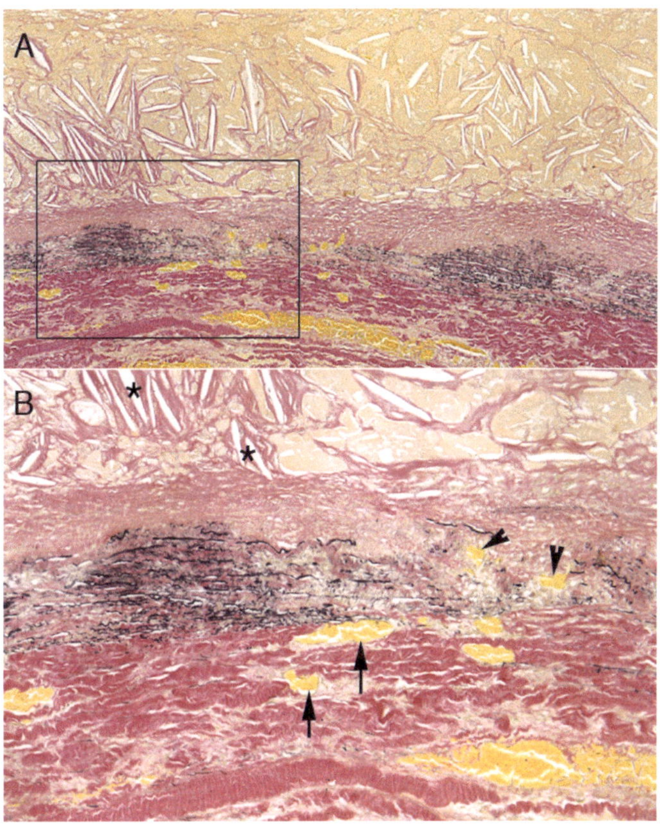

Fig. 9. Medial neovascularization. Histology of an abdominal aortic aneurysm (60-year male), showing a cholesterol crystal (*) rich intima with atrophy of the tunica media. Note the neovascularization of the media (arrowheads) originating from the adventitial vasa vasorum (arrows). Verhoeff's elastic tissue stain- van Gieson's counterstain (elastic tissue black, collagen red, Red blood cells orange). Original magnification A x13, B x66

The combined effects of intimal atherosclerosis and medial neovascularistion result in progressive medial atrophy (Crawford & Levene, 1953; Isner et al., 1986). This is associated with a loss of medial smooth muscle cells due to migration into the intima (Fig. 10) and increased cell death due to apoptosis (Lopez-Candales et al., 1997; Henderson et al., 1999; Boyle et al., 2001). This process can be demonstrated by quantifying the cellularity of the media within infrarenal aortae of varying diameters (Fig. 11). Large AAAs have approximately half the number of (smooth muscle) cells compared with normal sized aortae.

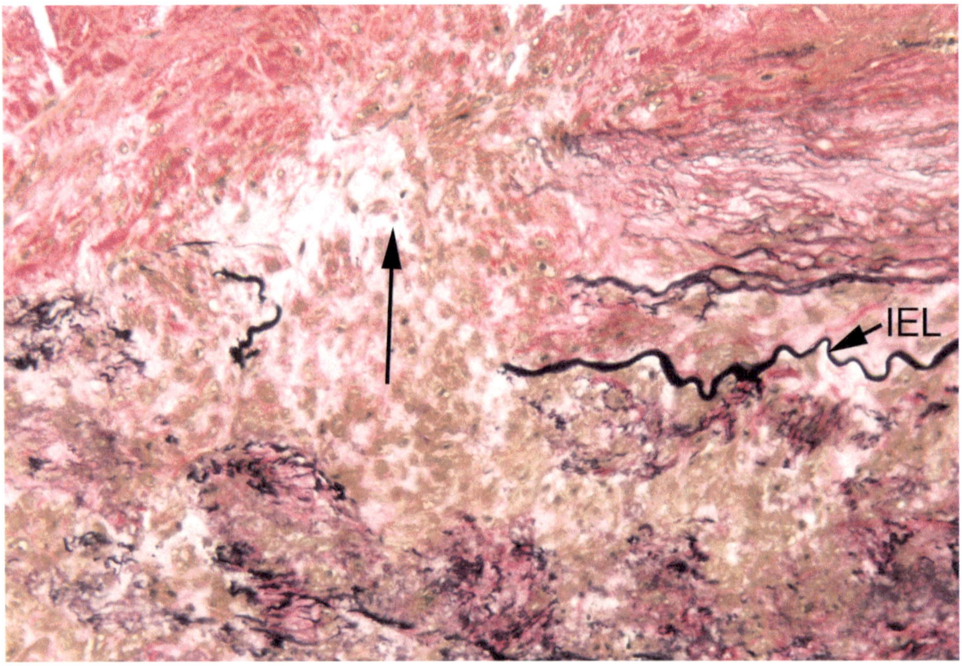

Fig. 10. Medial smooth muscle cell migration into the intima. Histology of the intimal-medial boundary in an 85-year old male. The closely packed medial smooth muscle cells (stained brown) are shown migrating (long arrow) into the intima through a disrupted internal elastic lamina (IEL). Within the intima they are loosely arranged and surrounded by abundant extracellular matrix (stained pink/red). Verhoeff's elastic tissue stain- van Gieson's counterstain. Original magnification x66.

2.5 Medial and peri-aortic inflammation

As described above, the formation of an atherosclerotic intima stimulates a neovascular response from the adventitia towards the intima. The presence of these new channels allows for direct recruitment of inflammatory cells, such as macrophages, plasma cells and T-lymphocytes, into the arterial wall. These cells secrete cytotoxic mediators, such as perforin, which induce smooth muscle apoptosis (Henderson et al., 1999; Lindeman et al., 2008) and further weakens the aortic wall. Moreover, these cells also release chemoattractants thereby stimulating further inflammatory recruitment and sustaining the inflammatory tissue reaction. In this way, medial and adventitial neovascularization establishes a chronic inflammatory state within the outer aortic wall (Figs 12 &13), resulting in continued matrix degradation and remodelling, propagating outward expansion of the aorta and consequent aneurysm formation.

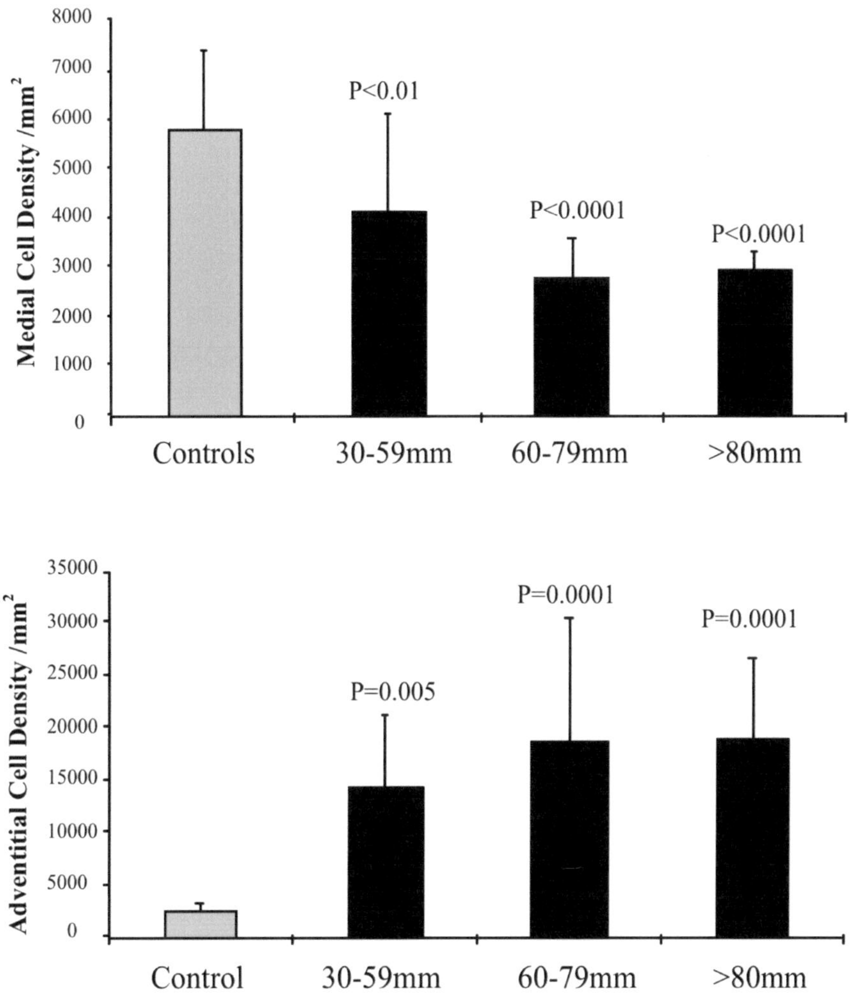

Fig. 11. Cell densities (number of nuclei) in different layers of the infrarenal aortic wall. Non-aneurysmal controls (n=11) were compared with AAAs of varying sizes (30-59mm n=7, 60-79mm n=12 and >80mm n=9). (Top) Within the degenerated media of aneurysms there is a progressive reduction in cell density to approximately half that of controls. (Bottom) In the adventitia there is a marked increase in cell density, vastly in the form of inflammatory cell infiltrate. *(Data courtesy of Dr Jun Li, Vascular Research Group, Dunedin School of Medicine).*

In a small but significant subset (3-10%) of AAA patients this process can become so extensive that the adventitia undergoes significant macroscopic thickening, developing peri-aortic (Fig 14) and retroperitoneal fibrosis and even adhesions of adjacent abdominal organs. These are typically referred to as inflammatory aneurysms (Tang et al., 2005), but it is generally accepted that, rather than representing a separate pathobiological entity, the inflammatory AAA is an extreme manifestation of the same medial and adventitia inflammation which characterizes all abdominal aneurysms (Koch et al., 1990). While there is a spectrum of inflammatory cell infiltration, ranging from minimal (Fig. 9), moderate (Fig. 12) to extensive (Figs. 13 &14), the adventitia cellularity tends to be increased in all aneurysms compared with non-aneurysm vessels (Fig 11). This is due a combination of both cells forming neovascular channels and variable degrees of associated inflammatory infiltrate.

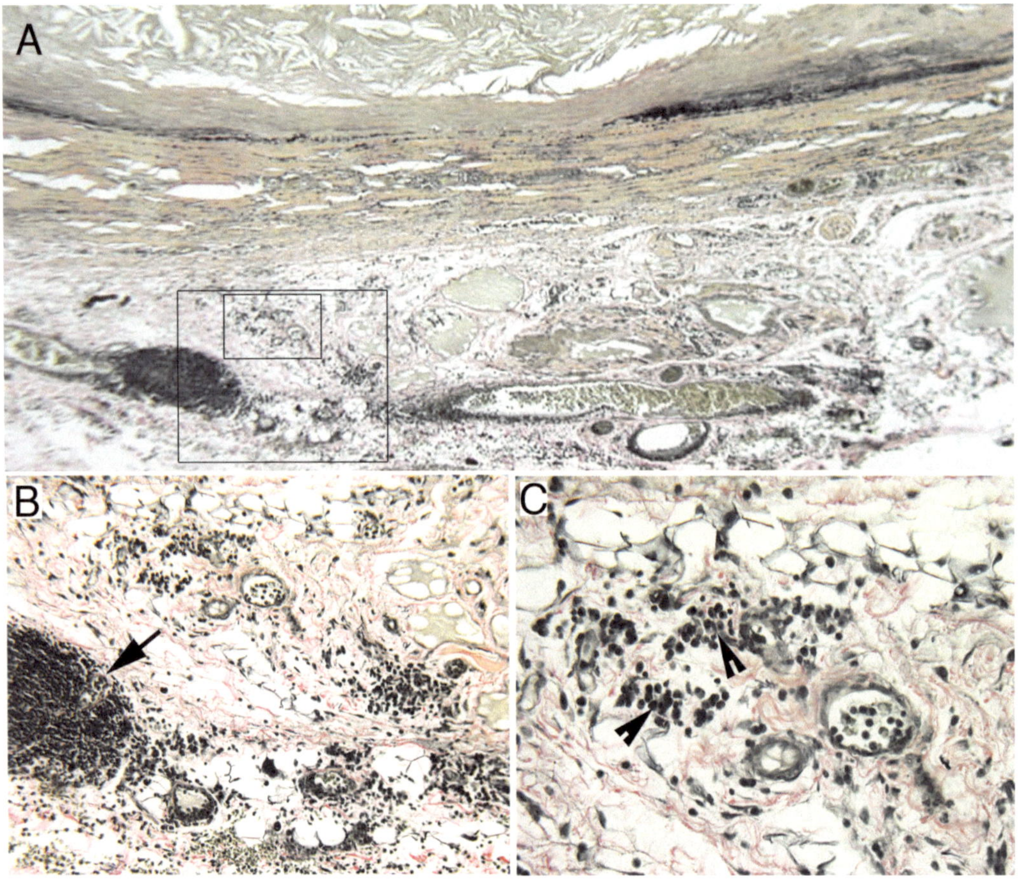

Fig. 12. Microscopic adventitial inflammation. A. Low magnification image of the aneurysm wall from an 82-year old female. (A) Magnified regions of the adventitia are indicated by boxes. Lymphocyte infiltrate forms either large aggregates surrounding blood vessels (arrow in B) or smaller diffuse collections within the extracellular matrix (arrowheads in C). Verhoeff's elastic tissue stain- van Gieson's counterstain. Magnification A x25, B x66, C x132

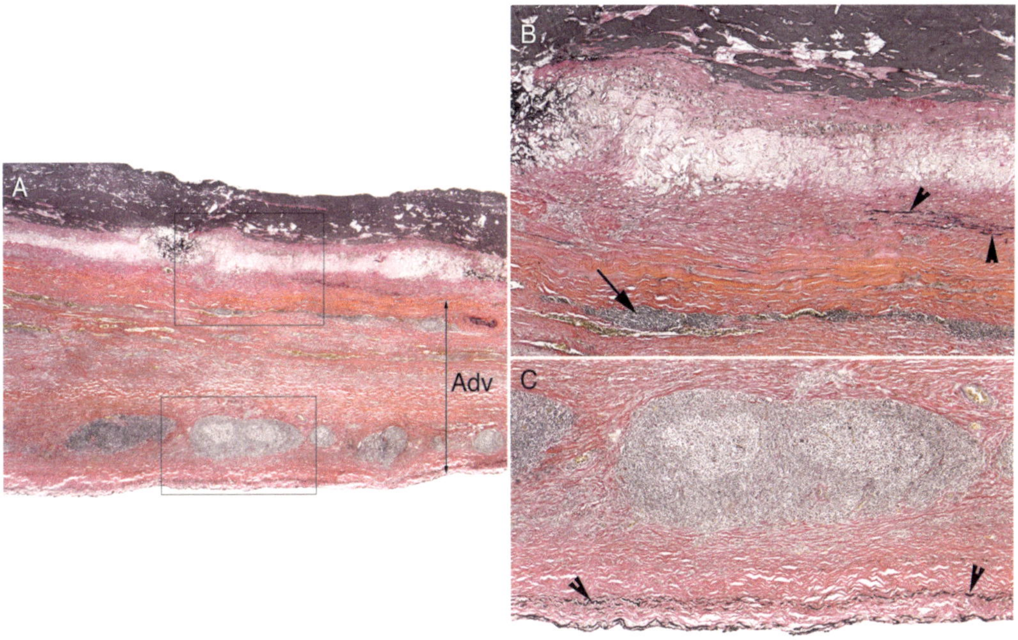

Fig. 13. Moderate adventitial inflammation. (A) Low magnification image of the AAA wall from an 77-year old male. (B & C) Higher magnification images of the boxed regions in A. The adventitia (Adv) is the thickest layer of the aneurysm wall with increased fibrosis and the formation of numerous lymphoid aggregates towards the outer adventitia (C). Regions of more diffuse inflammatory infiltrate are present within the inner adventitia and beneath the atherosclerotic core (arrows in B). Note the remnants of medial and adventitia elastic tissue (arrowheads in B and C respectively). Verhoeff's elastic tissue stain- van Gieson's counterstain. Magnification A x4, B x13, C x13

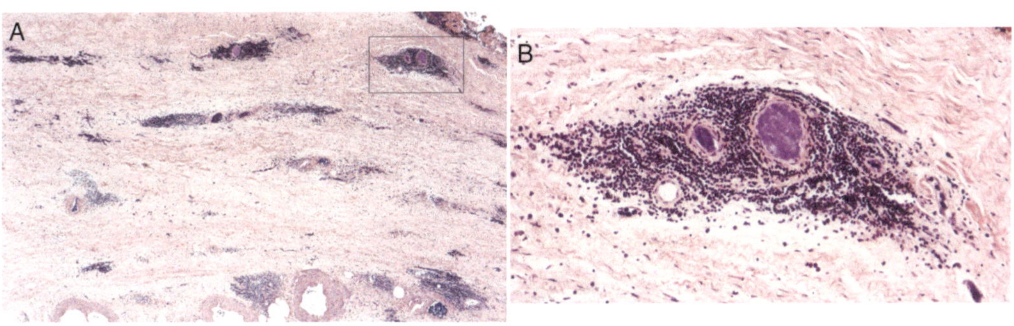

Fig. 14. Adventitia of an inflammatory AAA (female 77-years). (A) low magnification image of the thick adventitial layer. Part of the atrophic media is visible in the top right corner and large vasa vasorum are present towards the bottom. There is extensive fibrosis throughout the adventitia, largely consisting of fibrillar collagen bundles and lymphoid follicles. (B) higher magnification a small network of 3-4 vasa vasorum channels surrounded by a dense inflammatory infiltrate. PTAH Stain (nuclei blue, fibrin within the vasa vasorum blue, collagen red) Original magnification A x10, B x50.

2.6 Intraluminal thrombus

Blood flow studies suggest that the shape of an abdominal aortic aneurysm results in disordered flow, an increased wall tension and thrombus formation within the sac (Moore et al., 1992). Chronic intraluminal thrombus (ILT) forms as a mutli-layered structure, consisting of a luminal layer of fresh red clot, a middle laminated thrombus and an actively fibrinolysed ablumenal layer (Fig 15), with variable incorporation into the aortic intima, including regions of intramural haemorrhage. The presence of ILT contributes to aneurysm progression in multiple ways (Michel et al., 2011). Firstly, when present, ILT significantly thickens the aortic wall (Fig. 16) and acts as a barrier for oxygen transport, resulting in further hypoxia-associated degeneration (Vorp et al., 1998), as described above. Secondly, ILT is a rich source of proteases and their activators, including MMPs and urokinase-type plasminogen activator (Houard et al., 2007).

The luminal zone is enriched with neutrophils, due to these cells strong affinity for the fibrin-fibronectin network. Neutrophil proteases are centrifugally propelled towards the abluminal zone and underlying aortic wall through a network of canaliculi (Adolph et al., 1997). The plasmin within the fibrinolytic abluminal zone results in MMP activation and facilates the release of matrix sequestered growth factors such as transforming growth factor beta. An association between the presence of ILT and risk of AAA rupture (Fig 16B) has been suggest by many authors but the relationship remains controversial. Recent evidence suggests that a key factor may be the degree of ILT fissuring, leading to localised regions of increased wall stress (Polzer et al., 2011).

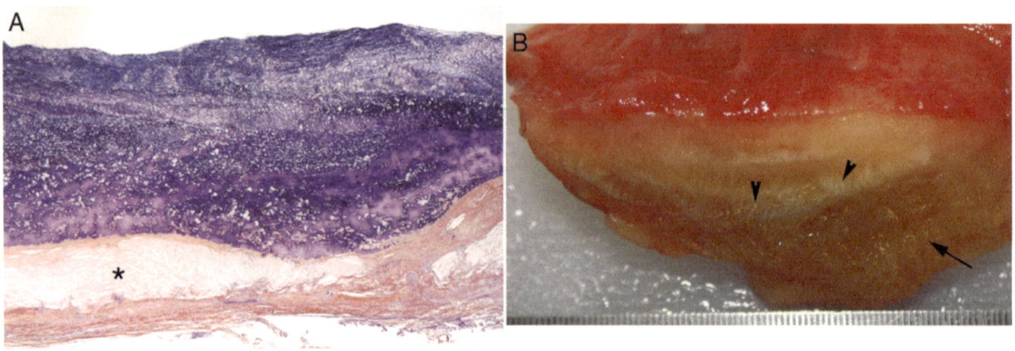

Fig. 15. Intraluminal thrombus. (A) Histology of a AAA (from an 71-year old male) stained with Phosphotungstic Acid Haematoxylin (PTAH). A thick layer of adherent thrombus (fibrin blue), is observed overlying an atheromatous intima (*), pronounced medial atrophy and adventitial collagen (red bands towards the bottom). Notice that the fibrinolytic abluminal zone stains a paler blue. Original magnification x4 (B) A gross thrombus specimen removed from the aneurysm sac of a 74-year old male. Notice the multiple layers consisting of fresh red thrombus on the luminal surface, an organized middle layer including lines of Zahn (arrowheads), and an abluminal fibrinolytic layer (arrow) adjacent to the aortic wall. Scale in millimeters.

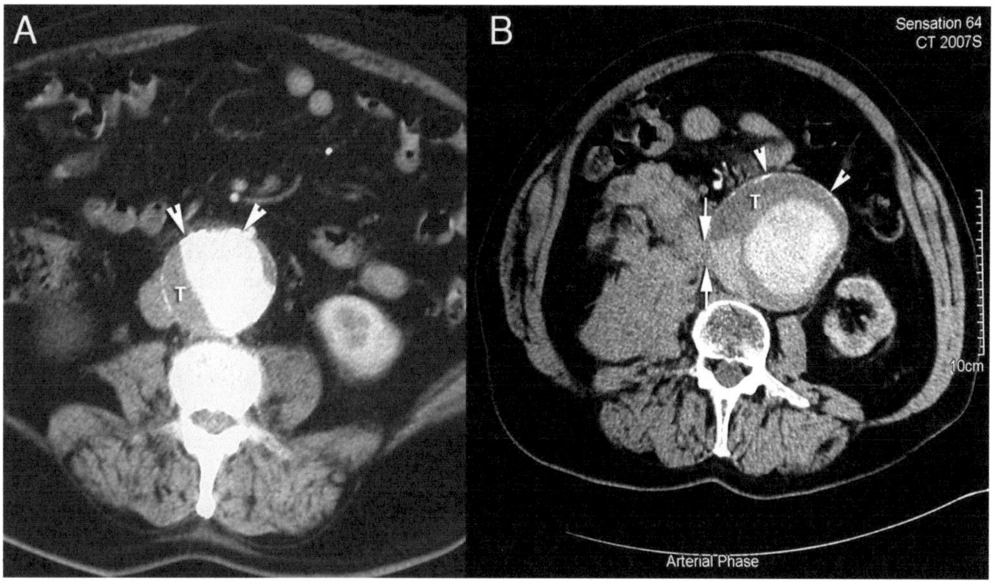

Fig. 16. Computed tomography of a (A) 6.5cm AAA in a 74-year old male and (B) ruptured 8.3cm AAA in a 79-year old male. The anterior aneurysm wall is calcified (arrowheads) in both cases. Notice the effect of adherent intraluminal thrombus (T) on total wall thickness. (B) the posterolateral (retroperitoneal) rupture site (arrows). This is a common site for AAA rupture.

3. Conclusion

The pathohistology of AAA involves the initial formation of intimal atherosclerosis followed by medial atrophy, neovascularisation, inflammatory cell infiltration and intraluminal thrombus formation. Elastic tissue fragility, both in terms of the initial intimal connective tissue degeneration and subsequent medial atrophy, along with the vascular inflammatory response to atherosclerosis appear to be key pathogenic features of AAA.

4. Acknowledgment

A special thanks to Professor Andre van Rij, Dr Ian Thomson, Professor Han-Seung Yoon and Dr Noelyn Hung for their assistance in obtaining specimens. The use of material from Dr Jun Li's BMedSci dissertation is acknowledged and much appreciated. A special thanks to Mrs Vicky Phillips and Ms Liz Girvan for their invaluable technical assistance. On going funding support provided by the Health Research Council of New Zealand is acknowledged.

5. References

Adams, C. W. M. & Tuqan, N. A. (1961). Elastic degeneration as source of lipids in the early lesion of atherosclerosis. *J Pathol Bacteriol* 82: 131-139.

Adolph, R., Vorp, D. A., Steed, D. L., Webster, M. W., Kameneva, M. V. & Watkins, S. C. (1997). Cellular content and permeability of intraluminal thrombus in abdominal aortic aneurysm. *J Vasc Surg* 25(5): 916-926.

Bobryshev, Y. V., Killingsworth, M. C., Lord, R. S. & Grabs, A. J. (2008). Matrix vesicles in the fibrous cap of atherosclerotic plaque: possible contribution to plaque rupture. *J Cell Mol Med* 12(5B): 2073-2082.

Boyle, J. J., Bowyer, D. E., Weissberg, P. L. & Bennett, M. R. (2001). Human blood-derived macrophages induce apoptosis in human plaque-derived vascular smooth muscle cells by Fas-ligand/Fas interactions. *Arterioscler Thromb Vasc Biol* 21(9): 1402-1407.

Crawford, T. & Levene, C. I. (1953). Medial thinning in atheroma. *J Pathol Bacteriol* 66(1): 19-23.

Davies, M. G. & Hagen, P.-O. (1994). Pathobiology of intimal hyperplasia. *Brit J Surg* 81: 1254-1269.

Dobrin, P. B. (1989). Pathophysiology and pathogenesis of aortic aneurysms. Current concepts. *Surg Clin North Am* 69(4): 687-703.

Gargiulo, M., Stella, A., Spina, M., Faggioli, G., Cenacchi, G., Degani, A., Guiducci, G., Tonelli, M., Bertoni, F. & D'Addato, M. (1993). Content and turnover of extracellular matrix protein in human "nonspecific" and inflammatory abdominal aortic aneurysms. *European Journal of Vascular Surgery* 7(5): 546-553.

Ge, J., Erbel, R., Zamorano, J., Koch, L., Kearney, P., Gorge, G., Gerber, T. & Meyer, J. (1993). Coronary artery remodeling in atherosclerotic disease: an intravascular ultrasonic study in vivo. *Coron Artery Dis* 4(11): 981-986.

Gillman, T., Penn, J., Bronks, D. & Roux, M. (1955). Abnormal elastic fibres. *Arch Pathol* 59: 733-749.

Grundy, S. M. (1995). Role of low-density lipoproteins in atherogenesis and development of coronary heart disease. *Clin Chem* 41: 139-146.

Guyton, J. R. (2001). Phospholipid hydrolytic enzymes in a 'cesspool' of arterial intimal lipoproteins: a mechanism for atherogenic lipid accumulation. *Arterioscler Thromb Vasc Biol* 21(6): 884-886.

He, C. M. & Roach, M. R. (1994). The composition and mechanical properties of abdominal aortic aneurysms. *J Vasc Surg* 20(1): 6-13.

Heistad, D. D. & Marcus, M. L. (1979). Role of vasa vasorum in nourishment of the aorta. *Blood Vessels* 16(5): 225-238.

Henderson, E. L., Geng, Y. J., Sukhova, G. K., Whittemore, A. D., Knox, J. & Libby, P. (1999). Death of smooth muscle cells and expression of mediators of apoptosis by T lymphocytes in human abdominal aortic aneurysms. *Circulation* 99(1): 96-104.

Hermiller, J. B., Tenaglia, A. N., Kisslo, K. B., Phillips, H. R., Bashore, T. M., Stack, R. S. & Davidson, C. J. (1993). In vivo validation of compensatory enlargement of atherosclerotic coronary arteries. *Am J Cardiol* 71(8): 665-668.

Holmes, D. R., Liao, S., Parks, W. C. & Thompson, R. W. (1995). Medial neovascularization in abdominal aortic aneurysms: a histopathologic marker of aneurysmal degeneration with pathophysiologic implications. *J Vasc Surg* 21(5): 761-771; discussion 771-762.

Houard, X., Rouzet, F., Touat, Z., Philippe, M., Dominguez, M., Fontaine, V., Sarda-Mantel, L., Meulemans, A., Le Guludec, D., Meilhac, O. & Michel, J. B. (2007). Topology of

the fibrinolytic system within the mural thrombus of human abdominal aortic aneurysms. *J Pathol* 212(1): 20-28.
Ikari, Y., McManus, B. M., Kenyon, J. & Schwartz, S. M. (1999). Neonatal intima formation in the human coronary artery. *Arterioscler Thromb Vasc Biol* 19(9): 2036-2040.
Isner, J. M., Donaldson, R. F., Fortin, A. H., Tischler, A. & Clarke, R. H. (1986). Attenuation of the media of coronary arteries in advanced atherosclerosis. *Am J Cardiol* 58(10): 937-939.
Jones, G. T., Jiang, F., McCormick, S. P. & Dusting, G. J. (2005). Elastic lamina defects are an early feature of aortic lesions in the apolipoprotein E knockout mouse. *J Vasc Res* 42(3): 237-246.
Jones, G. T. & Stehbens, W. E. (1995). The ultrastructure of arteries proximal to chronic experimental carotid-jugular fistulae in rabbits. *Pathology* 27(1): 36-42.
Jousilahti, P., Vartiainen, E., Tuomilehto, J. & Puska, P. (1999). Sex, age, cardiovascular risk factors, and coronary heart disease. A prospective follow-up study of 14786 middle-aged men and women in finland. *Circulation* 99: 1165-1172.
Kaiura, T. L., Itoh, H., Kubaska, S. M., 3rd, McCaffrey, T. A., Liu, B. & Kent, K. C. (2000). The effect of growth factors, cytokines, and extracellular matrix proteins on fibronectin production in human vascular smooth muscle cells. *J Vasc Surg* 31(3): 577-584.
Karrer, H. E. (1961). An electron microscope study of the aorta in young and in aging mice. *J Ultrastruct Res* 5: 1-27.
Keech, M. K. (1960). Electron microscope study of the normal rat aorta. *J Biophys Biochem Cytol* 7: 533-538.
Knox, J. B., Sukhova, G. K., Whittemore, A. D. & Libby, P. (1997). Evidence for altered balance between matrix metalloproteinases and their inhibitors in human aortic diseases. *Circulation* 95(1): 205-212.
Koch, A. E., Haines, G. K., Rizzo, R. J., Radosevich, J. A., Pope, R. M., Robinson, P. G. & Pearce, W. H. (1990). Human abdominal aortic aneurysms. Immunophenotypic analysis suggesting an immune-mediated response. *Am J Pathol* 137(5): 1199-1213.
Kojimahara, M. (1988). Intimal laminated elastosis in the intrarenal arteries. An electron microscopic study. *Acta Pathol Jpn* 38(3): 315-323.
Krettek, A., Sukhova, G. K. & Libby, P. (2003). Elastogenesis in human arterial disease: a role for macrophages in disordered elastin synthesis. *Arterioscler Thromb Vasc Biol* 23(4): 582-587.
Lederle, F. A., Johnson, G. R., Wilson, S. E., Chute, E. P., Hye, R. J., Makaroun, M. S., Barone, G. W., Bandyk, D., Moneta, G. L. & Makhoul, R. G. (2000). The aneurysm detection and management study screening program: validation cohort and final results. Aneurysm Detection and Management Veterans Affairs Cooperative Study Investigators. *Arch Intern Med* 160(10): 1425-1430.
Levene, C. I. (1956). The early lesions of atheroma in the coronary arteries. *J Pathol Bacteriol* 72: 79-83.
Lindeman, J. H., Abdul-Hussien, H., Schaapherder, A. F., Van Bockel, J. H., Von der Thusen, J. H., Roelen, D. L. & Kleemann, R. (2008). Enhanced expression and activation of pro-inflammatory transcription factors distinguish aneurysmal from atherosclerotic aorta: IL-6- and IL-8-dominated inflammatory responses prevail in the human aneurysm. *Clin Sci (Lond)* 114(11): 687-697.

Lopez-Candales, A., Holmes, D. R., Liao, S., Scott, M. J., Wickline, S. A. & Thompson, R. W. (1997). Decreased vascular smooth muscle cell density in medial degeneration of human abdominal aortic aneurysms. *Am J Pathol* 150(3): 993-1007.

Lusis, A. J. (2000). Atherosclerosis. *Nature* 407(6801): 233-241.

McMillan, W. D., Patterson, B. K., Keen, R. R., Shively, V. P., Cipollone, M. & Pearce, W. H. (1995). In situ localization and quantification of mRNA for 92-kD type IV collagenase and its inhibitor in aneurysmal, occlusive, and normal aorta. *Arteriosclerosis, Thrombosis & Vascular Biology* 15(8): 1139-1144.

Meyer, W. W. & Lind, J. (1972). Calcifications of iliac arteries in newborns and infants. *Arch Dis Child* 47(253): 364-372.

Meyer, W. W., Walsh, S. Z. & Lind, J. (1980). *Functional morphology of human arteries during fetal and post-natal development. Structure and function of the circulation.* C. J. Schwartz, N. T. Werthessen and S. Wolf. New York, Plenum Press. 1: 95-380.

Michel, J. B., Martin-Ventura, J. L., Egido, J., Sakalihasan, N., Treska, V., Lindholt, J., Allaire, E., Thorsteinsdottir, U., Cockerill, G. & Swedenborg, J. (2011). Novel aspects of the pathogenesis of aneurysms of the abdominal aorta in humans. *Cardiovasc Res* 90(1): 18-27.

Miller, E. J., Malcom, G. T., McMahan, C. A. & Strong, J. P. (1993). Atherosclerosis in young white males: arterial collagen and cholesterol. *Matrix* 13: 289-296.

Moon, H. D. (1957). Coronary arteries in fetuses, infants, and juveniles. *Circulation* 16(2): 263-267.

Moore, J. E., Jr., Ku, D. N., Zarins, C. K. & Glagov, S. (1992). Pulsatile flow visualization in the abdominal aorta under differing physiologic conditions: implications for increased susceptibility to atherosclerosis. *J Biomech Eng* 114(3): 391-397.

Moreno, P. R., Purushothaman, K. R., Sirol, M., Levy, A. P. & Fuster, V. (2006). Neovascularization in human atherosclerosis. *Circulation* 113(18): 2245-2252.

Nackman, G. B., Karkowski, F. J., Halpern, V. J., Gaetz, H. P. & Tilson, M. D. (1997). Elastin degradation products induce adventitial angiogenesis in the Anidjar/Dobrin rat aneurysm model. *Surgery* 122(1): 39-44.

Napoli, C., D'Armiento, F. P., Mancini, F. P., Postiglione, A., Witztum, J. L., Palumbo, G. & Palinski, W. (1997). Fatty streak formation occurs in human fetal aortas and is greatly enhanced by maternal hypercholesterolemia. Intimal accumulation of low density lipoprotein and its oxidation precede monocyte recruitment into early atherosclerotic lesions. *J Clin Invest* 100(11): 2680-2690.

Ogata, T., MacKean, G. L., Cole, C. W., Arthur, C., Andreou, P., Tromp, G. & Kuivaniemi, H. (2005). The lifetime prevalence of abdominal aortic aneurysms among siblings of aneurysm patients is eightfold higher than among siblings of spouses: an analysis of 187 aneurysm families in Nova Scotia, Canada. *J Vasc Surg* 42(5): 891-897.

Polzer, S., Gasser, T. C., Swedenborg, J. & Bursa, J. (2011). The Impact of Intraluminal Thrombus Failure on the Mechanical Stress in the Wall of Abdominal Aortic Aneurysms. *Eur J Vasc Endovasc Surg*.

Pugh, C. W. & Ratcliffe, P. J. (2003). Regulation of angiogenesis by hypoxia: role of the HIF system. *Nat Med* 9(6): 677-684.

Robert, L., Jacob, M. P. & Fulop, T. (1995). Elastin in blood vessels. *Ciba Foundation Symposium*(192): 286-299.

Robinet, A., Fahem, A., Cauchard, J. H., Huet, E., Vincent, L., Lorimier, S., Antonicelli, F., Soria, C., Crepin, M., Hornebeck, W. & Bellon, G. (2005). Elastin-derived peptides enhance angiogenesis by promoting endothelial cell migration and tubulogenesis through upregulation of MT1-MMP. *J Cell Sci* 118(Pt 2): 343-356.

Ross, R. (1993). The pathogenesis of atherosclerosis: a perspective for the 1990s. *Nature* 362(6423): 801-809.

Sakalihasan, N., Limet, R. & Defawe, O. D. (2005). Abdominal aortic aneurysm. *Lancet* 365(9470): 1577-1589.

Sandiford, P., Mosquera, D. & Bramley, D. (2011). Trends in incidence and mortality from abdominal aortic aneurysm in New Zealand. *Br J Surg*.

Schaefer, E. J., Lichenstein, A. H., Lamon-Fava, S., McNamara, J. R. & Ordovas, J. M. (1995). Lipoproteins, nutrition, aging and atherosclerosis. *Am J Clin Nutr* 61(Suppl): 726S-740S.

Schwartz, S. M. (1997). Smooth muscle migration in atherosclerosis and restenosis. *J Clin Invest* 100(11 Suppl): S87-89.

Scott, R. A., Wilson, N. M., Ashton, H. A. & Kay, D. N. (1995). Influence of screening on the incidence of ruptured abdominal aortic aneurysm: 5-year results of a randomized controlled study. *Br J Surg* 82(8): 1066-1070.

Shantikumar, S., Ajjan, R., Porter, K. E. & Scott, D. J. (2010). Diabetes and the abdominal aortic aneurysm. *Eur J Vasc Endovasc Surg* 39(2): 200-207.

Shapiro, S. D., Endicott, S. K., Province, M. A., Pierce, J. A. & Campbell, E. J. (1991). Marked longevity of human lung parenchymal elastic fibers deduced from prevalence of D-aspartate and nuclear weapons-related radiocarbon. *J Clin Invest* 87(5): 1828-1834.

Sims, F. H. (1985). Discontinuities in the internal elastic lamina: a comparison of coronary and internal mammary arteries. *Artery* 13(3): 127-143.

Singh, K., Bonaa, K. H., Jacobsen, B. K., Bjork, L. & Solberg, S. (2001). Prevalence of and risk factors for abdominal aortic aneurysms in a population-based study : The Tromso Study. *Am J Epidemiol* 154(3): 236-244.

Stary, H. C. (2000). Lipid and macrophage accumulations in arteries of children and the development of atherosclerosis. *Am J Clin Nutr* 72(5 Suppl): 1297S-1306S.

Stehbens, W. E. (1995). *Atherosclerosis and degenerative diseases of blood vessels. Vascular Pathology*. W. E. Stehbens and J. T. Lie. London, Chapman & Hall: 175-270.

Stehbens, W. E. (1997). Mechanisms underlying arterial fragility and the complications of atherosclerosis. *Pathobiology* 65(1): 1-13.

Strong, J. P. & Group, P. R. (1995). Natural history and risk factors of early human atherogenesis. *Clin Chem* 41: 134-138.

Tang, T., Boyle, J. R., Dixon, A. K. & Varty, K. (2005). Inflammatory abdominal aortic aneurysms. *Eur J Vasc Endovasc Surg* 29(4): 353-362.

Tangirala, R. K., Jerome, W. G., Jones, N. L., Small, D. M., Johnson, W. J., Glick, J. M., Mahlberg, F. H. & Rothblat, G. H. (1994). Formation of cholesterol monohydrate crystals in macrophage-derived foam cells. *J Lipid Res* 35(1): 93-104.

Tanimura, A., McGregor, D. H. & Anderson, H. C. (1983). Matrix vesicles in atherosclerotic calcification. *Proc Soc Exp Biol Med* 172(2): 173-177.

Thompson, R. W., Holmes, D. R., Mertens, R. A., Liao, S., Botney, M. D., Mecham, R. P., Welgus, H. G. & Parks, W. C. (1995). Production and localisation of 92-kilodalton gelatinase in abdominal aortic aneurysms. *J Clin Invest* 96: 318-326.

Thompson, R. W. & Parks, W. C. (1996). Role of matrix metalloproteinases in abdominal aortic aneurysms. *Annals of the New York Academy of Sciences* 800: 157-174.

Urry, D. W. (1975). Molecular aspects of the elastic fiber as a site of vascular pathology. *Alabama Journal of Medical Sciences* 12(4): 361-368.

Verloes, A., Sakalihasan, N., Koulischer, L. & Limet, R. (1995). Aneurysms of the abdominal aorta: familial and genetic aspects in three hundred thirteen pedigrees. *J Vasc Surg* 21(4): 646-655.

Vine, N. & Powell, J. T. (1991). Metalloproteinases in degenerative aortic disease. *Clinical Science* 81: 233-239.

Vorp, D. A., Wang, D. H., Webster, M. W. & Federspiel, W. J. (1998). Effect of intraluminal thrombus thickness and bulge diameter on the oxygen diffusion in abdominal aortic aneurysm. *J Biomech Eng* 120(5): 579-583.

Williams, K. J. & Tabas, I. (1995). The response-to-retention hypothesis of early atherogenesis. *Arterioscler Thromb Vasc Biol* 15(5): 551-561.

Willis, A. I., Pierre-Paul, D., Sumpio, B. E. & Gahtan, V. (2004). Vascular smooth muscle cell migration: current research and clinical implications. *Vasc Endovascular Surg* 38(1): 11-23.

Wolinsky, H. (1970). Comparison of medial growth of human thoracic and abdominal aortas. *Circulation Research* 27(4): 531-538.

Wolinsky, H. & Glagov, S. (1964). Structural Basis for the Static Mechanical Properties of the Aortic Media. *Circulation Research* 14: 400-413.

Wolinsky, H. & Glagov, S. (1969). Comparison of abdominal and thoracic aortic medial structure in mammals. Deviation of man from the usual pattern. *Circulation Research* 25(6): 677-686.

4

Actual Pharmacological Treatment to Reduce Growth of Small Abdominal Aneurysm

Guillermo Moñux Ducajú[1], Javier Modrego[2], Antonio López Farré[2] and Javier Serrano[1]
[1]*Vascular Surgery Department and Cardiovascular Research Unit,*
[2]*Hospital Clínico San Carlos, Madrid*
Spain

1. Introduction

Abdominal aortic aneurysm (AAA), defined as a permanent segmental dilatation of the abdominal aorta, is a pathology responsible for significant morbidity and mortality especially among adult population over 60 years of age. Indeed, AAA is one of the fifteen most frequent causes of death among men older than 55 years in Western societies (Lederle et al., 2000). However, despite of its importance, little is known about etiopathogenesis of AAA. The observation by non-invasive imaging methods of an abdominal aorta of 3 cm typically or large in maximal diameter is generally considered to indicate aneurysm formation (Lederle et al., 2000). Diagnosis is typically made by non-invasive imaging modalities such as ultrasound, computerized tomography scan or magnetic resonance imaging with formal aortic angiography utilized in special clinical scenarios. At present, surgical treatment, conventional or endovascular surgery of AAA are very effective to prevent AAA rupture in patients with large AAA, at least 5,5 cm in diameter, with high risk of rupture. However, despite AAA with diameter <5,5 cm (termed as small AAA) have a low risk of rupture there are non well-defined therapeutic strategies for them. Moreover, the group of patients with small AAA should wait expectantly for the aneurysm reaches the minimum size to undergo surgical treatment, living through those days with great anxiety. Many factors may contribute to AAA formation and rupture, there are mechanical and rupture factors among them. Indeed, ultrasound examination showed AAA in 5.8% of World War II amputees, compared with 1% of non-amputees related to asymmetrical flow pattern at the aortic bifurcation. Moreover, evidence of genetic predisposition to the development of AAA has been noteworthy with 19% of AAA patients reporting one or more first-degree relatives with an aneurysm. Therefore, it is important to understand and know the molecular mechanisms involved in AAA expansion and which pharmacological treatments may prevent and delay it.

2. Pathophysiology of AAA

Now, knowledge of the physiopathology of AAA is necessary to understand the mechanisms of action of drugs that are being used for trying to reduce the AAA growth. Moreover, investigations are needed to design new pharmacological approaches and to develop more effective new drugs. Although the cause of aneurismal degeneration is still non-well known, it is widely recognized that AAA are closely associated with chronic (transmural) inflammation and destruction of connective tissue proteins within the outer aortic wall. Indeed, the natural history of AAA could be summarized in three different steps. The first one is an increased production of inflammatory-related substances by the vascular wall (Figure 1). Until now, it has not been identified the triggers of this inflammatory reaction. The second step seems to be the release of molecular mediators by infiltrated cells. In addition, the third step is the release of metalloproteinases and their inhibitors in an unbalanced way mediated by the previously released inflammatory agents and infiltrated cells. Indeed, there is a reduction of the medial elastin and thinning of collagen within the media in the aortic wall .Then, it is important the role of infiltrated inflammatory cells in the degradation of the vascular wall. Indeed, activated macrophages segregate different proteases most of them members of the matrix metalloproteinase family (MMP). The increased MMP release, mainly MMP-9 and MMP-2, seem to be not compensated by an increased release of their specific inhibitors (TIMPs) (Brophy et al., 1991) favoring an unbalance between synthesis and degradation of connective tissue proteins. As mentioned before, this involves the destruction of collagen and elastin, two of the major structural components of the extracellular matrix, disrupting the orderly lamellar structure of the aortic media and then forming the aneurysm. Studies in human AAA tissue have shown extensive inflammatory infiltrates containing macrophages and lymphocytes in both the media and the adventitia. Indeed, increasing aneurysm diameter was associated with higher density of inflammatory cells in the adventitia (Freestone et al.,1995).

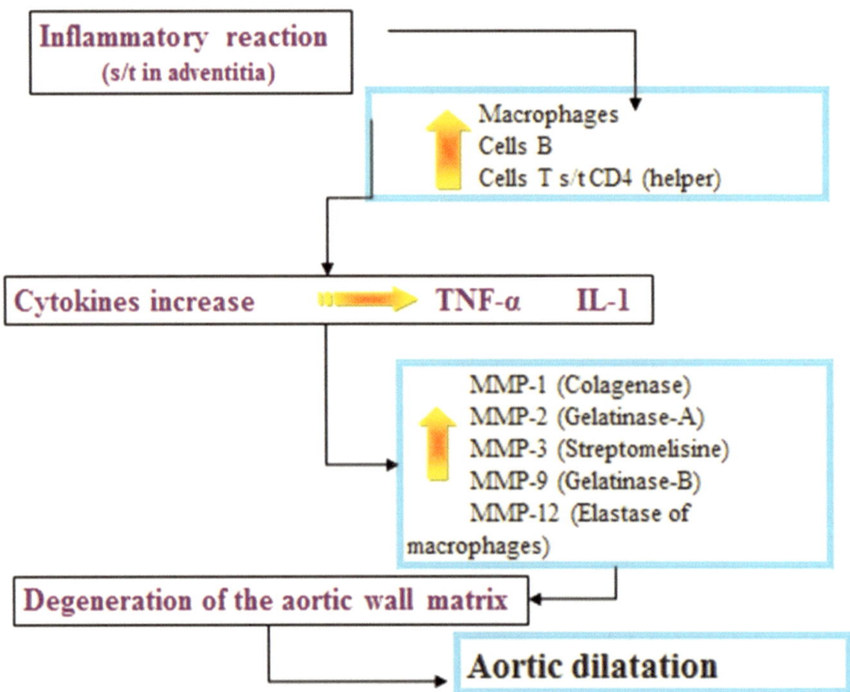

Fig. 1. Schematic representation of changes that occur in molecular mediators during abdominal aortic aneurysm formation.

Nowadays, the main research effort is focused on identifying new molecular pathways involved in expansion of small aneurysm. At present, drugs under investigation have been mainly designed to act on the third step of AAA formation, the inhibition of metalloproteinases system. In this regard, drugs like doxycyclins, statins and synthetic MMP inhibitors have been tested.

3. Novel drugs for AAA treatment

3.1 Doxycycline

In 1948, tetracyclines were discovered as a product of Streptomyces aureofaciens fermentation. Accordingly, with their origin, there are three different tetracyclines groups: natural products, semi-synthetic compounds and chemically modified tetracyclines (Nelson,1998). It is also known that tetracyclines have other effects besides the powerful antibiotic. These properties include (Sapadin & Fleischmajer,2006):

3.1.1 Inhibition of inflammation

Through the inhibition of neutrophil migration and chemotaxis, transmigration of T lymphocytes, etc (Brundula,2002;Kloppenburg,1994;Martin,1974).

3.1.2 Proteolysis

Tetracyclines and its analogues inhibit MMP (Golub,1983,1991).

3.1.3 Angiogenesis

Doxycycline inhibits MMP synthesis in endothelial cells. This inhibition promotes the decrease of both protein and mRNA MMP levels that may affect endothelial cells migration during angiogenesis (Hanemaaijer et al.,1998).

3.1.4 Apoptosis

Recent experiments have suggested antiapoptotic properties for tetracyclines (Yrjanheikii,1998,1999).

The use of tetracyclins in AAA was initially justified by the detection of microbacterial organism within the aortic aneurysm. In this regard, it has been suggested aneurysm progression associated with bacterial infection (Meijer et al.,1999). Other bacteries such as *Helicobacter pylori* and cytomegalovirus has also been linked to aortic pathology.

Tetracyclines are used as antibiotics to treat Chlamydia pneumonia-related infections but also they are non-specific inhibitors of MMPs (Ryan & Golub,2000). In this regard, AAA studies has been conducted with doxycycline. It has been shown that doxycycline decreased the protein expression of MMP-9 and MMP-2 in experimental animal models of AAA (Pyo et al.,2000). In this regard, in vitro incubation of AAA with doxycycline demonstrated inhibition of MMP-2 expression (17). It was also observed for MMP-9 production (Liu et al.,2003).

In a clinical trial, doxycycline treatment showed high tolerance and decreased MMP-9 serum levels although, did not decrease AAA size (Baxter et al.,2002). However, another clinical trial including thirty-two patients with AAA receiving doxycycline (150 mg daily) or placebo for 3 months demonstrated that AAA growth rate in doxycycline group was significantly lower than that in the placebo group (Mosorin et al.,2001).

It has been recently proposed local administration of doxycycline as a new possible therapeutic option for AAA treatment (Bartoli et al.,2006). In this regard, doxycycline administration by periaortic infusion decreased aneurysm growth as much than systemic administration of doxycycline (Bartoli et al.,2006). However in this study lower doses of local doxycycline was used with systemic doxycycline administration and, therefore, with lesser risk of adverse effects. Then, it may open the possibility to develop drug-eluting stents containing doxycycline to treat AAA.

3.2 Statins

Statins are hydroxymethylglutamyl-coenzyme A (HMG-CoA) inhibitors that are widely prescribed for their lipid-lowering effects. Although reduction of lipid levels prevents the progression of atherosclerosis, additional non-related lipid effects of statins have been also demonstrated and their have been termed as "pleiotropic statins effects". Between the pleiotropic effects of statins may be included anti-inflammatory effects, anti-oxidant effects and reduction of MMP secretion.

Several works have demonstrated the beneficial pleiotropic effects of statins to prevent AAA development. As example, it has been demonstrated for different statins including fluvastatin, pravastatin and simvastatin, reduction of MMP-9 production by AAA and even by the infiltrated inflammatory cells (Bellosta,1998;Kalela,2001;Paraskevas,2008). In experimental studies, simvastatin increased TIMP-1 production but it did not modify inflammatory cells infiltration into AAA; however, atorvastatin suppressed macrophage recruitment by inhibiting intercellular adhesion molecule-1 expression in the vascular wall, leading to MMP-12 inhibition (Shiraya,2009;Steinmetz,2005).

It is noteworthy that in human studies, some works have not observed effects of statins on AAA growth. In this regard, there was no association between statin prescription or serum low-density lipoprotein (LDL) concentration with AAA expansion. However, AAA growth was found positively associated with initial diameter and negatively associated with diabetes (Ferguson et al.,2010). Other studies were able to find beneficial effects of statins reducing or delaying AAA expansion in humans. In this regard, Feeney et al have recently reported that prehospital statin use appears to be associated with a significant survival benefit in the ruptured AAA population (Feeney et al.,2009). In addition, an observational study including 130 patients follow up for 2 years, no aneurysm expansion was observed in 75 patients taking statins (Baxter et al.,2008). Other studies have been also suggested that the aneurysm expansion rate was decreased in the patients who were taking statins compared with those not taking statins (Schouten et al.,2006).

Another important query is about the molecular pathways by which statins may affect AAA growth. As mentioned, some studies have shown that statins reduced the in vitro expression of MMPs. However, our group using human AAA explants observed that statins particularly pravastatin, failed to modify either total production of MMP-9 or the active fraction of MMP-9 (Mateos-Cáceres et al.,2008). However, pravastatin increased TIMP-1 content in human AAA explants (Mateos-Cáceres et al.,2008). The increased TIMP-1 expression in AAA by pravastatin was unrelated to HMG-CoA inhibition by this statin (Mateos-Cáceres et al.,2008). It is remarkable that the beneficial effects of increased TIMP-1 expression may not be limited to MMP-9 inhibition. In this regard, TIMP-1 may be also involved in other cellular processes including the prevention of apoptosis which it has been demonstrated increased in AAA (Lambert,2003;Liu,2005;Zhang,2003). Accordingly, in human AAA explants pravastatin increased the expression of the proto-oncogene Bax (associated with apoptosis induction) without modification in the expression of the anti-apoptotic proto-oncogene Bcl-2 (Mateos-Cáceres et al.,2008). However, Bax upregulation induced by pravastatin did not modify Bax/Bcl-2 ratio, an important apoptotic index, probably discarding that pravastatin may influence apoptotic status in AAA. Therefore, it is plausible that TIMP-1 may be involved in other biological functions such as growth factor-like activity, stimulation of aortic smooth cell proliferation and anti-inflammatory activity, which may all prevent AAA progression.

In summary, statins may be useful in controlling AAA growth, although the exact involved molecular mechanisms remained to be elucidated. However, many studies promote an pleiotropic effect of statins to prevent AAA growth which seem to be associated with reduction of inflammation in the aneurysmal wall, in addition to diminish MMP expression and/or enhance the synthesis of their inhibitors, TIMPs.

3.3 Synthetic inhibitors of MMPs

MMPs play a fundamental role in the development of aneurysm. Therefore, it is then plausible that the use of synthetic inhibitors may slow AAA growth. BB-94 (Batimastat) is a broad-spectrum inhibitor of metalloproteinases that has been effective in controlling inflammatory responses in rats (Rassmussen,1997;Taraboletti,1995).

BB-94 decreased the aneurysm expansion in rats (Bigatel et al.,1999). Researchers have also observed that BB-94 has effect not only as metalloproteinases inhibitor but also decreasing the inflammatory response to aneurysm. However, long-term used of BB-94 is at present limited by its lack of bioavalibility. Marimastat, a second generation of this type of drugs, it is active orally but it has been demonstrated 30% of musculoskeletal side effects. It has been studied in human experimental models of intima hyperplasia and aneurysms (Porter el al.,1998). These initially promising drugs have failed to show human therapeutic utility, and other drugs have overlooked them.

3.4 Angiotensin Converting Enzyme Inhibitors (ACEI) and angiotensin receptor blockers

ACEI are drugs used for blood pressure control. Several studies have shown that ACEI affect the natural evolution of aneurysms although their possible mechanisms of action are not well known. It has been observed that administration of Angiotensin-II to experimental animals decreased the content of elastin in the aortic wall including in AAA (Tham et al.,2002). Moreover, ACEI administration to patients with established AAA increased collagen production in the vascular wall and decreased the arterial wall size (Claridge et al.,2004). Liao et al demonstrated that differents ACEI could decreased elastin in AAA independently of their lowering arterial blood pressure effects and without changes in the inflammatory status of the aortic wall (Liao et al.,2001). Moreover, Alsac et al. have shown that perindopril, an ACEI, is able to reduce aneurysm growth in experimental models not only by changes in elastin levels but also by inhibiting MMPs synthesis (Alsac et al.,2011). In clinical trials, patients treated with ACEI before inclusion presented lesser aneurysm rupture than those not treated with ACEI. This effect was not observed in patients treated with other blood pressure lowering drugs including β-blockers, calcium channel blockers antagonists of angiotensin-II receptors and even diuretics (Hackam et al.,2006).

However, there are also studies demonstrating detrimental effects of ACEI on AAA growth. For example, a study performed with 1700 patients from UK showed that aneurysm growth

rate was higher in patients treated with ACEI compared with those without ACEI treatment (Sweeting et al.,2010). These findings support that are needed prospective randomized studies to clarify the real therapeutic benefits of ACEI for AAA.
There are also studies testing the effect of angiotensin II-receptor antagonists (ARBs) to prevent AAA growth. In experimental models based on the chronic release of angiotensin II into apolipoprotein deficient mice resulted in aortic dilation and eventual rupture, losartan administration prevented aneurysm formation (Fujiwara et al.,2008). Moreover, antagonism by losartan of transforming growth factor-B prevented progressive matrix degradation (Habashi et al.,2006). More studies, particularly clinical studies, are needed to assess the utility of ARBs to prevent AAA growth.

4. Conclusions

The study of AAA should be focused on the knowledge about the main causes that produces the inflammatory infiltrate resulting in the cascade of events that ends with aneurysm formation. Moreover, it is also important to delay AAA growth. In this regard, reduction in the expansion rate of AAA potentially increases the time of surgical intervention and in many cases, this delayed time may exceed life expectation for patients.
Larger multicenter studies are needed to fully elucidate the effect of the currently used drugs. Moreover, it is important the efforts in the research of this disease, focusing in the determination of mechanisms involved in the appearance of the inflammatory infiltrate. In this regard, protein expression studies may help us to identify new molecular mediators and pathways including oxidative-stress mediators, energetic metabolism targets and others involved in AAA formation and growth. This type of studies may open new knowledge about the disease, in addition to find new molecular targets to develop drugs and pharmacological treatments.

5. References

Alsac JM, Journe C, Louedec L, Dai J, Julia P, Fabiani JN & Michel JB. (2011). Downregulation of Remodelling Enzymatic Activity Induced by an Angiotensin-converting Enzyme Inhibitor (Perindopril) Reduces the Degeneration of Experimental Abdominal Aortic Aneurysms in a Rat Model. *Eur J Vasc Endovasc Surg* , doi:10.1016/j.ejvs.2010.12.007, ISSN: 1078-5884

Bartoli Ma., Parodi FE., Chu J., Pagano MB., Mao D., Baxter BT. (2006). Localized administration of doxicycline suppresses aortic dilatation in a experimental mose model of abdominal aortic aneuriysm. *Ann Vasc Surg* ; 20: 228-36, ISSN: 0890-5096

Baxter BT., Pearce WH, waltke EA., Littoy FN., Hallet JW, Ken KC. (2002). Prolonged administration of doxicicline in patients with small asymthomatic abdominal aortic aneurysms: repost of a prospective (phase II) multicenter study. *J Vasc Surg* ; 36: 1-12, ISSN: 0741-5214

Baxter BT, Terrin MC, Dalman RL. (2008) Medical management of small abdominal aortic aneurysms. *Circulation*;117:1883-9, ISSN: 0009-7322

Bellosta S., Via D., Canavesi M., Pfister P., Fumagalli R., Paoletti R., Bernini F. (1998). HMGCoA reductase inhibitors reduce MMP-9 secretion by macrophages. *Arterioescler Thromb Vasc Biol*; 18: 1671-8, ISSN: 1079-5642

Bigatel Da., Elmore JR., Carey DJ., Cizmeci G., Franklin DP., Youkey JR. (1999). The matrix metalloproteinases BB-94 limits expansion of experimental abdominal aortic aneurysms. *J vasc surg*; 29:130-9, ISSN: 0741-5214

Brophy CM., Marks WH, Reilly JM, Wilson MD. (1991). Decreased tissue inhibitor of metalloproteinase (TIMP) in abdominal aortic aneurysm tissue: a preliminary report. *J Surg Res*; 50: 653-657

Brundula V., Rewcastle NB., Metz LM., Bernard CC., Yong VW. Targeting leukocyte MMPs and transmigration: minocycline as a potential therapy for multiple sclerosis (2002). *Brain*; 125: 1297-308, ISSN: 0006-8950

Claridge MW, Hobbs SD, Quick CR, Day NE, Bradbury AW,Wilmink AB. ACE inhibitors increase type III collagen synthesis: a potential explanation for reduction in acute vascular events by ACE inhibitors (2004). *Eur J Vasc Endovasc Surg* ; 28: 67–70, ISSN: 1078-5884

Feeney JM, Burns K, Staff I, Bai J, Rodrigues N, Fortier J, Jacobs LM. (2009). Prehospital HMG Co-A reductase inhibitor use and reduced mortality in ruptured abdominal aortic aneurysm. *J Am Coll Surg.*; 209:41-6, ISSN: 1072-7515

Ferguson CD, Clancy P, Bourke B, Walker PJ, Dear A, Buckenham T, Norman P,Golledge J. (2010). Association of statin prescription with small abdominal aortic aneurysm progression. Am *Heart J.* ; 159:307-13, ISSN: 0002-8703

Freestone T, Turner RJ, Coady A, Higman DJ, Greenhalgh RM, Powell JT (1995). Inflammation and matrix metalloproteinases in the enlarging abdominal aortic aneurysm. *Arterioscler Thromb Vasc Biol.* ;15(8):1145-51, ISSN: 1079-5642

Fujiwara Y, Shiraya S, Miyake T, Yamakawa S, Aoki M, Makino H, Nishimura M, Morishita R. (2008). Inhibition of experimental abdominal aortic aneurysm in a rat model by the angiotensin receptor blocker valsartan. *Int J Mol Med.*; 22:703-8

Golub LM., Lee HM., Leher G., Nemiroff A., Mc Namara TF., Kaplan R. (1983) Minocycline reduces gingival collagenolytic activity during diabetes: preliminary observations and a proposed new mechanism of action. *J Periodont Res* ; 18: 516-26, ISSN: 0022-3484

Golub LM., Ramamurthy NS., McNamara TF., Grenwald RA., Rifkin BR. (1991). Tetracyclines inhibit connective tissue breakdown: new therapeutic implications. *Crit Rev Oral Biol Med*;2(3):297-321, ISSN: 1045-4411

Habashi JP, Judge DP, Holm TM, Cohn RD, Loeys BL, Cooper TK, Myers L, Klein EC, Liu G, Calvi C, Podowski M, Neptune ER, Halushka MK, Bedja D, Gabrielson K, Rifkin DB, Carta L, Ramirez F, Huso DL, Dietz HC (2006). Losartan, an AT1 antagonist, prevents aortic aneurysm in a mouse model of Marfan syndrome. *Science*; 312:117-21, ISSN: 0036-8075

Hackam DG, Thiruchelvam D, Redelmeier DA. (2006). Angiotensin-converting enzyme inhibitors and aortic rupture: a population-based case-control study. Lancet; 368:659-665, ISSN: 0099-5355

Hanemaaijer R., Visser H., Koolwijk P., sorsa T., Salo T., Golub LM. Inhibition of MMP synthesis by doxicycline and chemically modified tetracyclines (CMTs) in human endothelial cells (1998) *Adv Dent Res* ; 12: 114-18

Kalela A., Laaksonen R., Lehtimaki T., Koivu TA., Hoyhtya M., Janatuinen T. Effect of pravastatin in midly hypercholesterolemic young men on serum matrix metalloproteinases (2001) *Am J Cardiol*; 88: 173-5, ISSN: 0002-9149

Kloppenburg M., Breedweld FC., Terwiel J., Mallee C., Dijkmans BAC(1994). Minocycline in active rheumatoid artrhitis: a double blind, placebo controlled trial. *Arthritis reum;* 37: 629-36, ISSN: 0077-8923

Lambert E, Boudot C, Kadri Z, Soula-Rothhut M, Sowa ML, Mayeux P, Hornebeck W, Haye B, Petitfrere E (2003). Tissue inhibitor of metalloproteinases-1 signalling pathway lead up to erythroid cell survival. *J Biochem* : 372: 767-774, ISSN: 0264-6021

Lederle FA, Johnson GR, Wilson SE, Chute EP, Hye RJ, Makaroun MS, Barone GW, Bandyk D, Moneta GL, Makhoul RG (2000). The aneurysm detection and management study screening program: validation cohort and final results. Aneurysm Detection and Management Veterans Affairs Cooperative Study Investigators. *Arch Intern Med;* 160(10):1425-30, ISSN: 0003-9926

Liao S, Miralles M, Kelley BJ, et al (2001). Suppression of experimental abdominal aortic aneurysms in the rat by treatment with angiotensin-converting enzyme inhibitors. *J Vasc Surg;* 33:1057-1064, ISSN: 0741-5214

Liu J., Xiong W., Baca-Ragen L., Nagase H., Baxter BT (2003). Mechanism of inhibition of matrix metalloproteinase-2 expression by doxicicline in human aortic smooth muscle cells. *J Vasc Surg* ; 38: 1376-83, ISSN: 0741-5214

Liu XW, Taube ME, Jung KK, Dong Z, Lee YJ, Roshy S, Sloane BF, Fridman R, Kim HR (2005). Tissue inhibitor of metalloproteinase-1 protects human breast epithelial cells from extrusica cell death: a potential oncogenic activity of tissue inhibitor of metalloproteinase-1. Cancer Res. : 65: 898-906

Martin RR., Warr GA., Couch RB., Yeager H., Knight V (1974). Effects of Tetracyclines on leukotaxis. *J Infect Dis* ; 129: 110-116

Mateos-Cáceres PJ, López-Farré AJ, Morata PC, Ramos-Mozo P, Macaya C, Serrano FJ, Moñux G (2008). Pravastatin increases the expression of the tissue inhibitor of matrix metalloproteinase-1 and the oncogene Bax in human aortic abdominal aneurysms. *Can J Physiol Pharmacol.* Jul;86(7):431-7, ISSN: 1205-7541

Meijer A, van Der Vliet JA, Roholl PJ, Gielis-Proper SK, de Vries A,Ossewaarde JM (1999). Chlamydia pneumoniae in abdominal aortic aneurysms: abundance of membrane components in the absence of heat shock protein 60 and DNA. *Arterioscler Thromb Vasc Biol;* 19(11):2680-6, ISSN: 1079-5642

Mosorin M., Juvonen J., Biancari F., Satta J., Surcel HM., Leinonen M (2001). Use of doxicycline to decrease the growth rate of abdominal aortic aneurysms: a randomized double-blind placebo-controlled pilot study. *J Vasc Surg* ; 34: 606-10, ISSN: 0741-5214

Nelson ML. (1998) Chemical and biologycal dynamics of tetracyclines. *Adv Dent Res;* 12:5-11

Paraskevas KI, Liapis CD, Hamilton G, Mikhailidis DP. (2008) Are statins an option in the management of abdominal aortic aneurysms? *Vasc Endovascular Surg*; 42(2):128-34, ISSN: 1538-5744

Porter KE., Loftus MI., Peterson M., Bell PR., London NJ., Thomson MM. (1998) Marismastat inhibits neointimal thickening in a model of human vein graft stenosis. *Br J surg*; 85: 1373-77, ISSN: 0007-1323

Pyo R., Lee JK., Shipley JM., Curci JA, Mao D., Ziporin SJ. (2000) Targeted gene disruption of matrix metalloproteinase (geltinase B) supresses development of experimental abdominal aortic aneurysms. *J Clin Invest*; 105: 1641-9, ISSN: 0021-9738

Rassmussen HS., Mc cann PP. (1997) Matrix metalloproteases inhibition as a novel anticancer strategy: a review with special focus on batimastat and marimastat. *Pharmacol therapy*; 75:69-75, ISSN: 0163-7258

Ryan ME, Golub LM. (2000) Modulation of matrix metalloproteinase activities in periodontitis as a treatment strategy. Periodontol 2000; 24:226-38, ISSN: 0906-6713

Sapadin AN., Fleischmajer R. (2006) Tetracyclines : Nonantibiotic propeties and their clinical implications. *J Am Acad Dermatol*; 54:258-265, ISSN: 0190-9622

Schouten O., Van Laanen JHH., Boersma E., Vidakovic R., Feringa HHH. (2006) Dulkengrun M. Statins are associated with a reduced infrarenal abdominal aortic aneurysm growth. *Eur J Vasc Endovasc Surg*; 32: 21-26, ISSN: 1078-5884

Shiraya S, Miyake T, Aoki M, Yoshikazu F, Ohgi S, Nishimura M, Ogihara T, Morishita R. (2009) Inhibition of development of experimental aortic abdominal aneurysm in rat model by atorvastatin through inhibition of macrophage migration. *Atherosclerosis*; 202:34-40, ISSN: 0021-9150

Steinmetz EF., Buckley C., Shames ML., Ennis TL., Vanvickle-Chavez SJ., Mao D. (2005) Treatment with simvastatin supresses the development of experimental abdominal aortic aneurysms in normal and hypercholesterolemic mice. *Ann Surg*; 241: 92-101, ISSN: 0003-4932

Sweeting MJ, Thompson SG, Brown LC, Greenhalgh RM, Powell JT. (2010) Use of angiotensin converting enzyme inhibitors is associated with increased growth rate of abdominal aortic aneurysms. *J Vasc Surg*;52:1-4, ISSN: 0741-5214

Taraboletti G., Garofalo A., Belotti D. (1995) Inhibition of angiogenesisand murine hemangioma growth by batismastat a synthetic inhibitor of matrix metalloproteinases. . *J Natl Cancer inst*; 87:293-98, ISSN: 0027-8874

Tham DM, Martin-McNulty B, Wang YX, et al. (2002) Angiotensin II injures the arterial wall causing increased aortic stiff ening in apolipoprotein E-defi cient mice. *Am J Physiol Regul Integr Comp Physiol*; 283:R1442–49

Yrjanheikki J., Keinamen R., Pellikka M., Hokfelt T., Koistinaho J. (1998) Tetracyclines inhibit microglial activation and are neuroprotective in global brain ischaemia. *Proc Natl Acad Sci USA*; 95: 12769-74, ISSN: 0027-8424

Yrjanheikki J., Tikka T., Keinanen R., Goldstein G., Chan PH., Koistihaho J. (1999). A tetracycline derivate, minocycline, reduces inflammation and protects against focal cerebral ischemia with a wide therapeutic window. *Proc Natl Acad Sci USA*; 96: 13496-500

Zhang J, Schmidt J, Ryschich E, Schumacher H, Allenberg JR. (2003) Increased apoptosis and decreased density of medial smooth muscle cells in human abdominal aortic aneurysms. *Chin Med*: 116: 1549-1552

5

Diagnosis of Aortic Aneurysm

Serosha Mandika Wijeyaratne
University of Colombo,
Sri Lanka

1. Introduction

For most of its course the aorta lies in front of the vertebral bodies, well away from the anterior abdominal wall and is not visible or palpable unless it is significantly dilated. The physician, during routine abdominal palpation or less commonly the patient him/ herself may note abnormal and excessively prominent upper abdominal pulsations that will point to the possibility of an abdominal aortic aneurysm. More frequently, an uncomplicated aortic aneurysm comes to light as an incidental finding during radiologic imaging as part of a routine health check or investigation for other conditions.

The aortic wall per se is insensate and its gradual stretching is not perceived, which explains the clinical silence in the uncomplicated state. Pain is experienced only when adjacent sensitive structures such the pleura or peritoneum comes into contact with blood or the adjacent vertebral structures are compressed and eroded. Thus aortic aneurysms become clinically apparent only when such complications set in. Clinical presentation with complications is characterized by severe pain and shock, where the severity depends on the magnitude of the bleed. Other rare complications include rupture into the adjacent intestinal tract or cava, aneurysm occlusion due to thrombosis, distal embolisation, and consumptive coagulopathy. In most instances, these complications cause death over a short time interval. Thus an accurate clinical diagnosis without delay becomes crucial.

However clinical diagnosis is in no way straightforward and has become a major challenge to clinicians. Understanding the reasons for this is important in overcoming the problem. An aortic aneurysm is often impalpable and symptoms and signs of complications non specific. Clinical presentation of aneurysm complications often mimic other more common conditions and this is the main reason for not suspecting the diagnosis. This chapter examines the frequency with which different presentations occur and the reliability of individual symptoms and signs.

It may be perceived that modern imaging would overcome clinical deficiencies in diagnosing aneurysm complications. This again is incorrect in some instances. Haemodynamic instablility at presentation is common and this does not allow time for imaging. In instances where imaging is feasible results may be equivocal and clinical judgment must take over.

Ultrasound, computerized tomography and magnetic resonance are all being used to confirm the presence of an aneurysm, its location, physical dimensions and morphology. These parameters are assuming greater importance today with the emergence of endovascular stent repair of aneurysms. Furthermore, these modalities contribute to the diagnosis of complications and the relative merits of each of these will be discussed.

2. Methods

Method: A review of literature, to determine the evidence base on the accuracy of diagnostic modalities commonly used in the diagnosis of aortic aneurysm, was performed using MEDLINE from 1966 and EMBASE from 1988 to the present. This was supplemented by a bibliographic search of papers identified by hand searching publications on vascular surgery.

3. Uncomplicated aneurysm

Most aortic aneurysms are uncomplicated and asymptomatic. Aneurysms that produce symptoms are at increased risk for rupture. Abdominal or back pain and tenderness are the two main clinical features suggestive of either recent expansion or a leak. Complications are often life threatening, and can occur over a short time span. Therefore the challenge is to diagnose prior to onset of symptoms. Asymptomatic aneurysms are often detected incidentally, during physical examination when a pulsatile mass is felt at or above the umbilicus (the aorta bifurcates at the level of the umbilicus) or during imaging for other reasons. This was confirmed by Kakos et al in a study based in a district general hospital where 48% of abdominal aortic aneurysms were discovered clinically compared with 37.4% radiologically, and 14.6% at laparotomy (Karkos, Mukhopadhyay et al. 2000). Of those diagnosed radiologically, subsequent physical examination showed that one third were palpable but missed at presentation. This suggests that there is greater room for improvement in the clinical detection of asymptomatic abdominal aortic aneurysms. The average size of those discovered clinically (6.48 cm ±1.32 cm) was significantly larger than those discovered either radiologically (5.37 cm ±1.44 cm, $P<0.001$) or at laparotomy (5.43 cm ±1.48 cm, $P = 0.039$) (Karkos, Mukhopadhyay et al. 2000). Of course it seems easier to detect large aneurysms, particularly those occurring in slim persons. Even the most experienced clinician might miss an abdominal aortic aneurysm at palpation when there is abdominal obesity, abdominal distention, or inability to relax the anterior abdominal wall musculature during the examination (Sabiston and Townsend 2008). This explains the wide variation in sensitivity of physical examination in the detection of abdominal aortic aneurysms. The documented sensitivity of clinical detection of aneurysms ranges from 22 to 96 percent, reflecting differences in the populations screened (Houston, Elster et al. 1998).

In a blinded assessment of abdominal palpation in detecting aortic aneurysms >3cms among 200 subjects over the age of 50 years with and without an aneurysm, the sensitivity and specificity for abdominal palpation was 68 and 75 percent respectively. The positive likelihood ratio, defined as the increase in the odds of having the disease when the finding is positive (sensitivity/1-specificity), was 2.7 and the negative likelihood ratio, defined as the decrease in odds of having the disease when the finding is negative (1-sensitivity/specificity), was 0.43. Sensitivity increases with increasing aortic diameter, from 61% for those of between 3.0 and 3.9 cm to 69% for those between 4.0 and 4.9 cm, and 82% for those that are 5.0 cm or greater. A 1.0 cm increase in abdominal aortic aneurysm diameter doubles the odds of detecting it on clinical examination. An additional factor that was found to affect the detection rate was abdominal girth. A girth less than 100cm (40 cm in waistline) increases sensitivity from 52% to 91%(Fink, Lederle et al. 2000). In a further analysis of pooled data from 15 studies of patients not previously known to have an aneurysm who were screened by both abdominal palpation and ultrasound, the sensitivity of abdominal palpation increased significantly with the abdominal aortic aneurysm diameter; the sensitivities for aneurysms 3 to 3.9, 4 to 4.9, and ≥ 5.0 cm were 29, 50, and 76 percent respectively ($p<0.001$). The reviewers concluded that palpation was moderately sensitive for detecting an aneurysm that is large enough to be referred for surgery (Lederle and Simel 1999).

Awareness of the high risk groups for aortic aneurysms, i.e. ≥65 years, peripheral atherosclerotic vascular disease, smoking, chronic obstructive pulmonary disease, hypertension ("Screening for abdominal aortic aneurysm: recommendation statement" 2005) and Marfan and Ehlers-Danlos syndromes or having an affected first-degree relative, may help anticipate and improve sensitivity to palpation. It is disappointing that there have been no large scale community studies on this subject. It is worth emphasizing that palpation of abdominal aortic aneurysms is safe and has not been reported to precipitate rupture. It must be noted that during palpation a tortuous aorta or other retroperitoneal mass lesions can sometimes be confused with an aneurysm. However, the borders of a tortuous aorta can usually be distinguished, and pulsating peri-aortic retroperitoneal masses are not expansile. A false positive physical exam is usually harmless and can easily be clarified by imaging. Finally the vascular examination should include auscultation of the abdomen. The presence of a bruit may indicate aortic or visceral arterial atherosclerotic disease, turbulence within an aneurysm or an aorto-caval fistula. Such a finding would warrant imaging to clarify the situation.

3.1 Imaging studies

The diagnostic drawback due to the limited sensitivity of abdominal palpation in the detection of abdominal aortic aneurysms has been largely overcome by easy access to and a low threshold for imaging. The incidental finding of an asymptomatic abdominal aortic aneurysm has become commonplace, largely due to the increased use of abdominal ultrasound, computed tomography and magnetic resonance imaging for most abdominal symptoms and during preoperative staging and follow up of abdominal malignancies. Furthermore, an aneurysm may be incidentally noted during left sided cardiac catheterization.

An abdominal aortic aneurysm may be suspected on plain x-ray studies, when there is curvilinear calcification outlining both opposing aortic walls. Nevertheless, in more than 50% of cases the calcification is inadequate and does not mark opposing walls. In such instances a tortuous, calcified aorta may in fact mimic an AAA. The lack of overlying bony structures in the lateral projection may allow clearer definition of an aneurysm. However, real-time ultrasonography is the preferred modality for the initial assessment and follow up of abdominal aortic aneurysms because of its portability, easy availability, lack of ionizing radiation, low cost and a sensitivity and specificity approaching 100 percent (LaRoy, Cormier et al. 1989)), (Lindholt, Vammen et al. 1999). Routine sonographic evaluation of an abdominal aortic aneurysm involves measuring the anteroposterior, longitudinal, and transverse dimensions of the aorta. Echo dense calcifications in or adjacent to the aortic wall also may be visualized. Patients are asked to undergo the examination after fasting to reduce the presence of overlying bowel gas which can obscure the aorta. Potential problems with abdominal ultrasonography are that it is operator dependent and frequently does not give an accurate depiction of the iliac arteries which also may be aneurismal. In addition, in approximately 1 to 2 percent of cases, the aorta cannot be imaged because of technical difficulty such as overlying bowel gas or obesity (Scott, Ashton et al. 1991).

If the aneurysm is approaching 5 cm or more or if rapid enlargement is seen on serial US images, a computed tomography (CT) or CT angiography (CTA) scan should be obtained, to better determine the size, presence of dissection and mural thrombus and delineate the extent of disease, prior to conventional surgery or treatment with the insertion of an endovascular graft. Disadvantages of CT scan compared to ultrasound include greater cost, significant irradiation, the requirement for contrast, failure to provide clear visualization of aortic branch vessel origins, and in some cases inaccuracy localizing the aneurysm neck as compared with contrast angiography (Ernst 1993). In patients whose renal function does not permit the administration of iodinated contrast material, magnetic resonance imaging (MRI) and magnetic resonance angiography (MRA) provide good alternatives. Nevertheless, MRI has several absolute contraindications, including cardiac pacemakers and intracranial aneurysm clips. Claustrophobia and a patient's inability to remain motionless are likely to yield a non-diagnostic study. Finally access to MRI is less than that for other modalities (Ernst 1993; Petersen, Cambria et al. 1995). Angiography is invasive and has greater risks to the patient. The true size of the aneurysm may not be discernible because of a mural thrombus; therefore, underestimation of the true extent of the aneurysm is common and it has no place in the diagnosis of aortic aneurysms. The role of angiography is in planning surgical or endovascular repair.

Clinical examination plays an important part in the detection of abdominal aortic aneurysm and has moderate overall sensitivity; however, it cannot be relied upon to exclude them, especially if rupture is a possibility. Larger abdominal aortic aneurysms are usually palpable and more likely to be detected on clinical examination, particularly in patients who do not have a large abdominal girth. Ultrasound is accurate in the detection of non-ruptured abdominal aortic aneurysms, with a sensitivity and specificity approaching 100%.

4. Complicated aortic aneurysms

Complications are symptomatic and life threatening. These include acute rupture into the retroperitoneal (85.3%) or peritoneal space (7.1%), or gastrointestinal tract (1.8%) (Miani, Mingazzini et al. 1984). Such ruptures typically cause exsanguinating hemorrhage and profound, unstable hypotension leading to death. In contrast some ruptures do not have an acute presentation, but are slow and contained, presenting with chronic low grade symptoms. Additionally rupture could also occur into major abdominal and pelvic veins (5.8%). Other complications include acute thrombotic occlusion of the aneurysm, distal thromboembolism and disseminated intravascular coagulation.

4.1 Rupture of aortic aneurysms

4.1.1 Acute rupture of abdominal aortic aneurysms

Rupture into the retroperitoneum typically originates from the left posterior aspect of the abdominal aortic aneurysm, whereas intra peritoneal rupture tends to occur from the right anterior aspect (Bergan and Thompson 1987). Whenever the hemorrhage is tamponaded by the surrounding retroperitoneum and temporarily contained, hemodynamic compensatory mechanisms are able to maintain vital organ perfusion allowing the patient time to reach the hospital. Clinical suspicion of aneurysm rupture is therefore crucial for rational management and to prevent death.

Clinically, hypotension, pulsatile abdominal mass, and flank or back pain constitutes the classic triad for the diagnosis of abdominal aortic aneurysm rupture. However, this triad may be incomplete in as many as 50% of patients contributing to misdiagnoses in 24-42%. The patient's blood pressure often recovers and stabilizes giving normal vital signs at examination. An important clue to the diagnosis of rupture, a syncopal attack at the outset indicative of hypotension, may be easily overlooked. Abdominal obesity and muscle guarding contribute to impalpability of an aneurysm. Furthermore, when hypotensive, the aneurysm may become less pulsatile making it more difficult to detect. More than 80% of patients with ruptured abdominal aortic aneurysm present without a previous diagnosis of an aneurysm. Even when it is known that there is an abdominal aneurysm, only 25% of vascular surgeons are able to palpate it at the time of preparation of the patient for surgery. Despite the incomplete triad, a correct and early diagnosis of rupture can still be made in the majority of cases, enabling prompt surgical or endovascular intervention. In the remainder, rupture of aneurysms of the abdominal aorta simulates other clinical conditions, where symptoms are related to impingement of the hematoma on adjacent structures.

These include renal colic, acute cholecystitis, acute diverculitis of the sigmoid colon, and other gastrointestinal pathology that may delay the correct diagnosis and reduce the patient's chance of survival.

In most instances the obvious clinical feature of rupture is severe abdominal or back ache in an elderly male. This clinical picture is easily confused with several other abdominal emergencies. The leading misdiagnosis is renal colic (Marston, Ahlquist et al. 1992). Blood dissects out into the perirenal space and tracks down the iliac fossa to the groin mimicking the loin to groin radiation of a renal colic. Concomitant dissection of the renal artery may contribute to flank pain and cause hematuria (Eckford and Gillatt 1992).*70*

Right sided aneurysm leaks often cause right upper quadrant pain which could easily be misinterpreted as biliary colic or acute cholecystitis. It is interesting that the well known physicist, Albert Einstein, died from rupture of abdominal aortic aneurysm that simulated acute cholecystitis, and this symptomatology was subsequently described as Einstein's sign (Solberg 1998; Treska 2003). Retroperitoneal hematoma in the left iliac fossa mimics acute diverticulitis with an inflammatory mass (Lederle, Parenti et al. 1994).

Other reported conditions that mimic a leaking or ruptured abdominal aortic aneurysms include ureteral obstruction (Tejada, Becker et al. 1990),*13* obstruction of the left colon (Politoske 1990), *85*upper gastrointestinal obstruction from compression of the third portion of the duodenum (Pal and Cameron 2009), hiccoughs (Stine and Trued 1979) and haematuria (Fetting, Eagan et al. 1973).

An irreducible inguinal mass is commonly due to an incarcerated hernia and the diagnosis is usually straightforward and correct. Rarely this simple presentation may be the external manifestation of a high volume retroperitoneal hematoma which has extended to the extremes of its anatomical boundaries that includes the inguinal canal. There are several reports of ruptured aneurysms presenting as irreducible symptomatic inguinal masses often diagnosed as complicated inguinal hernia (Abulafi, Mee et al. 1991; Grabowski and Pilcher 1981; Khaw, Sottiurai et al. 1986; Louras and Welch 1984; Owen and Klark 1990; Villegas-Cabello and Siller 1999). Therefore, the presence of haematoma within the inguinal canal warrants further exploration to identify the primary cause.

Retroperitoneal acute rupture with blood tracking inferiorly between the iliacus and psoas, may cause acute femoral nerve compression neuropathy (L2, 3, 4) with quadriceps weakness and anterior thigh pain (Fletcher and Frankel 1976). It may irritate the ilioinguinal nerve (L1) causing groin pain (Lynch 2002), irritate the femoral branch of the genitofemoral nerve (L1) causing testicular pain (O'Keefe and Skiendzielewski 1989) or irritate the lateral cutaneous

nerve of thigh (L2, 3) causing lateral thigh pain. Finally, the posterior cutaneous nerve of the thigh (L2, L3) or the origin of the sciatic nerve (L4- S3) may be irritated by retroperitoneal blood, presenting as pain in the hip or buttock (Mahmood, Ahsan et al. 2005). Any one of these presentations may or may not be associated with thigh ecchymoses, abdominal pain or palpable masses. The only clue to the diagnosis of aneurysm rupture could be a syncopal attack pointing to acute circulatory collapse at the very outset which may have been ignored because of subsequent recovery and dominant extra-abdominal symptoms.
Marston and co-workers(Marston, Ahlquist et al. 1992) catalogued the initial erroneous diagnosis in 46 of 152 retrospectively reviewed cases of ruptured abdominal aortic aneurysm as shown in in Table 1 below.

Initial Diagnosis	Misdiagnosed Cases %	Average Delay, Hours
Renal Colic	24	15
Diverticulitis	13	79
GI Hemorrhage	13	17
Acute MI	8.7	13
Back pain	8.7	18
Motor vehicle accidents	6.5	15
Sepsis	6.5	26
Other GI problems	6.5	4
Other diagnoses	13	18

Table 1. Percentage misdiagnosis and delay in diagnosis

Misdiagnosis in the case of atypical presentations is the main cause of treatment delays leading to increased mortality. The inclusion of abdominal aortic aneurysm in the differential diagnosis of a wide spectrum of symptoms should lead to a low threshold for confirmatory diagnostic imaging that would minimize treatment delays and improve outcomes.

4.1.2 Chronic contained rupture of aneurysms

Although aortic aneurysm ruptures usually present with acute symptoms requiring emergency treatment, in rare instances these get localized to the retroperitoneum and present with chronic compressive symptoms of hematoma which are more subtle and include months of back pain. Other symptoms have been described, including obturator neuropathy, obstructive jaundice and groin hernia (Caynak, Onan et al. 2008; Saiki, Urata et al. 2006). Chronic contained aneurysms represent only 4% of all ruptured aortic aneurysms

(Bansal, Thukral et al. 2006) and 2.7% of operated infrarenal abdominal aortic aneurysms (Jones, Reilly et al. 1986).
The descriptive criteria of chronic contained rupture includes a known history of AAA, pain that radiates to the lower back, a stable condition and normal hematocrit value, radiologic findings of retroperitoneal hematoma, and pathologic confirmation of an organized hematoma. Retroperitoneal hematoma can lead to vertebral erosion in 30% of cases (Booth and Galland 2002).
Symptoms are attributable to tissue compression or erosion and are most often found in the workup of back pain or an abdominal problem. The differential diagnosis includes primary and metastatic spinal tumors, retroperitoneal tumors, iliopsoas muscle abscess, rheumatoid arthritis, osteoporosis, and osteomalacia.
A thorough clinical and radiological workup is required, and the radiological examination should involve a careful look at all structures surrounding the vertebral body. CT scans or magnetic resonance imaging provide a rapid and noninvasive approach for the diagnosis and the extent of bony destruction (Ando, Igari et al. 2003)

4.1.3 Imaging for rupture

Although the imaging findings of abdominal aortic aneurysm rupture are usually obvious, small ruptures can be mistaken for unopacified bowel, lymph node enlargement, or perianeurysmal fibrosis. Careful examination of the morphology of the aneurysm may aid in detecting subtle ruptures.
In a retrospective study (Siegel, Cohan et al. 1994) that evaluated CT scans of patients with ruptured and non ruptured abdominal aortic aneurysms to determine whether a number of morphologic features were associated with rupture, the length of the aneurysm was not significantly different between the rupture and control groups. The ruptured aneurysms had significantly larger anteroposterior and transverse dimensions. The two groups had similar rates of lumen irregularity. Ruptured aneurysms contained a lesser amount of thrombus than aneurysms that were not ruptured. Thrombus calcification was seen more commonly in non ruptured aneurysms, which was thought to be related to the greater amount of thrombus in the non ruptured aneurysms.
Attenuation characteristics of the thrombus that were not associated with rupture included the homogeneous, diffusely heterogeneous, and low-attenuation periluminal halo patterns (Siegel, Cohan et al. 1994). High-attenuation crescents within the mural thrombus were seen only in ruptured aneurysms (Siegel, Cohan et al. 1994). Mural calcification patterns were also evaluated, and a focal discontinuity in otherwise circumferential calcification was rare and seen only in ruptured aneurysms. It was noted, however, that mural calcification was often discontinuous, and the discontinuity was most useful when shown to be new compared with a prior scan (Siegel, Cohan et al. 1994).
There are several studies that have examined hyperattenuating crescents as a sign of impending rupture. It has been reported that thrombus transformation with contrast extravasation into the thrombus and lumen irregularity signify impending rupture (Pillari, Chang et al. 1988). Mehard et al reported a significant correlation between impending rupture and high-attenuating crescents in the wall of abdominal aortic aneurysms on unenhanced CT scans (Mehard, Heiken et al. 1994). In this retrospective study, the high-attenuating crescents were present in 77% of patients with complicated aneurysms, with complications including intramural hematoma, contained rupture, and frank rupture. The

specificity of the "high-attenuating crescent" sign was 93%. For a crescent to be considered high attenuation, the crescent needed to be well defined and of higher attenuation than the psoas muscle on enhanced scans or of higher attenuation than that of the patent lumen on unenhanced scans. In another study, crescents of increased attenuation were present in 21% of ruptured aneurysms and in none of the patients with intact aneurysms (Siegel, Cohan et al. 1994).

Hyperattenuating crescents have been attributed histopathologically to hemorrhage into the mural thrombus or into the aneurysm wall, with clefts of blood seeping from the lumen into the thrombus. The hemorrhage later penetrates the aneurysm wall, which weakens the wall. This places the aneurysm at risk for frank rupture, and prompt surgical consultation should be obtained (Arita, Matsunaga et al. 1997).

4.1.3.1 Imaging in chronic contained rupture

The following criteria have been proposed to enable diagnosis of chronic contained ruptures: known abdominal aortic aneurysm, previous pain symptoms that may have resolved, stable hemodynamic status with a normal hematocrit, CT scans showing retroperitoneal hemorrhage, and pathologic confirmation of organized hematoma (Jones, Reilly et al. 1986). Draping of the posterior aspect of the aorta over the adjacent vertebral body is an indicator of aortic wall insufficiency and contained rupture. Even in the absence of retroperitoneal hemorrhage associated vertebral body erosion may be seen (Halliday and al-Kutoubi 1996).

However, in urgent situations in which the clinical diagnosis is fairly certain and the patient is unstable, there is no place for confirmatory imaging. In such instances the diagnosis is confirmed at open surgery or during angiography as part of endovascular stenting.

4.2 Rupture elsewhere

Aneurysm rupture is not limited to the retroperitoneum or the general peritoneal cavity alone. Rarely an aneurysm may rupture into an adjacent structure and manifest with clinical features pointing towards a primary lesion in that particular viscus. Examples are ruptures into the gastrointestinal tract (aortoenteric fistula) causing gastrointestinal bleeding and rupture into an adjacent vein (cava, renal, lumbar, or common iliac vein) causing hematuria, priapism or lower extremity swelling.

4.2.1 Aortoenteric fistula

Primary aortoenteric fistula (PAEF) is a potentially fatal condition which poses a considerable diagnostic challenge because of its infrequency and the nonspecific presentation. Such fistulae may involve any part of the aorta, with the intestinal tract from the esophagus to the colon, the esophagus and the duodenum being most common (Song, Liu et al. 2008). Secondary fistulae are more common after previous open or endovascular aortic interventions (Saratzis, Saratzis et al. 2008) and mycotic aneurysms (Bunt 1983).

Although rare, primary fistulae from fusiform aortic aneurysms must be considered when the combination of gastrointestinal bleeding and aortic aneurysm coexist (Wijeyeratne SM, Ubayasiri R et al. 2009). Disappointingly, the combination of a pulsatile abdominal mass and gastrointestinal bleeding has been reported in only 23% (Sweeney and Gadacz 1984) to 27.8% (Song, Liu et al. 2008) for aortoduodenal fistulae. These proportions would in fact increase with the use of ultrasound and computerized tomography. Even in such instances the common assumption is that the bleed is from either diverticuli, ulcers or varices (Jiao, Zong et al. 2009; Senadhi, Brown et al. 2010; Thomson, Gopinath et al. 2009) and the aneurysm is usually considered an incidental finding.

The pattern of bleeding from an aortoenteric fistula (AEF) is of interest. A "herald" hemorrhage is followed hours, days, or weeks later by catastrophic hemorrhage and this is characteristic of an AEF (Song, Liu et al. 2008). This initial self limiting bleed is the result of a small fistula occluded by thrombus. Since 70% survive at least 6 hours (Sweeney and Gadacz 1984) and up to 50% for 24 hours (Steffes and O'Leary 1980) after the initial bleed, a "herald" hemorrhage should be viewed as an opportunity for prompt surgical intervention. Hence clinical awareness is crucial and should be broad based, particularly among emergency care specialists, gastroenterologists, general surgeons and physicians.

Endoscopy is the cornerstone in the diagnostic work up for haematemesis. Nevertheless the detection of non bleeding erosions, ulcers, varices or polyps may be misleading (Jiao, Zong et al. 2009) and negative endoscopy does not rule out an AEF as the length of the endoscope does not allow visualization of the distal duodenum where AEFs commonly occur (Brand, Sivak et al. 1979).

Although no single imaging modality demonstrates the condition with sufficient sensitivity and specificity, computed tomography (CT), owing to its widespread availability and high efficiency, has become the imaging modality of choice for evaluations in the emergency setting. CT has widely variable sensitivity (40%-90%) and specificity (33%-100%) for the diagnosis of aortoenteric fistulae. To use this modality effectively for the initial diagnostic examination, radiologists must be familiar with the spectrum of CT appearances. Mimickers of aortoenteric fistulae include retroperitoneal fibrosis, infected aortic aneurysm, infectious aortitis, and perigraft infection without fistulization. Differentiation is aided by the observation of ectopic gas, loss of the normal fat plane, extravasation of aortic contrast material into the enteric lumen, or leakage of enteric contrast material into the paraprosthetic space; these features are highly suggestive of aortoenteric fistula in a patient with bleeding into the gastrointestinal tract (Daly, Nott et al. 1997; Vu, Menias et al. 2009). But the absence of these features in the presence of an AEF is not unusual and one must be aware of its limited negative predictive value (Ranasinghe, Loa et al. 2011). This awareness would help in justifying proceeding with interventions based on high clinical suspicion when there is uncontrolled bleeding.

It must also be remembered that percutaneous angiography is of little value since the need for it coincides with the need for immediate surgery (Yeong 1995). Despite technological advances in endoscopy and imaging, the cornerstone in the diagnosis of an AEF remains clinical suspicion (Mehmood, Mushtaq et al. 2007; Wijeyeratne SM, Ubayasiri R et al. 2009)

4.2.2 Aortocaval fistula

Aortocaval fistula is a rare complication of AAA, involving less than 1% of all aortic aneurysms. The diagnosis is dependent on recognition of its clinical features. The dramatic picture of a patient with pain, a large pulsatile abdominal mass, a machinery-like abdominal bruit, and acute dyspnea is pathognomic for an aortocaval fistula and has been well described (Bednarkiewicz, Pretre et al. 1997). However, classic features may be absent in up to one half of patients (Reckless, McColl et al. 1972). Absence of characteristic findings together with the rarity of such lesions and resultant lack of awareness may lead to delay in diagnosis.

Several factors may contribute to misdiagnosis. Failure to auscultate the abdomen for a bruit is probably a key reason for non diagnosis before surgery (Brewster, Cambria et al. 1991) and underscores the importance of routine auscultation of the abdomen in all patients with an aneurysm.

In some instances the diagnosis may be missed despite detecting the abdominal bruit because of the inability to detect a palpable pulsatile abdominal mass, more so in those patients with isolated iliac aneurysms. Finally the mural thrombus within the aneurysm sac may partially or totally obstruct the fistula and obliterate the typical continuous bruit (Baker, Sharzer et al. 1972; Dardik, Dardik et al. 1976; Weinbaum, Riles et al. 1984).

Although the principal hemodynamic effects of left-to-right AV shunts have been well characterized in general, the specific clinical features of large vessel central AV fistulas may be quite variable. Factors influencing the clinical manifestations of such lesions include the size, and location of the fistula as well as its duration. In addition, differences in patient age, preexistent cardiopulmonary or renal disease, and possible associated retroperitoneal blood loss at the time of fistula occurrence can markedly alter the manner of clinical presentation in individual patients.

In the case of high output fistulae, a sensation of fullness in the chest, and that the heart is about to burst, the aptly named "bursting heart " syndrome has been reported (Leigh-Smith and Smith 2000). Chest pain in such instances are often misdiagnosed as angina (Beierlein, Walker et al. 2002) and acute coronary syndrome (Vigna, Santoro et al. 2008). Decompensated high-output cardiac failure, occurring when the increased venous return overwhelms cardiac compensatory mechanisms, has often been emphasized as the predominant clinical feature (Brewster, Cambria et al. 1991). Predisposition to cardiac failure would depend on available cardiac reserve, fistula size and duration of illness (Kazmier and Harrison 1973; Nennhaus and Javid 1968; Reckless, McColl et al. 1972).

Caval compression by the adjacent aortic aneurysm tends to minimize flow towards the heart and augment peripheral venous flow and pressure. Diversion of most shunted blood toward the pelvis and extremities produces marked *regional* venous hypertension and accounts for many of the symptoms and findings, which may confuse or obscure correct diagnosis (Brewster, Cambria et al. 1991).

Regional venous hypertension is responsible for the often marked swelling of the lower extremities frequently seen and explains the often striking contrast of bluish, congested lower extremities and the presence of cool, pale, ischemic upper extremities and trunk. Distended veins in the lower abdomen and legs in the lying down position and even with leg elevation are diagnostic. Careful examination may detect pulsation. The presence of long saphenous bruits suggests saphenofemoral incompetence due to arterialised, reversed venous flow dynamics and strengthens the clinical diagnosis of aortocaval fistula (Phillips, Chaudhuri et al. 2006).

Phlegmasia cerulea dolens, characterized by the triad of limb swelling, cyanosis, and acute ischemic pain, usually arises because of acute massive thrombosis of major deep, collateral, and superficial veins of an extremity. A similar clinical picture has been reported following aneurysm rupture into the cava (Myers, Kalangos et al. 2008) .

Transmission of such venous hypertension to the pelvic venous system may also lead to hematuria, which may cause diagnostic confusion. Hematuria has been reported in 17% to 24% of patients with an aortocaval fistula (Brewster, Cambria et al. 1991; Crawford, Turell et al. 1963; Nennhaus and Javid 1968; van Driel, van Gelder et al. 1984). The presence of hematuria in a patient suffering from an abdominal aortic aneurysm is an indication for imaging to rule out an aortocaval fistula (Salo, Verkkala et al. 1990). Prompt clearing of hematuria with repair of the fistula, supports the key role of pelvic venous hypertension (Brewster, Cambria et al. 1991).

Rupture of distended superficial colorectal mucosal veins may cause rectal bleeding (Doty, Wright et al. 1978; van Driel, van Gelder et al. 1984). A similar mechanism accounts for reported cases of painless priapism thus indicating high flow as the cause in the case of an aortocaval fistula (Gordon, Marsh et al. 2004).

Aortocaval fistula may also present primarily with renal insufficiency, manifesting with oliguria or anuria and acidosis, and cause diagnostic confusion. Spontaneous aortocaval fistula can also present with acute liver and renal failure (Kanbay, Gur et al. 2004). Furthermore the rapid increase of intra-abdominal blood volume due to a massive fistula has been reported to cause acute abdominal compartment syndrome leading to multi-organ dysfunction (Music, Radevic et al. 2006).

Abdominal color doppler ultrasonography is useful in establishing the diagnosis, which will show the jet effect of aortic flow into the IVC. Characteristic findings for the CT diagnosis include early synchronous and equivalent enhancement of the IVC and aorta and dilatation of IVC and pelvic veins. Furthermore CT angiography would help in the delineation of anatomy that may be particularly important for its management.

4.3 Acute thrombosis

Thrombosis of an abdominal aortic aneurysm is a rare (0.6-1.8%, less than 60 reported cases) (Bolduc, Clayson et al. 1989; Fairhead, Phillips et al. 2005; Hachiro, Kawaharada et al. 2004; Hirose, Takagi et al. 2000; Shnacker, Witz et al. 2001; Suliman, Raffetto et al. 2003) yet devastating complication with an estimated mortality rate of 50%. Unlike AAA rupture, the risk of developing an AAA thrombosis is independent of the size of the aneurysm (Beach and Manthey 1998; Hachiro, Kawaharada et al. 2004).

The usual presentation of AAA thrombosis is that of abrupt vascular compromise of the lower extremities, with absent distal pulses (68%), pain (45.7%) involving lower extremities, coolness (31.4%), numbness (34.3%) and mottled skin below the umbilicus (42.9%) being the most frequent findings (Hachiro, Kawaharada et al. 2004; Suliman, Raffetto et al. 2003). Some motor disturbance is found in 22.9% of these cases (Hachiro, Kawaharada et al. 2004).

The differential diagnosis for AAA thrombosis includes aortic dissection and AAA rupture. Abdominal pain is more indicative of AAA rupture, whereas AAA thrombosis usually has severe lower limb pain (Hachiro, Kawaharada et al. 2004).

Hypertension can be associated with both AAA thrombosis and aortic dissection, and an initial presentation of paralysis has also been documented with aortic dissection (Ayerdi, Gupta et al. 2002). Usually chest or upper back pain will be expected with aortic dissection in addition to the paralysis. When the thrombus obstructs the artery of Adamkiewicz, the main blood supply to the lower spinal cord, spinal ischemia and paralysis can occur without pain or other features of limb ischaemia (Bogie, Willigendael et al. 2008; Bolduc, Clayson et al. 1989; Lo, Vallee et al. 2002; van Zyl 2005). Rarely an abdominal aortic aneurysm may thrombose without causing acute limb ischaemia (Brandao, Simoes et al. 2009; Moulakakis, Maras et al. 2010).

4.4 Coagulopathy as a form of presentation of aortic aneurysms

Infrequently, a large abdominal aortic aneurysm is associated with clinically overt disseminated intravascular coagulation causing a consumptive coagulopathy and hemorrhagic and thrombotic complications; the reported incidence being as high as 3 to 4 percent (Aboulafia and Aboulafia 1996; Fisher, Yawn et al. 1983).

In the majority of cases, consumptive coagulopathy is asymptomatic and has a chronic course, but in 0.5-4% of patients it is clinically overt and may be the presenting feature leading to the diagnosis of a previously unknown aortic aneurysm (Peters, Triolo et al. 2005; Trelinski, Stelagowski et al. 2009) .

4.5 Inflammatory aortic aneurysms

In contrast with atherosclerotic aortic aneurysms, the majority of patients with an intact inflammatory aneurysm are symptomatic (Goldstone, Malone et al. 1978). The most common symptom is abdominal and/or back pain while anorexia and weight loss are frequent associates. Ureteric entrapment causing colic is another unique feature (Crawford, Stowe et al. 1985). Interestingly the majority (85%) of these aneurysms are palpable at the time of diagnosis while one fourth are tender and have a bruit. There are several reports of these patients having a moderate rise in the erythrocyte sedimentation rate (Bainbridge and Woodward 1982; Darke, Glass et al. 1977; Pennell, Hollier et al. 1985) and this would further strengthen the accuracy of diagnosis of inflammatory aneurysms in symptomatic patients.

Nevertheless the classic triad of chronic abdominal or back pain, elevated ESR, and weight loss is rare, implying a low diagnostic sensitivity but has high specificity for inflammatory aneurysms. When ureteric obstruction is added the diagnostic accuracy increases further.

Although preoperative clinical diagnosis of an inflammatory aneurysm was infrequent in the past, routine preoperative imaging since of late has significantly facilitated the diagnosis. The thickening of the aortic wall occurs in the anterior and lateral walls. This can be demonstrated by both CT scan and ultrasonography. The ultrasound scan shows an echolucent halo anteriorly and laterally with clear definition of the posterior aortic wall (Bundy and Ritchie 1984; Pennell, Hollier et al. 1985; Walker, Bloor et al. 1972). The diagnostic accuracy is greater with CT scanning. The characteristic findings are a preaortic retroperitoneal soft tissue density that is sometimes enhanced with intravenous contrast (Pahira, Wein et al. 1979; Vint, Usselman et al. 1980). It must be noted that these features could easily be mistaken for those from a leaking aneurysm with retroperitoneal hematoma (Aiello and Cohen 1980; Pang, Chan et al. 2010; Pennell, Hollier et al. 1985) Medial ureteral deviation or obstruction on CT ureterography in a patient with an aneurysm strongly suggests the inflammatory variety. Although lateral ureteral deviation may be seen with large atherosclerotic aneurysms, ureteral obstruction is very rare (Culp and Bernatz 1961).

5. Conclusion

Typically uncomplicated aortic aneurysms are asymptomatic and discovered incidentally, but abdominal pain and back pain are the most common symptoms and point to complications which are often life threatening.

Diagnosis relies on clinical suspicion confirmed by imaging. Ultrasound remains the definitive test for initial diagnosis and screening. CT scan is typically required for confirmation of rupture in stable patients and for preoperative planning in uncomplicated cases. In the case of complications with hemodynamic instability there is no time for imaging and one must proceed with definitive care based on clinical judgment alone.

6. Acknowledgement

Sara Mohammed Jinnah

7. References

Aboulafia, D. M. and E. D. Aboulafia (1996). "Aortic aneurysm-induced disseminated intravascular coagulation." *Ann Vasc Surg* 10(4): 396-405.ISSN 0890-5096.

Abulafi, A. M., W. M. Mee, et al. (1991). "Leaking abdominal aortic aneurysm presenting as an inguinal mass." *Eur J Vasc Surg* 5(6): 695-696.ISSN 0950-821X

Aiello, M. R. and W. N. Cohen (1980). "Inflammatory aneurysm of the abdominal aorta." *J Comput Assist Tomogr* 4(2): 265-267.ISSN 0363-8715

Ando, M., T. Igari, et al. (2003). "CT features of chronic contained rupture of an abdominal aortic aneurysm." *Ann Thorac Cardiovasc Surg* 9(4): 274-278.ISSN 1341-1098.

Arita, T., N. Matsunaga, et al. (1997). "Abdominal aortic aneurysm: rupture associated with the high-attenuating crescent sign." *Radiology* 204(3): 765-768.ISSN 0033-8419

Ayerdi, J., S. K. Gupta, et al. (2002). "Acute abdominal aortic thrombosis following the Heimlich maneuver." *Cardiovasc Surg* 10(2): 154-156.ISSN 0967-2109

Bainbridge, E. T. and D. A. Woodward (1982). "Inflammatory aneurysms of the abdominal aorta with associated ureteric obstruction or medial deviation." *J Cardiovasc Surg (Torino)* 23(5): 365-370.ISSN 0021-9509

Baker, W. H., L. A. Sharzer, et al. (1972). "Aortocaval fistula as a complication of abdominal aortic aneurysms." *Surgery* 72(6): 933-938.ISSN 0039-6060

Bansal, M., B. B. Thukral, et al. (2006). "Contained rupture of a thoracoabdominal aortic aneurysm presenting as a back mass." *J Thorac Imaging* 21(3): 219-221.ISSN 0883-5993

Beach, C. and D. Manthey (1998). "Painless acute aortic dissection presenting as left lower extremity numbness." *Am J Emerg Med* 16(1): 49-51.ISSN 0735-6757

Bednarkiewicz, M., R. Pretre, et al. (1997). "Aortocaval fistula associated with abdominal aortic aneurysm: a diagnostic challenge." *Ann Vasc Surg* 11(5): 464-466.ISSN 0890-5096

Beierlein, W., T. Walker, et al. (2002). "[Angina pectoris as initial clinical manifestation of ruptured abdominal aortic aneurysm with aortocaval fistula]." *Med Klin (Munich)* 97(6): 357-360.ISSN 0723-5003

Bergan, J. J. and J. E. Thompson (1987). "The ruptured abdominal aortic aneurysm. In: Bergan JJ, Yao JT, eds. ." *Vascular Surgical Emergencies*: 285-297.ISSN.

Bogie, R., E. M. Willigendael, et al. (2008). "Acute thrombosis of an abdominal aortic aneurysm: a short report." *Eur J Vasc Endovasc Surg* 35(5): 590-592.ISSN 1532-2165

Bolduc, M. E., S. Clayson, et al. (1989). "Acute aortic thrombosis presenting as painless paraplegia." *J Cardiovasc Surg (Torino)* 30(3): 506-508.ISSN 0021-9509

Booth, M. I. and R. B. Galland (2002). "Chronic contained rupture of an abdominal aortic aneurysm: a case report and review of the literature." *Eur J Vasc Endovasc Surg* Extra(3): 33-35.

Brand, E. J., M. V. Sivak, Jr., et al. (1979). "Aortoduodenal fistula: endoscopic diagnosis." *Dig Dis Sci* 24(12): 940-944.ISSN 0163-2116

Brandao, D., J. C. Simoes, et al. (2009). "Occlusion of inferior vena cava: a singular presentation of abdominal aortic aneurysm." *Case Report Med* 2009: 827954.ISSN 1687-9635

Brewster, D. C., R. P. Cambria, et al. (1991). "Aortocaval and iliac arteriovenous fistulas: recognition and treatment." *J Vasc Surg* 13(2): 253-264; discussion 264-255.ISSN 0741-5214

Bundy, A. L. and W. G. Ritchie (1984). "Inflammatory aneurysm of the abdominal aorta." *J Clin Ultrasound* 12(2): 102-104.ISSN 0091-2751

Bunt, T. J. (1983). "Synthetic vascular graft infections. II. Graft-enteric erosions and graft-enteric fistulas." *Surgery* 94(1): 1-9.ISSN 0039-6060

Caynak, B., B. Onan, et al. (2008). "Vertebral erosion due to chronic contained rupture of an abdominal aortic aneurysm." *J Vasc Surg* 48(5): 1342.ISSN 1097-6809

Crawford, E. S., D. J. Turell, et al. (1963). "Aorto-inferior vena caval fistula of neoplastic origin. Hemodynamic and coronary blood flow studies." *Circulation* 27: 414-421.ISSN 0009-7322

Crawford, J. L., C. L. Stowe, et al. (1985). "Inflammatory aneurysms of the aorta." *J Vasc Surg* 2(1): 113-124.ISSN 0741-5214

Culp, O. and P. E. Bernatz (1961). "Urologic aspects of lesions in the abdominal aorta." *J Urol* 86: 189-195.ISSN 0022-5347

Daly, C. A., D. M. Nott, et al. (1997). "Aortoduodenal fistula: appearances on computed tomography." *Aust N Z J Surg* 67(10): 745-746.ISSN 0004-8682

Dardik, H., I. Dardik, et al. (1976). "Intravenous rupture of arteriosclerotic aneurysms of the abdominal aorta." *Surgery* 80(5): 647-651.ISSN 0039-6060

Darke, S. G., R. E. Glass, et al. (1977). "Abdominal aortic aneurysm: Perianeurysmal fibrosis and ureteric obstruction and deviation." *Br J Surg* 64(9): 649-651.ISSN 0007-1323

Doty, D. B., C. B. Wright, et al. (1978). "Aortocaval fistula associated with aneurysm of the abdominal aorta: current management using autotransfusion techniques." *Surgery* 84(2): 250-252.ISSN 0039-6060

Eckford, S. D. and D. A. Gillatt (1992). "Abdominal aortic aneurysms presenting as renal colic." *Br J Urol* 70(5): 496-498.ISSN 0007-1331

Ernst, C. B. (1993). "Abdominal aortic aneurysm." *N Engl J Med* 328(16): 1167-1172.ISSN 0028-4793

Fairhead, J. F., D. Phillips, et al. (2005). "Embolic spinal cord infarction as a presentation of abdominal aortic aneurysm." *J R Soc Med* 98(2): 59-60.ISSN 0141-0768

Fetting, J. H., J. W. Eagan, Jr., et al. (1973). "Hematuria due to an abdominal aortic aneurysm leaking into a ureteral stump." *Johns Hopkins Med J* 133(6): 339-342.ISSN 0021-7263

Fink, H. A., F. A. Lederle, et al. (2000). "The accuracy of physical examination to detect abdominal aortic aneurysm." *Arch Intern Med* 160(6): 833-836.ISSN 0003-9926

Fisher, D. F., Jr., D. H. Yawn, et al. (1983). "Preoperative disseminated intravascular coagulation associated with aortic aneurysms. A prospective study of 76 cases." *Arch Surg* 118(11): 1252-1255.ISSN 0004-0010

Fletcher, H. S. and J. Frankel (1976). "Ruptured abdominal aneurysms presenting with unilateral peripheral neuropathy." *Surgery* 79(1): 120-121.ISSN 0039-6060

Goldstone, J., J. M. Malone, et al. (1978). "Inflammatory aneurysms of the abdominal aorta." *Surgery* 83(4): 425-430.ISSN 0039-6060

Gordon, S., P. Marsh, et al. (2004). "Priapism as the presenting symptom of an aortocaval fistula." *Emerg Med J* 21(2): 265.ISSN 1472-0213

Grabowski, E. W. and D. B. Pilcher (1981). "Ruptured abdominal aortic aneurysm manifesting as symptomatic inguinal hernia." *Am Surg* 47(7): 311-312.ISSN 0003-1348

Hachiro, Y., N. Kawaharada, et al. (2004). "[Thoracoabdominal aortic aneurysm repair after detection of the Adamkiewicz artery by magnetic resonance angiography; a way to shorten operating time and improve outcome]." *Kyobu Geka* 57(4): 280-283.ISSN 0021-5252

Halliday, K. E. and A. al-Kutoubi (1996). "Draped aorta: CT sign of contained leak of aortic aneurysms." *Radiology* 199(1): 41-43.ISSN 0033-8419

Hirose, H., M. Takagi, et al. (2000). "Acute occlusion of an abdominal aortic aneurysm--case report and review of the literature." *Angiology* 51(6): 515-523.ISSN 0003-3197

Houston, T. P., A. B. Elster, et al. (1998). "The U.S. Preventive Services Task Force Guide to Clinical Preventive Services, Second Edition. AMA Council on Scientific Affairs." *Am J Prev Med* 14(4): 374-376.ISSN 0749-3797

Jiao, Y., Y. Zong, et al. (2009). "Aortoesophageal fistula: a case misdiagnosed as esophageal polyp." *World J Gastroenterol* 15(47): 6007-6009.ISSN 1007-9327

Jones, C. S., M. K. Reilly, et al. (1986). "Chronic contained rupture of abdominal aortic aneurysms." *Arch Surg* 121(5): 542-546.ISSN 0004-0010

Kanbay, M., G. Gur, et al. (2004). "Spontaneous aortocaval fistula presenting with acute liver and renal failure: a case report." *Turk J Gastroenterol* 15(3): 169-172.ISSN 1300-4948

Karkos, C. D., U. Mukhopadhyay, et al. (2000). "Abdominal aortic aneurysm: the role of clinical examination and opportunistic detection." *Eur J Vasc Endovasc Surg* 19(3): 299-303.ISSN 1078-5884

Kazmier, F. J. and C. E. Harrison, Jr. (1973). "Acquired aortocaval fistulas." *Am J Med* 55(2): 175-183.ISSN 0002-9343

Khaw, H., V. S. Sottiurai, et al. (1986). "Ruptured abdominal aortic aneurysm presenting as symptomatic inguinal mass: report of six cases." *J Vasc Surg* 4(4): 384-389.ISSN 0741-5214

LaRoy, L. L., P. J. Cormier, et al. (1989). "Imaging of abdominal aortic aneurysms." *AJR Am J Roentgenol* 152(4): 785-792.ISSN 0361-803X

Lederle, F. A., C. M. Parenti, et al. (1994). "Ruptured abdominal aortic aneurysm: the internist as diagnostician." *Am J Med* 96(2): 163-167.ISSN 0002-9343

Lederle, F. A. and D. L. Simel (1999). "The rational clinical examination. Does this patient have abdominal aortic aneurysm?" *JAMA* 281(1): 77-82.ISSN 0098-7484

Leigh-Smith, S. and R. C. Smith (2000). "Aorto caval fistula--the "bursting heart syndrome"." *J Accid Emerg Med* 17(3): 223-225.ISSN 1351-0622

Lindholt, J. S., S. Vammen, et al. (1999). "The validity of ultrasonographic scanning as screening method for abdominal aortic aneurysm." *Eur J Vasc Endovasc Surg* 17(6): 472-475.ISSN 1078-5884

Lo, D., J. N. Vallee, et al. (2002). "Unusual origin of the artery of Adamkiewicz from the fourth lumbar artery." *Neuroradiology* 44(2): 153-157.ISSN 0028-3940

Louras, J. C. and J. P. Welch (1984). "Masking of ruptured abdominal aortic aneurysm by incarcerated inguinal hernia." *Arch Surg* 119(3): 331-332.ISSN 0004-0010

Lynch, R. M. (2002). "Ruptured abdominal aortic aneurysm presenting as groin pain." *Br J Gen Pract* 52(477): 320-321.ISSN 0960-1643

Mahmood, F., F. Ahsan, et al. (2005). "Ruptured abdominal aortic aneurysm presenting as buttock pain." *Emerg Med J* 22(6): 453-454.ISSN 1472-0213

Marston, W. A., R. Ahlquist, et al. (1992). "Misdiagnosis of ruptured abdominal aortic aneurysms." *J Vasc Surg* 16(1): 17-22.ISSN 0741-5214

Mehard, W. B., J. P. Heiken, et al. (1994). "High-attenuating crescent in abdominal aortic aneurysm wall at CT: a sign of acute or impending rupture." *Radiology* 192(2): 359-362.ISSN 0033-8419

Mehmood, R. K., A. Mushtaq, et al. (2007). "Clinical presentation of a missed primary aorto-enteric fistula." *J Pak Med Assoc* 57(12): 616-618.ISSN 0030-9982

Miani, S., P. Mingazzini, et al. (1984). "Influence of the rupture site of abdominal aortic aneurysms with regard to postoperative survival rate." *J Cardiovasc Surg (Torino)* 25(5): 414-419.ISSN 0021-9509

Moulakakis, K. G., D. Maras, et al. (2010). ""Silent" thrombosis of an abdominal aortic aneurysm not producing acute limb ischemia." *Vasa* 39(3): 265-267.ISSN 0301-1526

Music, D., B. Radevic, et al. (2006). "[Abdominal compartment syndrome caused by ruptured abdominal aortic aneurysm in vena cava]." *Vojnosanit Pregl* 63(9): 843-846.ISSN 0042-8450

Myers, P. O., A. Kalangos, et al. (2008). "Ruptured aortic aneurysm masquerading as phlegmasia cerulea." *Am J Emerg Med* 26(9): 1067 e1061-1062.ISSN 1532-8171

Nennhaus, H. P. and H. Javid (1968). "The distinct syndrome of spontaneous abdominal aortocaval fistula." *Am J Med* 44(3): 464-473.ISSN 0002-9343

O'Keefe, K. P. and J. J. Skiendzielewski (1989). "Abdominal aortic aneurysm rupture presenting as testicular pain." *Ann Emerg Med* 18(10): 1096-1098.ISSN 0196-0644

Owen, E. R. and A. E. Klark (1990). "Irreducible inguinal hernia as a presentation of ruptured abdominal aortic aneurysm." *J R Coll Surg Edinb* 35(6): 399.ISSN 0035-8835

Pahira, J. J., A. J. Wein, et al. (1979). "Bilateral complete ureteral obstruction secondary to an abdominal aortic aneurysm with perianeurysmal fibrosis: diagnosis by computed tomography." *J Urol* 121(1): 103-106.ISSN 0022-5347

Pal, A. and A. E. Cameron (2009). "Superior mesenteric artery syndrome in association with an abdominal aortic aneurysm." *Ann R Coll Surg Engl* 91(7): W6-7.ISSN 1478-7083

Pang, Y. C., Y. C. Chan, et al. (2010). "Tender inflammatory infrarenal aortic aneurysm simulating acute rupture." *Asian Cardiovasc Thorac Ann* 18(2): 180-182.ISSN 1816-5370

Pennell, R. C., L. H. Hollier, et al. (1985). "Inflammatory abdominal aortic aneurysms: a thirty-year review." *J Vasc Surg* 2(6): 859-869.ISSN 0741-5214

Peters, K. A., P. T. Triolo, et al. (2005). "Disseminated intravascular coagulopathy: manifestations after a routine dental extraction." *Oral Surg Oral Med Oral Pathol Oral Radiol Endod* 99(4): 419-423.ISSN 1079-2104

Petersen, M. J., R. P. Cambria, et al. (1995). "Magnetic resonance angiography in the preoperative evaluation of abdominal aortic aneurysms." *J Vasc Surg* 21(6): 891-898; discussion 899.ISSN 0741-5214

Phillips, A. W., A. Chaudhuri, et al. (2006). "Bilateral long saphenous bruits: a marker of aortocaval fistula." *Eur J Vasc Endovasc Surg* 32(5): 529-531.ISSN 1078-5884

Pillari, G., J. B. Chang, et al. (1988). "Computed tomography of abdominal aortic aneurysm. An in vivo pathological report with a note on dynamic predictors." *Arch Surg* 123(6): 727-732.ISSN 0004-0010

Politoske, E. J. (1990). "Ruptured abdominal aortic aneurysm presenting as an obstruction of the left colon." *Am J Gastroenterol* 85(6): 745-747.ISSN 0002-9270

Ranasinghe, W., J. Loa, et al. (2011). "Primary aortoenteric fistulae: the challenges in diagnosis and review of treatment." *Ann Vasc Surg* 25(3): 386 e381-385.ISSN 1615-5947

Reckless, J. P., I. McColl, et al. (1972). "Aorto-caval fistulae: an uncommon complication of abdominal aortic aneurysms." *Br J Surg* 59(6): 461-462.ISSN 0007-1323

Sabiston, D. C. and C. M. Townsend (2008). *Sabiston textbook of surgery : the biological basis of modern surgical practice*. Saunders/Elsevier,ISBN 9781416036753

Saiki, M., Y. Urata, et al. (2006). "Chronic contained rupture of an abdominal aortic aneurysm with vertebral erosion: report of a case." *Ann Thorac Cardiovasc Surg* 12(4): 300-302.ISSN 1341-1098

Salo, J. A., K. A. Verkkala, et al. (1990). "Hematuria is an indication of rupture of an abdominal aortic aneurysm into the vena cava." *J Vasc Surg* 12(1): 41-44.ISSN 0741-5214

Saratzis, N., A. Saratzis, et al. (2008). "Aortoduodenal fistulas after endovascular stent-graft repair of abdominal aortic aneurysms: single-center experience and review of the literature." *J Endovasc Ther* 15(4): 441-448.ISSN 1526-6028

Scott, R. A., H. A. Ashton, et al. (1991). "Abdominal aortic aneurysm in 4237 screened patients: prevalence, development and management over 6 years." *Br J Surg* 78(9): 1122-1125.ISSN 0007-1323

"Screening for abdominal aortic aneurysm: recommendation statement." (2005). *Ann Intern Med* 142(3): 198-202.ISSN 1539-3704

Senadhi, V., J. C. Brown, et al. (2010). "A Mysterious Cause of Gastrointestinal Bleeding Disguising Itself as Diverticulosis and Peptic Ulcer Disease: A Review of Diagnostic Modalities for Aortoenteric Fistula." *Case Rep Gastroenterol* 4(3): 510-517.ISSN 1662-0631

Shnacker, A., M. Witz, et al. (2001). "Acute thrombosis of an aortic aneurysm." *J Cardiovasc Surg (Torino)* 42(1): 111-113.ISSN 0021-9509

Siegel, C. L., R. H. Cohan, et al. (1994). "Abdominal aortic aneurysm morphology: CT features in patients with ruptured and nonruptured aneurysms." *AJR Am J Roentgenol* 163(5): 1123-1129.ISSN 0361-803X

Solberg, S. (1998). "[Curriculum vitae aortae]." *Tidsskr Nor Laegeforen* 118(30): 4644-4647.ISSN 0029-2001

Song, Y., Q. Liu, et al. (2008). "Diagnosis and management of primary aortoenteric fistulas--experience learned from eighteen patients." *Surgery* 143(1): 43-50.ISSN 1532-7361

Steffes, B. C. and J. P. O'Leary (1980). "Primary aortoduodenal fistula: a case report and review of the literature." *Am Surg* 46(3): 121-129.ISSN 0003-1348

Stine, R. J. and S. J. Trued (1979). "Hiccups: an unusual manifestation of an abdominal aortic aneurysm." *JACEP* 8(9): 368-370.ISSN 0361-1124

Suliman, A. S., J. D. Raffetto, et al. (2003). "Acute thrombosis of abdominal aortic aneurysms--report of two cases and review of the literature." *Vasc Endovascular Surg* 37(1): 71-75.ISSN 1538-5744

Sweeney, M. S. and T. R. Gadacz (1984). "Primary aortoduodenal fistula: manifestation, diagnosis, and treatment." *Surgery* 96(3): 492-497.ISSN 0039-6060

Tejada, E., G. J. Becker, et al. (1990). "Two unusual manifestations of aortic aneurysms." *Clin Cardiol* 13(2): 132-135.ISSN 0160-9289

Thomson, V. S., K. G. Gopinath, et al. (2009). "Primary aorto-enteric fistula: a rare complication of abdominal aortic aneurysm." *J Postgrad Med* 55(4): 267-269.ISSN 0022-3859

Trelinski, J., M. Stelagowski, et al. (2009). "[Disseminated intravascular coagulation in abdominal aortic aneurysm--case report]." *Pol Merkur Lekarski* 27(158): 116-118.ISSN 1426-9686

Treska, V. (2003). "[The Einstein sign]." *Rozhl Chir* 82(2): 73-74.ISSN 0035-9351

van Driel, M., B. van Gelder, et al. (1984). "Hematuria as a presenting symptom of an aortic-vena caval fistula from ruptured aortic aneurysm." *J Urol* 132(4): 774-775.ISSN 0022-5347

van Zyl, H. P. (2005). "Paralysis: a rare presentation of abdominal aortic aneurysm thrombosis." *CJEM* 7(6): 420-422.ISSN 1481-8035

Vigna, C., T. Santoro, et al. (2008). "Aortocaval fistula mimicking an acute coronary syndrome." *J Cardiovasc Med (Hagerstown)* 9(11): 1138-1139.ISSN 1558-2027

Villegas-Cabello, O. and J. Siller (1999). "Asymptomatic rupture of an aortoiliac aneurysm." *Tex Heart Inst J* 26(3): 219-222.ISSN 0730-2347

Vint, V. C., J. A. Usselman, et al. (1980). "Aortic perianeurysmal fibrosis: CT density enhancement and ureteral obstruction." *AJR Am J Roentgenol* 134(3): 577-580.ISSN 0361-803X

Vu, Q. D., C. O. Menias, et al. (2009). "Aortoenteric fistulas: CT features and potential mimics." *Radiographics* 29(1): 197-209.ISSN 1527-1323

Walker, D. I., K. Bloor, et al. (1972). "Inflammatory aneurysms of the abdominal aorta." *Br J Surg* 59(8): 609-614.ISSN 0007-1323

Weinbaum, F. I., T. S. Riles, et al. (1984). "Asymptomatic vena caval fistulization complicating abdominal aortic aneurysm." *Surgery* 96(1): 126-128.ISSN 0039-6060

Wijeyeratne SM, Ubayasiri R, et al. (2009). "Haematemesis due to primary aortic aneurysm-duodenal fistula - clinical suspicion is the cornerstone of diagnosis: a case report." *Cases J* 2(7803).ISSN 1757-1626-2-7803.

Yeong, K. Y. (1995). "Angiographic demonstration of primary aorto-enteric fistula--a case report." *Ann Acad Med Singapore* 24(3): 467-469.ISSN 0304-4602

6

Ultrasound in Abdominal Aortic Aneurysm

Reidar Brekken[1,2], Torbjørn Dahl[1,3] and Toril A. N. Hernes[1,2]
[1]*Norwegian University of Science and Technology, Dept. Circulation and Medical Imaging*
[2]*SINTEF, Dept. Medical Technology*
[3]*St. Olav's Hospital, The University Hospital of Trondheim*
Norway

1. Introduction

Formation and growth of abdominal aortic aneurysms (AAA) may lead to rupture resulting in life threatening haemorrhage. Elective treatment of asymptomatic AAA, either as open surgery or endovascular repair, is recommended when the maximum diameter of the aneurysm exceeds 50-55mm or increases rapidly (Brewster et al., 2003), whereas smaller aneurysms are recommended kept under surveillance. Risk factor modification, such as cessation of smoking, treatment of hypertension and pharmaceutical inhibition of inflammation and protease, could reduce growth in aneurysms kept under surveillance (Baxter et al., 2008; Chaikof et al., 2009; Moll et al., 2011).
The size and growth of the aneurysm is monitored using different radiological imaging modalities. Imaging is also important during image guided endovascular repair, and in follow-up examinations after treatment. In this chapter, we describe how ultrasound is currently used in management of abdominal aortic aneurysm, and discuss future potential and challenges of ultrasound for assisting in improved clinical management with regard to patient selection, treatment alternatives and follow-up.

2. Ultrasound

Ultrasound does not depend on ionizing radiation, and it is relatively inexpensive compared with other imaging modalities. Ultrasound equipment is also portable, and can be used both bedside as well as outside of hospitals. Ultrasound is a fast imaging modality, and presents images in real-time. Therefore, in addition to imaging anatomical structures, ultrasound can also be used for studying function by investigating blood flow or organ motion, e.g. dynamics of the heart. Being a real-time imaging modality, ultrasound further provides an opportunity to interactively investigate the anatomy and potential pathologies. Ultrasound has a certain operator dependency; specifically that it requires skills both to obtain good images, and to interpret the images. Also, in some cases, the image quality suffers from limited view due to bowel gas or obesity. Practical training and knowledge of principles and artefacts is therefore beneficial for successful application of ultrasound.
The physical foundation for medical ultrasound is high frequency waves that are transmitted into the body. The waves are reflected from structures within the body, and the echoes are analysed for retrieving diagnostic information. **Structural imaging** was first obtained using amplitude (A) mode, directly visualizing the amplitude of the echo as a

function of depth. Brightness (B)-line displays the amplitudes as grayscale values. In motion (M) mode imaging, several B-lines in the same direction are drawn consecutively as a function of time for examination of dynamical properties. By combining spatially adjacent B-lines, two-dimensional (2D) B-mode images are obtained and can be visualized in real time. More recently, new ultrasound probes and visualization techniques have made three-dimensional (3D) imaging of anatomical structures possible. 3D images (or volumes) are obtained either by mechanically sweeping the scanplane in the elevation direction to cover a 3D sector, or in real-time by steering the ultrasound beam in 3D using 2D transducer arrays.

In addition to structural imaging, ultrasound can be used for extracting information about function. One example is imaging of blood flow. The **Doppler** effect can be measured with ultrasound to quantify the velocity of blood and moving tissue. In short, the Doppler effect refers to a shift in frequency of a signal that is transmitted (or reflected) from a moving object. The frequency shift is proportional to the velocity of the moving object. By detecting the shift in frequency content of a reflected ultrasound signal relative to the transmitted signal, the velocity of the moving object can therefore be estimated. The velocity information can be presented either by visualizing the Doppler frequency spectrum as a function of time, or by visualizing the velocity as a colour-coded overlay on the B-mode image (Colour Doppler or Duplex imaging). Another example of functional imaging is **strain imaging or elastography**, which displays a quantitative measure of the response of tissues under compression (Garra, 2007; Ophir et al., 1991). The compression can be due to natural motion, e.g. heart contractions or pulsating arteries, or enforced by an external compression, e.g. movement of the ultrasound probe. The ultrasound pulse itself can also be used for enforcing compression, in which case the method is often referred to as artificial radiation force imaging (ARFI) (Nightingale et al., 2002). Clinical applications of strain imaging and elastography include assessment of left ventricular myocardial function, and differentiation of stiff tumours from surrounding normal tissues. Examples of B-mode and colour Doppler images of an abdominal aorta are shown in Fig. 1.

For some applications, it is beneficial to use contrast imaging by injecting **contrast agents** (microbubbles) in the blood to increase the echo obtained from blood. The microbubbles respond differently than human tissue under influence of the ultrasound pulse, thus allowing for specialized detection methods separating the contrast agents from surrounding tissues (Frinking et al., 2000; Hansen & Angelsen, 2009). Contrast agents may provide better images of the ventricles of the heart and larger blood vessels as well as visualization of microcirculation, which is interesting for detection of e.g. myocardial perfusion (Lindner et al., 2000). Targeted microbubbles that attach to specific molecular signatures may provide new possibilities for diagnosis of various diseases, e.g. tumours or atherosclerosis (Anderson et al., 2011; ten Kate et al., 2010).

Ultrasound is most commonly used for diagnostic purposes, but may also be used therapeutically. One application is ultrasound imaging for guidance during surgery, biopsy or needle insertion. Another therapeutic use of ultrasound is **high intensity focused ultrasound (HIFU)**, exploiting that ultrasound, being mechanical waves, can be used for focused delivery of high energies. Sonic waves (extracorporeal shock wave lithotripsy) can be used for destruction of kidney stones (Gallucci et al., 2001). Other applications include focused ultrasound surgery (FUS), thrombolysis and hemostasis (Kim et al., 2008; Vaezy et al., 2001). Burgess et al. (2007) reported HIFU for hemostasis in the posterior liver of 17 pigs. The probe was placed on the anterior surface of the liver and aimed at the bleeding. 17 became hemostatic, whereas 7 controls (sham-HIFU) did not become hemostatic, illustrating the potential of HIFU as a pro-coagulant. Local treatment of various diseases may be possible by using nanotechnology for producing targeted microbubbles, which may be loaded with drugs or genes. The microbubbles can be monitored by ultrasound and destructed for local drug release. Bio-effects of the destruction can be used for disrupting cell membranes for killing malicious cells, or for increased drug uptake.

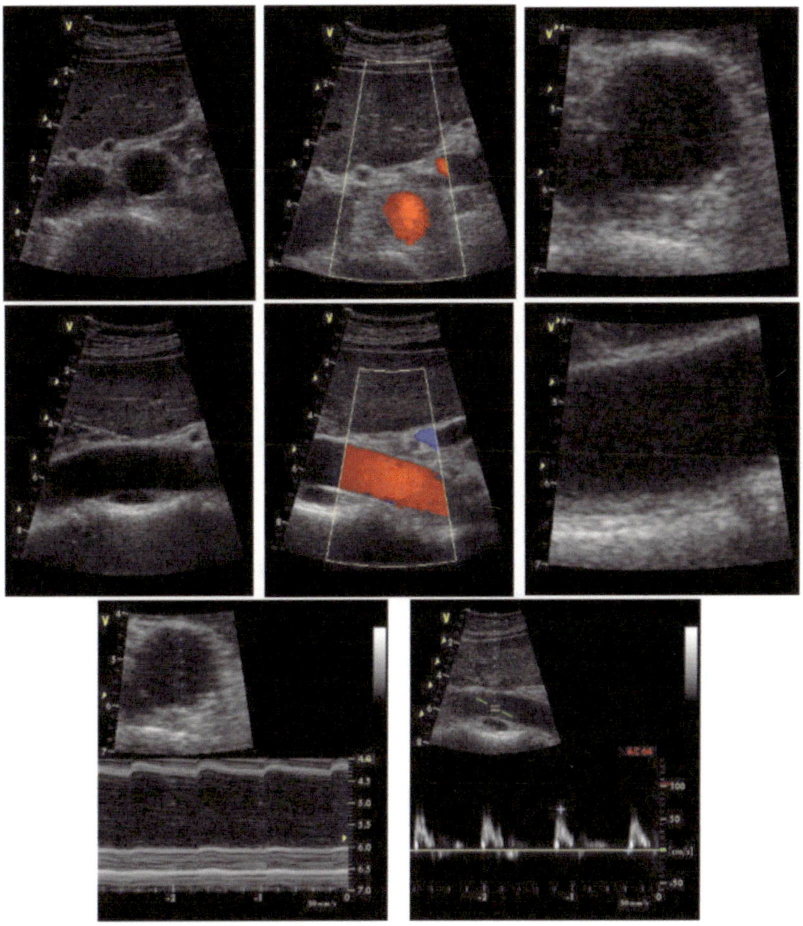

Fig. 1. Ultrasound images of abdominal aorta. Upper row: Cross-sectional view, 2D B-mode, colour Doppler (duplex) and zoomed B-mode image, respectively. Mid row: Same as upper row, but with longitudinal view. Lower row: M-mode (left) and Doppler velocity spectrum.

3. Ultrasound in AAA management

Use of ultrasound in the management of AAA was reported in the late 1960ies. Segal et al. (1966) published a case report of ultrasound for detection and size measurement of an AAA, and Goldberg et al. (1966) investigated 10 normal and 10 aneurysmal aortas. It was recognized that ultrasound could be used for detection of AAA, determination of size and monitoring of growth. During the following decade, several reports demonstrated favourable results for ultrasound in assessment of AAA, including analysis of pulsation, detection of aneurysms, measurement of diameter and amount of thrombus (Brewster et al., 1977; Hassani & Bard, 1974; Lee et al., 1975; McGregor et al., 1975; Mulder et al., 1973; Wheeler et al., 1976; Winsberg & Cole, 1972). Bernstein et al. (1976) used ultrasound for studying growth rates of small AAA. During the recent decades, ultrasound has been dramatically improved through development of new technology and processing methods assisting in improved patient management in several clinical areas. We present an overview of the current clinical use, and discuss potential future use related to ultrasound in detection and monitoring of AAA, prediction of growth and rupture, and treatment and follow-up.

3.1 Detection and monitoring

AAA is most often asymptomatic until rupture, and coincidentally detected during examination for other diseases. Ultrasound has been recommended for detection of AAA in symptomatic patients and for asymptomatic patients in risk groups. A number of studies suggest that population screening reduces AAA mortality in subgroups with increased AAA susceptibility (Cosford & Leng, 2007; Ferket et al., 2011; Takagi et al., 2010). Screening may still represent an ethical dilemma because growth and rupture is difficult to predict, and it is therefore disputable when to recommend repair on a patient-specific basis, considering the risk involved in surgical or endovascular treatment.

High degree of validity of ultrasound for detection of AAA has been reported. Numbers indicate a sensitivity and specificity of almost 100% (Cosford & Leng, 2007; Lindholt et al., 1999). The accuracy and operator dependencies of size measurements are especially important in order to reliably monitor growth. Fig. 2 shows cross-sectional and longitudinal images of AAA. Singh et al. (1998) reported intra- and inter-observer variability less than 4mm, and concluded that maximal diameter could be measured by ultrasound with high degree of accuracy. Also Thomas et al. (1994) concluded that ultrasound diameter measurements were reproducible between ultrasonographers. However, compared to measurements from X-ray computed tomography (CT), ultrasound was found to consistently give lower values for maximum AAA diameter, with a mean underestimation of 4.4mm. Similar results were reported using duplex ultrasound (Dalainas et al., 2006; Manning et al., 2009). Sprouse et al. (2004) suggested that ultrasound is more accurate than axial CT in determining the true perpendicular diameter. This was based on use of orthogonally reconstructed CT, which varied insignificantly from US, while axial CT overestimated the diameter when the aortic angulation was high. It has also been noted that the variation using internal or external wall diameter would give discrepancies of 5-6mm (Thapar et al., 2010). It is important that measurements be carried out consistently, and being aware of differences between imaging modalities compared to evidence from different clinical trials (Lederle et al., 1995). When care is taken to adjust the critical limits for intervention for a modality, reproducibility is the most important characteristic.

Detection of AAA in emergencies

Emergency ultrasound is becoming more widespread as the development in ultrasound technology provides more portable and even handheld ultrasound scanners at an affordable cost. Ultrasound can be used bedside or in the ambulance for fast examination and early decision making. This development has a potential for reducing AAA mortality by early detection of ruptured (or otherwise symptomatic) aneurysms, allowing early surgery without having to use time for additional examinations in the emergency entrance. Sebesta et al. (1998) investigated the importance of fast treatment of ruptured aneurysms by studying 103 patients with ruptured AAA. They concluded that "delay in surgical treatment caused both by time consuming confirmative evaluation and patient's lengthy transfers is responsible for ominous protraction of the original shock". Further, renal failure was found to be a leading cause of postoperative mortality. In combination with hemorrhagic shock, it should be considered that X-ray contrast material cause additional burden to renal function.

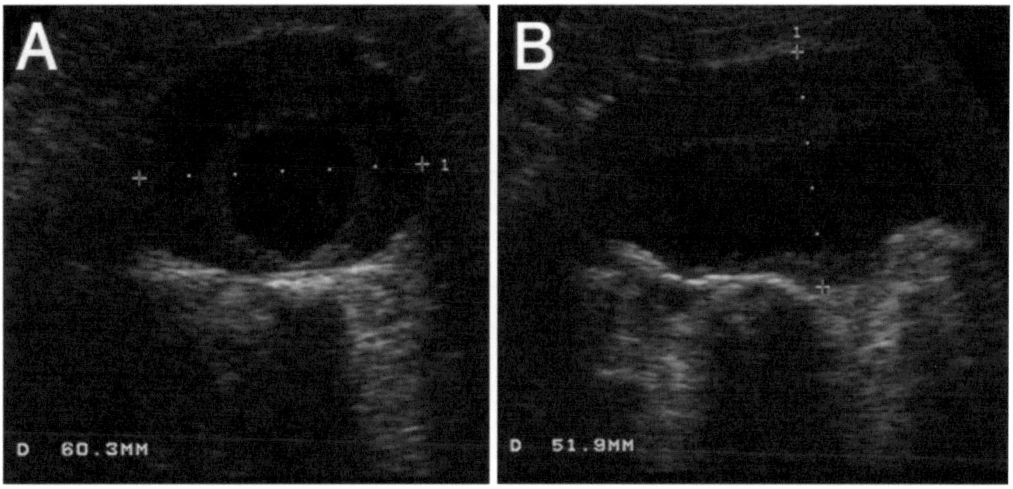

Fig. 2. Ultrasound images of AAA. Cross-sectional (A) and longitudinal (B) views. Courtesy of Asbjørn Ødegård, St. Olav's Hospital, Trondheim, Norway.

The sensitivity and specificity of detection of AAA in emergency medicine ultrasound is almost 100% (Kuhn et al., 2000). With appropriate training, emergency residents accurately determine both presence as well as size of AAA (Bentz & Jones, 2006; Costantino et al., 2005). Hoffmann et al. (2010) concluded that more experienced emergency department sonographers perform better in detecting aneurysms, and suggested training on more than 25 cases, including technically difficult cases, for credentialing personnel for the process. Although rupture of AAA could be indirectly diagnosed from clinical signs and symptoms and presence of an aneurysm, B-mode ultrasound can also reveal direct and indirect signs of rupture (Catalano & Siani, 2005a). Also, Catalano et al. (2005b) further examined 8 ruptured AAA using contrast-enhanced ultrasound, concluding that contrast-enhanced ultrasound may be as effective as CT in detecting rupture, and does not delay surgery significantly. Further considerations on AAA emergency ultrasound can be found in Reardon et al. (2008). The appearance of rupture in different modes of ultrasound images is shown in Fig. 3.

3.2 Prediction of growth and rupture

The validity of aneurysm size and growth as prognostic parameters has been questioned. Specifically, rupture does occur in aneurysm with diameter less than 5 to 5.5 cm, while on the other hand, several aneurysms with diameter larger than 5.5 cm are observed without rupture. Brewster et al. (2003) summarized findings from several studies, and estimated annual rupture risk versus size to be 0% (<4cm), 0.5-5% (4-5cm), 3-15% (5-6cm), 10-20% (6-7cm), 20-40% (7-8cm) and 30-50% (>8cm). Women appeared to have higher risk of rupture for a given diameter. These population-based values should be balanced against the expected risk associated with repair to determine appropriate time for intervention.

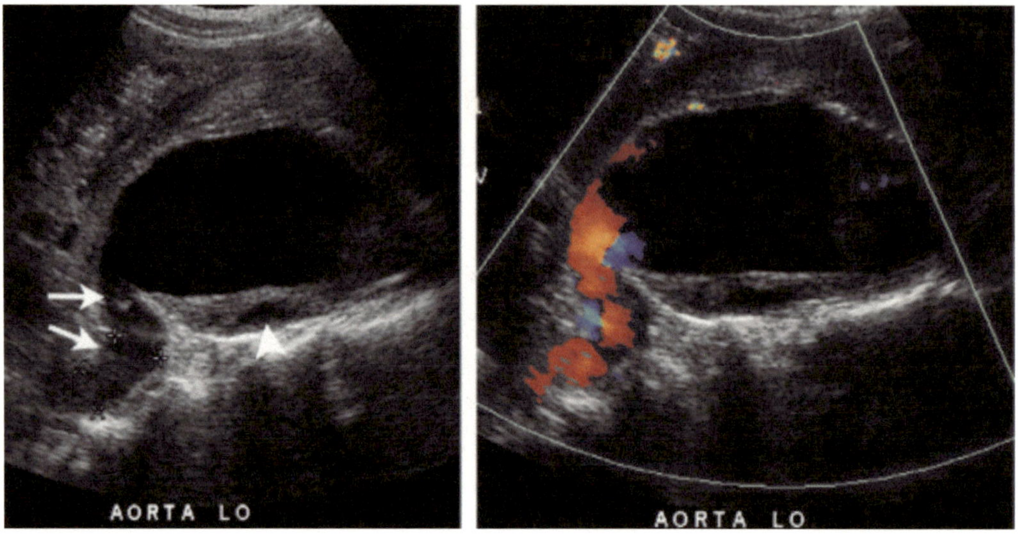

Fig. 3. Ultrasonic appearance of rupture. Left: Longitudinal B-mode image demonstrating a "tubular hypoechoic structure (arrows), which is continuous with the lumen of the aneurysm sac". The hypoechoic area in the thrombus (arrowhead) is a sign of aortic wall rupture. Right: Corresponding duplex image demonstrating an active bleeding. *In Bhatt et al. (2007), used with permission.*

Although diameter is currently the dominating population based indicator of rupture risk, additional indicators are warranted to predict rupture on an individual level. Improved patient specific assessment of rupture risk would provide better patient selection and reduce harm to patients as well as reducing societal cost. In a study by Hafez et al. (2008), 4308 patients were followed for research purpose after ultrasound screening showing a normal aorta. 3.9% (166/4308) were found to later develop AAA. Improved prediction of growth and rupture (prognostic monitoring) would 1) reduce the number of unnecessary examinations and interventions, and 2) make screening programs more favourable. Both would contribute to reduce AAA mortality.

Substantial efforts have been devoted to improved selection of patients for AAA repair through systematic assessment of risk factors of AAA growth and rupture, as well as individualized risk associated with repair. In this text, we will focus on image-based assessment of growth and rupture risk, specifically ultrasound imaging. Several groups have for more than a decade developed increasingly sophisticated numerical simulation tools for analysing the mechanical state of aneurysms, based on patient specific geometries. By applying solid-state stress analysis, Fillinger et al. (2003) found that peak wall stress was a better predictor of rupture than was maximum diameter. Further details on biomechanical analysis of AAA can be found in e.g. the reviews by Malkawi et al. (2010) and Vorp (2007).

Patient specific geometries applied for numerical analysis are most often based on CT, which is easily obtainable for AAA patients, and gives a good representation of the full 3D geometry of the aneurysm and blood vessels. Ultrasound imaging may be beneficial for early and consecutive measurements (i.e. screening/ detection and repeated monitoring). Real time 3D ultrasound imaging is used in cardiology, but gives a limited sector, and is not yet adapted to abdominal imaging. A possible alternative would be to obtain 3D volume by reconstruction of 2D ultrasound slices acquired with position tracking (Solberg et al., 2007).

An interesting application of ultrasound in analysis of AAA mechanics is due to the dynamical properties of ultrasound. Ultrasound is a fast imaging modality, which makes it possible to study the dynamical behaviour of the aneurysm when exposed to the blood pulse. Imura et al. (1986) presented a method using ultrasound for tracking the dynamic diameter of the abdominal aorta over the cardiac cycle in order to quantify the elastic properties of human abdominal aorta in vivo.

Analysis of the dynamical properties of the AAA may be motivated by the association between evolution of aneurysms and alteration of the elastic properties of the vessel wall. This alteration has been linked to matrix-metalloproteinase (MMP) activity (Freestone et al., 1995). It has been suggested that growth is associated with degradation of elastin, whereas rupture may be caused by degradation of collagen (Petersen et al., 2002). Consistent with this, it has been shown that aneurysm tissue is stiffer than normal tissue, but that softer aneurysm tissue is more prone to rupture than stiff aneurysm tissue (Di Martino et al., 2006). Several authors have used ultrasound to study the elastic properties of AAA by tracking dynamical change in diameter over the cardiac cycle, and obtained interesting, but to some extent diverging, results. Wilson et al. (1998) reported results that might support the hypothesis of aneurysms being stiffer than normal tissue, while less stiff aneurysms may be more prone to rupture. Later studies reported that large aneurysms tended to be stiffer than smaller, but with large variations for equally sized aneurysms (Wilson et al., 1999), and that increased distensibility over time (compared to baseline) indicated significantly reduced time to rupture (Wilson et al., 2003). However, Long et al. (2005) used tissue Doppler imaging, and reported a trend toward increased distensibility with increased AAA diameter. Ultrasonic tracking of diameter has demonstrated that the aorta is stiffer in men than age-matched women, that stiffness increases with age, and that aneurysm tissue is much stiffer than normal aorta (Länne et al., 1992; Sonesson et al., 1993). However, Sonesson et al. (1999) studied 285 AAA patients and found no difference in "aneurysmal aortic wall mechanics in those AAAs that subsequently ruptured compared with electively operated AAAs. The results indicate that it is not possible to use aneurysmal aortic wall stiffness as a predictor of rupture."

Measuring the dynamical change in diameter over the cardiac cycle gives a stiffness measure representing an average over the cross section of the aneurysm wall. The mechanical properties of the wall are however known to vary heterogeneously over the wall (Thubrikar et al., 2001). Ultrasound strain imaging estimates local deformation of tissue due to applied load, and may therefore have a potential for better assessment and characterization of the local properties of the wall. In a study by Brekken et al. (2006), 2D cross-sectional ultrasound data with high frame rate (~40-50 fps, depending on the size of the aneurysm) was used to derive patient-specific information about in-vivo elastic properties of the aneurysm wall of 10 patients. For each dataset, points were semi-automatically selected along the aneurysm circumference in one ultrasound image. These points were then automatically traced over the cardiac cycle. A measure of cyclic circumferential strain was estimated by calculating the time varying distance between the points relative to the initial (diastolic) distance. (Fig. 4.) The preliminary patient study showed that the strain values were inhomogeneous along the circumference, thus indicating that additional information could be obtained as compared to maximum diameter alone. Further clinical trials are necessary to investigate the method's potential for improved prediction of growth and rupture.

In addition to potentially carry clinically relevant information in itself, the strain estimates could be integrated with computational methods to contribute to more patient specific analysis of wall stress. In order to relate the strain estimates to the geometry of the aneurysm, and hence relate to biomechanical simulations based on 3D geometries, Brekken et al. (2007) reported attachment of a positioning sensor to the ultrasound probe for placing the ultrasound cross-section in a 3D space. The ultrasound data were then registered to CT data from the same patient, and strain was visualized together with the 3D geometry segmented from the CT data. (Fig. 5.) This allows for direct comparison of ultrasound based strain measurements with biomechanical simulations, and opens for more patient specific simulations by including elasticity measures from ultrasound.

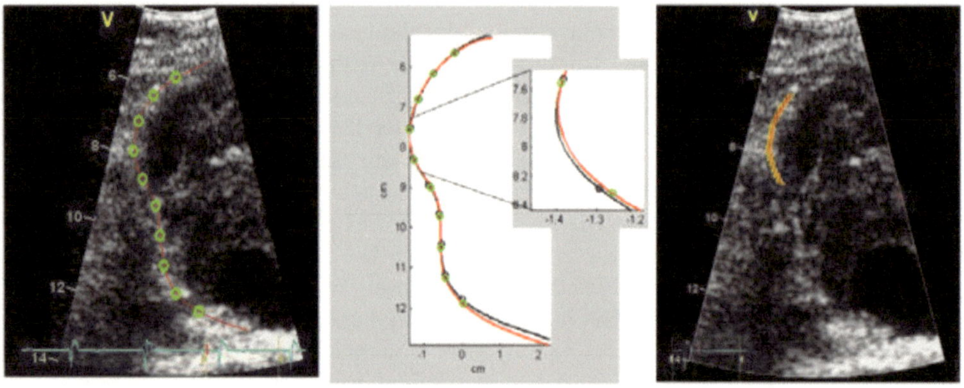

Fig. 4. Strain processing and ultrasound strain. Left: The aneurysm wall is manually identified (red line). A number of points (green) are placed equidistantly along the curve, and automatically traced over the cardiac cycle. Mid: Illustrating the points in diastole and systole. Right: Colour-coded strain in systole relative to diastole. It is noted that one part of the wall experiences elevated cyclic strain. *In Brekken et al. (2006), used with permission.*

Future research should be aimed at investigation also of longitudinal strain, and eventually estimation of full 3D strain, e.g. by developing probes and methods for 3D ultrasound acquisition and analysis. Also, low signal-to-noise ratio in abdominal ultrasound images reduces accuracy of tracking and thus strain estimation. Methods for noise reduction should therefore be explored. In addition, use of ultrasound Doppler for blood velocity estimation could provide further information to be used as input to patient specific simulations.

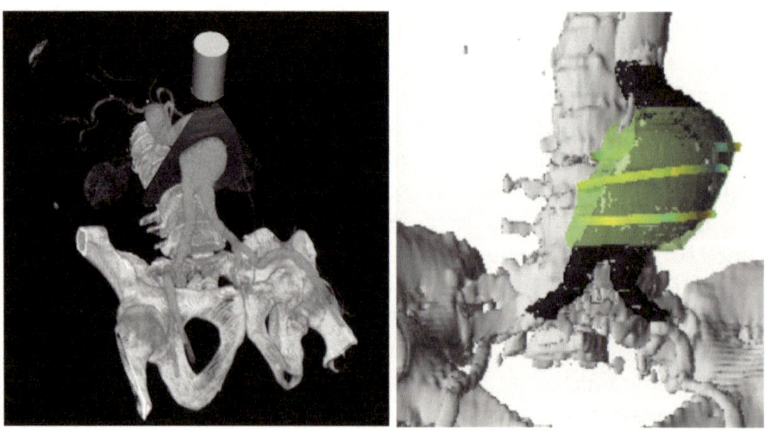

Fig. 5. Left: CT and ultrasound in the same scene. Right: 3D visualization of strain. *In Brekken et al. (2007), used with permission.*

3.3 Endovascular treatment and follow-up

Ultrasound in endovascular treatment

Radiological imaging is used in pre-operative planning of endovascular aneurysm repair (EVAR) and for intra-operative guidance and control. In pre-operative planning, imaging is used to get a measure of the 3D anatomy for investigating eligibility of EVAR and for choosing or customizing stentgrafts. A common imaging modality for this purpose is CT angiography (Broeders & Blankensteijn, 1999). CT has the advantage of visualizing the entire anatomical area of interest. Transabdominal 3D ultrasound offers only a limited sector, and, in addition, parts of the relevant anatomy will be obscured by acoustical shadows or absorption.

Some of these challenges are avoided in intravascular ultrasound (IVUS). IVUS has been used for pre-operative planning in combination with CT, for guidance and for control after device placement. (Fig. 6.) Several authors have concluded that IVUS gave accurate and reproducible measurements of the geometry of the aneurysm, and assisted in correct selection of stentgraft or final correction of stentgraft diameter or length. IVUS further assisted in rapid identification of fixation sites, and assessment of accuracy and patency of device placement (Eriksson et al., 2009; Garret et al., 2003; Tutein et al., 2000; van Essen et al., 1999; White et al., 1997; Zanchetta et al., 2003).

Ultrasound guidance during minimally invasive therapy has been reported and is in regular use within some clinical applications. Especially within neurosurgery ultrasound has been found beneficial for intra-operative imaging (Unsgaard et al., 2011). Intra-operative guidance during EVAR is usually performed with X-ray fluoroscopy. Both intraoperative CT (Dijkstra et al., 2011) as well as fluoroscopy in combination with navigation using electromagnetic sensors (Manstad-Hulaas et al., 2007) has been investigated for guiding insertion of fenestrated grafts. Some investigators have also reported transabdominal ultrasound for guidance of EVAR. Lie et al. (1997) studied the use of 2D transabdominal ultrasound during EVAR. They found that ultrasound could be useful for guiding the insertion of guidewire and control the wire position before connecting second graft limb to the main limb of bifurcated grafts (Fig. 6.). Kaspersen et al. (2003) reported a feasibility study registering ultrasound acquired during EVAR to pre-acquired CT data. This may be useful for updating the CT data used for navigation due to e.g. respiratory motion and deformation of the blood vessels during the procedure. With recent advances in ultrasound technology, we believe that real-time 3D ultrasound has potential for further advancing insertion of stentgraft, especially delivery of fenestrated stentgrafts. Specifically, it is easier to track e.g. the tip of guidewires in 3D, while simultaneously visualizing a focused area of the 3D anatomy in real-time, perhaps in combination with CT. Contrast-enhanced ultrasound has also been used intraoperatively for localization of fixation sites and identification of endoleaks (Kopp et al., 2010). The fixation sites were visualized in >80% of the 17 patients investigated with contrast-enhanced ultrasound, and more endoleaks were detected than with conventional EVAR. It was noted that ultrasound was especially beneficial in case of patients with contraindications for usage of X-ray contrast material.

Percutaneous EVAR, i.e. minimally invasive femoral access, is an alternative to open femoral access. A systematic review by Malkawi et al. (2010) concluded that percutaneous EVAR was associated with fewer access related complications and reduced operating time. In a study by Arthurs et al. (2008), it was shown that use of ultrasound guided access significantly reduced access-related complications compared to percutanous access without ultrasound guidance. Successful ultrasound guidance in secondary interventions, for sealing endoleak after EVAR, has also been reported. Boks et al. (2005) described transabdominal embolization using duplex ultrasound guidance, and Kasthuri et al. (2005) used ultrasound for guiding percutaneous thrombin injection.

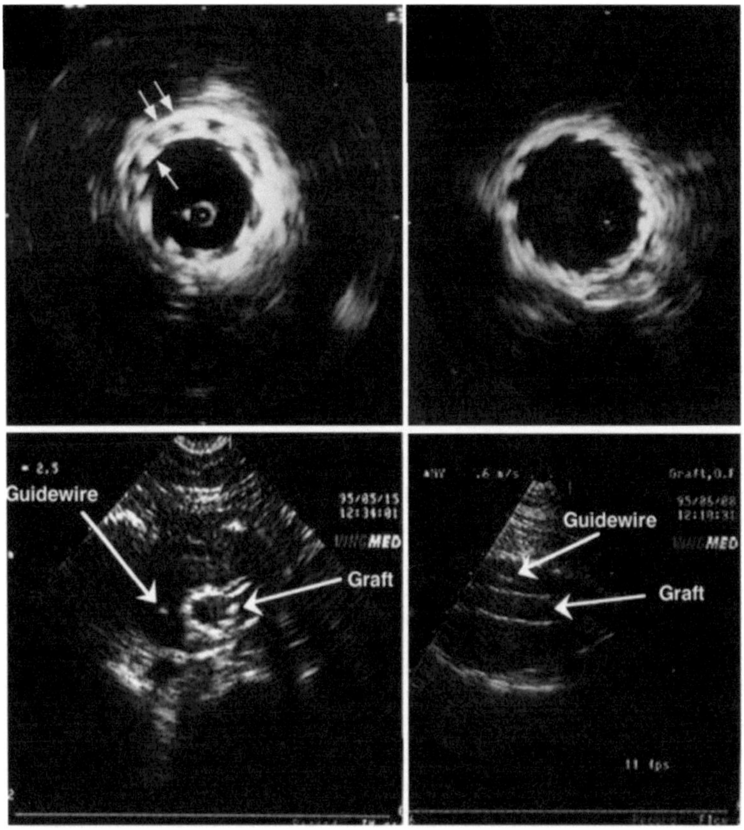

Fig. 6. Upper: IVUS during EVAR, left: incomplete stent expansion, right: stent correctly placed after additional dilation. *In White et al. (1995), used with permission.* Lower: Transabdominal ultrasound guidance during EVAR. Guidewire and stentgraft is visible inside the aneurysm. *In Lie et al. (1997), used with permission.*

Ultrasound in post-operative surveillance

Due to incidences of complications such as endoleak or continued growth after EVAR, it is necessary to conduct long-term follow-up. CT is in widespread use, but due to the repeated investigations, there is a significant radiation dose involved. Also, for some patients, the use of X-ray contrast material may cause allergic reactions or impair the renal function. Ultrasound has been suggested as an alternative that reduces these risks as well as the cost associated with follow-up of EVAR patients.

Several authors have investigated duplex ultrasound for detection of endoleak. In comparison with CT, duplex ultrasound is by some authors considered not to be sensitive or specific enough for replacing CT (Mirza et al., 2010; Sun, 2006). Other authors have found that duplex ultrasound may be sufficient in groups of patients, specifically those with a stable aneurysm (Bargellini et al., 2009; Chaer et al., 2009; Nagre et al., 2011). Patel & Carpenter (2010) suggested that duplex ultrasound could be sufficient for long-term follow-up if the initial postoperative CT angiogaphy was normal. Collins et al. (2007) also compared duplex ultrasound with CT, and found that three endoleaks determined from CT could not be seen with ultrasound due to bowel gas, body habitus or hernia, whereas out of 41 endoleaks discovered by ultrasound, only 14 were visible on a CT scan. A number of studies have reported use of contrast-enhanced ultrasound for detection of endoleaks. Generally, it is considered to be more accurate than ultrasound without contrast, and similar to magnetic resonance imaging (MR) and CT (Cantisani et al., 2011; Iezzi et al., 2009; Mirza et al., 2010; Sun 2006). McWilliams et al. (2002) investigated 53 patients and found contrast enhanced ultrasound to be more sensitive than unenhanced ultrasound in detection of endoleak when compared to CT, but concluded that ultrasound (with or without contrast) was less reliable than CT. On the contrary, several other authors have concluded that contrast enhanced ultrasound may perform better than CT in detection of endoleak (Carrafiello et al., 2006; Clevert et al., 2008; Henao et al., 2006; Ten Bosch et al., 2010). Bakken & Illig (2010) presented a review summarizing use of ultrasound for detection of endoleak. They concluded that ultrasound was suitable for "monitoring the evolution of aneurysm sac post-EVAR and, in combination with endoleak evaluation, seems to provide follow-up comparable to CT and sufficient to identify complications requiring intervention". In addition to capture the majority of endoleaks, the authors suggested that ultrasound could also provide better characterization and localization of the endoleak than with CT. The sensitivity of ultrasound for endoleak detection is likely to be underestimated by comparing it to CT as the reference standard because some endoleaks are missed also by CT. Therefore, the validity of ultrasound for endoleak detection should ideally be tested against clinically relevant outcome measures rather than to CT. Operator dependency of ultrasound may be an additional cause for diverging results. The introduction of 3D ultrasound could provide simpler protocols for detection of endoleak, and reduce user dependency. Fig. 7 shows examples of endoleak appearance in duplex and contrast-enhanced ultrasound.

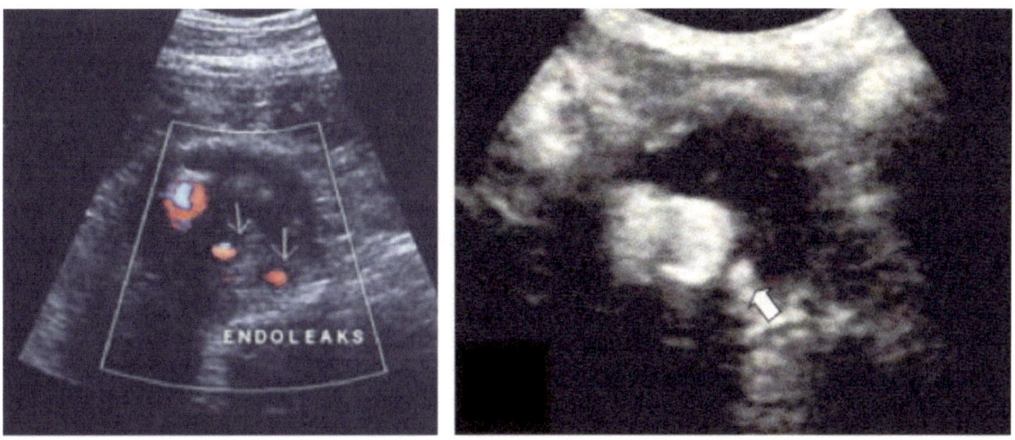

Fig. 7. Ultrasound for detection of endoleak. Left: Type II endoleaks with duplex ultrasound. *In Beeman et al. (2010), used with permission.* Right: Contrast-enhanced ultrasound illustrating flow inside the aneurysmal sac. *In Henao et al. (2006), used with permission.*

Another use of ultrasound in follow-up after EVAR is to study the pulsatile diameter. Malina et al. (1998) found that pulsatile wall motion was significantly reduced after EVAR as compared to before, and that endoleak was associated with smaller reduction. However, Lindblad et al. (2004) reported a similar study with more patients, and concluded that the reduction in pulsatile motion was not significantly different in the presence of endoleak. Using the ultrasound strain method previously described, Brekken et al. (2008) measured strain before and after insertion of stentgraft, confirming that the method detected a reduction in strain after endovascular repair. Pulsatility was observed after EVAR, and the strain values were heterogeneous along the circumference also after EVAR. It remains to investigate if the method is sensitive and accurate enough for detecting possible changes due to endoleak. Also, some aneurysms continue to grow without evidence of endoleak (Gilling-Smith et al., 2000). It is uncertain whether this is because of imaging modalities not being sensitive enough to detect all endoleaks, or other reasons. Therefore, in addition to monitor size, it is worth investigating if ultrasound strain could be used to predict growth or rupture, with or without endoleak, during follow-up after endovascular repair.

3.4 Functional and molecular imaging

The main pathophysiological mechanisms in development and progression of AAA are inflammation, proteolysis and apoptosis (Zankl et al., 2007). As these mechanisms and their role in AAA become more clear, new alternatives for detection, risk prediction and treatment may become available.

Compared to traditional imaging modalities, there is a need for alternative imaging to investigate pathophysiological mechanisms in-vivo, which could eventually identify high risk patients and monitor results of treatment. Hong et al. (2010) reviewed different modalities for imaging of AAA. They classified the modalities into anatomical, functional and molecular imaging. Anatomical imaging displays the structure of organs, whereas functional imaging can reveal physiological activities by detecting "changes in the metabolism, blood flow, regional chemical composition and absorption". Molecular imaging "introduces molecular agents (probes) to determine the expression of indicative molecular markers at different stages of disease." Functional and molecular imaging may be performed using SPECT, optical imaging and PET in combination with the appropriate contrast agents.

In addition to imaging functional properties using ultrasound Doppler or strain imaging, the use of ultrasound contrast agents constitutes a research area of great interest for imaging both functional and molecular properties. By injection of microbubbles in the blood stream, microcirculation has been imaged for investigation of myocardial perfusion and detection of neovascularization in relation to tumours and atherosclerosis (Fig. 8). (Anderson et al., 2011; Lindner et al., 2000 ; ten Kate et al., 2010). Staub et al. (2010a) demonstrated that adventitial vasa vasorum and plaque neovascularization of the carotid artery correlated with cardiovascular disease and past cardiovascular events using contrast-enhanced ultrasound in a retrospective study of 147 patients. Neovascularization or angiogenesis is also found in relation to AAA (Herron et al., 1991; Holmes et al., 1995; Thompson et al., 1996). Choke et al. (2006) found that rupture of AAA was associated with increased medial neovascularization. Assessment of neovascularization by contrast enhanced ultrasound may therefore have a significant potential for assisting in more accurate prediction of rupture.

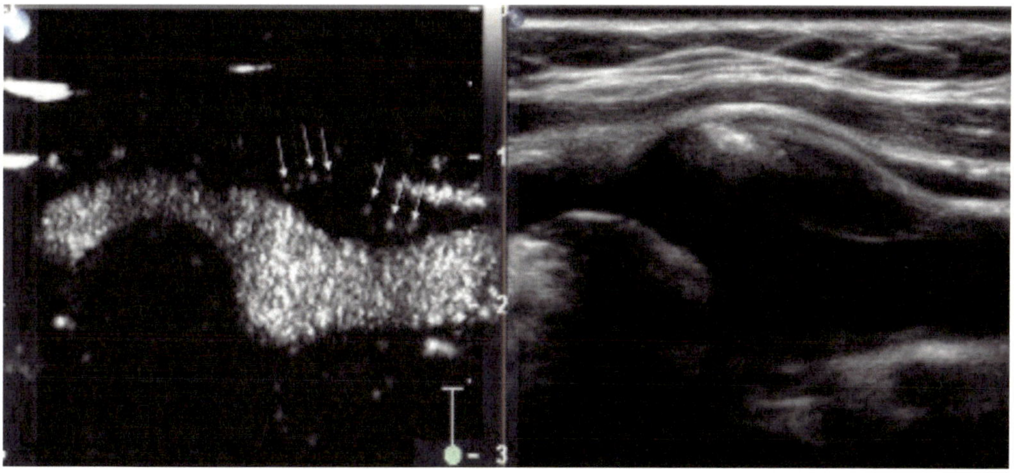

Fig. 8. Left: Contrast-enhanced ultrasound showing neovascularization in carotid artery plaque. Microbubbles within the plaque are indicated by arrows. Right: Corresponding B-mode ultrasound image without contrast. *In Staub et al. (2010b), used with permission.*

With recent advances in nanotechnology (nanomedicine), it is possible to produce targeted contrast agents, which connect to specific receptors. Due to current investigation of markers associated with AAA, targeted ultrasound imaging may be a future option (Moxon et al., 2010; Villanueva 2008). With increased knowledge of pathophysiological mechanisms, pharmacotherapy or gene therapy may be available for stabilization of aneurysms (Baxter et al., 2008; Cooper et al., 2009; Golledge et al., 2009; Raffetto & Khalil, 2008; Twine & Williams, 2011). It may then be interesting to apply drug- or gene-loaded contrast agents, which could be monitored and destructed using ultrasound for local drug delivery. Targeted drug delivery might benefit higher doses (locally) without increased risk of side effects.

4. Conclusions

The general aim of AAA research is to provide cost effective management for reducing mortality of AAA. Management includes screening/detection, monitoring, risk prediction, treatment and follow-up. We have described current and future potential of ultrasound for assisting in clinical management of AAA. Advantages of using ultrasound are that it is inexpensive, safe and portable, and allows for real-time dynamic imaging. New techniques, along with more widespread use of ultrasound, could contribute in several manners to improved AAA management.

Ultrasound is highly suitable for detection and monitoring of AAA size for screening and surveillance. In emergencies, ultrasound should be used for AAA detection and assessment of rupture as early as possible and preferably pre-hospital. Contrast enhanced ultrasound may be beneficial in detection of ruptured aneurysms. Early detection can provide early treatment and thereby reduce mortality of ruptured AAA. Ultrasound, and especially contrast enhanced ultrasound, is also a good alternative for detection of endoleak after EVAR. Ultrasound is cost-effective, does not include ionizing radiation or X-ray contrast material, and sensitivity may be better than CT. IVUS may be beneficial during EVAR for optimal measurement of stentgraft diameter, length and fixation site, as well as for post-operative control. Further research may find both IVUS and 3D transabdominal real-time

ultrasound guidance during EVAR to be useful in insertion of stentgrafts, especially fenestrated grafts. Ultrasound could also be used for guiding access to femoral artery in percutanuos EVAR.
A potential new application is to use ultrasound for analysing in-vivo mechanical properties of the aneurysm wall. This could provide additional parameters in predicting growth and rupture, or contribute to more patient-specific adaptation of numerical simulations both before and after EVAR. Improved prediction of growth and rupture would reduce the number of unnecessary examinations and interventions, reduce mortality and further benefit screening for detection of AAA. Another potential use of ultrasound in AAA management is in detection of neovascularization or other relevant markers by using general or targeted contrast agents. Contrast agents may also have a potential in treatment as drug carriers. Drug-loaded contrast agents can be monitored and destructed using ultrasound for local drug-delivery.
Obstacles for further use of ultrasound may be that ultrasound to some extent is operator dependent, and that abdominal ultrasound often is obscured from bowel gas, obesity and noise due to ultrasound propagation through the abdominal wall. Technology development will hopefully advance ultrasound image quality. An improvement was obtained with the introduction of tissue harmonic imaging (Caidahl et al., 1998). Several research groups are working on techniques for further improving quality of ultrasound images, such as suppression of reverberation and aberration correction. Due to operator dependencies, it might be necessary to investigate validity of ultrasound in the individual clinical surroundings before implementation in AAA management. Further, for ultrasound to become a widespread useful tool for AAA assessment, health personnel should be trained in focused assessment of presence and size of aneurysms, and detection of rupture and endoleak. Experts should be trained for more sophisticated examinations, such as analysis of wall mechanics and studies of microcirculation using contrast agents.

5. Acknowledgment

This work was funded by the Liaison Committee between the Central Norway Regional Health Authority and the Norwegian University of Science and Technology, SINTEF Department of Medical Technology and the National Centre for 3D Ultrasound in Surgery.

6. References

Anderson CR, Hu X, Zhang H, Tlaxca J, Declèves AE, Houghtaling R, Sharma K, Lawrence M, Ferrara KW, Rychak JJ. (2011). Ultrasound molecular imaging of tumor angiogenesis with an integrin targeted microbubble contrast agent. *Invest Radiol.* Vol.46, No.4, (April), pp. 215-224.

Arthurs ZM, Starnes BW, Sohn VY, Singh N, Andersen CA. (2008). Ultrasound-guided access improves rate of access-related complications for totally percutaneous aortic aneurysm repair. *Ann Vasc Surg.* Vol.22, No.6, (Nov), pp. 736-741.

Bakken AM, Illig KA. (2010). Long-term follow-up after endovascular aneurysm repair: is ultrasound alone enough? *Perspect Vasc Surg Endovasc Ther.* Vol.22, No.3, (Sep), pp. 145-151.

Bargellini I, Cioni R, Napoli V, Petruzzi P, Vignali C, Cicorelli A, Sardella S, Ferrari M, Bartolozzi C. (2009). Ultrasonographic surveillance with selective CTA after endovascular repair of abdominal aortic aneurysm. *J Endovasc Ther*. Vol.16, No.1, (Feb), pp. 93-104.

Baxter BT, Terrin MC, Dalman RL. (2008) Medical management of small abdominal aortic aneurysms. *Circulation*. Vol.117, No.14, (Apr), pp. 1883-1889.

Beeman BR, Murtha K, Doerr K, McAfee-Bennett S, Dougherty MJ, Calligaro KD. (2010). Duplex ultrasound factors predicting persistent type II endoleak and increasing AAA sac diameter after EVAR. *J Vasc Surg*.Vol.51, No.5, (Nov), pp. 1147-1152.

Bentz S, Jones J. (2006). Towards evidence-based emergency medicine: best BETs from the Manchester Royal Infirmary. Accuracy of emergency department ultrasound scanning in detecting abdominal aortic aneurysm. *Emerg Med J*. Vol.23, No.10, (Oct), pp. 803-804.

Bernstein EF, Dilley RB, Goldberger LE, Gosink BB, Leopold GR. (1976). Growth rates of small abdominal aortic aneurysms. *Surgery*. Vol.80, No.6, (Dec), pp. 765-773.

Bhatt S, Ghazale H and Dogra VS. (2007). Sonographic Evaluation of the Abdominal Aorta. *Ultrasound Clin*. Vol.2, No.3, (Jul), pp. 437-453.

Boks SS, Andhyiswara T, de Smet AA, Vroegindeweij D. (2005). Ultrasound-guided percutaneous transabdominal treatment of a type 2 endoleak. *Cardiovasc Intervent Radiol*. Vol.28, No.4, (Jul-Aug), pp. 526-529.

Brekken R, Bang J, Ødegård A, Aasland J, Hernes TA, Myhre HO. (2006). Strain estimation in abdominal aortic aneurysms from 2D Ultrasound. *Ultrasound Med Biol*. Vol.32, No.1, (Jan), pp. 33-42.

Brekken R, Dahl T, Hernes TAN, Myhre HO. (2008). Reduced strain in abdominal aortic aneurysms after endovascular repair. *J Endovasc Ther*. Vol. 15, No.4, (Aug), pp. 453-461.

Brekken R, Kaspersen JH, Tangen GA, Dahl T, Hernes TAN, Myhre HO. (2007). 3D visualization of strain in abdominal aortic aneurysms based on navigated ultrasound imaging. *Proceedings of SPIE Medical Imaging: Physiology, Function, and Structure from Medical Images*, 65111H, San Diego, CA, USA, February 18, 2007.

Brewster DC, Cronenwett JL, Hallett JW Jr, Johnston KW, Krupski WC & Matsumura JS. (2003). Guidelines for the treatment of abdominal aortic aneurysms. Report of a subcommittee of the Joint Council of the American Association for Vascular Surgery and Society for Vascular Surgery. *J Vasc Surg*. Vol.37, No.5 (May), pp. 1106-1117.

Brewster DC, Darling RC, Raines JK, Sarno R, O'Donnell TF, Ezpeleta M, Athanasoulis C. (1977). Assessment of abdominal aortic aneurysm size. *Circulation*. Vol.56, No.3S, (Sep), pp. II164-II169.

Broeders IA, Blankensteijn JD. (1999). Preoperative imaging of the aortoiliac anatomy in endovascular aneurysm surgery. *Semin Vasc Surg*. Vol.12, No.4, (Dec), pp. 306-314.

Burgess S, Zderic V, Vaezy S. (2007). Image-guided acoustic hemostasis for hemorrhage in the posterior liver. *Ultrasound Med Biol*. Vol.33, No.1, (Jan), pp. 113-119.

Caidahl K, Kazzam E, Lidberg J, Neumann Andersen G, Nordanstig J, Rantapää Dahlqvist S, Waldenström A, Wikh R. (1998). New concept in echocardiography: harmonic imaging of tissue without use of contrast agent. *Lancet*. Vol.352, No.9136, (Oct), pp. 1264-1270.

Cantisani V, Ricci P, Grazhdani H, Napoli A, Fanelli F, Catalano C, Galati G, D'Andrea V, Biancari F, Passariello R. (2011). Prospective Comparative Analysis of Colour-

Doppler Ultrasound, Contrast-enhanced Ultrasound, Computed Tomography and Magnetic Resonance in Detecting Endoleak after Endovascular Abdominal Aortic Aneurysm Repair. *Eur J Vasc Endovasc Surg*. Vol. 41, No.2, (Feb), pp. 186-192.

Carrafiello G, Laganà D, Recaldini C, Mangini M, Bertolotti E, Caronno R, Tozzi M, Piffaretti G, Genovese EA, Fugazzola C. (2006). Comparison of contrast-enhanced ultrasound and computed tomography in classifying endoleaks after endovascular treatment of abdominal aorta aneurysms: preliminary experience. *Cardiovasc Intervent Radiol*. Vol.29, No.6, (Nov-Dec), pp. 969-974.

Catalano O and Siani A. (2005a). Ruptured Abdominal Aortic Aneurysm: Categorization of Sonographic Findings and Report of 3 New Signs. *J Ultrasound Med*. Vol.24, No.8, (Aug), pp. 1077-1083.

Catalano O, Lobianco R, Cusati B, Siani A. (2005b). Contrast-Enhanced Sonography for Diagnosis of Ruptured Abdominal Aortic Aneurysm. *Am J Roentgenol*. Vol.184, No.2, (Feb), pp. 423-427.

Chaer RA, Gushchin A, Rhee R, Marone L, Cho JS, Leers S, Makaroun MS. (2009). Duplex ultrasound as the sole long-term surveillance method post-endovascular aneurysm repair: a safe alternative for stable aneurysms. *J Vasc Surg*. Vol.49, No.4, (Apr), pp. 845-849.

Chaikof EL, Brewster DC, Dalman RL, Makaroun MS, Illig KA, Sicard GA, Timaran CH, Upchurch GR Jr, Veith FJ. (2009). The care of patients with an abdominal aortic aneurysm: the Society for Vascular Surgery practice guidelines. *J Vasc Surg*. Vol.50, No.4S, (Oct), pp. S2-S49.

Choke E, Thompson MM, Dawson J, Wilson WR, Sayed S, Loftus IM, Cockerill GW. (2006). Abdominal aortic aneurysm rupture is associated with increased medial neovascularization and overexpression of proangiogenic cytokines. *Arterioscler Thromb Vasc Biol*. Vol.26, No.9, (Sep), pp. 2077-2082.

Clevert DA, Minaifar N, Weckbach S, Kopp R, Meimarakis G, Clevert DA, Reiser M. (2008). Color duplex ultrasound and contrast-enhanced ultrasound in comparison to MS-CT in the detection of endoleak following endovascular aneurysm repair. *Clin Hemorheol Microcirc*. Vol.39, No.1-4, pp. 121-132.

Collins JT, Boros MJ, Combs K. (2007). Ultrasound surveillance of endovascular aneurysm repair: a safe modality versus computed tomography. *Ann Vasc Surg*. Vol.21, No.6, (Nov), pp. 671-675.

Cooper DG, King JA, Earnshaw JJ. (2009). Role of medical intervention in slowing the growth of small abdominal aortic aneurysms. *Postgrad Med J*. Vol.85, No.1010, (Dec), pp. 688-692.

Cosford PA, Leng GC. (2007). Screening for abdominal aortic aneurysm. *Cochrane Database Syst Rev*. Vol.18, No.2, (Apr), CD002945.

Costantino TG, Bruno EC, Handly N, Dean AJ. (2005). Accuracy of emergency medicine ultrasound in the evaluation of abdominal aortic aneurysm. *J Emerg Med*. Vol.29, No.4, (Nov), pp. 455-460.

Dalainas I, G. Nano, P. Bianchi, R. Casana, T. Lupattelli and S. Stegher, Malacrida G, Tealdi DG. (2006). Axial computed tomography and duplex scanning for the determination of the maximal abdominal aortic diameter in patients with abdominal aortic aneurysms. *Eur Surg*. Vol. 38, No.4, pp. 312-314.

Di Martino ES, Bohra A, Vande Geest JP, Gupta N, Makaroun MS,Vorp DA. (2006). Biomechanical properties of ruptured versus electively repaired abdominal aortic aneurysm wall tissue. *J Vasc Surg*. Vol.43, No.3, (Mar), pp. 570-576.

Dijkstra ML, Eagleton MJ, Greenberg RK, Mastracci T, Hernandez A. (2011). Intraoperative C-arm cone-beam computed tomography in fenestrated/branched aortic endografting. *J Vasc Surg*. Vol.53, No.3, (Mar), pp. 583-590.

Eriksson MO, Wanhainen A, Nyman R. (2009). Intravascular ultrasound with a vector phased-array probe (AcuNav) is feasible in endovascular abdominal aortic aneurysm repair. *Acta Radiol*. Vol.50, No.8, (Oct), pp. 870-875.

Ferket BS, Grootenboer N, Colkesen EB, Visser JJ, van Sambeek MR, Spronk S, Steyerberg EW, Hunink MG. (2011). Systematic review of guidelines on abdominal aortic aneurysm screening. *J Vasc Surg*. Epub: Feb 14.

Fillinger MF, Marra SP, Raghavan ML, Kennedy FE. (2003). Prediction of rupture risk in abdominal aortic aneurysm during observation: wall stress versus diameter. *J Vasc Surg*. Vol.37, No.4, (Apr), pp. 724-732.

Freestone T, Turner RJ, Coady A, Higman DJ, Greenhalgh RM, Powell JT. (1995). Inflammation and matrix metalloproteinases in the enlarging abdominal aortic aneurysm. *Arterioscler Thromb Vasc Biol*. Vol.15, No.8, (Aug), pp. 1145-1151.

Frinking PJ, Bouakaz A, Kirkhorn J, Ten Cate FJ, de Jong N. (2000). Ultrasound contrast imaging: current and new potential methods. *Ultrasound Med Biol*. Vol.26, No.6, (Jul), pp. 965-975.

Gallucci M, Vincenzoni A, Schettini M, Fortunato P, Cassanelli A, Zaccara A. (2001). Extracorporeal shock wave lithotripsy in ureteral and kidney malformations. *Urol Int*. Vol.66, No.2, pp. 61-65.

Garra BS. (2007). Imaging and estimation of tissue elasticity by ultrasound. *Ultrasound Q*. Vol.23, No.4, (Dec), pp. 255-268.

Garret HE Jr, Abdullah AH, Hodgkiss TD, Burgar SR. (2003). Intravascular ultrasound aids in the performance of endovascular repair of abdominal aortic aneurysm. *J Vasc Surg*. Vol.37, No.3, (Mar), pp. 615-618.

Gilling-Smith GL, Martin J, Sudhindran S, Gould DA, McWilliams RG, Bakran A, Brennan JA, Harris PL. (2000). Freedom from endoleak after endovascular aneurysm repair does not equal treatment success. *Eur J Vasc Endovasc Surg*. Vol.19, No.4, (Apr), pp. 421-425.

Goldberg BB, Ostrum BJ, Isard HJ. (1966). Ultrasonic aortography. *JAMA*. Vol.198, No.4, (Oct), pp. 353-358.

Golledge J, Dalman RL, Norman PE. (2009). Developments in non-surgical therapies for abdominal aortic aneurysm. *Curr Vasc Pharmacol*. Vol.7, No.2, (Apr), pp. 153-158.

Hafez H, Druce PS, Ashton HA. (2008). Abdominal aortic aneurysm development in men following a "normal" aortic ultrasound scan. *Eur J Vasc Endovasc Surg*. Vol.36, No.5, (Nov), pp. 553-558.

Hansen R, Angelsen BA. SURF imaging for contrast agent detection. (2009). *IEEE Trans Ultrason Ferroelectr Freq Control*. Vol.56, No.2, (Feb), pp. 280-290.

Hassani S, Bard R. (1974). Ultrasonic diagnosis of abdominal aortic aneurysms. *J Natl Med Assoc*. Vol.66, No.4, (Jul), pp. 298-299.

Henao EA, Hodge MD, Felkai DD, McCollum CH, Noon GP, Lin PH, Lumsden AB, Bush RL. (2006). Contrast-enhanced Duplex surveillance after endovascular abdominal aortic aneurysm repair: improved efficacy using a continuous infusion technique. *J Vasc Surg*. Vol.43, No.2, (Feb), pp. 259-264.

Herron GS, Unemori E, Wong M, Rapp JH, Hibbs MH, Stoney RJ. (1991). Connective tissue proteinases and inhibitors in abdominal aortic aneurysms. Involvement of the vasa vasorum in the pathogenesis of aortic aneurysms. *Arterioscler Thromb*. Vol.11, No.6, (Nov-Dec), pp. 1667-1677.

Hoffmann B, Bessman ES, Um P, Ding R, McCarthy ML. (2010). Successful sonographic visualisation of the abdominal aorta differs significantly among a diverse group of credentialed emergency department providers. *Emerg Med J*. Epub: Aug 2.

Holmes DR, Liao S, Parks WC, Thompson RW. (1995). Medial neovascularization in abdominal aortic aneurysms: a histopathologic marker of aneurysmal degeneration with pathophysiologic implications. *J Vasc Surg*. Vol.21, No.5, (May), pp. 761-771.

Hong H, Yang Y, Liu B, Cai W. (2010). Imaging of Abdominal Aortic Aneurysm: the present and the future. *Curr Vasc Pharmacol*. Vol.8, No.6, (Nov), pp. 808-819.

Iezzi R, Basilico R, Giancristofaro D, Pascali D, Cotroneo AR, Storto ML. (2009). Contrast-enhanced ultrasound versus color duplex ultrasound imaging in the follow-up of patients after endovascular abdominal aortic aneurysm repair. *J Vasc Surg*. Vol.49, No.3, (Mar), pp. 552-560.

Imura T, Yamamoto K, Kanamori K, Mikami T, Yasuda H. (1986). Non-invasive ultrasonic measurement of the elastic properties of the human abdominal aorta. *Cardiovasc Res*. Vol.20, No.3, (Mar), pp. 208-214.

Kaspersen JH, Sjølie E, Wesche J, Asland J, Lundbom J, Odegård A, Lindseth F, Nagelhus Hernes TA. (2003). Three-dimensional ultrasound-based navigation combined with preoperative CT during abdominal interventions: a feasibility study. *Cardiovasc Intervent Radiol*. Vol.26, No.4, (Jul-Aug), pp. 347-356.

Kasthuri RS, Stivaros SM, Gavan D. (2005). Percutaneous ultrasound-guided thrombin injection for endoleaks: an alternative. *Cardiovasc Intervent Radiol*. Vol.28, No.1, (Jan-Feb), pp. 110-112.

Kim YS, Rhim H, Choi MJ, Lim HK, Choi D. (2008). High-intensity focused ultrasound therapy: an overview for radiologists. *Korean J Radiol*. Vol.9, No.4, (Aug), pp. 291-302.

Kopp R, Zürn W, Weidenhagen R, Meimarakis G, Clevert DA. (2010). First experience using intraoperative contrast-enhanced ultrasound during endovascular aneurysm repair for infrarenal aortic aneurysms. *J Vasc Surg*. Vol.51, No.5, (May), pp. 1103-1110.

Kuhn M, Bonnin RLL, Davey MJ, Rowland JL, Langlois S. (2000). Emergency Department Ultrasound Scanning for Abdominal Aortic Aneurysm: Accessible, Accurate, and Advantageous. *Ann Emerg Med* Vol.36, No.3, (Sep), pp. 219-223.

Länne T, Sonesson B, Bergqvist D, Bengtsson H, Gustafsson D. (1992). Diameter and compliance in the male human abdominal aorta: influence of age and aortic aneurysm. *Eur J Vasc Surg*. Vol.6, No.2, (Mar), pp. 178-184.

Lederle FA, Wilson SE, Johnson GR, Reinke DB, Littooy FN, Acher CW, Messina LM, Ballard DJ, Ansel HJ. (1995).Variability in measurement of abdominal aortic aneurysms. Abdominal Aortic Aneurysm Detection and Management Veterans Administration Cooperative Study Group. *J Vasc Surg*. Vol.21, No.6, (Jun), pp. 945-952.

Lee KR, Walls WJ, Martin NL, Templeton AW. (1975). A practical approach to the diagnosis of abdominal aortic aneurysms. *Surgery*. Vol.78, No.2, (Aug), pp. 195-201.
Lie T, Lundbom J, Hatlinghus S, Grønningsaeter A, Ommedal S, Aadahl P, Saether OD, Myhre HO. (1997). Ultrasound imaging during endovascular abdominal aortic aneurysm repair using the Stentor bifurcated endograft. *J Endovasc Surg*. Vol.4, No.3, (Aug), pp. 272-278.
Lindblad B, Dias N, Malina M, Ivancev K, Resch T, Hansen F, Sonesson B. (2004). Pulsatile wall motion (PWM) measurements after endovascular abdominal aortic aneurysm exclusion are not useful in the classification of endoleak. *Eur J Vasc Endovasc Surg*. Vol.28, No.6, (Dec), pp. 623-628.
Lindholt JS, Vammen S, Juul S, Henneberg EW, Fasting H. (1999). The validity of ultrasonographic scanning as screening method for abdominal aortic aneurysm. *Eur J Vasc Endovasc Surg*. Vol.17, No.6, (Jun), pp. 472-475.
Lindner JR, Villanueva FS, Dent JM, Wei K, Sklenar J, Kaul S. (2000). Assessment of resting perfusion with myocardial contrast echocardiography: theoretical and practical considerations. *Am Heart J*. Vol.139, No.2pt1, (Feb), pp. 231-240.
Long A, Rouet L, Bissery A, Rossignol P, Mouradian D, Sapoval M. (2005). Compliance of abdominal aortic aneurysms evaluated by tissue Doppler imaging: correlation with aneurysm size. *J Vasc Surg*. Vol.42, No.1, (Jul), pp. 18-26.
Malina M, Länne T, Ivancev K, Lindblad B, Brunkwall J. (1998). Reduced pulsatile wall motion of abdominal aortic aneurysms after endovascular repair. *J Vasc Surg*. Vol.27, No.4, (Apr), pp. 624-631.
Malkawi AH, Hinchliffe RJ, Holt PJ, Loftus IM, Thompson MM. (2010). Percutaneous access for endovascular aneurysm repair: a systematic review. *Eur J Vasc Endovasc Surg*. Vol.39, No.6, (Jun), pp. 676-682.
Malkawi AH, Hinchliffe RJ, Xu Y, Holt PJ, Loftus IM, Thompson MM. (2010). Patient-specific biomechanical profiling in abdominal aortic aneurysm development and rupture. *J Vasc Surg*. Vol.52, No.2, (Aug), pp. 489-488.
Manning BJ, Kristmundsson T, Sonesson B, Resch T. (2009). Abdominal aortic aneurysm diameter: a comparison of ultrasound measurements with those from standard and three-dimensional computed tomography reconstruction. *J Vasc Surg*. Vol.50, No.2, (Aug), pp. 263-268.
Manstad-Hulaas F, Ommedal S, Tangen GA, Aadahl P, Hernes TN. (2007). Side-branched AAA stent graft insertion using navigation technology: a phantom study. *Eur Surg Res*. Vol.39, No.6, (), pp. 364-371.
McGregor JC, Pollock JG, Anton HC. (1975). The value of ultrasonography in the diagnosis of abdominal aortic aneurysm. *Scott Med J*. Vol.20, No.3, (May), pp. 133-137.
McWilliams RG, Martin J, White D, Gould DA, Rowlands PC, Haycox A, Brennan J, Gilling-Smith GL, Harris PL. (2002). Detection of endoleak with enhanced ultrasound imaging: comparison with biphasic computed tomography. *J Endovasc Ther.*.9, No.2, (Apr), pp. 170-179.
Mirza TA, Karthikesalingam A, Jackson D, Walsh SR, Holt PJ, Hayes PD, Boyle JR. (2010). Duplex ultrasound and contrast-enhanced ultrasound versus computed tomography for the detection of endoleak after EVAR: systematic review and bivariate meta-analysis. *Eur J Vasc Endovasc Surg*. Vol.39, No.4, (Apr), pp. 418-428.

Moll FL, Powell JT, Fraedrich G, Verzini F, Haulon S, Waltham M, van Herwaarden JA, Holt PJ, van Keulen JW, Rantner B, Schlösser FJ, Setacci F, Ricco JB. (2011). Management of abdominal aortic aneurysms clinical practice guidelines of the European society for vascular surgery. *Eur J Vasc Endovasc Surg*. Vol.41, No.S1, (Jan), pp. S1-S58.

Moxon JV, Parr A, Emeto TI, Walker P, Norman PE, Golledge J (2010). Diagnosis and Monitoring of Abdominal Aortic Aneurysm: Current Status and Future Prospects. *Curr Probl Cardiol*. Vol.35, No.10, (Oct), pp. 512-548.

Mulder DS, Winsberg F, Cole CM, Blundell PE, Scott HJ. (1973). Ultrasonic "B" scanning of abdominal aneurysms. *Ann Thorac Surg*. Vol.16, No.4, (Oct), pp. 361-367.

Nagre SB, Taylor SM, Passman MA, Patterson MA, Combs BR, Lowman BG, Jordan WD Jr. (2011). Evaluating outcomes of endoleak discrepancies between computed tomography scan and ultrasound imaging after endovascular abdominal aneurysm repair. *Ann Vasc Surg*. Vol.25, No.1, (Jan), pp. 94-100.

Nightingale K, Soo MS, Nightingale R, Trahey G. (2002). Acoustic radiation force impulse imaging: in vivo demonstration of clinical feasibility. *Ultrasound Med Biol*. Vol.28, No.2, (Feb), pp. 227-235.

Ophir J, Céspedes I, Ponnekanti H, Yazdi Y, Li X. (1991). Elastography: a quantitative method for imaging the elasticity of biological tissues. *Ultrason Imaging*. Vol.13, No.2, (Apr), pp. 111-134.

Patel MS, Carpenter JP. (2010). The value of the initial post-EVAR computed tomography angiography scan in predicting future secondary procedures using the Powerlink stent graft. *J Vasc Surg*. Vol.52, No.5, (Nov), pp. 1135-1139.

Petersen E, Wagberg F, Angquist KA. (2002). Proteolysis of the abdominal aortic aneurysm wall and the association with rupture. *Eur J Vasc Endovasc Surg*. Vol.23, No.2, (Feb), pp. 153-157.

Raffetto JD, Khalil RA. (2008). Matrix metalloproteinases and their inhibitors in vascular remodeling and vascular disease. *Biochem Pharmacol*. Vol.75, No.2, (Jan), pp. 346-359.

Reardon, RF; Cook, T; Plummer, D (2008). Abdominal aortic aneurysm, In *Emergency Ultrasound 2nd Edition*, O.J. Ma; J.R. Mateer; M. Blaivas (Eds), 149-167. The McGraw-Hill Companies, Inc. ISBN 978-0-07-147904-2. China.

Sebesta P, Klika T, Zdrahal P, Kramar J. (1998). Ruptured abdominal aortic aneurysm: role of initial delay on survival. *J Mal Vasc*. Vol.23, No.5, (Dec), pp. 361-367.

Segal BL, Likoff W, Asperger Z, Kingsley B. (1966). Ultrasound diagnosis of an abdominal aortic aneurysm. *Am J Cardiol*. Vol.17, No.1, (Jan), pp. 101-103.

Singh K, Bønaa KH, Solberg S, Sørlie DG, Bjørk L. (1998). Intra- and interobserver variability in ultrasound measurements of abdominal aortic diameter. The Tromsø Study. *Eur J Vasc Endovasc Surg*. Vol.15, No.6, (Jun), pp.497-504.

Solberg OV, Lindseth F, Torp H, Blake RE, Nagelhus Hernes TA. (2007). Freehand 3D ultrasound reconstruction algorithms--a review. *Ultrasound Med Biol*. Vol.33, No.7, (Jul), pp. 991-1009.

Sonesson B, Hansen F, Stale H, Länne T. (1993). Compliance and diameter in the human abdominal aorta--the influence of age and sex. *Eur J Vasc Surg*. Vol.7, No.6, (Nov), pp. 690-697.

Sonesson B, Sandgren T, Länne T. (1999). Abdominal aortic aneurysm wall mechanics and their relation to risk of rupture. *Eur J Vasc Endovasc Surg*. Vol.18, No.6, (Dec), pp. 487-493.

Sprouse L.R., G.H. Meier, F.N. Parent, R.J. DeMasi, M.H. Glickman and G.A. Barber. (2004). Is ultrasound more accurate than axial computed tomography for determination of maximal abdominal aortic aneurysm diameter? *Eur J Vasc Endovasc Surg*. Vol.28, No.1, (Jul), pp. 28-35.

Staub D, Patel MB, Tibrewala A, Ludden D, Johnson M, Espinosa P, Coll B, Jaeger KA, Feinstein SB. (2010a). Vasa vasorum and plaque neovascularization on contrast-enhanced carotid ultrasound imaging correlates with cardiovascular disease and past cardiovascular events. *Stroke*. Vol.41, No.1, (Jan), pp. 41-7.

Staub D, Schinkel AF, Coll B, Coli S, van der Steen AF, Reed JD, Krueger C, Thomenius KE, Adam D, Sijbrands EJ, ten Cate FJ, Feinstein SB. (2010b). Contrast-enhanced ultrasound imaging of the vasa vasorum: from early atherosclerosis to the identification of unstable plaques. *JACC Cardiovasc Imaging*. Vol.3, No.7, (Jul), pp. 761-771.

Sun Z. (2006). Diagnostic value of color duplex ultrasonography in the follow-up of endovascular repair of abdominal aortic aneurysm. *J Vasc Interv Radiol*. Vol.17, No.5, (May), pp. 759-764.

Takagi H, Goto SN, Matsui M, Manabe H, Umemoto T. (2010). A further meta-analysis of population-based screening for abdominal aortic aneurysm. *J Vasc Surg*. Vol.52, No.4, (Oct), pp. 1103-1108.

Ten Bosch JA, Rouwet EV, Peters CT, Jansen L, Verhagen HJ, Prins MH, Teijink JA. (2010). Contrast-enhanced ultrasound versus computed tomographic angiography for surveillance of endovascular abdominal aortic aneurysm repair. *J Vasc Interv Radiol*. Vol.21, No.5, (May), pp. 638-643.

ten Kate GL, Sijbrands EJ, Valkema R, ten Cate FJ, Feinstein SB, van der Steen AF, Daemen MJ, Schinkel AF. (2010). Molecular imaging of inflammation and intraplaque vasa vasorum: a step forward to identification of vulnerable plaques? *J Nucl Cardiol*. Vol.17, No.5, (), pp. 897-912.

Thapar A, Cheal D, Hopkins T, Ward S, Shalhoub J, Yusuf SW. (2010). Internal or external wall diameter for abdominal aortic aneurysm screening? *Ann R Coll Surg Engl*. Vol.92, No.6, (Sep), pp. 503-505.

Thomas PR, Shaw JC, Ashton HA, Kay DN, Scott RA. (1994). Accuracy of ultrasound in a screening programme for abdominal aortic aneurysms. *J Med Screen*. Vol.1, No.1, (Jan), pp. 3-6.

Thompson MM, Jones L, Nasim A, Sayers RD, Bell PR. (1996). Angiogenesis in abdominal aortic aneurysms. *Eur J Vasc Endovasc Surg*. Vol.11, No.4, (May), pp. 464-469.

Thubrikar MJ, Labrosse M, Robicsek F, Al-Soudi J, Fowler B. (2001). Mechanical properties of abdominal aortic aneurysm wall. *J Med Eng Technol*. Vol.25, No. 4, (Jul-Aug), pp. 133-142.

Tutein Nolthenius RP, van den Berg JC, Moll FL. (2000). The value of intraoperative intravascular ultrasound for determining stent graft size (excluding abdominal aortic aneurysm) with a modular system. *Ann Vasc Surg*. Vol.14, No.4, (Jul), pp. 311-317.

Twine CP, Williams IM. (2011). Systematic review and meta-analysis of the effects of statin therapy on abdominal aortic aneurysms. *Br J Surg*. Vol.98, No.3, (Mar), pp. 346-353.

Unsgård G, Solheim O, Lindseth F, Selbekk T. (2011). Intra-operative imaging with 3D ultrasound in neurosurgery. *Acta Neurochir Suppl*. Vol.109, pp. 181-186.

Vaezy S, Martin R, Crum L. (2001). High intensity focused ultrasound: a method of hemostasis. *Echocardiography*. Vol.18, No.4, (May), pp. 309-315.

van Essen JA, Gussenhoven EJ, van der Lugt A, Huijsman PC, van Muiswinkel JM, van Sambeek MR, van Dijk LC, van Urk H. (1999). Accurate assessment of abdominal aortic aneurysm with intravascular ultrasound scanning: validation with computed tomographic angiography. *J Vasc Surg*. Vol.29, No.4, (Apr), pp. 631-638.

Villanueva FS. (2008). Molecular imaging of cardiovascular disease using ultrasound. *J Nucl Cardiol*. Vol. 15, No.4, (Jul-Aug;). pp. 576-586.

Vorp DA. (2007). Biomechanics of abdominal aortic aneurysm. *J Biomech*. Vol.40, No.9, (), pp. 1887-1902.

Wheeler WE, Beachley MC, Ranniger K. (1976). Angiography and ultrasonography. A comparative study of abdominal aortic aneurysms. *Am J Roentgenol*. Vol.126, No.1, (Jan), pp. 95-100.

White RA, Donayre C, Kopchok G, Walot I, Wilson E, de Virgilio C. (1997). Intravascular ultrasound: the ultimate tool for abdominal aortic aneurysm assessment and endovascular graft delivery. *J Endovasc Surg*. Vol.4, No.1, (Feb), pp. 45-55.

White RA, Verbin C, Kopchok G, Scoccianti M, de Virgilio C, Donayre C. (1995). The role of cinefluoroscopy and intravascular ultrasonography in evaluating the deployment of experimental endovascular prostheses. *J Vasc Surg*. Vol.21, No.3, (Mar), pp. 365-74.

Wilson K, Bradbury A, Whyman M, Hoskins P, Lee A, Fowkes G, McCollum P, Ruckley CV. (1998). Relationship between abdominal aortic aneurysm wall compliance and clinical outcome: a preliminary analysis. *Eur J Vasc Endovasc Surg*. Vol.15, No.6, (Jun), pp. 472-477.

Wilson K, Whyman M, Hoskins P, Lee AJ, Bradbury AW, Fowkes FG, Ruckley CV. (1999). The relationship between abdominal aortic aneurysm wall compliance, maximum diameter and growth rate. *Cardiovasc Surg*. Vol.7, No.2, (Mar), pp. 208-213.

Wilson KA, Lee AJ, Lee AJ, Hoskins PR, Fowkes FG, Ruckley CV, Bradbury AW. (2003). The relationship between aortic wall distensibility and rupture of infrarenal abdominal aortic aneurysm. *J Vasc Surg*. Vol.37, No.1, (Jan), pp. 112-117.

Winsberg F, Cole CM. (1972). "Continuous ultrasound visualization of the pulsating abdominal aorta. *Radiology*. Vol.103, No.2, (May), pp. 455-457.

Zanchetta M, Rigatelli G, Pedon L, Zennaro M, Ronsivalle S, Maiolino P. (2003). IVUS guidance of thoracic and complex abdominal aortic aneurysm stent-graft repairs using an intracardiac echocardiography probe: preliminary report. *J Endovasc Ther*. Vol.10, No.2, (Apr), pp. 218-226.

Zankl AR, Schumacher H, Krumsdorf U, Katus HA, Jahn L, Tiefenbacher CP. (2007). Pathology, natural history and treatment of abdominal aortic aneurysms. *Clin Res Cardiol*. Vol.96, No.3, (Mar), pp-140-151.

7

Motion Calculations on Stent Grafts in AAA

Almar Klein[1], W. Klaas Jan Renema[2], J. Adam van der Vliet[3],
Luuk J. Oostveen[2], Yvonne Hoogeveen[2],
Leo J. Schultze Kool[2] and Cornelis H. Slump[1]
[1]*Institute of Technical Medicine, University of Twente.*
[2]*Dept. of Radiology, Radboud University Nijmegen Medical Center.*
[3]*Dept. of Surgery, Radboud University Nijmegen Medical Center.*
The Netherlands

1. Introduction

Although endovascular aortic replacement (EVAR) has been proven to be successful (Blankensteijn et al., 2005; Zarins et al., 1999), due to the need for reintervention it does not have a significant advantage over open repair on the long term (Bruin et al., 2010; Investigators, 2010). Late stent graft failure is therefore a serious complication in endovascular repair of aortic aneurysms (Cao et al., 2009; Demirci et al., 2009; Jacobs et al., 2003; Li & Kleinstreuer, 2006; Mattes et al., 2005; Roos et al., 2005). Examples are metal fatigue, stent graft migration (Koning et al., 2006; Li & Kleinstreuer, 2006), and the formation of endoleaks (Lu et al., 2008; Stavropoulos & Charagundla, 2007).

The long-term durability of stent grafts is affected by the stresses and hemodynamic forces applied to them, which may be reflected by the movements of the stent graft itself during the cardiac cycle. Studying the dynamic behavior of stent grafts can therefore give a better understanding of their motion characteristics, and can give insights into how these motion characteristics relate to certain stent-related problems. This information will be beneficial for designing future devices and can be valuable in predicting stent graft failure in individual patients (Langs et al., 2007).

Motions of (stent grafts in) AAA can be measured using fluoroscopic roentgenographic stereophotogrammetric analysis (FRSA) (Koning et al., 2007), dynamic magnetic resonance imaging (van Herwaarden, Muhs, Vincken, van Prehn, Teutelink, Bartels, Moll & Verhagen, 2006), and ECG-gated CT (Teutelink et al., 2007). Although ultrasound is also used (van der Laan et al., 2003), it does not produce the three dimensional images that are required for the quantitative analysis of the whole stent graft. ECG-gated CT has the advantage of having high contrast for metal objects. Furthermore, ECG-gated CT is widely available, easily accessible, and can easily be applied in a post-operative setting.

To study the motions quantitatively, and to process the large datasets associated with ECG gating, automated processing is required. We divide the processing in two steps: segmentation of the stent, and calculating the motions of the stent[1].

---

[1] A stent graft consists of a metal frame surrounded by blood-proof material (the graft). When we only use the word "stent", we refer to the metallic frame: the graft is not visible on a CT scan.

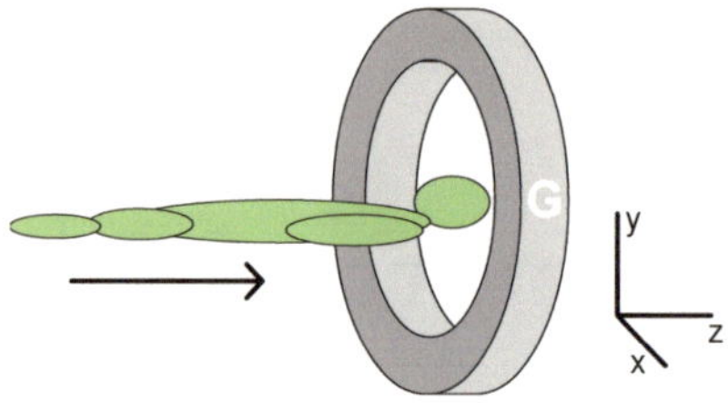

Fig. 1. Illustration of the orientation of the patient with respect to the CT scanner. The ring indicated by 'G' represents the gantry of the CT scanner.

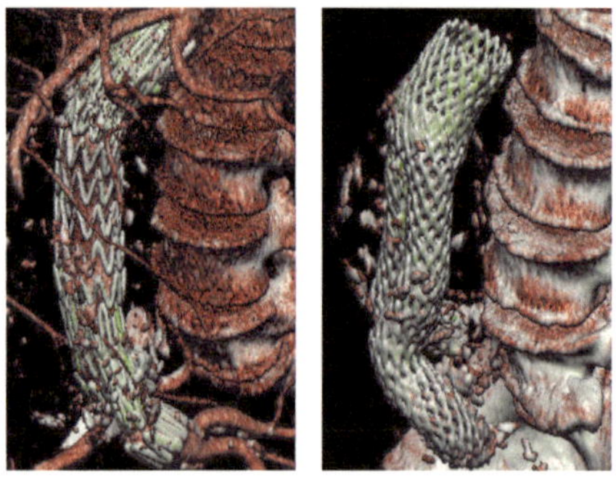

Fig. 2. Illustration of iso surfaces rendered from CT data of two types of stent grafts.

2. ECG-gated CT

In computed tomography (CT) a three-dimensional image of an object is constructed by a computer from a series of images obtained using roentgen radiation (Figure 1, Figure 2). In current CT scanners the x-ray source rotates around the object while the object is moved through the scanner in the *z*-direction. This enables scanning the complete object in one continuous (helical) motion (Kalender, 2005).

In recent years there have been major advancements in CT. Shorter rotation times and the development of multi detector CT (MDCT) enabled the technique of ECG gating, often referred to as cardiac CT (Fuchs et al., 2000). With this technique, the patient's ECG signal is measured during the scan. It is then possible to divide the raw scan data into bins that correspond to consecutive phases of the heart beat. The data in each bin is then reconstructed into a three-dimensional image (i.e. a volume), and the final result is a sequence of volumes, each corresponding to a different phase of the heart cycle (Figure 3). This allows 4D visualization of the scanned object and enables investigation to its temporal behavior (Fuchs et al., 2000; Ohnesorge et al., 2000). ECG-gated CT enables measuring motions that are synchronous with the patient's heart beat; other motions, such as those caused by breathing result in motion artifacts. The number of volumes that is reconstructed per scan is in the order of 8-20 (Hazer et al., 2009; Teutelink et al., 2007).

2.1 Dose and the noisy nature of CT data

One of the major downsides of CT in general is the exposure of the patient to ionizing radiation, which can have negative effects on the long term health of the patient (Fazel et al., 2009; Prokop, 2005). The dose should therefore be kept as low as reasonably achievable. However, this results in higher noise levels and more image artifacts, which can cause

problems for automatic image analysis algorithms that often need high quality data to operate. Algorithms that can perform their task on low dose data can therefore contribute to better patient safety.
In ECG-gated CT, multiple volumes are produced from the same amount of raw data. Assuming that the dose is kept the same, the amount of noise in each volume is therefore significantly larger than in volumes reconstructed using conventional CT.

2.2 Combining the volumes

The clinic sometimes also requires the result of a non-gated scan because of its lower levels of noise. Unfortunately, not all scanners are capable of producing a non-gated three-dimensional image in case ECG-gated scanning was used. Scanning patients twice is not an option considering the extra dose this would imply.
Averaging the data of the volumes off-line (i.e. not on the scanner's reconstruction computer) also produces a 3D dataset. This is a straightforward process, yet fundamentally different from combining the raw data (sinogram) before the filtered back-projection reconstruction (as happens for a non-gated scan). Due to non-linearities in the reconstruction process of the scanner, the results may be similar but will never be exactly the same.
In a study on phantom data acquired with a 64-slice Siemens Somatom CT scanner it was found that averaging the volumes in this way does not have negative effects on image quality in terms of noise, frequency response and motion artifacts (Klein, Oostveen, Greuter, Hoogeveen, Kool, Slump & Renema, 2009b). Rather, the noise was found to be slightly lower, and motion artifacts were found to be less severe.
For the purpose of segmentation, combining the volumes can also be advantageous. It has been shown that combining a subset of all volumes in the sequence can produce better results due to a more optimal compromise between noise and motion blur [Accepted for publication in Medical Image Analysis].

2.3 The effect of the patient's heart rate

While the patient is moved through the scanner (i.e. along the z-axis), data is collected and the patient's ECG-signal is measured (Figure 1). To construct a single volume with full coverage in the z-direction, data is collected from multiple heart beats (Figure 3). The table speed, rotation time of the scanner, and the heart beat of the patient together determine the amount of overlap in the z-direction. Negative overlap signifies a volume gap (Figure 3(b)), which is expressed as extremely noisy bands (Figure 4) that propagate through the data (the exact effects can differ per scanner). The data inside these gaps is completely unreliable (even if the scanner tries to interpolate it) because data at these positions is simply not available (Klein, Oostveen, Greuter, Hoogeveen, Kool, Slump & Renema, 2009a).
It can be shown theoretically, and it has been verified in an experiment (Klein, Oostveen, Greuter, Hoogeveen, Kool, Slump & Renema, 2009a), that there is a minimum required heart beat in order to obtain images without volume gaps. This minimum heart beat can be calculated as follows:

$$B_{min} = \frac{60 \cdot p}{T_{rot}}, \tag{1}$$

where p is the pitch factor, T_{rot} the rotation time, and B_{min} the minimum required heart rate in beats per minute. For a typical setup with $T_{rot} = 0.37$ and $p = 0.34$ the minimum required heart beat $B_{min} = 55$ bpm.

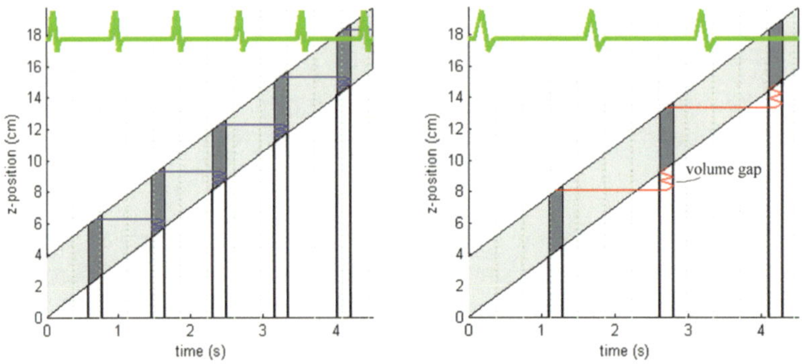

(a) 70 bpm (b) 40 bpm

Fig. 3. Diagram illustrating the process of ECG-gating. The light grey band indicates the covered z-positions of the detector during the scan. The dark grey patches represent parts of the phase in each heart beat.

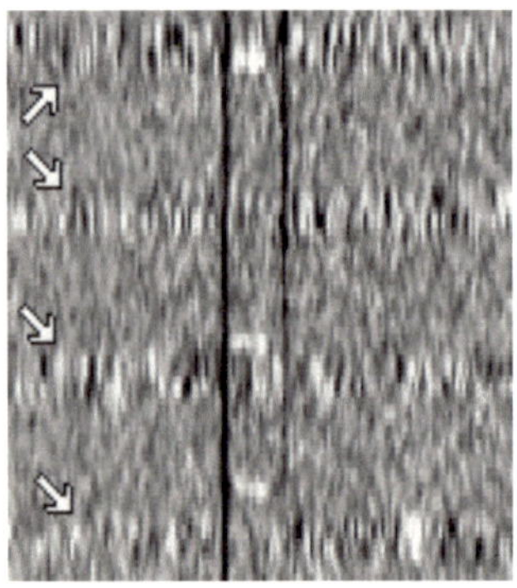

Fig. 4. Illustration of the noise bands in the CT images caused by the volume gaps due to a too low heart rate (45 bpm) during scanning. Shown is an image of a phantom which has small metal bars embedded at regular intervals. It can be seen how the second bar from the top is hidden by a noise band (i.e. volume gap).

It is noteworthy that a too high heart rate should also be avoided, since this leads to increased motion artifacts.

2.4 Temporal resolution

The temporal resolution of the technique of ECG gating consists of two parts (Figure 5): the first is the width of each phase T_w, which is fully determined by the rotation time and reconstruction algorithm. Its value determines to what extent motion causes artifacts in the resulting data. Since T_w depends on the applied reconstruction algorithm, which is often chosen by the manufacturer, this value is often unknown. In Klein, Oostveen, Greuter, Hoogeveen, Kool, Slump & Renema (2009a) a simple experiment is described to measure the value of T_w empirically.

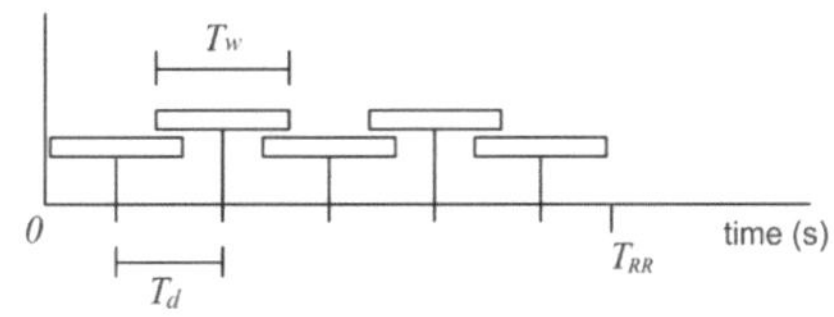

Fig. 5. Diagram illustrating the two aspects of temporal resolution. T_w is determined by the rotation time and reconstruction algorithm. T_d is determined by the heart rate and the number of reconstructed phases (five in this example).

The second part is the (temporal) distance between phases T_d, which is determined by the number of phases and the heart rate. It represents the sampling rate of the technique. If more phases are reconstructed, T_d decreases and the overlap between phases increases.
In an ideal scenario, T_w should be as low as possible to be least affected by motion artifacts, and T_d should be approximately equal such that the sampling frequency is high enough to prevent aliasing, with a minimal number of phases.

2.5 Application

ECG-gated CT is extensively used in cardiac exams (Albers et al., 2003; Manzke et al., 2004; Williamson et al., 2008), especially for the assessment of coronary arteries (Chartrand-Lefebvre et al., 2007; Dewey et al., 2008; Greuter et al., 2005). The goal in most of these studies is to limit the effect of motion rather than to examine the motion itself for which the technique can also be utilized.
Recently, ECG-gated CT was used to study the pulsating motion of AAA (Teutelink et al., 2007), and the motion of the renal arteries (Muhs, Teutelink, Prokop, Vincken, Moll & Verhagen, 2006).
The abdominal aorta is constantly in motion caused by the pressure waves from the contracting heart. However, the dynamics of this motion are more subtle than the motions present in the heart itself. It has been shown that the order of magnitude of these motions is in the order of 2 mm (Muhs, Vincken, van Prehn, Stone, Bartels, Prokop, Moll & Verhagen, 2006; Teutelink et al., 2007). It is reported that the limits of the motion that can be detected in clinical practice by ECG gating are slightly less than the spacing between the voxels (usually in the order of 0.5 mm), and that for a typical setup frequency components up to 2.7 Hz can be accurately detected (Klein, Oostveen, Greuter, Hoogeveen, Kool, Slump & Renema, 2009a). This makes ECG-gated CT a suitable technique for studying motions in AAA.

3. Segmentation of the stent graft

Segmentation of the stent graft is performed on a three-dimensional image. Depending on how the data is processed further, the segmentation is applied to all volumes in the sequence, or to a single volume obtained by combining the volumes in the sequence.
Several studies have been published on the segmentation of blood vessels in 3D, which have correspondences with the wires of the frame of the stent and may therefore be of interest (see Lesage et al. (2009) and Kirbas & Quek (2004) for an overview of vessel segmentation methods). Methods that fit a series of spheres or ellipsoids to the vessel (Beck et al., 2009; Zhou et al., 2008), and methods that segment the contour in slices perpendicular to the vessel centerline (Hernandez-Hoyos et al., 2002; Lee et al., 2007) assume a solid vessel with a diameter of several voxels. Due to the small diameter of stent wires (1 to 3 voxels) and their

sharp corners, these methods are not suitable for the segmentation of stents. Region growing methods (Bock et al., 2008) have problems with leaks and gaps and need a second stage to find the geometry from the segmented voxels. A common method is the two-step approach (Freiman et al., 2009; Kaftan et al., 2009; Manduca et al., 2009; Worz et al., 2009), which first segments the vessel using a vessel measure (Frangi et al., 1998) followed by centerline tracking. This method, however, is known to have difficulties where the structure is not tubular, such as in crossings and sharp corners in the stent's frame.

A related method is used by Langs et al. (2011) for the segmentation of stent grafts in the aortic arch. Interest points are extracted that are located on the center line of the stent determined by a skeletonization of the volume thresholded at 2000 Hounsfield units (HU) and weighted by its vesselness measure (Frangi et al., 1998). The result is a dense set of points that lie on the frame of the stent.

Unfortunately, the *quality of the data*—defined as how well the frame of the stent is distinguishable in the data—is not always sufficient for such a method to fully segment the stent's frame (Klein et al., 2008). This quality depends on the combination of used dose, stent wire diameter, material properties of the stent (i.e. absorption coefficient), and patient anatomy. The stent can consist of CT values as low as 300 HU (Klein et al., 2008). There are also reports of some stent types being barely distinguishable, whereas other stent types are well visible in data obtained using the same scanner settings [Submitted to Medical Image Analysis].

In addition to the bad visibility of the frame of the stent, several problems can be identified for (low dose) CT data. Firstly, the data is relatively noisy. Secondly, streak artifacts occur where the stent's metal frame is thick or where a coil is present next to the stent graft. Thirdly, contrast agent injected in the blood results in CT-values close to the range of CT-values seen for most stents. Fourthly, due to image artifacts, the wire of the stent sometimes contains gaps.

In this section, we discuss a way to model the stent graft, and two approaches to obtain such a model from the volumetric CT data in ways that are relatively robust for the aforementioned problems.

3.1 Modeling the stent

Most studies related to the motion of stent grafts focus on measuring the stent's diameter changes (van Herwaarden, Bartels, Muhs, Vincken, Lindeboom, Teutelink, Moll & Verhagen, 2006) or determining the motion at a sparse set of points on the stent (Langs et al., 2007). A model that enables capturing material properties and high level knowledge regarding the stent graft characteristics would be valuable to gain more insight in the stent's in vivo behavior (Langs et al., 2007). Furthermore, such a model can also help in performing more reliable (fluid dynamics) simulations, which is important for improving current stent designs (Cebral et al., 2009; Kleinstreuer et al., 2007).

In [submitted to Medical Image Analysis] a geometric model is proposed that represents the wire frame of the stent as an undirected graph, with nodes placed at the corners and crossings of the frame, and the edges between the nodes representing the wires (Figure 6). This model can be applied to different stent types, and represents the topology of the stent's frame in a concise and natural way.

3.2 Segmentation of the stent graft via centerline tracking

A stent has a tubular structure, sometimes with branches, and can be approximated by a series of stacked contours which are orthogonal to the centerline (Figure 7). An approach

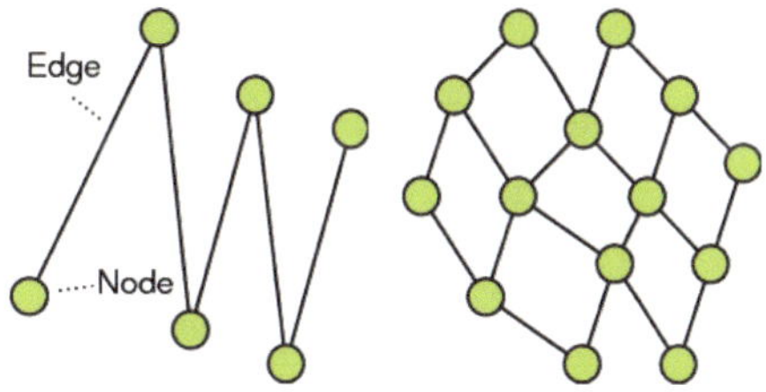

(a) (b)

Fig. 6. Example graphs that describe a geometric model of a stent frame. The edges between the nodes represent the physical wire frame of the stent. Nodes are placed at corners (a) and crossings (b).

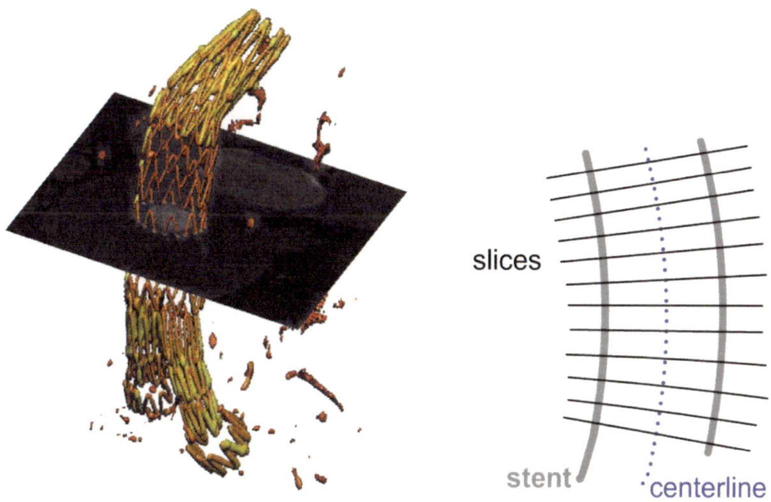

Fig. 7. Illustration of how the stent can be approximated as a series of stacked contours. (a) shows a volume rendering of the stent and a slice orthogonal to its centerline. (b) shows a schematic illustration of contours perpendicular to the stent's centerline.

published by Klein et al. (2008) is to segment the stent in 2D images sampled perpendicular to its centerline. Regions with high CT-values (typically above 500 HU) exist where the metallic frame of the stent penetrates the image. These regions have high CT-values and—due to their "pointy" structure—well suited for point detection.

The approach to segment the stent in these 2D images is to first detect a set of interest points, after which a clustering algorithm is applied to find the points that are on the wire of the stent. This process is then repeated in an iterative fashion, while tracking along the centerline of the stent. At the end of this process, a 3D geometric model of the stent is obtained.

An advantage of this approach is that part of the algorithm is 2D, which makes visualization and algorithm design easier. A disadvantage is that modeling the stent as a series of stacked contours causes difficulties at bifurcations and when parts of the frame of the stent overlap.

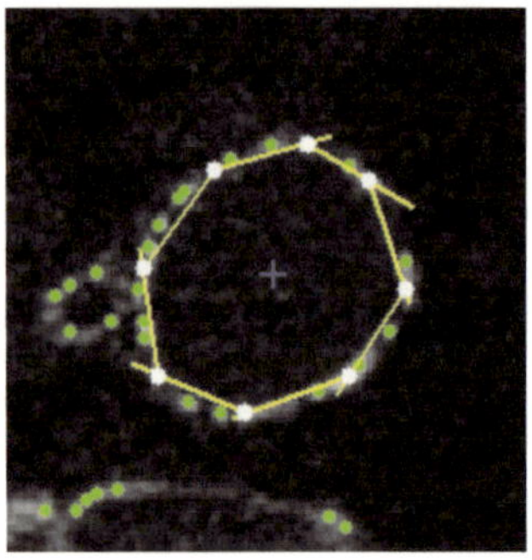

Fig. 8. Example of the clustering algorithm after finding a coarse contour.

3.2.1 Point detection

Four different point detection algorithms were taken into consideration and tested in an experiment. An algorithm based on the product of Eigenvalues was found to work the best. This measure, also known as the Gaussian curvature, can be expressed using image derivatives: $\frac{\partial^2 L}{\partial x^2} \cdot \frac{\partial^2 L}{\partial y^2}$, where L is the 2D image. Other methods taken into consideration were a static threshold, a dynamic threshold, and the Laplacian (the sum of Eigenvalues).

3.2.2 Clustering

Four different clustering algorithms were taken into consideration and tested in an experiment. The best method was found to be a custom method that uses a virtual stick to select the stent-points in an iterative fashion. By selecting points from the inside of the contour, spurious points outside of the contour are ignored (Figure 8). Other clustering methods taken into consideration were circle fitting, ellipse fitting, and GVF snakes (Xu & Prince, 1998).
The result of the clustering method is a set of points that represent the contour of the stent. By fitting a circle on these points, an estimate of the radius and center position can be obtained, which are used during centerline tracking.

3.2.3 Centerline tracking and modeling

Starting from a manually selected seed point, the algorithm tracks the stent in both directions. Starting from a coarse estimate of the centerline orientation, slices are sampled, to which the aforementioned algorithms are applied. The center position found at each slice is used to estimate the next centerline position. For the method to be less sensitive to noise present on the center estimate (caused by the discrete nature of the contour points), a smoothness constraint is adopted. Bifurcations are detected when a significant change in the diameter estimate is encountered. Subsequently, both branches of the bifurcations are tracked individually.
To deal with the gaps between the different parts of the stent graft that are present in some stent types (Figure 7(a)), the tracking will proceed in the last known direction if no contour could be found. When no contour is found along a predefined distance, it is assumed that the end of the stent is reached, and the tracking stops.
During centerline tracking the contour points in the current slice are matched to the contour points of the previous slice. In this fashion the individual wires are tracked too. The positions where two wires meet—which represent the corners and crossings of the stent's frame—are detected, and nodes are created at these positions to build the geometric model (Figure 9).

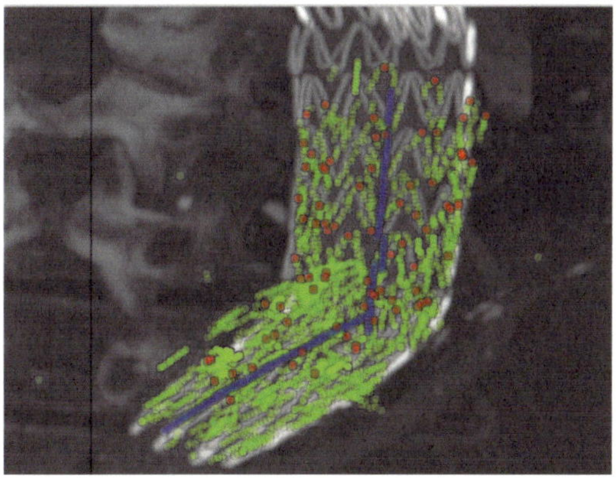

Fig. 9. Illustration of the centerline tracking algorithm in progress. The blue dots indicates the found centerline. The green dots indicate the found stent points, and the larger red dots indicate the found nodes which will be connected to form a geometrical model.

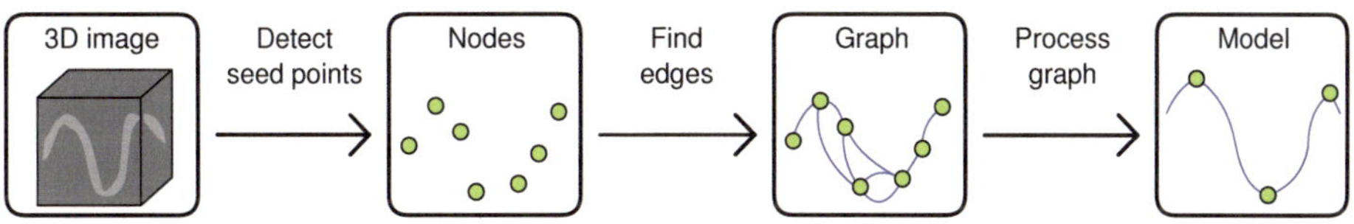

Fig. 10. Flowchart illustrating the three processing steps of the MCP-based algorithm to extract a geometrical model from the CT data.

3.3 Segmentation of the stent graft via the minimum cost path method

A method to segment the stent graft in 3D by finding the optimal paths between a large set of automatically detected seed points is proposed in [submitted to Medical Image Analysis]. The method can be divided into three steps, which are illustrated in the flow chart in Figure 10.

3.3.1 Detection of seed points

In the first step, a set of seed points is found by searching the volume for voxels subject to three criteria: 1) The voxel intensity must be a local maximum. 2) The voxel intensity must be higher than a predefined threshold value. 3) The voxel must have a direct neighbor with an intensity also above this threshold value.

3.3.2 Finding the optimal paths

In the second step, the seed points are connected using a modified version of the minimum cost path (MCP) method. The MCP method can be used for segmentation of vessels and other structures (e.g. (Cohen & Deschamps, 2007; Deschamps & Cohen, 2000; Fahmi et al., 2008; Gülsün & Tek, 2008; Jandt et al., 2009; Quek & Kirbas, 2001; Wink et al., 2004)). It is a level set method in which a front is propagated monotonically following a (non-negative) cost function. The advantages of this method are that it can be implemented in a computationally efficient way, and that it can easily be modified to make it more suitable for a specific problem, see for example Klein, Renema, Kool & Slump (2009) and Cohen & Deschamps (2007).
To use the MCP method for stent segmentation, it is modified such that the fronts evolve from all the seed points found in the seed point detection step. Connections between the nodes

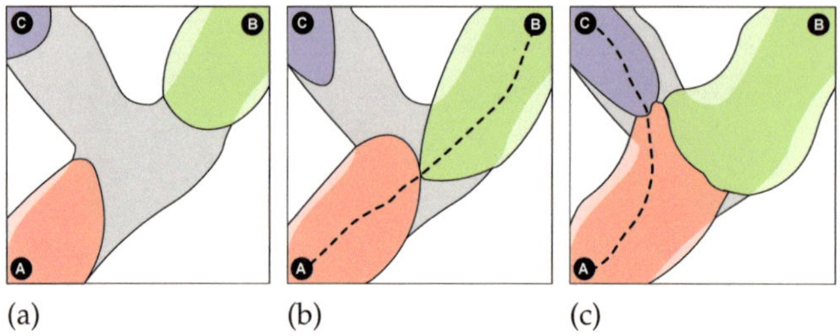

Fig. 11. Illustration of three meeting fronts in the MCP algorithm. The black circular shapes indicate seed points A, B and C. In (a) the fronts do not yet meet. In (b) front A meets front B, and the path is traced. A few iterations later, in (c) a third front meets with the first, connection seed points A and C.

are detected when two fronts collide, and the paths between the points are found using a backtrace map that is maintained during the evolution of the front.

The result of the MCP algorithm is a graph consisting of nodes (the seed points) connected by edges. Each edge is associated with a path of voxels connecting one node to another. However, many of these edges are false edges and have to be removed.

3.3.3 Graph processing

In the third step, the false edges are removed using graph processing techniques. For this purpose, two scalar values are associated with each edge. The first is α, the maximum cumulative cost on the path. It represents the *weakness* (i.e. inverse strength) of the edge. This value is used to establish the order of the edges; a stronger connection (lower α) is preferred over a weaker one. The second scalar value is β, the minimum intensity (the CT-value in Hounsfield Units) on the path. Due to the definition of CT-values (-1000 representing air and 0 representing water) this value has a physical meaning and represents the *quality* of the edge; it is used to determine whether an edge should be removed or not.

The processing of the graph occurs in multiple different passes. Firstly, weak edges are removed based on the expected number of edges for each node. This value depends on the specific stent type being segmented. The weakness value α is used to establish the weakest edges to consider for removal, and the quality measure β is used to determine whether an edge should be removed. Secondly, a clean-up pass is performed to remove redundant edges; an edge is found redundant if there is a path of one or two stronger (i.e. lower α) edges that connect the same nodes. Thirdly, corners are detected in the wire, and nodes are placed at the positions that have the highest curvature. Hereafter the graph is cleaned up again. Fourthly, crossings are detected and nodes are added to represent them. Finally, after a final clean-up step, all the paths are smoothed.

3.3.4 Experiments and results

To evaluate the quality of the geometric model produced by this method, experiments were performed in which the model was compared with a reference model annotated by three experts. By counting the number of corresponding edges, a similarity measure was obtained. A training set was used to obtain the optimal parameter values of the algorithm, and using a test set the final performance of the method was evaluated.

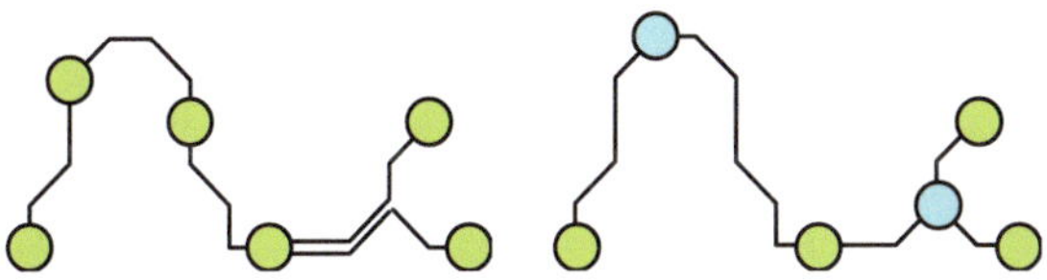

(a) Before (b) After

Fig. 12. Illustration of adding corners and nodes. In (b) two nodes were removed and a node was placed at the corner. Another node was inserted at the crossing.

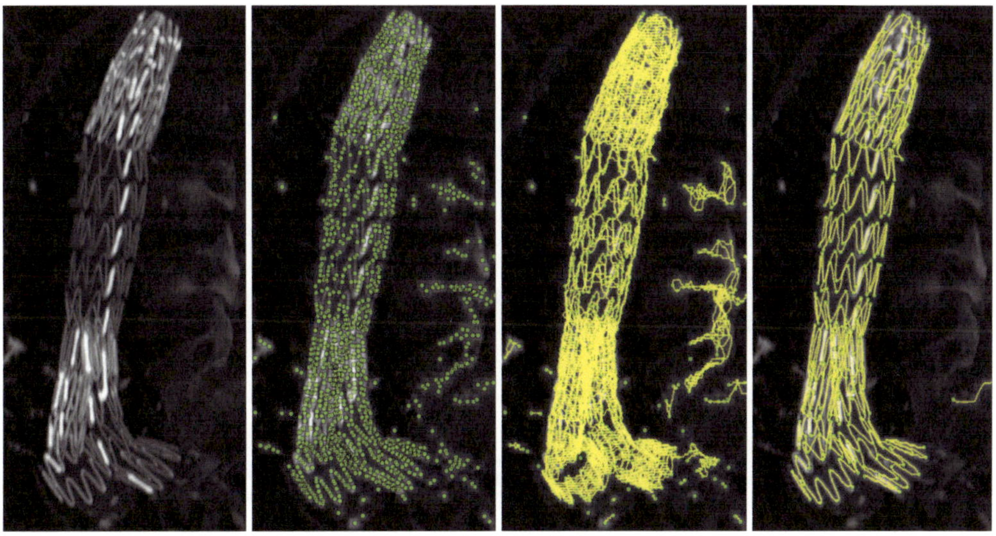

(a) MIP of the CT data (b) 1732 seed points (c) 4963 initial edges (d) 531 final edges

Fig. 13. Illustration of the different algorithm steps. Shown are a Maximum Intensity Projection (MIP) of the original data (a), the detected seed points (b), the found edges (c), the result after processing the graph (d).

The algorithm was found to be robust for variations in its parameter values, and for the high noise levels present in the data. The found similarity with the reference data was found to be 96% and 92% for the two stent types considered in the experiments. Visual inspections of the results showed that most errors were present in difficult areas of the stent, such as bifurcations and narrow legs where the wire has relatively sharp corners.
An example of the results after each processing step is shown in Figure 13. In Figure 14 lit surface renders are shown for the found geometric models of three datasets.

4. Calculating motions and forces of the stent graft

When the geometric model of the stent is obtained, it can be used as a tool to study the motions of the stent graft. For this purpose, motion is applied to the model. In the first part of this section we discuss how this can be done, following the ideas presented in [Accepted for publication in Medical Image Analysis]. In the second part of this section we discuss an alternative method that uses active shape models to study stent graft motions.

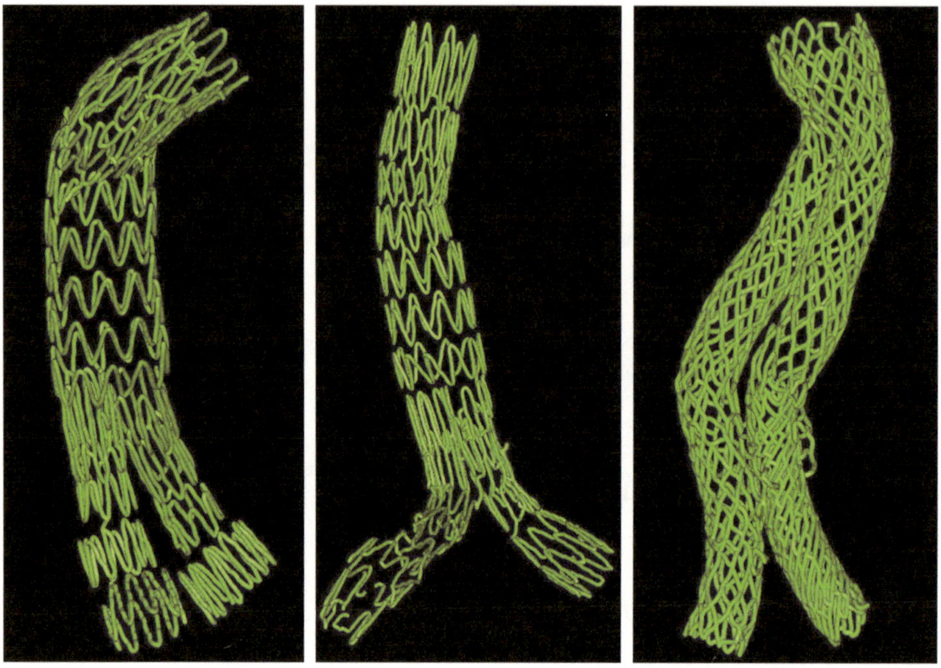

Fig. 14. Illustration of lit surface renders of the geometric models for three example stent grafts.

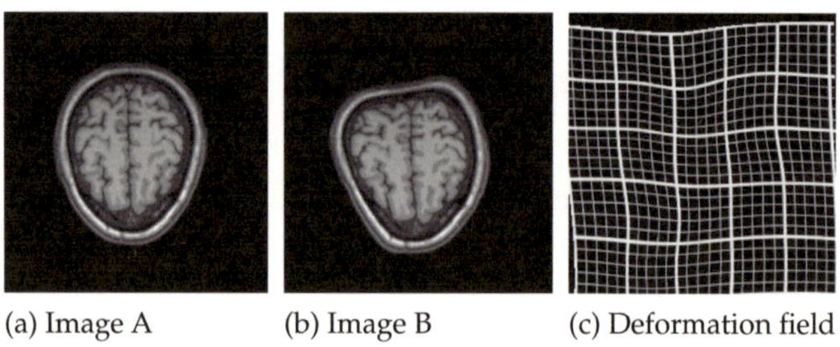

Fig. 15. An example of registering two images, and the resulting deformation field.

4.1 Motion analysis using a geometric model

The motion of interest is obtained from the sequence of CT volumes using a registration algorithm. The purpose of a registration algorithm is to (elastically) align two images; the result is a deformation field that describes how one image should be deformed to align it with the second (Figure 15). This deformation field can be applied to the geometric model to enable studying the motions.

4.1.1 Image registration

The current range of common region based image registration algorithms can be divided into two classes. Both classes usually adopt a multiscale approach in order to prevent finding a local minimum, and to speed up the registration process. The first class employs a B-spline grid to describe the deformation field, which is optimized by minimizing/maximizing a

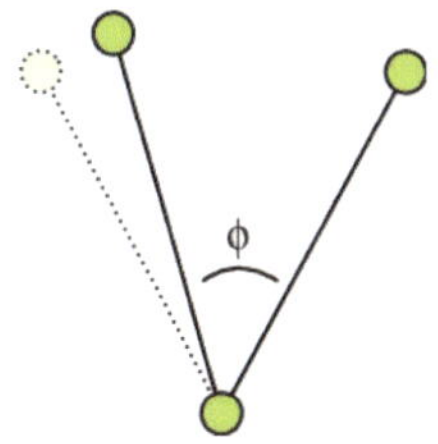

Fig. 16. Illustration of how the (change of) angle ϕ can be used to a estimate the force present in the node when motion is applied to the model.

similarity measure. Using Mutual Information (MI) as a similarity measure, these methods have been shown to be robust for differences in the appearance between the images (Maintz & Viergever, 1998; Rueckert et al., 1999; Wells et al., 1996). While the use of a B-spline grid can cause problems when describing rotational deformations (Kroon & Slump, 2009), it has the advantage that the deformations are described in an efficient way and are physically realistic (Noblet et al., 2006). Additionally, the deformations can be regularized in various ways, for example by minimizing bending energies or penalizing small Jacobians (Rueckert et al., 1999). The second class uses image forces calculated at the pixels/voxels to drive the registration process. A popular example is the Demons algorithm (Thirion, 1998), which is related to optical flow. The deformation is obtained for each pixel individually by calculating image forces, and regularization of the deformation field is performed by Gaussian diffusion. The Demons algorithm is capable of handling extreme deformations, which can also be a downside, since such deformations are usually not physically realistic. Another problem with the Demons algorithm is that it assumes pixel intensities in corresponding regions between images to be similar, which causes problems in images containing much noise or artifacts such as bias fields (Noblet et al., 2006).
It is of importance to select the right registration algorithm for each problem, and to choose the best parameters, of which most registration algorithms have many (Klein et al., 2010). In the case of registering the different volumes obtained by ECG-gated CT, the used registration algorithm should be accurate in order to deal with the small motions present in AAA, and should be robust for noise and other artifacts associated with low dose CT. Which algorithms qualify for this task is currently being investigated.

4.1.2 Analysis of motion and forces

The result of the registration algorithm is a deformation field that describes the deformation for each voxel in the volume. To study the motions of a stent, the deformation field is applied to the nodes of the geometric model: for each node the deformation is applied that corresponds to its location in the volume. This will allow quantitative studies to the motion patterns of individual stents, and allows comparison between patients.
Because the topology of the stent is fully captured by the geometric model, the forces acting on the stent's frame can be estimated by incorporating material properties such as stiffness, and by calculating the change of the angle between two edges (Figure 16).

4.2 Motion analysis using active shape models

A technique of interest for the evaluation of motions of stent grafts is that of Langs et al. (2011). Their application is for stent grafts in the aortic arch to treat aortic ruptures caused by trauma. In Langs et al. (2007) a method for the unsupervised learning of models from sets of

interest points was proposed. It is based on minimum description length (MDL) group-wise registration (Thodberg, 2003). The global and local deformation are captured using a statistical deformation model that is built during registration of a sparse set of interest points. No a priori annotation, or definition of topological properties of the structure is necessary.
Instead of deforming the whole volume they search for correspondences between finite lists of interest points and local features in the data. This has a few advantages: 1) The algorithm can omit variations that are not relevant to the model. 2) The approach is not constrained to an a priori topological class because it does not rely on a mapping to a reference image. 3) No prior segmentation of the object is necessary, only the interest point extraction method has to be chosen according to the structure of interest. A disadvantage of this approach, however, is that it is less accurate than texture-based registration with which registration errors smaller than the voxel size can be obtained (Klein et al., 2011; Murphy et al., 2011). This can be a problem for stent grafts in AAA, because—due to the larger distance from the heart—the motions are smaller than in the aortic arch.

4.2.1 MDL registration

First a set of interest points is detected in each volume of the ECG-gate sequence. These points are treated as landmarks candidates; each landmark is associated with a position (x, y, z) and local features (such as image intensity and steerable filters). The registration is initialized by pairwise matching of a subset of the interest points. Starting from these correspondences group-wise registration is performed by minimizing a criterion function that captures the compactness of the model comprising the variation of landmark positions and local feature variation at the landmark positions. The minimum description length criterion accounts for the fact that the landmarks located on the stent move in a highly correlated manner during the cardiac cycle.
The registration is optimized by a combination of k-D trees and genetic-optimization, and is followed by a refinement using a direct search. The optimization process results in a shape variation model, which is then used to study the motions of the stent.

4.2.2 Motion analysis

The analysis of the stent deformation during the cardiac cycle is performed using the shape model that results from the group wise registration (Figure 17). For each landmark the positions in all volumes in the sequence are known. Three measurements can be obtained for each landmark: 1) The modes of variation of the statistical shape model, which capture the correlation between landmark movements. 2) The displacement of the landmarks, which reflect the absolute movement in the anatomical environment. 3) The compactness of the local shape model build with the closest landmarks, which gives an indication about the complexity of the local deformation. This last measure is particularly of interest, since it is well suited to show regions of potential stress to the material.

5. Outlook

An automated method to quantitatively study the motions and forces of stent grafts in vivo enables studying the motion patterns of individual patients, relate them to data of a previous date, or relate them to the motion patterns of other patients.
It would also be interesting to study the range of motion patterns of stent grafts in patients without problems, and compare them to the motions in patients who do have problems. Such

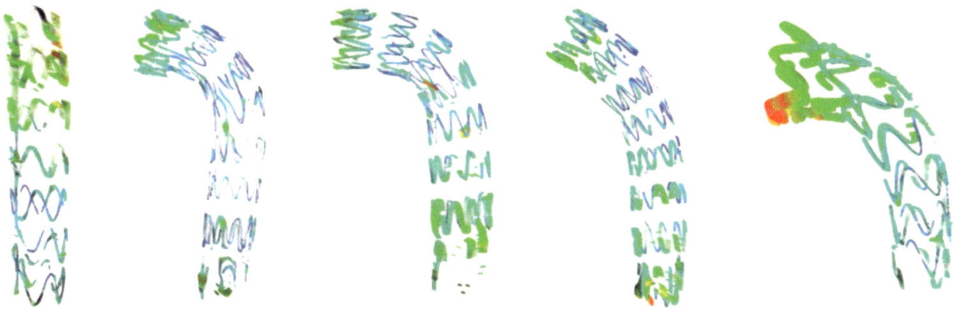

Fig. 17. Global deformation (color-coded) for a few stent grafts. (Image courtesy of G. Langs from Langs et al. (2011).)

studies would, however, require large datasets to incorporate all the variabilities in motion patterns, particularly because problems with stent grafts are relatively rare. Nevertheless, we believe that such studies can help our understanding of the dynamics and failure of stent grafts, and can thereby help in designing better stent grafts in the future. Further, we hope that we are able to correlate certain distinct motion patterns to specific stent-related problems, so that this technique can be used for diagnostic purposes and prediction of stent failure.

6. Conclusion

Using ECG-gated CTA, information about the motion of stent grafts in AAA can be obtained. Using segmentation methods, a geometric model of the stent can be obtained that describes the topology of the stent in a compact way. Using registration techniques, the deformation field can be found, which can then be applied to the found geometric model. Thereby the motions of the stent graft are known in great detail, and enables calculating the forces acting on the stent. Both parameters (motion and force) provide new information that can be used in further analysis of in vivo stent graft behavior and future device design.

7. References

Albers, J., Boese, J. M., Vahl, C. F. & Hagl, S. (2003). In vivo validation of cardiac spiral computed tomography using retrospective gating, *The Annals of Thoracic Surgery* 75: 885—889.

Beck, T., Biermann, C., Fritz, D., Dillmann, R., Pluim, J. P. W. & Dawant, B. M. (2009). Robust model-based centerline extraction of vessels in CTA data, *Proc. of SPIE*, Vol. 7259, Lake Buena Vista, FL, USA, p. 72593O.

Blankensteijn, J. D., de Jong, S. E., Prinssen, M., van der Ham, A. C., Buth, J., van Sterkenburg, S. M., Verhagen, H. J., Buskens, E., Grobbee, D. E. & the Dutch Randomized Endovascular Aneurysm Management (DREAM) Trial Group (2005). Two-Year outcomes after conventional or endovascular repair of abdominal aortic aneurysms, *N Engl J Med* 352(23): 2398–2405.

Bock, S., Kuhhnel, C., Boskamp, T. & Peitgen, H. (2008). Robust vessel segmentation, *Proc. of SPIE*, Vol. 6915, San Diego, CA, USA, p. 691539.

Bruin, J. L. D., Baas, A. F., Buth, J., Prinssen, M., Verhoeven, E. L., Cuypers, P. W., van Sambeek, M. R., Balm, R., Grobbee, D. E., Blankensteijn, J. D. & the DREAM Study Group

(2010). Long-Term outcome of open or endovascular repair of abdominal aortic aneurysm, *N. Engl. J. Med.* 362(20): 1881–1889.

Cao, P., Rango, P. D., Parlani, G. & Verzini, F. (2009). Durability of abdominal aortic endograft with the talent unidoc stent graft in common practice: Core lab reanalysis from the TAURIS multicenter study, *J. Cardiovasc. Surg.* 49(4): 859–865.

Cebral, J., Mut, F., Appanaboyina, S., Lohner, R., Miranda, C., Escrivano, E., Lylyk, P., Putman, C., Hu, X. P. & Clough, A. V. (2009). Image-based analysis of blood flow modification in stented aneurysms, *Proc. of SPIE*, Vol. 7262, Lake Buena Vista, FL, USA, p. 72621G.

Chartrand-Lefebvre, C., Cadrin-Chenevert, A., Bordeleau, E., Ugolini, P., Ouellet, R., Sablayrolles, J. & Prenovault, J. (2007). Coronary computed tomography angiography: Overview of technical aspects, current concepts, and perspectives, *Canadian Association of Radiology* 58: 92—108.

Cohen, L. D. & Deschamps, T. (2007). Segmentation of 3D tubular objects with adaptive front propagation and minimal tree extraction for 3D medical imaging, *Comput Methods Biomech Biomed Engin* 10(4): 289.

Demirci, S., Manstad-Hulaas, F., Navab, N., Miga, M. I. & Wong, K. H. (2009). Quantification of abdominal aortic deformation after EVAR, *Proc. of SPIE*, Vol. 7261, Lake Buena Vista, FL, USA, p. 72611U.

Deschamps, T. & Cohen, L. D. (2000). Fast extraction of minimal paths in 3D images and applications to virtual endoscopy, *Med Image Anal* 5: 281—299.

Dewey, M., Teige, F., Rutsch, W., Schink, T. & Hamm, B. (2008). CT coronary angiography: Influence of different cardiac reconstruction intervals on image quality and diagnostic accuracy, *European Journal of Radiology* 67: 92—99.

Fahmi, R., Jerebko, A., Wolf, M. & Farag, A. A. (2008). Robust segmentation of tubular structures in medical images, *Proc. of SPIE*, San Diego, CA, USA, p. 691443.

Fazel, R., Krumholz, H. M., Wang, Y., Ross, J. S., Chen, J., Ting, H. H., Shah, N. D., Nasir, K., Einstein, A. J. & Nallamothu, B. K. (2009). Exposure to Low-Dose ionizing radiation from medical imaging procedures, *New England Journal of Medicine* 361(9): 849–857.

Frangi, A. F., Niessen, W. J., Vincken, K. L. & Viergever, M. A. (1998). Multiscale vessel enhancement filtering, *Lect Notes Comput Sci* 1496: 130—137.

Freiman, M., Joskowicz, L., Sosna, J., Miga, M. I. & Wong, K. H. (2009). A variational method for vessels segmentation: algorithm and application to liver vessels visualization, *Proc. of SPIE*, Vol. 7261, SPIE, Lake Buena Vista, FL, USA, p. 72610H.

Fuchs, T. O., Kachelriess, M. & Kalender, W. A. (2000). System performance of multislice spiral computed tomography, *IEEE Eng Med Biol Mag* 19: 63—70.

Greuter, M. J. W., Dorgelo, J., Tukker, W. G. J. & Oudkerk, M. (2005). Study on motion artifacts in coronary arteries with an anthropomorphic moving heart phantom on an ECG-gated multidetector computed tomography unit, *European Radiology* 5: 995—1007.

Gülsün, M. A. & Tek, H. (2008). Robust vessel tree modeling, *Med Image Comput Comput Assist Interv* 11: 602–611.

Hazer, D., Finol, E. A., Kostrzewa, M., Kopaigorenko, M., Richter, G., Dillmann, R., Hu, X. P. & Clough, A. V. (2009). Computational biomechanics and experimental validation of vessel deformation based on 4D-CT imaging of the porcine aorta, *Proc. of SPIE*, Vol. 7262, Lake Buena Vista, FL, USA, p. 72621F.

Hernandez-Hoyos, M., Orkisz, M., Puech, P., Mansard-Desbleds, C., Douek, P. & Magnin, I. E. (2002). Computer-assisted analysis of three-dimensional MR angiograms, *Radiographics* 22(2): 421—436.

Investigators, T. U. K. E. T. (2010). Endovascular versus open repair of abdominal aortic aneurysm, *N. Engl. J. Med.* 362(20): 1863–1871.

Jacobs, T. S., Won, J., Gravereaux, E. C., Faries, P. L., Morrissey, N., Teodorescu, V. J., Hollier, L. H. & Marin, M. L. (2003). Mechanical failure of prosthetic human implants: A 10-year experience with aortic stent graft devices, *J. Vasc. Surg.* 37(1): 16–26.

Jandt, U., Schäfer, D., Grass, M. & Rasche, V. (2009). Automatic generation of 3D coronary artery centerlines using rotational x-ray angiography, *Med Image Anal* 13(6): 846–858.

Kaftan, J. N., Tek, H., Aach, T., Pluim, J. P. W. & Dawant, B. M. (2009). A two-stage approach for fully automatic segmentation of venous vascular structures in liver CT images, *Proc. of SPIE*, Vol. 7259, Lake Buena Vista, FL, USA, p. 725911.

Kalender, W. A. (2005). *Computed Tomography*, Publicis Corporate Publishing, Erlangen.

Kirbas, C. & Quek, F. (2004). A review of vessel extraction techniques and algorithms, *ACM Comput. Surv.* 36(2): 81–121.

Klein, A., Kroon, D., Hoogeveen, Y., Kool, L. J. S., Renema, W. K. & Slump, C. H. (2011). Multimodal image registration by edge attraction and regularization using a b-spline grid, *Proc. of SPIE*, Orlando, USA, pp. 7962–71.

Klein, A., Oostveen, L. J., Greuter, M. J. W., Hoogeveen, Y., Kool, L. J. S., Slump, C. H. & Renema, W. K. J. (2009a). Detectability of motions in AAA with ECG-gated CTA: a quantitative study, *Medical Physics* 36(10): 4616–4624.

Klein, A., Oostveen, L. J., Greuter, M. J. W., Hoogeveen, Y., Kool, L. J. S., Slump, C. H. & Renema, W. K. J. (2009b). Diagnostic quality of time-averaged ECG-gated CT data, *Proceedings of SPIE*, Lake Buena Vista, FL, USA, pp. 725836–725836-6.

Klein, A., Renema, W. K., Kool, L. J. S. & Slump, C. H. (2009). Initial steps towards automatic segmentation of the wire frame of stent grafts in CT data, *Proc. of IEEE-EMBS Benelux Chapter*, Enschede, The Netherlands, pp. 116—119.

Klein, A., Renema, W. K., Oostveen, L. J., Kool, L. J. S. & Slump, C. H. (2008). A segmentation method for stentgrafts in the abdominal aorta from ECG-gated CTA data, *Proc. of SPIE*, San Diego, CA, USA, p. 69160R.

Klein, S., Staring, M., Murphy, K., Viergever, M. & Pluim, J. (2010). elastix: A toolbox for Intensity-Based medical image registration, *Medical Imaging, IEEE Transactions on* 29(1): 196–205.

Kleinstreuer, C., Li, Z. & Farber, M. A. (2007). Fluid-Structure interaction analyses of stented abdominal aortic aneurysms, *Annu Rev Biomed Eng* 9: 169—204.

Koning, O. H. J., Kaptein, B. L., Garling, E. H., Hinnen, J. W., Hamming, J. F., Valstar, E. R. & van Bockel, J. H. (2007). Assessment of three-dimensional stent-graft dynamics by using fluoroscopic roentgenographic stereophotogrammetric analysis, *Journal of Vascular Surgery: Official Publication, the Society for Vascular Surgery [and] International Society for Cardiovascular Surgery, North American Chapter* 46(4): 773–779.

Koning, O. H., Oudegeest, O. R., Valstar, E. R., Garling, E. H., van der Linden, E., Hinnen, J. W., Hamming, J. F., Vossepoel, A. M. & van Bockel, J. H. (2006). Roentgen stereophotogrammetric analysis: An accurate tool to assess Stent-Graft migration, *Journal of Endovascular Therapy* 13(4): 468—475.

Kroon, D. & Slump, C. H. (2009). MRI modalitiy transformation in demon registration, *Proceedings of the Sixth IEEE international conference on Symposium on Biomedical Imaging: From Nano to Macro*, IEEE Press, Boston, Massachusetts, USA, pp. 963–966.

Langs, G., Paragios, N., Desgranges, P., Rahmouni, A. & Kobeiter, H. (2011). Learning deformation and structure simultaneously: In situ endograft deformation analysis, *Medical Image Analysis* 15(1): 12–21.

Langs, G., Paragios, N., Donner, R., Desgranges, P., Rahmouni, A. & Kobeiter, H. (2007). Motion analysis of endovascular Stent-Grafts by MDL based registration, *Proc IEEE Int Conf Comput Vis*, pp. 1–8.

Lee, J., Beighley, P., Ritman, E. & Smith, N. (2007). Automatic segmentation of 3D micro-CT coronary vascular images, *Med Image Anal* 11: 630—647.

Lesage, D., Angelini, E. D., Bloch, I. & Funka-Lea, G. (2009). A review of 3D vessel lumen segmentation techniques: Models, features and extraction schemes, *Med Image Anal* 13(6): 819–845.

Li, Z. & Kleinstreuer, C. (2006). Analysis of biomechanical factors affecting stent-graft migration in an abdominal aortic aneurysm model, *J Biomech* 39: 2264—2273.

Lu, J., Egger, J., Wimmer, A., Grosskopf, S., Freisleben, B., Miga, M. I. & Cleary, K. R. (2008). Detection and visualization of endoleaks in CT data for monitoring of thoracic and abdominal aortic aneurysm stents, *Proc. of SPIE*, Vol. 6918, SPIE, San Diego, CA, USA, p. 69181F.

Maintz, A. J. B. & Viergever, M. A. (1998). A survey of medical image registration, *Medical Image Analysis* 2(1): 1—37.

Manduca, A., Fletcher, J. G., Wentz, R. J., Shields, R. C., Vrtiska, T. J., Siddiki, H., Nielson, T., Hu, X. P. & Clough, A. V. (2009). Reproducibility of aortic pulsatility measurements from ECG-gated abdominal CTA in patients with abdominal aortic aneurysms, *Proc. of SPIE*, Vol. 7262, SPIE, Lake Buena Vista, FL, USA, p. 72620L.

Manzke, R., Kohler, T., Nielsen, T., Hawkes, D. & Grass, M. (2004). Automatic phase determination for retrospectively gated cardiac CT, *Medical Physics* 31: 3345—3362.

Mattes, J., Steingruber, I., Netzer, M., Fritscher, K., Kopf, H., Jaschke, W. & Schubert, R. (2005). Spatio-temporal changes and migration of stent grafts after endovascular aortic aneurysm repair, *Int. Congr. Ser.* 1281: 393–397.

Muhs, B. E., Teutelink, A., Prokop, M., Vincken, K. L., Moll, F. L. & Verhagen, H. J. M. (2006). Endovascular aneurysm repair alters renal artery movement: a preliminary evaluation using dynamic CTA, *Journal of Endovacular Therapy* 13(4): 476—480.

Muhs, B. E., Vincken, K. L., van Prehn, J., Stone, M. K., Bartels, L. W., Prokop, M., Moll, F. L. & Verhagen, H. J. (2006). Dynamic Cine-CT angiography for the evaluation of the thoracic aorta; insight in dynamic changes with implications for thoracic endograft treatment, *Eur J Vasc Endovasc Surg* 32(5): 532—536.

Murphy, K., van Ginneken, B., Klein, S., Staring, M., de Hoop, B., Viergever, M. & Pluim, J. (2011). Semi-automatic construction of reference standards for evaluation of image registration, *Medical Image Analysis* 15(1): 71–84.

Noblet, V., Heinrich, C., Heitz, F. & Armspach, J. (2006). Retrospective evaluation of a topology preserving non-rigid registration method, *Medical Image Analysis* 10(3): 366–384.

Ohnesorge, B., Flohr, T., Becker, C., Kopp, A. F., Schoepf, U. J., Baum, U., Knez, A., Klingenbeck-Regn, K. & Reiser, M. F. (2000). Cardiac imaging by means of electrocardiographically gated multisection spiral CT: initial experience, *Radiology* 217: 564—571.

Prokop, M. (2005). New challenges in MDCT, *European Journal of Radiology* 15: 35—45.

Quek, F. & Kirbas, C. (2001). Vessel extraction in medical images by wave-propagation and traceback, *IEEE Trans Med Imaging* 20(2): 117–131.

Roos, J. E., Hellinger, J. C., Hallet, R., Fleischmann, D., Zarins, C. K. & Rubin, G. D. (2005). Detection of endograft fractures with multidetector row computed tomography, *J. Vasc. Surg.* 42(5): 1002–1006.

Rueckert, D., Sonoda, L., Hayes, C., Hill, D., Leach, M. & Hawkes, D. (1999). Nonrigid registration using free-form deformations: application to breast MR images, *Medical Imaging, IEEE Transactions on* 18(8): 712–721.

Stavropoulos, S. W. & Charagundla, S. R. (2007). Imaging techniques for detection and management of endoleaks after endovascular aortic aneurysm repair, *Radiology* 243(3): 641—655.

Teutelink, A., Muhs, B., Vincken, K. L., Wartels, L. W., Cornelissen, S. A., van Herwaarden, J. A., Prokop, M., Moll, F. L. & Verhagen, H. J. M. (2007). Use of dynamic computed tomography to evaluate pre- and postoperative aortic changes in AAA patients undergoing eneurysm repair, *J. Endovasc. Ther.* 14(1): 44–49.

Thirion, J. P. (1998). Image matching as a diffusion process: an analogy with maxwell's demons, *Medical Image Analysis* 2(3): 243–60.

Thodberg, H. H. (2003). Minimum description length shape and appearance models, *IN IMAGE PROCESSING MEDICAL IMAGING, IPMI* pp. 51—62.

van der Laan, M. J., Teutelink, A., Meijer, R., Wixon, C. L. & Blankensteijn, J. D. (2003). Noninvasive evaluation of the effectiveness of endovascular AAA exclusion, *Journal of Endovascular Therapy: An Official Journal of the International Society of Endovascular Specialists* 10(3): 458–462. PMID: 12932156.

van Herwaarden, J. A., Bartels, L. W., Muhs, B. E., Vincken, K. L., Lindeboom, M. Y., Teutelink, A., Moll, F. L. & Verhagen, H. J. (2006). Dynamic magnetic resonance angiography of the aneurysm neck: Conformational changes during the cardiac cycle with possible consequences for endograft sizing and future design, *J. Vasc. Surg.* 44(1): 22—28.

van Herwaarden, J. A., Muhs, B. E., Vincken, K. L., van Prehn, J., Teutelink, A., Bartels, L. W., Moll, F. L. & Verhagen, H. J. (2006). Aortic compliance following EVAR and the influence of different endografts: determination using dynamic MRA, *Journal of Endovascular Therapy* 13(3): 406—414.

Wells, W. M., III, Viola, P. & Kikinis, R. (1996). Multi-Modal volume registration by maximization of mutual information.

Williamson, E. E., Kirsch, J., Araoz, P. A., Edmister, W. B., Borgeson, D. D., Glockner, J. F. & Breen, J. F. (2008). ECG-Gated cardiac CT angiography using 64-MDCT for detection of patent foramen ovale, *American Journal of Roentgenology* 190: 929—933.

Wink, O., Niessen, W. & Viergever, M. (2004). Multiscale vessel tracking, *IEEE Trans Med Imaging* 23(1): 130–133.

Worz, S., Godinez, W. J., Rohr, K., Pluim, J. P. W. & Dawant, B. M. (2009). Segmentation of 3D tubular structures based on 3D intensity models and particle filter tracking, *Proc. of SPIE*, Vol. 7259, Lake Buena Vista, FL, USA, p. 72591P.

Xu, C. & Prince, J. L. (1998). Snakes, shapes and gradient vector flow, *IEEE Transactions on Image Processing* 7(3): 359—369.

Zarins, C. K., White, R. A., Schwarten, D., Kinney, E., Diethrich, E. B., Hodgson, K. J. & Fogarty, T. J. (1999). AneuRx stent graft versus open surgical repair of abdominal aortic aneurysms: multicenter prospective clinical trial, *J. Vasc. Surg.* 29(2): 292–305.

Zhou, C., Chan, H., Chughtai, A., Patel, S., Agarwal, P., Hadjiiski, L. M., Sahiner, B., Wei, J., Ge, J., Kazerooni, E. A., Giger, M. L. & Karssemeijer, N. (2008). Automated segmentation and tracking of coronary arteries in ECG-gated cardiac CT scans, *Proc. of SPIE*, Vol. 6915, San Diego, CA, USA, p. 69150O.

8

A Prospective Clinical Economic and Quality of Life Analysis of Open Repair, Endovascular Aortic Repair and Best Medical Treatment in High Risk Patients with AAA

Sherif Sultan and Niamh Hynes
Western Vascular Institute, University College Hospital Galway and Galway Clinic
Ireland

1. Introduction

There is consensus that endovascular aneurysm repair (EVAR) offers several benefits when compared to open repair of abdominal aortic aneurysm (AAA). Although originally introduced for patients considered unfit for major surgery. (Parodi, 1991) EVAR has been used increasingly in patients judged fit for open repair (OR). Results of randomized trials demonstrated that the 30-day mortality in such patients is 2%. (EVAR trial 1 participants, 2005; Prinssen 2004)

The results of the EVAR-2 trial stunned the vascular community. The high mortality rates (9% at 30 days and 64% at 4 years) in the EVAR arm elicited trepidation that the minimally invasive approach may afford no benefit compared with the natural history of untreated AAAs in high-risk patients. (EVAR trial 2 participants, 2005) However, subsequent data from the Society for Vascular Surgery (SVS) Lifeline Registry (Sicard, 2006) and the Veterans Affairs National Surgical Quality Improvement Program (Bush, 2007) have shown that EVAR benefits many patients who fulfilled the EVAR-2 high-risk criteria by curtailing perioperative sequelae.

All of these published studies used objective endpoints of morbidity and mortality. However, in a high-risk cohort, the issue of quality of life in terms of years gained needs to be addressed, as well as the broader issue of the cost to society. There are also questions as to which patients are going to die from something else before they benefit from the aneurysm repair, which patients should not be treated, and what happens to patients who choose non-interventional management. These are complex issues, so it is necessary to approach optimizing AAA treatment of high-risk patients from a number of perspectives. Clinically, we need to verify the efficacy and safety of each treatment option and identify if a subgroup exists in which repair poses more of a risk than a benefit. Secondly, from the patient's viewpoint, what price is he/she willing to pay for quality of life? Finally, how much is the healthcare system keen to invest for optimal AAA treatment?

The aim of our study was to scrutinize EVAR as a feasible treatment option for high risk patients and elucidate whether it can enhance survival and quality of life in a cost-effective manner.

2. Methods

2.1 Study design

In 2002, a prospective study was designed to compare EVAR to open repair or best medical therapy (BMT) in high-risk AAA patients with aneurysms deemed suitable for EVAR. Patients with AAAs >4.5 cm on the initial duplex ultrasound had computed tomographic angiograms (CTA), which were scored for anatomical severity and EVAR suitability using guidelines from the Society for Vascular Surgery/American Association for Vascular Surgery (SVS/ AAVS). (Chaikof, 2002) Based on these recommendations, patients were assigned co-morbidity scores and classified as high risk if they were >60 years old and had at least one of the following co-morbidities:

- symptomatic congestive heart failure,
- valvular heart disease,
- cardiac arrhythmia,
- chronic obstructive pulmonary disease, or
- chronic kidney disease (kidney damage, a glomerular filtration rate,60 mL/min/1.73 m2 for 3 or more months regardless of the underlying etiology, or serum creatinine .200 mmol/L).

The decision on the management modality took into consideration life expectancy, operative risk, and risk of rupture, (Dorros, 1997; Sultan , 2001) but the ultimate decision was made by the patient after an adequate understanding of each procedure's risks and benefits had been discussed with the patient, the family, and the primary care physician.

Eligible patients electing BMT received a statin, a cardioselective beta-blocker, aspirin (300 mg/d), and clopidogrel (75 mg/d). Patients opting for intervention were also prescribed this pharmacological combination; however, clopidogrel was introduced only postoperatively. (Oaikhinan, 2004).

It is our policy that once a patient is deemed very high risk for elective AAA repair, the risk of survival following emergent repair does not warrant an attempt at surgery. Therefore, once a decision not to operate was taken, a red label was placed on the patient's hospital chart indicating that a decision not to operate had been made should the patient present to our Accident and Emergency Department with rupture. (Hynes, 2005)

2.2 Patient enrollment

Between January 2002 and January 2007, 1083 patients were referred to our tertiary care university center for evaluation of their aortic disease. Of these, 162 patients (119 men; mean age 76 years) were classified as high risk and had aneurysms anatomically suitable for EVAR. Fifty-two patients (36 men; mean age 74.6+/-7.3 years) had open repair, 66 (52 men; mean age 72.6+/-6.3 years) underwent EVAR, and 44 (31 men; mean age 80.9+/-6.7 years) were managed medically. All patients had the treatment that was originally decided upon.

All patients were classified as ASA (American Society of Anesthesiologists) III or IV; more than half (54%) of the OR group were ASA IV compared to 62% of the EVAR group and 80% of the non-operative group.

2.3 Follow-up protocols

EVAR patients had a plain abdominal radiograph (anteroposterior and lateral views) and color duplex ultrasound prior to discharge. They had a repeat color duplex ultrasound and

radiograph at 6 weeks, 3 months, 6 months, and 6-month intervals thereafter. CT scans were performed at 6 months and then yearly, unless there was evidence of sac expansion or substantial endoleak on duplex ultrasound or migration was noted on the radiograph.
Following open repair, patients were seen at 6 weeks, at 6-month intervals for 18 months, and yearly thereafter. OR patients had clinical examination and ankle-brachial index measurements at 6 weeks and clinical examination at subsequent visits. Duplex ultrasound or CT examination was performed if clinically indicated or the patient became symptomatic. BMT patients were followed at 6-month intervals with color duplex ultrasound at each visit.

2.4 Endpoints

The primary clinical endpoint was survival without aneurysm-related death. Cause of death was obtained from primary healthcare physicians if the death occurred outside our hospital or from medical records if the death occurred in hospital. All ruptures were confirmed by CT and/or autopsy. Secondary endpoints were freedom from all-cause mortality, secondary intervention, and major adverse clinical events (death, myocardial infarction, major amputation, cerebrovascular accident, respiratory morbidity requiring reintubation with/without tracheostomy, or renal failure requiring dialysis).
The two quality-of-life endpoints were cost per QALY (quality-adjusted life years) and TWIST (time spent without symptoms of disease and toxicity of treatment), a special QALY endpoint incorporating both length and quality of life. (Gelber, 1989) TWIST was useful for treatment comparison by compensating for situations when differences in aneurysm-related mortality were statistically significant but overall survival differences were not, since it acknowledges that extensions to disease-free time may be at the expense of treatment toxicity. To integrate quality and quantity of life, the quality-adjusted time with and without symptoms or toxicity (Q-TWIST) was used as a natural extension of the quality-of-life- oriented TWIST endpoint. QTWIST was an adaptation of the concept of QALYs; the methodology was extended so that periods spent with toxicity or relapses were included in the analysis but weighted to represent their quality value relative to TWIST. This allowed us to look at the intervention and the health effects persisting beyond the perioperative period.
In this study, the Q-TWIST was the sum of the quality-adjusted time (u) spent undergoing treatment and experiencing toxicity (TOX, i.e., hospital stay associated with the primary intervention including perioperative morbidity and mortality) plus the time spent free of disease in perfect health (TWIST), plus the time spent experiencing symptoms of disease relapse (REL, i.e., hospital stay associated with any secondary intervention including perioperative morbidity and mortality). In the formula for Q-TWIST (utTOX + TWIST + urREL), the utility values ut and ur associated with the periods of survival for both EVAR (ut50.7, ur50.7) and open repair (ut50.56, ur50.7) were based on sensitivity values from the Interim Report on the Cost-Effectiveness of Elective Endovascular Repair Compared to Open Surgical Repair of Abdominal Aortic Aneurysms prepared for the Ontario Ministry of Health and Long-term Care. (Bowen, 2005) The quality adjusted time utility for the BMT group in this study was u50.56.

2.5 Statistical analysis

The anatomical severity scores were correlated with technical success, endoleak rate, migration, conversion rate, and the need for secondary intervention. Prediction of perioperative outcome was assessed using the Kertai customized probability model based on a combination of clinical predictors, type of vascular surgery, and concomitant medication use. (Kertai, 2005)

Cumulative rates for survival without aneurysm-related or all-cause death were estimated using Kaplan-Meier analysis; curves were compared using the log-rank test. Due to the risks of informative censoring and biased Kaplan-Meier estimates of the survival function, a partitioned survival analysis was performed.(Glasziou, 1998) Overall survival was partitioned into the time spent in each health state, i.e., time spent without symptoms or toxicity from treatment was separated from time spent with toxicity of treatment and with secondary intervention. The mean duration in each state for each group was combined as a weighted sum according to the Q-TWIST model. Weighting the time spent in each health state at the group level, rather that at the individual level, avoided the need to weigh censored survival times and thus overcame the problem of informative censoring. Kaplan-Meier survival curves corresponding to each transition time were overlaid on one graph to show the partitioning of overall survival. The upper time limit for the analysis, 48 months, was based on the follow-up time of the study cohort and was chosen to reduce censoring.

The influence of co-morbid factors on outcome was determined using Cox proportional hazards models. The risk of a complication after open repair was compared with that after EVAR; the results are presented as risk ratios (RR) with 95% confidence intervals (CI). Differences among treatment groups were evaluated with ANOVA and the Mann-Whitney U test for continuous variables or Fisher exact test for proportions. Differences among groups were taken as significant if $p<0.05$.

2.6 Cost analysis

The total costs per procedure, inclusive of follow-up, were calculated to estimate the cost per QALY and the incremental cost-effectiveness ratio of an EVAR program relative to the standard open repair program. The incremental cost effectiveness ratio was determined by measuring the incremental benefits (in life years) for the new intervention (EVAR) and dividing it by the incremental cost relative to current practice (cost of open repair).

A relative value unit (RVU) cost accounting system, which included both direct and indirect expenses, was used at our hospital. (Finkler, 1999; West, 1996) Individual charge items were assigned a weight or RVU. Expenses from revenue generating centers were allocated to each of the charge items within a department according to category, such as labor, supplies, equipment depreciation, and overhead. The cost per category was derived from each charge item on the basis of its RVU. Mean hospital costs and mean diagnostic-related group (DRG)-weighted payments were analyzed to determine net profit or loss for the hospital. The DRG codes for AAA repair were F08A (major reconstruct vascular procedures without cardiopulmonary bypass pump with catastrophic CC) and F08B (major reconstruct vascular procedures without cardiopulmonary bypass pump without catastrophic CC).

Data from our cost analysis were correlated with allocations to our hospital by the National Health Service Executive for the relevant DRG codes. The RVU used for a DRG was based on amalgamated data from the 9 main Irish National University Teaching Hospitals.

3. Results

Although patients in the BMT group were on average older ($p<0.0001$), there was no significant difference in the proportion of patients with major cardiac ($p=0.104$), pulmonary ($p=0.170$), or renal ($p=0.108$) diseases among the 3 groups (Table 1).

	OR	EVAR	BMT	p
Number	52	66	44	
Aneurysm Diameter, cm	6.2+/-1.6	5.4+/-1.1	6.2+/-1.7	**0.005***
Age, y	74.6+/-7.3	72.6+/-6.3	80.9+/-6.7	**<0.0001***
Cardiac	27 (51.9%)	38 (57.6%)	32 (72.3%)	0.104
Ischaemic Heart Disease	25 (48.1%)	39 (59.1%)	36 (68.2%)	0.137
Congestive Cardiac Failure	19 (36.5%)	34 (51.5%)	27 (61.4%)	**0.047***
Respiratory Disease	23 (44.3%)	40 (60.6%)	26 (59.1%)	0.170
Renal Impairment	18 (34.6%)	25 (37.9%)	24 (54.6%)	0.108
Hypertension	34 (65.4%)	45 (68.2%)	28 (63.6%)	0.881
Cerebrovascular Disease	12 (23.1%)	17 (25.8%)	8 (18.2%)	0.654
Mean SVS combined Co-morbidity Severity Score	7.75	9.89	11.1	0.057
Mean Kertai Customised Probability Index	28.0	34.4	35.6	0.070

Continuous data are presented as means ± standard deviation; categorical data are given as counts (percentages).
BMT: best medical treatment; EVAR: endovascular aneurysm repair; OR: open repair

Table 1. Demographics and Risk Factors for the 3 Treatment Groups

The mean aneurysm size was smaller in the EVAR group (mean 5.4±1.1cm; $p=0.005$) versus OR (mean 6.2±1.6cm) or BMT (mean 6.2±1.7cm). There were also no significant differences in the proportions of hypertensive patients ($p=0.881$).
All patients were anatomically suitable for EVAR, and the proportion of patients at moderate to severe risk of access failure, endograft limb obstruction, or embolisation was not statistically different among the groups (Table 2). However, using the strict SVS/AAVS scoring system, the proportion of patients at moderate to severe risk of endoleak was zero in the EVAR group ($p=0.008$), while the proportion of patients at moderate to severe risk of failed deployment was highest in the BMT group ($p=0.015$).

	OR	EVAR	BMT	
Global score for risk of major morbidity and mortality after endograft repair ≥2	39%	57%	65%	P=0.079
Anatomic score of risk of access failure or endograft limb obstruction ≥2	76%	57%	86%	***P=0.008****
Anatomic score of risk of embolization ≥2	85%	77%	95%	P=0.053
Anatomic score of risk of endoleak ≥2	30%	0%	56%	***P<0.0001****
Anatomic score of risk of failed deployed ≥2	39%	43%	79%	***P=0.0003****

BMT: best medical treatment; EVAR: endovascular aneurysm repair; OR: open repair

Table 2. Anatomical Severity Scores

3.1 Initial outcomes

In the EVAR group, all but 2 procedures were completed satisfactorily. An 82-year-old man with severely calcified iliac arteries was converted to open repair following right common iliac artery perforation and a 79 year-old woman implanted with a Quantum device that failed to deploy properly was treated with a silver-impregnated Dacron graft.

Insofar as operative details are concerned, the mean length of the operation was considerably reduced in the EVAR group (169 minutes) compared to the open repair group (193 minutes; p=0.04). The need for blood transfusions was also significantly lower in the EVAR group (mean 0.6 units) versus the open group (mean 1.8 units; p=0.015).

There was no significant difference in the mean rise in postoperative creatinine between the groups (p=0.845).

Mean lengths of hospital and intensive care unit (ICU) stay were reduced with EVAR (10.2 and 0.5 days, respectively) compared with OR (20.4 and 6.8 days, respectively; p<0.0001 for both). In the EVAR group, 11 type II endoleaks were noted on postoperative duplex and/or CT scans; all resolved spontaneously.

3.2 Clinical endpoints

Compared to open repair, the 30-day morbidity was significantly improved for EVAR patients (6% versus 23%; p=0.007), but 30-day mortality was not different between EVAR (3.0%) and OR (5.8%; p=0.653).

At 30 days, freedom from MACE was similar for EVAR (95.5%) and OR (88.5%; p=0.173, RR=0.39, 95% CI 0.10 to 1.46). At 4 years, freedom from MACE was significantly improved with EVAR (77.5%) compared with BMT (27.9%; p=0.001, RR=0.32, 95% CI 0.17 to 0.61) and similar to OR (75.4%; p=0.519, RR=0.76, 95% CI 0.33 to 1.73).

Mean follow-up was 22.7+/-16.1 months; no patient was lost to follow-up. There were 2 (3.0%) aneurysm-related deaths in the EVAR group, while in the BMT group, 11 (25%) ruptures occurred over the study period, 5 within 6 months of diagnosis. Nine of these BMT rupture patients presented to the hospital, and each had a CT scan that confirmed rupture; none of these patients was operated upon. The 2 remaining patients died in the community, and autopsy reports cited AAA rupture as the cause of death.

At 1 year, the chance of survival without aneurysm-related death was 12.2% higher in the EVAR group compared to the BMT group (p=0.049, RR=0.23, 95% CI 0.06 to 0.94). This survival benefit increased with time, and at 4 years, the survival without aneurysm-related death (Figure 1) was significantly greater in the EVAR group (96.7%) compared to BMT (66.8%; p=0.002, RR=0.08, 95% CI 0.02 to 0.26), but it was not statistically different from OR (93.9%; p=0.483, RR 0.53, 95% CI 0.09 to 3.09).

Only 2 factors were found to adversely influence survival without aneurysm-related death (Table 3): age (p=0.034, RR=1.09, 95% CI 1.01 to 1.18) and aneurysm size (p=0.004, RR=1.51, 95% CI 1.14 to 2.00).

Four-year cumulative survival without death from any cause (Figure. 2) following EVAR (78.8%) was not statistically different from OR (84.9%; p=0.590, RR=1.30, 95% CI 0.50 to 3.36), but was significantly improved compared to BMT (27.9%; p<0.001, RR=0.30, 95% CI 0.16 to 0.57). As with aneurysm-related mortality, only age (p=0.014, RR=1.06, 95% CI 1.01 to 1.10) and aneurysm size (p=0.001, RR=1.35, 95% CI 1.13 to 1.62) were found to influence freedom from all-cause mortality (Table 4).

Risk Factor	Risk Ratio	95% CI	p
Age	**1.0889**	**1.0066 to 1.1780**	**0.0337***
Male	1.8064	0.5052 to 6.4596	0.3630
Cardiac	1.9562	0.4893 to 7.8202	0.3426
Respiratory	2.0177	0.5885 to 6.9174	0.2641
Renal	1.9054	0.6416 to 5.6588	0.2457
Hypertension	1.1772	0.3613 to 3.8357	0.7866
Diabetes	1.2693	0.4514 to 3.5691	0.6512
Smoking	0.6712	0.2459 to 1.8323	0.4365
Aneurysm Diameter	**1.5098**	**1.1410 to 1.9977**	**0.0039***

CI: confidence interval.

Table 3. Results of the Cox Proportional Hazards Model for Aneurysm-Related Mortality

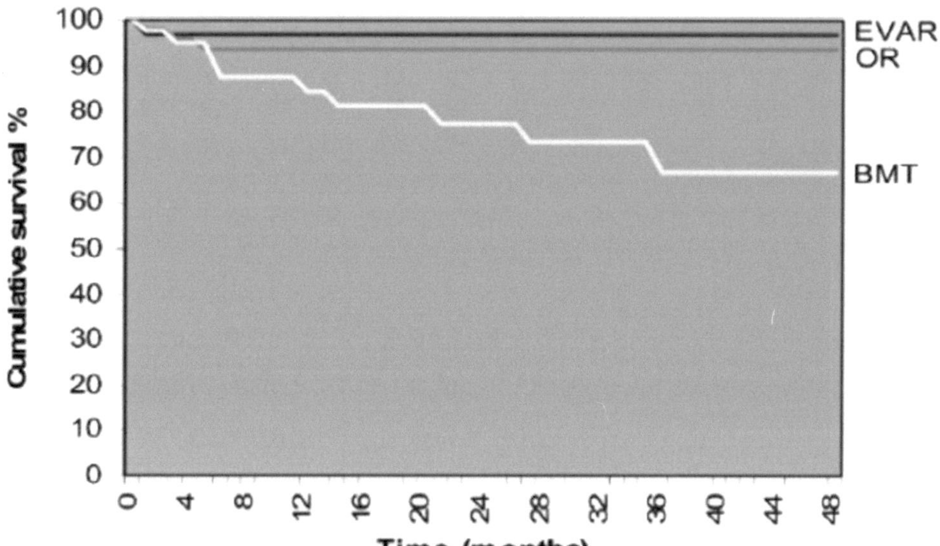

Patients at risk													
EVAR	66	54	44	40	37	31	23	17	12	4	2	1	1
OR	52	45	41	38	37	35	32	27	18	11	10	8	5
BMT	44	37	32	30	24	22	20	17	11	11	7	4	3

At 4 years, EVAR (96.7%) vs. OR (93.9%; p50.483, RR50.53, 95% CI 0.09 to 3.09) or vs. BMT (66.8%; p50.0021, RR50.08, 95% CI 0.02 to 0.26).
BMT: best medical treatment; EVAR: endovascular aneurysm repair; OR: open repair

Fig. 1. Aneurysm-related Kaplan-Meier survival curves.

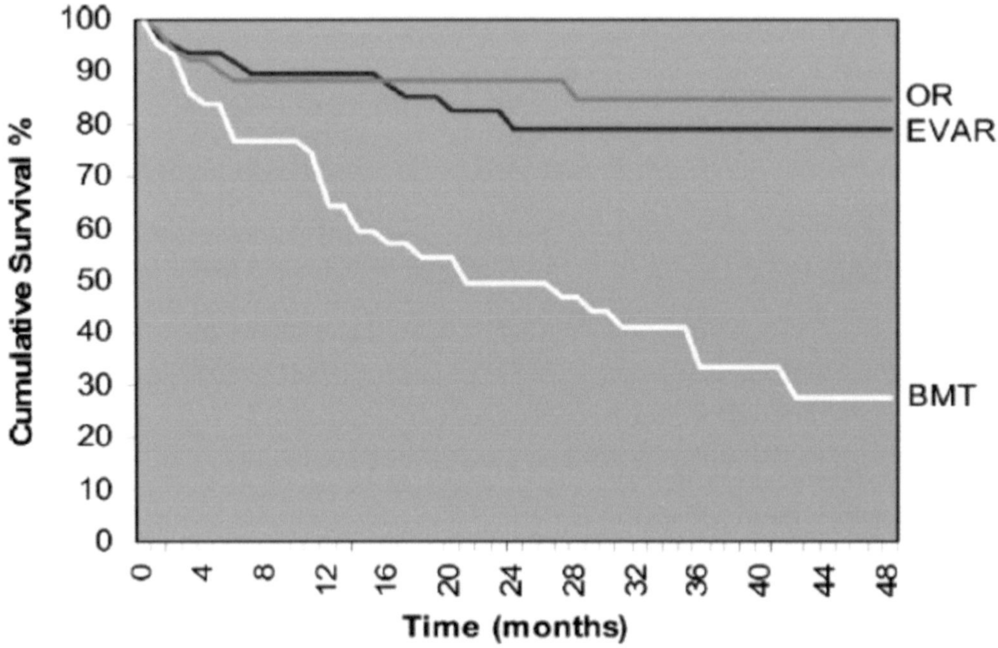

Patients at risk

EVAR	66	54	44	40	37	31	23	17	12	4	2	1	1
OR	52	45	41	38	37	35	32	27	18	11	10	8	5
BMT	44	37	32	30	24	22	20	17	11	11	7	4	3

Fig. 2. All-cause Kaplan-Meier survival curves. At 4 years, EVAR (78.8%) vs. OR (84.9%; P=0.59, RR=1.3, 95% CI 0.50 to 3.36) or vs. BMT (27.9%; p=0.0005, RR=0.30, 95% CI 0.16 to 0.57).

Risk Factor	Risk Ratio	95% CI	p
Age	**1.0555**	**1.0109 to 1.1020**	**0.0141***
Male	1.7141	0.8223 to 3.5731	0.1505
Cardiac	1.3501	0.6614 to 2.7559	0.4097
Respiratory	1.3264	0.6781 to 2.5942	0.4093
Renal	1.3485	0.7273 to 2.5002	0.3426
Hypertension	1.2164	0.6265 to 2.3616	0.6605
Diabetes	1.3173	0.7217 to 2.4045	0.3693
Smoking	1.2317	0.6749 to 2.2479	0.4972
Aneurysm Diameter	**1.3495**	**1.1276 to 1.6151**	**0.0011***

CI: confidence interval.

Table 4. Results of the Cox Proportional Hazards Model for All-Cause Mortality

3.3 Secondary interventions

Over the observation period, there were 3 secondary interventions in the EVAR group versus 1 among the OR patients. Thus, at 4 years, the intervention-free survival rate for EVAR (94.5%) was similar to OR (98.1%, p=0.410, HR=2.51, 95% CI 0.35 to 18.0). In the OR group, an 80-year-old woman suffered distal embolization; femoral thromboembolectomy, endarterectomy, and femorofemoral bypass grafting were done 72 hours postoperatively.
Two EVAR patients had limb sequelae: a 76-year-old man had a kink develop in the contralateral limb due to aneurysm tortuosity and an 83-year-old man had a thrombosed left graft limb 1 year post EVAR. Both were treated with endovascular techniques and recovered. The third secondary procedure was done in an 82-year-old woman with a type III endoleak diagnosed on the postoperative duplex scan. An aortic cuff and iliac extension were placed 3 days after her primary procedure.

3.4 Quality of life assessment

Over a 4-year follow-up period, the QTWIST was 3.64 years for EVAR and 3.60 years for OR. The 28% 4-year freedom from all-cause mortality in the BMT group resulted in only a 2.22-year Q-TWIST for every 4 years of treatment. Sensitivity analysis showed that Q-TWIST was significantly improved with EVAR compared to OR over a full range of utility values between 0 and 1 (p<0.003; Table 5).

EVAR vs. Open Repair					
	Utility for TOX				
Utility for Relapse	0	0.25	0.50	0.75	1.0
0	0.0029	0.0028	0.0027	0.0026	0.0025
0.25	0.0030	0.0028	0.0027	0.0027	0.0026
0.50	0.0030	0.0029	0.0028	0.0027	0.0026
0.75	0.0031	0.0029	0.0028	0.0027	0.0027
1.0	0.0031	0.0030	0.0029	0.0027	0.0027
EVAR vs. Best Medical Therapy					
	Utility for TOX				
Utility for Relapse	0	0.25	0.50	0.75	1.0
0	0.039	0.044	0.05	0.057	0.064
0.25	0.040	0.045	0.05	0.057	0.064
0.50	0.040	0.045	0.05	0.059	0.066
0.75	0.041	0.046	0.05	0.059	0.066
1.0	0.041	0.046	0.05	0.060	0.067

Table 5. Threshold Utility Analyses

3.5 Cost analysis

In the analysis of costs (Table 6), 52 high-risk patients were treated with OR over a 5-year period (2002–2007) at a total inpatient cost of €1,257,457. The 66 patients treated with EVAR (14 patients more than OR) incurred a lower cost of €1,129,138. If the cost of follow-up over 4 years was included, the mean costs per patient were €18,476 for EVAR and €24,252 for OR, a savings of €5,776 per patient treated with EVAR. The in-hospital costs were €17,108 for EVAR and €24,182 for OR. For the F08A code, our hospital was assigned a RVU of 5.44 and was allocated €23,453 in our budget. For the F08B code, our hospital was assigned a RVU 2.44, providing a budgetary allocation of €10,625. Thus, for AAA repair, EVAR generated a net profit of € 6345 per case for the hospital, while OR was done at a net loss of €729 per case.

Costs		EVAR (n=66)	OR (n=52)	BMT (n=44)
Pre-op work-up				
CTAngiogram	€600	€39,600	€31,200	€26,400
Chest X-ray	€88	€5,779	€4,553	€3,853
Duplex Screening	€185	€12,210	€9,620	€8,140
Echocardiogram	€145	€9,570	€7,540	€6,380
Pulmonary function Tests	€125	€8,250	€6,500	€5,500
Pharmacy, transfusion and Laboratory costs	€305-€415	€27,390	€21,580	€13,420
Accomodation				
Hospital Bed *per diem*	€540	€348,300	€382,860	€23,760
ICU Bed *per diem*	€1,646	€51,018	€582,592	
Theatre				
Per diem Theatre Overheads (inc. Staffing, Radiology etc)	€6,402	€105,630	€166,447	
Equipment				
Graft (Intervascular)	€915	€1,830	€47,580	
Graft (Dynaflo)	€625	€11,250	€625	
Endograft	€7,000	€462,000		
Catheters/Wires/Balloons etc	€635	€41,941		
Embolisation				
Coils	€554	€1,659		
Catheters/Wires/Balloons etc	€359	€1,077		
Bed Stay	€545	€1,635		
Total-In-Patient Cost		**€1,129,138**	**€1,257,457**	**€87,453**
Follow-up				
Vascular Laboratory	€150	€33,150	€3,640	€23,350
PFA	€88	€19,351		
CTA	€300	€37,800		
Total Cost		**€1,219,439**	**€1,261,097**	**€110,803**
Mean Cost per Patient		€18,476	€24,252	€2,518
Q-TWiST		3.64years	3.60years	2.22years
QALY		0.91	0.90	0.56
Cost per QALY		**€5,076**	**€6,737**	**€1,134**

Table 6. Cost Analysis

Treatment with EVAR cost €5076 per QALY, which was €1661 less than OR, giving a negative incremental cost-effectiveness ratio (ICER) for EVAR versus OR of €144,388 per QALY gained. EVAR was €3,942 more expensive per QALY than BMT alone; the ICER was €45,595 per QALY gained with EVAR versus BMT.

4. Dicussion

At present, considerable controversy exists in the vascular community regarding optimum management of high-risk patients with large AAAs. There has been a remarkable convergence of data from randomized trials giving level-1 evidence that EVAR reduces operative mortality by two thirds compared with open repair; the survival benefit is sustained over intermediate-term follow-up in low- to intermediate risk patients.(EVAR trial-1 participants, 2005; Prinssen, 2004) However, the results of these trials cannot be generalized to patients who are at high risk for open repair. The patients in EVAR 2 (EVAR trial-2 participants, 2005) were older and had more cardiovascular co-morbidities; this was reflected in the high 9% 30-day mortality rate and a 4-year survival of only 36%. Moreover, there was considerable crossover between the trial groups and after randomization to the non-intervention group, 20% of patients subsequently underwent elective repair of their aneurysm. Furthermore, the trial was not limited to an objective list of high-risk criteria, which led to a lack of objectivity and uniformity in what is truly a high-risk patient. This biased the study against EVAR and weakened the investigators conclusions that prophylactic operations designed to improve survival cannot be effective in patients with short life expectancy. They concluded that EVAR is much more costly than no intervention, without a survival benefit in high-risk patients.

Our results show that EVAR can be safely performed in high-risk patients. Our 30-day perioperative mortality (3%) rate was considerably lower than the EVAR-2 trial. However, although we saw a clear advantage at 4 years with EVAR versus BMT, we did not see a clear benefit in terms of all-cause mortality for EVAR versus open repair. When interpreting these results, one has to question the merits of using all-cause mortality as a primary endpoint for a study on a specific treatment. All-cause mortality is an extremely important variable, but it is a metric of limited value when assessing a disease-specific treatment in a senior citizen population. This is best illustrated if you consider that 48 patients in EVAR 1 (EVAR trial-1 participants, 2005) died from cancer, representing about one third of the overall mortality over the study period. These cancer deaths diluted the overall survival benefit conferred by EVAR over open repair. It appeared more logical to us to use survival without aneurysm-related death as our primary endpoint, but here too, the difference between EVAR and OR was not significant, likely due to our high OR survival rate and low morbidity in the context of high-risk patients. This means that a large cohort is needed to show statistical significance without risk of a type II error. However, it confirms that high-risk patients can still experience low perioperative morbidity and high midterm survival if they are treated in centers with high-volume practice and appropriate preoperative patient assessment, optimal selection of operative strategy, careful intraoperative anesthetics management, meticulous attention to operative technical detail, and skilled postoperative management.

At 6 months, a significant 9.3% survival benefit was seen with EVAR compared to BMT. Fully half of the deaths in the non-operative group were due to rupture, and 50% of the ruptures occurred within the first 9 months, which helped to increase the benefit with EVAR to 30% at 4 years. The survival curves for EVAR and non-operative management continue to diverge after 4 years, which contrasts to the EVAR-2 trial, (EVAR trial-2 participants, 2005) in which a high operative mortality rate meant that no late difference in aneurysm related mortality and no difference in overall survival were seen despite more deaths occurring from aneurysm rupture in the non-intervention group. We are not alone in establishing that favorable outcomes are possible in high-risk patients. In an attempt to address some of the issues with EVAR 2, the SVS Outcomes Committee analyzed their Lifeline Registry (Sicard, 2006) and found that 565 of the ,3000 patients in the registry met the high-risk criteria set out in EVAR 2, far exceeding the number of patients in the EVAR 2 trial. Sicard et al. reported that there was a significant difference in 30-day mortality (2.9%) in the investigational device exemption (IDE) trial registries compared to 9% in EVAR 2. Moreover, the 4-year survival rate for the IDE group was 56% (based on all-cause mortality, not just aneurysm-related mortality), versus 36% in EVAR 2, so there was a difference of 20 percentage points between the 2 trials. One explanation for the large difference in both aneurysm-related and all-cause mortality rates between EVAR 2 and the US IDE data is that the EVAR-2 trial was dealing with sicker patients. Another possible explanation is that the actual medical care of these patients was different. The EVAR-2 trial participants explained the long delay between randomization and treatment because of the need to manage patient co-morbidities; they emphasized the need for optimization of the patient before the intervention. Despite a mean aneurysm diameter of 6.7 cm, EVAR was not done until a median of 57 days after randomization. During this time, 9 aneurysms ruptured, causing nearly half of the 20 aneurysm-related deaths in the EVAR group. Once the decision to intervene was taken in our study, the procedure was performed within 14 days, and despite 5 ruptures occurring in the non-operative group within the first 6 months, no ruptures occurred preoperatively in the EVAR or open repair groups. It could then be argued that if patients are anatomically suitable for EVAR, they should be treated without delay. However, it is extremely important to adequately assess and improve patient fitness before intervention, which is especially true in very high-risk patients. All our patients were given best medical treatment, (Oaikhinan, 2004) and every effort was made to optimize cardio-respiratory and renal function preoperatively, which our extended mean length of hospital stay reflects.

4.1 Benefit to the individual

The debate over the relative long- or intermediate- term risks and benefits associated with intervention versus observation is especially pertinent in the context of high-risk patients. The improvement in QALY in the immediate postoperative period for both EVAR and OR in most studies reflects the relief a patient must feel at overcoming intervention and escaping a potentially lethal disease. (Malina, 2007; UK Small Aneurysm Trial Participants, 1998) For some patients, the knowledge that they have a large or expanding aneurysm and the realization that outcomes following ruptured AAA repair are bleak may cause considerable psychological stress and impact significantly on their quality of life.

Most studies have shown that quality of life is improved in the perioperative period following EVAR compared to OR, which is a reflection of the shorter hospital stay, reduced blood loss, early improvements in physical mobility and pain, as well as a likelihood for a patient to be discharged to home rather than to an institution. (Geraghty, 2003; Lee, 2004) However, most studies demonstrated no difference in QALY when patients are surveyed at remote time points.(EVAR trial-2 participants, 2005; Lottman, 2004; Prinssen, 2004) On the other hand, Aljabri et al. (Aljabri, 2006) and the DREAM trial investigators (Prinssen, 2004) reported that EVAR patients had a lower QALY 6 months after surgery than in OR patients.

Much criticism has been directed toward EVAR because of the impression that the need for long-term surveillance and risk of secondary interventions will reduce future quality of life. The DREAM investigators (Blankensteijn, 2005) reported that the rate of reintervention after EVAR in the first 9 months after randomization was almost 3 times the rate after open repair. High reintervention rates were a problem in EVAR 1 (EVAR trial-1 participants, 2005) and are most certainly due to poor preoperative estimation of anatomical suitability. In EVAR 1, 54% of potentially eligible patients were found to be anatomically "suitable" for EVAR, but this proportion ranged from 6% to 100% across the 34 centers, illustrating the variation in assessing this important variable. In our study, the intervention-free survival rates at 4 years were similar for EVAR and OR.

Our low secondary reintervention rate most certainly impacted positively on our quality of life analysis. We had only 3 reinterventions in our EVAR patients, 2 for type III endoleak. None of the 11 type II endoleaks required treatment. In our experience, complete obliteration of all patent branches is not warranted. (Dias, 2004; van Marrewijk, 2004) Our policy is not to intervene either prophylactically or therapeutically for type II endoleaks unless there is a persistent increase in sac diameter .5 mm for 3 months; all of the type II endoleaks in this study resolved within 3 months, and there was no increase in sac diameter.

4.2 Benefit to society

The EVAR-1 investigators showed that aneurysm-related mortality stayed 3% lower with EVAR throughout the 4-year follow-up period. (EVAR trial-1 participants, 2005) However, obtaining this benefit required a 33% increase in hospital costs without a sustained benefit in quality of life. Rationing parameters for healthcare resources are admittedly controversial and generate ethical dilemmas. It has been suggested that perhaps EVAR should be restricted to those patients who are "fit" for surgery, by whatever definition deemed appropriate, as the procedure, the endovascular devices, the continuing need for surveillance imaging, and possible secondary re-interventions are costly.

To the contrary, we have shown that EVAR can be performed with clinical equivalence and enhances quality of life in high-risk patients. However, the benefit to the individual cannot be at the expense of the healthcare system. A report commissioned by the Belgian government and published in 2005 found that EVAR was not cost effective. (Bonneux, 2005) Multiple authors have reported that hospitals lose money on EVAR compared to earning significant profits from OR. In a comprehensive cost analysis, Bertges et al. (Bertges, 2003) analyzed the costs associated with EVAR in 221 Medicare patients and found that "mean total hospital cost was $22,999, and mean reimbursement, weighted by case mix, was $20,837, resulting in a net loss of $2162" per case. However, Patel et al. (Patel, 1999) in a hypothetical Markov model concluded that EVAR was cost effective, with a mean endograft cost of >$13,000 and overhead of an additional $1100. They used a baseline mortality rate of 4.8% for OR and concluded that if OR could be done with comparable morbidity and mortality to EVAR, the cost-effectiveness of EVAR ceased to exist. Similarly, the Belgian report recommended that long-term mortality and morbidity must be lower to make EVAR a cost-effective alternative to OR. (Bonneux, 2005) The Belgian report found that although the endograft contributed most to the cost disparity between OR and EVAR, CT follow-up was the second most important determinant, contributing more to cost than secondary interventions or procedure-related complications.

Contrary to the predictions of Patel et al. (Patel, 1999) and the Belgian report, (Bonneux, 2005) we found that despite no benefit in terms of freedom from MACE, EVAR was cost-effective compared to OR even in this high-risk cohort. We used a comprehensive analysis of the cost benefit ratio of EVAR on a real patient cohort in an attempt to validate the cost-effectiveness of EVAR. We found that the mean cost, including 4-year follow-up, was >€5,000 less with EVAR, giving a negative incremental cost-effectiveness ratio of €144,388 per QALY gained. This is in part due to a financial deal with our graft providers, reduced hospital stay, minimal need for ICU facilities, increasing use of duplex in follow-up, and a low secondary reintervention rate. However, to ensure cost-effectiveness and to guarantee maximum impact of this technology, we believe it must be performed in high-volume centers, which is in line with recommendations from the Belgian report. (Bonneux)

If we minimize perioperative problems, then the question that we really need to ask ourselves is which patients are going to die from something else before they benefit from the aneurysm repair? This question has not yet been answered by any trials or datasets and is fundamental to the treatment of aneurysm disease. From our data, the only factors that we identified as having a negative impact on both all-cause and aneurysm specific mortality were advanced age and large aneurysm diameter.

The physician and patient must decide on an individual basis whether any aneurysm repair should be undertaken, or as EVAR 2 might suggest, whether the patient is so ill that treating the aneurysm would not confer any survival benefit. We reported our results over 48 months, and although the 95% confidence intervals might suggest these to be simple speculative estimations, we strongly believe that our results reflect the reality that endovascular specialists face continually when dealing with high-risk patients. Our study may be underpowered due to the small sample size; however, the patient and family did take the lead in deciding which treatment best suited them.

4.3 Conclusion

We have shown that EVAR significantly reduces both long-term aneurysm-related and all-cause mortality, with minimal operative mortality risk and a low secondary intervention rate. High-risk patients ought to be managed in high-volume centers where they can benefit from specialized multidisciplinary care with low perioperative morbidity and mortality rates. EVAR and OR options are plausible and both can be tailored to the patient. In financial terms, our hospital has profited from our EVAR program. High patient turnover rates and low use of ICU facilities have certainly contributed to its profitability and overall benefit to the individual, health economy, and the community as a whole. We have shown EVAR to be a safe, durable, and feasible option for high-risk patients. It significantly improves quality of life compared to open repair or best medical therapy and can be performed with minimal risk of major complications or secondary intervention. The results of EVAR are exceptional and have positively influenced the choices available to the patients and their referring primary physicians.

5. References

Aljabri B, Al Wahaibi K, Abner D, et al. Patientreported quality of life after abdominal aortic aneurysm surgery: a prospective comparison of endovascular and open repair. J Vasc Surg. 2006;44:1182–1187.

Bertges DJ, Zwolak RM, Deaton DH, et al. Current hospital costs and Medicare reimbursement for endovascular abdominal aortic aneurysm repair. J Vasc Surg. 2003;37:272–279.

Blankensteijn JD, de Jong SE, Prinssen M, et al. Two-year outcomes after conventional or endovascular, repair of abdominal aortic aneurysms. N Engl J Med. 2005;352:2398–2405.

Bonneux L, Cleemput I, Vrijens F, et al. KCE report 23: Elective endovascular treatment of the abdominal aortic aneurysm (AAA). Brussels, Belgium: Belgium Health Care Knowledge Center; 2005.

Bowen J, De Rose G, Hopkins R, et al. Systematic review and cost-effectiveness analysis of elective endovascular repair compared to open surgical repair of abdominal aortic aneurysms. Interim Report for the Ontario Ministry of Health and Longterm Care. Hamilton, ON: Program for Assessment of Technology in Health, McMaster University; July 2005.

Bush RL, Johnson ML, Hedayati N, et al. Performance of endovascular aortic aneurysm repair in high-risk patients: results from the Veterans Affairs National Surgical Quality Improvement Program. J Vasc Surg. 2007;45:227–235.

Chaikof EL, Fillinger MF, Matsumura JS, et al. Identifying and grading factors that modify the outcome of endovascular aortic aneurysm repair. J Vasc Surg. 2002;35:1061–1066.

Dias NV, Ivancev K, Malina M, et al. Intraaneurysm sac pressure measurements after endovascular aneurysm repair: differences between shrinking, unchanged, and expanding aneurysms with and without endoleaks. J Vasc Surg. 2004;39:1229–1235.

Dorros G, Parodi J, Schonholz C, et al. Evaluation of endovascular abdominal aortic aneurysm repair: anatomical classification, procedural success, clinical assessment, and data collection. J Endovasc Surg. 1997;4:203–225.

EVAR trial participants. Endovascular aneurysm repair versus open repair in patients with abdominal aortic aneurysm (EVAR trial 1): randomised controlled trial. Lancet. 2005;365:2179–2186.

EVAR trial participants. Endovascular aneurysm repair and outcome in patients unfit for open repair of abdominal aortic aneurysm (EVAR trial 2): randomised controlled trial. Lancet. 2005;365:2187–2192.

Finkler SA, Ward DM. Cost Accounting for Health Care Organizations: Concepts and Applications, 2nd ed. Gaithersburg, MD: Aspen Publishers; 1999.

Gelber RD, Gelman RS, Goldhirsh A. A qualityof- life-orientated endpoint for comparing therapies. Biometrics. 1989;45:781–795.

Geraghty PJ, Sicard GA. Abdominal aortic aneurysm repair in high-risk and elderly patients. J Cardiovasc Surg (Torino). 2003;44:543–547.

Glasziou PP, Cole BF, Gelber RD, et al. Quality adjusted survival analysis with repeated quality of life measures. Stat Med. 1998;17:1215- 1229.

Hynes N, Koh N, Sultan S. Abdominal aortic aneurysm repair in octogenarians versus younger patients in a tertiary referral center. Vascular. 2005;13:1–11.

Kertai MD, Boersma E, Klein J, et al. Optimizing the prediction of perioperative mortality in vascular surgery by using a customized probability model. Arch Intern Med. 2005;165:898- 904.

Lee WA, Carter JW, Upchurch G, et al. Perioperative outcomes after open and m endovascular repair of intact abdominal aortic aneurysms in the United States during 2001. J Vasc Surg. 2004;39:491–496.

Lottman PE, Laheij RJ, Cuypers PW, et al. Health-related quality of life outcomes following elective open or endovascular AAA repair: a randomized controlled trial. J Endovasc Ther. 2004;11:323–329.

Malina M, Nilsson M, Brunkwall J, et al. Quality of life before and after endovascular and open repair of asymptomatic AAAs: a prospective study. J Endovasc Ther. 2000;7:372–379.

Oaikhinan K, Sultan S. An observational parallel group comparative study with and without the "Magic Bullet" (MB: Aspirin, cardio selective beta-blocker, Pravastatin and Clopidogrel) in the perioperative and postoperative period for abdominal aortic aneurysms surgery and femoral-popliteal segment revascularisation. Does the "Magic Bullet" improve the 30-day morbidity and mortality outcome? Br J Surg. 2004;91:113–114.

Parodi JC, Palmaz JC, Barone HD. Transfemoral intraluminal graft implantation for abdominal aortic aneurysms. Ann Vasc Surg. 1991;5:491–499.

Patel ST, Haser PB, Bush HL, et al. The costeffectiveness of endovascular repair versus open surgical repair of abdominal aortic aneurysms: a decision analysis model. J Vasc Surg. 1999;29:958–972.

Prinssen M, Verhoeven EL, Buth J, et al. A randomized trial comparing conventional and endovascular repair of abdominal aortic aneurysms. N Engl J Med. 2004;351:1607–1618.

Prinssen M, Buskens E, Blankensteijn JD. On behalf of the DREAM trial participants. Quality of life after endovascular and open AAA repair. Results of a randomized trial. Eur J Vasc Endovasc Surg. 2004;27:121–127.

Sicard GA, Zwolak RM, Sidawy AN, et al. Endovascular abdominal aortic aneurysm repair: long-term outcome measures in patients at high-risk for open surgery. J Vasc Surg. 2006;44:229–236.

Sultan S, Moore D, Shanik G. Endoluminal stent grafts in the management of infrarenal abdominal aortic aneurysms: a realistic assessment. Eur J Vasc Endovasc Surg. 2001;21:70–74.

UK Small Aneurysm Trial Participants Health service costs and quality of life for early elective surgery or ultrasonographic surveillance for small abdominal aortic aneurysms.. Lancet. 1998;352:1656–1660.

van Marrewijk CJ, Fransen G, Laheij RJ, et al. Is a type II endoleak after EVAR a harbinger of risk? Causes and outcome of open conversion and aneurysm rupture during follow-up. Eur J Vasc Endovasc Surg. 2004;27:128–137.

West TD, Balas EA, West DA. Contrasting RCC, RVU, and ABC for managed care decisions. A case study compares three widely used costing methods and finds one superior. Healthc Financ Manage. 1996;50:54–61.

9

Incidence and Predictors of Clinical Failures Following Catheter-Based Treatment of Abdominal Aortic Aneurysms

Daniel R. Watson, Angela Kruse, Jeffrey Weiner and Christina Prabhu
Riverside Methodist Hospital
United States

1. Introduction

An abdominal aortic aneurysm (AAA) is a balloon-like bulge or weakened area in the wall of aorta. The larger the aneurysm becomes, the more likely it will rupture which could lead to life-threatening bleeding, and potentially death. Surgical repair of the aneurysm prior to rupture is often life-saving. This can be performed either as an open procedure or endoluminal with a stent graft.

The management of abdominal aortic aneurysms (AAA), whether discovered incidentally on imaging studies or by an astute physician on physical exam, continues to have a huge impact on clinical practice and the lives of patients. Through research, the art of medicine, and extensive patient counseling, surveillance versus elective repair continues to be a dynamic and changing science. When indications for elective repair arise, such as worsening symptoms, increased or rapid growth of the aneurysm, or a diameter greater than 5 cm is present, a decision regarding surgical options are brought to the forefront.

Open AAA repair was the sole form of surgical treatment until endoluminal repair was introduced into practice in 1991. Much research has been publicized supporting the decreased recovery time and the short term morbidity of endoluminal repair compared to open repair. However, some authors suggest that the benefits of endoluminal repair with respect to mortality rate achieved in the early postoperative period disappear in the long term recovery scheme (Zeebregts et al., 2004).

The controversies surrounding endoluminal repair of AAA have involved defining the ideal candidate based on risk factor stratification and overcoming challenging anatomy of the aorta. According to Steinmetz et al, "the ideal candidate for endovascular repair [is] still to be defined" (Steinmetz et al., 2010). However, with new improvements to detect complications intraoperatively, and advances in technology to prevent/treat migration and endoleaks, the quest to determine the ideal candidate may be unnecessary. The presence of an intraoperative endoleak may increase the likelihood of an endoleak being seen during the follow-up period, but not necessarily the likelihood of an additional reintervention or operative procedure (Sampaio et al., 2009). The ultimate goal is to enable the applicability of this elective, minimally invasive approach to prevent the catastrophic event of a ruptured AAA to be widespread.

Endoluminal AAA repair obviates the three major physiologic insults associated with open repair laparotomy, aortic cross-clamping, and ischemia reperfusion injury (Halak et al.,

2007). In addition, the majority of the patients undergoing endovascular aneurysmal repair (EVAR) had regional anesthesia, thus reducing perioperative morbidity associated with sedative medication utilization in patients with multiple co-morbidities. Furthermore, this study determined that the duration of operation was shorter, blood loss was significantly less, and there was decreased hospital stay in the EVAR verses open repair (Zeebregts et al., 2004).

For these reasons, uncertainty remains regarding the long-term effectiveness of endoluminal AAA repair and its proper role in the management of patients with AAA. In particular, debate continues as to whether or not younger patients at good risk should be treated in this fashion or whether small aneurysms should be treated at an earlier interval in a more aggressive approach with stent grafts. To examine outcome data that might impact decisions on these issues, we reviewed a 12-year experience with 807 primary AAA endografts to determine the frequency of beneficial outcome and the incidence and causes of clinical failures of endovascular repair.

2. Materials and methods

Over 12 years ending in 2010, 807 patients underwent endovascular repair of infrarenal AAA. Five devices were used over this period: Ancure (Guidant, Menlo Park, Calif), AneuRx (Medtronic/AVE, Santa Rosa, Calif), Excluder (W. L. Gore, Flagstaff, Ariz), Quantum (Cordis Corp., NJ) and Zenith (Cook Inc, Bloomington, Ind). All procedures were performed in a Hybrid operating room environment, where Radiologic imaging was performed with a high-quality, fixed C-arm fluoroscopic unit with digital imaging and road mapping capability on a radiolucent operating room table with movable top.

Patient selection for the procedure and decisions regarding devices used were based on radiologic imaging studies. Preoperative helical computed tomography (CT) was performed with 3 mm axial reconstruction. If initial measurements and morphology of the aneurysm were favorable for endovascular repair, multiplanar contrast angiography was performed with a special catheter with radiopaque markers at 1-cm intervals (Cook, Inc) to allow for precise length measurements and assessment of renal and pelvic anatomy, particularly in regard to device access and deployment. Intravascular ultrasound studies were also performed when measurements were deemed inaccurate on the basis of these studies, or in the presence of suspected renal or iliac occlusive disease. Except in patients with contraindications to contrast material, postoperative CT scans included non-contrast-enhanced, contrast- enhanced, and 3-minute to 5-minute delayed post-contrast-enhanced images.

Outcome was assessed with physical examination, lower extremity arterial studies, plain abdominal radiography, and computed tomography at discharge, at 1, 6, and 12 months postoperatively, and annually thereafter.

Data were collected from a review of operative imaging reports and physician chart notes. Any significant discrepancy between these two data sources prompted an interrogation of the source imaging studies. Outcome reporting adhered to the standards outlined by the Ad Hoc Committee for Standardized Reporting Practices in Vascular Surgery of The Society for Vascular Surgery/American Association for Vascular Surgery (SVS/AAVS) (Chaikof et al., 2002)

Clinical failures of endovascular AAA repair were defined as the following events: peri-procedural death (<30 days), late (>30 days) or late conversion of endograft repair to conventional open surgical repair, increase in maximal AAA sac diameter of 5 mm or greater after endograft exclusion, and AAA rupture after endoluminal aneurysm treatment. All perioperative deaths occurred as a result of aneurysm rupture or after a primary or secondary procedure directed at treating the aneurysm or complications thereof.

Secondary procedures were defined as any subsequent procedure (exclusive of diagnostic angiography), whether percutaneous or open surgical, related to aneurysm repair or complications thereof. While procedures performed because of wound complications were tabulated for descriptive purposes, they were excluded from statistical analysis.

Endoleak was classified on the basis of serial imaging studies. CT findings, although most influential, composed only one factor. Presumed type I leak observed on CT scans was invariably followed up with angiographic confirmation. A leak was considered type II when the contrast collection was posterior or at the orifice of the inferior mesenteric artery. Type II and IV endoleaks noted only on an intraoperative or predischarge imaging study were excluded from analysis. Leakage through enlarged suture holes or fabric tears was classified as type III endoleak, as were defects related to separation of modular components. An endoleak was suspected to be type III when it directly abutted the graft fabric or was associated with obvious disunion of components; half of these were confirmed at angiography or at open surgical conversion.

Migration was defined with clinical and radiographic parameters, as suggested by the SVS/AAVS document on endovascular reporting standards (Chaikof et al., 2002). Migration included caudal movement of the proximal attachment site or cranial movement of a distal attachment site. A device was considered to have migrated when at least 1 cm of movement was noted relative to anatomic landmarks, when the patient experienced symptoms, or when an intervention was undertaken to treat migration, irrespective of distance.

Aneurysm shrinkage or growth was determined with a pre-procedural CT scan performed 3 months or less before the date of the procedure as the baseline. A predischarge imaging study was used as the reference scan when a preoperative study was not available. Size measurements were made on the CT scan with the greatest minor sac dimension on any axial image. Aneurysm shrinkage was defined as decrease of 5 mm or more in the minor dimension of the sac; enlargement was defined as increase of 5 mm or more in this dimension.

The individual clinician responsible for the patient's determined the need for secondary procedures. Certain clinical events mandated intervention, including post-implant aneurysm rupture or symptomatic graft limb occlusion. Most, however, were less catastrophic, and the need for secondary intervention was subjective. Basic treatment paradigms were, however, standard at the institution.

Treatment of types I and III endoleaks was always recommended. Type II endoleak was treated when the aneurysm sac was observed to enlarge over time. As well, patients with type II leak received treatment when the aneurysm failed to contract despite observation for more than 12 months after the initial endovascular repair. Type II leak in patients with a shrinking sac was not treated. Device migration was treated when it was associated with a type I leak or when the remaining length of sealing was deemed inadequate, usually when reduced to less than 10 mm.

3. Results

Eighty percent of treated patients were men. The mean age was 72.6 years (range, 44 to 87 years), and the mean AAA sac maximal diameter was 5.7 cm (range, 4.1 to 10.2 cm). Risk

factors and co-morbidities were typical of patients undergoing vascular surgical procedures. Patient demographics are displayed in Table 1.
In the 12-year experience, one or more clinical failures, as defined previously, were observed in a total of 74 patients (9.2%). Because some patients had more than one adverse event denoting failure, the number of such events exceeded the number of patients sustaining them.

Patient Demographics (n = 807)	**Mean/n (range/%)**
Age (years)	72.6 (range 44-87)
Gender	
Male	646 (80)
Female	161 (20)
Average sac diameter (cm)	5.7 (range 4.1-10.2)
Comorbidities	
HTN	480 (59)
CAD	451 (56)
Tobacco use	407 (50)
Diabetes	159 (20)
Hyperlipidemia	255 (32)
COPD	201 (25)
Renal insufficiency	79 (10)
Notes: HTN = Hypertension, CAD = coronary artery disease; COPD = chronic obstructive pulmonary disease	

Table 1. Patient demographics

3.1 Operative deaths

Eight periprocedural deaths (1%) occurred in the total of 807 AAA stent graft repairs (Table 2.) One death occurred as the result of an acute myocardial infarction on day 3 after implant in a patient with a symptomatic AAA at high risk with known extensive coronary artery disease not amenable to surgical or catheter-based repair. This mortality occurred early in our experience after the procedure had been prolonged with a series of vascular access, device introduction, and deployment difficulties. Although eventually a technically successful implant was achieved, in retrospect, more prompt conversion to standard open repair would likely have resulted in a more favorable outcome.

Diffuse atheroembolization was the most common cause of death in our series after endoluminal stent graft placement. Uniformly, the 4 patients afflicted by this complication expired secondary to severe multisystem organ failure. All patients had significant thrombus burden within either the proximal landing zone or suprarenal aorta (or both). The complication was seen irrespective of graft type or fixation mechanism. In each case the potential for this complication had been recognized preoperatively. However, endoluminal therapy was chosen for AAA repair due to patient/family demand (2 cases), hostile abdominal status for open repair (1 case), or severe concomitant pulmonary disease which precluded the likelihood of postoperative extubation (1 case). In three cases the primary inciting event was the discovery of inoperable small bowel (2 cases) or colonic (1 case) ischemia. All patients had arteriographic demonstration of proximal, branch vessel patency when the complication was initially suspected. But the distal vascular "pruning" was resistant to all attempts at pharmacologic rescue. In the remaining case the insult was rendered to the parenchyma of a lone kidney. The family refused dialysis and withdrew supportive care 10 days after surgery.

One sudden early death occurred at home 8 days after discharge and was presumed to be the result of rupture of a large symptomatic AAA. No evidence of a proximal attachment leak had been suspected on predischarge CT scanning, but the patient had a short, angulated proximal AAA neck and was high-risk for graft migration. We elected to schedule this patient for frequent surveillance for a period of several months. Although no autopsy was performed to confirm rupture, this seems the likely cause, as the patient had severe back and abdominal pain before collapse.

Another patient became hypotensive in the hospital 12 hours after an endoluminal repair during which a persistent endoleak was evident at the distal fixation zone. The leak appeared resistant to all conventional means of resolution (ballooning, additional cuff, stents, etc) and it was elected to inject biologic glue into the coaptation zone. Emergency CT scan showed complete thrombsis of the entire pelvic vasculature, emanating from the affected internal iliac artery in the landing zone. Limb and lower extremity ischemia ensued soon thereafter. Despite operative exploration and fem-fem bypass, the patient died of renal and pulmonary insufficiency after a prolonged and complex 2-week postoperative course. In retrospect, more prompt conversion to standard open repair would likely have undoubtedly resulted in a more favorable outcome.

The remaining early death occurred after an early complication of attempted sheath insertion for endograft implantation, resulting in external iliac rupture and severe retroperitoneal hemorrhage. Attempt at open repair failed due to prolific calcification throughout the patient's aorto-iliac system, confounding conventional attempts at vascular clamping or suture repair.

A common thread in most of these cases was technical complications occurring in patients who were elderly, fragile, and at high risk for perioperative morbidity.

Cause	n (%)
MI after surgery	1 (0.1)
Massive atheroemboli	4 (0.4)
Died at home 8 days after discharge	1 (0.1)
Limb /pelvic thrombosis-rhabdomyolysis	1 (0.1)
Avulsion EIA	1(0.1)
Notes: MI=myocardial infarction, EIA=external iliac artery	

Table 2. Perioperative deaths (30 days)

3.2 Early conversions

During the 12-year study period, twelve patients (1.5%) needed early conversion to open repair within the first 48 hours after the procedure. Successful endograft implantation was achieved in the remaining 795 patients, for an overall procedural technical success rate of 98.5%.

Two patients treated early in our experience had small, calcified iliac arteries that sustained severe traumatic injury during attempted passage of large-caliber stents or devices. In retrospect, these cases were examples of inappropriate judgments and poor patient selection, typical of grappling with a formidable "learning curve" associated with a new, paradigm-changing technology. One of the patients had a 360-degree twist in the limbs of an unsupported Ancure bifurcated device (Guidant, Santa Clara, Calif) that could not be corrected, requiring fem-fem bypass. Another patient needed immediate conversion when acute migration of the proximal attachment system occurred in a short and heavily calcified aortic neck, resulting in the endograft falling into the AAA sac. Seven patients required fem-fem bypass for access site complications ranging from uncontrollable hemorrhage to occlusion, not amenable to conventional repair secondary to vessel fragility, small size, or calcification. The final patient in this subgroup had acute rupture of his aneurysm on postoperative day 8, as already described in the previous section detailing periprocedural deaths.

3.3 Late conversions

Nine patients (1.1%) needed late (30 days) conversion to standard open graft repair for a variety of clinical scenarios. Conversions were performed at a mean of 20 months after the original endograft procedure (range, 9 to 32 months).

Six of nine conversions in our series were caused by AAA sac growth with demonstrated endoleak ("endotension"). Two endoluminal grafts needed late conversion as the result of graft infection. Both were presumed to be caused by septicemic seeding of the endoluminal device. Although these cases might conceivably be the result of primary endograft infections, this is much less likely in our opinion. One conversion in our series was caused by continued AAA sac growth *without* demonstrated endoleak. At the time of laparotomy and explantation, numerous small leaks were evident at the suture-fixation points of the stents to the graft.

As outlined above, conversion was necessary in seven patients because of continued AAA growth. Endoleak was present in all but one patient in this subgroup. One patient had a persistent proximal type 1 attachment leak, four had persistent type 2 leaks from lumbar arteries, and one patient an acute late type 3 endoleak caused by a fabric hole erosion in a Zenith endograft implanted 20 months previously. The patient had done well, with sac shrinkage and no demonstrable endoleak, up to the 6-month interval. The patient then was seen with sudden back pain, and CT scanning showed a type 3 leak with acute sac re-expansion. Emergent open operation and repair proceeded uneventfully.

One patient did well until 32 months after the original procedure when he was seen at an outside facility with a septic left ankle joint. The patient underwent treatment with drainage and antibiotics. Within several months, however, the patient returned again with bilateral septic hips and septic shoulder joint. Blood cultures grew methicillin-resistant Staphylococcus aureus. The patient again underwent treatment with drainage and antibiotics. Despite this, al psoas muscle abscess developed that was drained percutaneously. However, subsequent CT scans showed communication with the endograft and the area of abscess.

Further, evidence of bone destruction developed of vertebral bodies lumbar 3 and 4. Subsequently, the patient underwent a staged procedure of axillobifemoral bypass grafting followed by removal of the infected endograft with radical debridement of vertebral body osteomyelitis. The patient was discharged from the hospital after a prolonged hospital course.

One patient needed late conversion at 27 months for acute thrombosis of the entire endograft, resulting in severe lower extremity ischemia. Prior follow-up CT scans had shown good AAA exclusion, with sac shrinkage and no endoleak. However, distortion and slight kinking of the endograft limbs was noted and believed attributable to the morphologic sac changes caused by its shrinkage. The patient was asymptomatic with intact pulses, so observation and continued surveillance was elected. Presumably, limb kinking increased, resulting in thrombosis. Emergent axillobifemoral bypass grafting was performed, with a satisfactory result.

3.4 Sac growth

In the series, follow-up CT imaging revealed 82 patients with sac growth of the aneurysm of 5 mm or greater, despite endoluminal repair of the AAA.

All of these patients had at least 90 days of follow-up. Of the 82 patients, 64 thus far have undergone successful treatment with endovascular therapies. Further secondary interventions are planned for most of the remaining patients with AAA sac growth but had not yet been performed when the study period was terminated. Such secondary procedures included a variety of catheter-based therapies, including insertion of proximal or distal extender cuffs, branch or sac embolization, or related interventions as deemed appropriate with angiography or other diagnostic methods. None of the patients with sac growth are symptomatic, and no ruptures, thromboses, or conversions have occurred in this cohort.

3.5 Ruptures

During the 12-year experience, seven patients (0.9%) are believed to have had AAA rupture after their endoluminal repair. five patients, all with unproven but presumed rupture at home at varying intervals (5-17 months) after surgery and a sixth with post-discharge rupture on postoperative day 5 have already been described previously in the sections detailing periprocedural deaths and early conversions.

A final rupture occurred at 2 years after the original endovascular procedure.

The patient had undergone three interval CT scans that had shown no leak and a decrease in maximal AAA diameter from 5 to 4.6 cm. Shortly after the most recent follow-up CT scan, the patient was seen acutely with abdominal and back pain. Emergency CT scan showed a large endoleak and acute re-expansion of the AAA sac to greater than the original 6-cm diameter, with an adjacent retroperitoneal hematoma. At emergency operation, acute detachment of the proximal stent attachment mechanism was found, with the distal endograft lying free in the AAA sac. We presumed the shrinking AAA sac wall had become atretic and ruptured when acutely repressurized. The patient survived operative conversion to open repair. After a prolonged hospitalization, the patient was discharged to a rehabilitation facility.

Despite often extensive and emergent operations needed for late conversion of endovascular to open repairs, no deaths occurred as a result of such procedures in our series.

3.6 Secondary reinterventions

A variety of problems after endograft repair were identified at various intervals during clinical and radiologic postimplant follow-up surveillance. These included persistent primary endoleaks, late secondary leaks, instances of graft migration, kinking, or thrombosis, and other problems that were believed to threaten endoluminal repair and expose the patient to possible conversion or rupture or both. For this reason, reinterventions were believed necessary.

During the 12-year study period, 81 patients (10%) needed a total of 109 secondary procedures. The vast majority of these were catheter-based reinterventions , including percutaneous angioplasty, pharmacologic lysis of limb thrombosis, insertion of additional vascular stents in native vessels, proximal or distal extensions of the original stent graft device, embolization of branch vessels or the AAA sac itself, or similar related procedures. These were judged clinically effective in correcting or eliminating the problem needing reintervention in 94% (n=76) of the 81 patients. Patients who underwent such success reinterventions were not classified as having clinical failures but rather as having assisted-primary successes.

4. Discussion

This series summarizes the data from our 12-year experience with 807 patients with AAAs treated with endoluminal stent graft repair.

Our results confirm an extensive number of reports from other centers that clearly document that endovascular AAA repair is safe and can be successfully performed in patients with suitable anatomy (Blum et al., 1997; Brewster et al., 1998; Brewster et al., 2003; Dillavou et al., 2006; May et al., 1998; Moore et al., 1999; Moore et al., 2001; Zarins et al., 1999).

The implant success in most centers, as in our series, is now approaching 99%. This and other outcome parameters are likely to further improve with newer generation devices, namely as such devices involve lower profile technology and the bulk of our complications stemmed from access challenges. In addition to low mortality and only a 1% early conversion rate, our results document quite effective treatment of the AAA relative to its anticipated natural history, albeit with a relatively short 2.5-year mean follow-up period. The AAA has remained stable in size or actually diminished in maximal diameter in 92% of cases, and serious late problems, such as conversion to open repair and AAA rupture, remain infrequent.

The mortality rate of our series was 1%. The less invasive characteristics of endoluminal repair are clearly reflected by this as well as the low morbidity and mortality rates reported in the aforementioned series. Although this rate is not significantly different from results from several high-volume single institution reports involving traditional open repair, we believe many of the patients in our series who underwent endoluminal repair were frail, high-risk patients, often with advanced cardiopulmonary problems or other comorbidities, who would very likely have had considerably higher mortality rates if treated with conventional open operation.

This contention remains unproven, of course, because no truly randomized prospective studies exist in this regard. It is worthwhile emphasizing that most of the deaths in our series occurred after procedural challenges during the endovascular stent access, introduction or deployment. These difficulties invariably occurred in elderly, fragile patients with adverse and challenging anatomic features. We believe this underscores the need for careful patient selection and adherence to accepted anatomic selection criteria.

The presence of endoleaks, defined as a failure to totally exclude the AAA from continued perfusion and pressurization, may be associated with the subsequent expansion of the aneurysm and possible rupture. However, the patient is unaware of an endoleak and not really concerned unless an undesirable outcome results. Thus, endoleaks remain a potential concern, but we have not regarded these as a mode of clinical failure unless adverse sequelae, such as continued AAA enlargement, AAA rupture, or other problems, resulted. This position may be challenged by some who believe that any demonstrated endoleak is a criteria of failure. Indeed, the clinical significance of endoleak remains uncertain and poorly understood (Chuter et al., 2001; Makaroun et al., 1999; Matsumura & Moore, 1998; Steinmetz et al., 2004; Timaran et al., 2005).

Two factors indendently favored an increased incidence of endoleak in our series: advanced age and female gender. Increasing age may be associated with more complex anatomy, although none of the anatomic variables investigated were found to be predictive of endoleaks. The higher incidence of endoleak associated with female gender may be related to as yet undetermined factors, intrinsic to the aneurysm, to the vessel wall, or to the blood. In addition, the coagulation profile, on which we have no information in this study, may be a significant factor, especially with respect to type 2 endoleaks. Importantly, many authorities believe the most common variety of endoleak (type 2 retrograde branch leak) rarely causes clinical consequences, and several studies have shown poor correlation between endoleak and outcome. (Baum et al., 2002; Gilling-Smith et al., 2000; Jones et al., 2007; Resch et al., 1998; Velazquez et al., 2000; Zarins et al., 2000).

However, it should be acknowledged that almost all type III endoleaks will need some form of reintervention or conversion and that type I attachment leaks are well recognized as more hazardous in terms of AAA enlargement and rupture risk. Further, it should be noted that, in our series, all patients with AAA sac growth resulting in conversion to open repair did have some type of endoleak, including one patient with a type II branch leak alone, which was visualized at open repair. Our conclusion, that endoleak is not a desirable or benign phenomenon seems justified, but we do not regard its presence alone as reliable prognostic predictor or a clear-cut indicator of clinical failure of endoluminal repair.

Similarly, in our opinion, an indicator of clinical failure of endoluminal AAA repair should not be the need for limited secondary reinterventions on this patient population. As illustrated by our series in which a relatively modest 10% of patients needed secondary procedures, almost all catheter-based endovascular interventions rather than surgical procedures, the vast majority were believed clinically successful in correcting the presumed cause of sac growth or other clinical problems, thereby maintaining the integrity and success of the endograft repair. Similar success rates have been reported by other investigators with respect to secondary interventions (Dattilo et al., 2002; Giles et al., 2011; Hobo et al., 2006; Laheij et al., 2000; May et al., 2000).

As long as successful endovascular treatment of their aneurysm can be maintained and major surgical repair avoided, we believe the concept of primary-assisted success, achieved by means of such limited re-interventions, is valid and well accepted by patients.

Although our re-intervention rate was a 10%, our relatively short mean follow-up period of 33 months must be recognized. In the large European collaborative registry (Eurostar) experience of more than 1000 patients followed for 12 or more months, 18% have needed secondary interventions at a mean follow-up interval of 20 months (Laheij et al., 2000). It appears reasonable to assume that secondary interventions will be necessary within this patient population at a cumulative rate of approximately 10-20% per year. Similar Eurostar data have emphasized the ongoing and cumulative incidence of both late conversions and aneurysm rupture, noting cumulative rates of approximately 2%/year for conversion to open repair and a rupture risk of approximately 1%/year (Harris et al., 2000).

Application of this procedure has increased rapidly in many centers around the world, and many investigators now urge more widespread use. The less invasive nature of this approach, and the generally good and beneficial early results of treatment, clearly have made endovascular AAA repair an appealing, if not compelling, therapeutic alternative to many patients with AAA. Some regard it as the procedure of choice for all AAAs that are anatomically suitable and believe it is reasonable to use even in young patients at good risk. Other advocates urge prophylactic repair of small (5 cm) AAA, with the belief that the safer and less invasive treatment would justify earlier treatment and potentially improve long-term outcomes (Becquemin et al., 2000; Holzenbein et al., 2001; Ouriel et al., 2003; Peppelenbosch et al., 2004; Zarins et al., 2006).

Thoughtful concern in this regard should be considered, given that long-term effectiveness and durability of endovascular repair clearly appears to be less than that anticipated by most surgeons after standard open operative repair. This is supported by our results, as well as the mid-term results reported by other investigators. (Bush et al., 2001; Buth & Laheij, 2000; Chaikof et al., 2009; Crawford et al., 1981; Hallett et al., 1997; Johnston, 1994).

Although it must be acknowledged that conventional surgical repair is rarely subjected to the intense scrutiny and post-implant surveillance common to endovascular repair, nonetheless long-term effectiveness of endograft repair as we now know cannot match the late outcome and reliability of standard AAA operative repair, based on the finding of the aforementioned investigators.

Theoretically, newer-generation, lower profile devices may improve endoluminal outcomes. Further, future device advances and improvements may reduce device structural failures and may enable the endoluminal grafts to better accommodate to morphologic AAA sac changes that have been recognized by many authorities and that contribute to late failures by causing endograft kinking, migration, component separation, and other adverse consequences. However, this remains to be established. Most series to date, including this report, are dominated by results of earlier, first-generation endografts. (Beebe et al., 2001; Chaikof et al., 2009; Harris et al., 1999; Rutherford & Krupski, 2004).

We believe the clinical implications of our study are several. First, endoluminal AAA repair has clearly been a major advance in the treatment of aortic aneurismal disease. Its safety, efficacy, feasablility and generally good early and mid-term results have been well shown in our series and many other published reports. It appears particularly advantageous to more elderly patients at high risk and patients with hostile abdominal characteristics, many of whom may have previously been denied repair. In such patients with suitable vascular anatomy for delivery and deployment, it is reasonable and appropriate in our opinion to consider endovascular repair the procedure of choice (Brewster, 2001; Dattilo et al., 2002; Visser et al., 2006).

However, it should be recognized that the actual definition of "high-risk" remains debatable and not well defined in the literature. Further, endoluminal repair seems advantageous in patients with a "hostile" abdomen because of a variety of factors and also an appealing and likely beneficial option in patients with other unusual conditions that may cause technical difficulties and challenges for conventional open repair, such as para-anastomotic aneurysms after previous aortic surgery, AAA in the presence of a horseshoe kidney, and AAA in patients with prior renal transplants.

Secondly, because of current concerns related to device structural stability and long-term reliability of this form of repair, in our opinion, more widespread use of endografts to repair small AAA cannot be supported (Finlayson et al., 1999).

Similarly, because failure modes of endoluminal repair such as endoleak, graft migration, and other are much more frequent in patients with adverse anatomy, this procedure should not be used in a wonton fashion in patients who do not have well-defined appropriate aneurysmal anatomic features for potential rupture. This is particularly true in patients at very high risk because the need for conversion in these circumstances is likely to be associated with truly excessive morbidity and mortality rates (Cuypers et al., 2000; Goodney et al., 2010; May et al., 1997; Starnes et al., 2006).

5. Conclusion

Despite the minimal invasive nature of endovascular aneurysm repair, a variety of complications do occur with considerable frequency. The patient's age, anatomy, and cardiac and general medical status have a compelling influence on the risk of morbidity and mortality. The experience of the operating team is an important factor influencing the risk of device-related or procedure-related adverse events. These findings underline the importance of adequate training and may help to guide the selection of patients and devices for endovascular AAA repair in the future. One cannot overemphasize the importance of proper and appropriate patient selection to ensure procedural success.

6. Acknowledgment

Thanks to John O. Elliott for editorial assistance.

7. References

Baum, R. A., Carpenter, J. P., Golden, M. A., Velazquez, O. C., Clark, T. W., Stavropoulos, S. W., et al. (2002). Treatment of type 2 endoleaks after endovascular repair of abdominal aortic aneurysms: Comparison of transarterial and translumbar techniques. *Journal of Vascular Surgery,* Vol. 35, No.1, pp. 23-29, ISSN 0741-5214

Becquemin, J., Bourriez, A., D'Audiffret, A., Zubilewicz, T., Kobeiter, H., Allaire, E., et al. (2000). Mid-term results of endovascular versus open repair for abdominal aortic aneurysm in patients anatomically suitable for endovascular repair. *European Journal of Vascular and Endovascular Surgery,* Vol.19, No.6, pp. 656-661, ISSN 1078-5884

Beebe, H. G., Cronenwett, J. L., Katzen, B. T., Brewster, D. C., Green, R. M., & Vanguard Endograft Trial Investigators. (2001). Results of an aortic endograft trial: Impact of device failure beyond 12 months. *Journal of Vascular Surgery,* Vol.33, No.2 (Suppl), pp. S55-63, ISSN 0741-5214

Blum, U., Voshage, G., Lammer, J., Beyersdorf, F., Tollner, D., Kretschmer, G., et al. (1997). Endoluminal stent-grafts for infrarenal abdominal aortic aneurysms. *The New England Journal of Medicine,* Vol.336, No.1, pp. 13-20, ISSN 0028-4793

Brewster, D. C. (2001). Presidential address: What would you do if it were your father? Reflections on endovascular abdominal aortic aneurysm repair. *Journal of Vascular Surgery,* Vol.33, No.6, pp. 1139-1147, ISSN 0741-5214

Brewster, D. C., Cronenwett, J. L., Hallett, J. W.,Jr, Johnston, K. W., Krupski, W. C., Matsumura, J. S., et al. (2003). Guidelines for the treatment of abdominal aortic aneurysms. Report of a subcommittee of the joint council of the American association for vascular surgery and society for vascular surgery. *Journal of Vascular Surgery,* Vol.37, No.5, pp. 1106-1117, ISSN 0741-5214

Brewster, D. C., Geller, S. C., Kaufman, J. A., Cambria, R. P., Gertler, J. P., LaMuraglia, G. M., et al. (1998). Initial experience with endovascular aneurysm repair: Comparison of early results with outcome of conventional open repair. *Journal of Vascular Surgery,* Vol.27, No.6, pp. 992-1003; discussion pp. 1004-1005, ISSN 0741-5214

Bush, R. L., Lumsden, A. B., Dodson, T. F., Salam, A. A., Weiss, V. J., Smith, R. B.,3rd, et al. (2001). Mid-term results after endovascular repair of the abdominal aortic aneurysm. *Journal of Vascular Surgery,* Vol.33, No.2 (Suppl), pp. S70-76, ISSN 0741-5214

Buth, J., & Laheij, R. J. (2000). Early complications and endoleaks after endovascular abdominal aortic aneurysm repair: Report of a multicenter study. *Journal of Vascular Surgery,* Vol.31, No.1 (Pt 1), pp. 134-146, ISSN 0741-5214

Chaikof, E. L., Blankensteijn, J. D., Harris, P. L., White, G. H., Zarins, C. K., Bernhard, V. M., et al. (2002). Reporting standards for endovascular aortic aneurysm repair. *Journal of Vascular Surgery,* Vol.35, No.5, pp. 1048-1060, ISSN 0741-5214

Chaikof, E. L., Brewster, D. C., Dalman, R. L., Makaroun, M. S., Illig, K. A., Sicard, G. A., et al. (2009). The care of patients with an abdominal aortic aneurysm: The society for vascular surgery practice guidelines. *Journal of Vascular Surgery,* Vol.50, No.4 (Suppl), pp. S2-49, ISSN 0741-5214

Chuter, T. A., Faruqi, R. M., Sawhney, R., Reilly, L. M., Kerlan, R. B., Canto, C. J., et al. (2001). Endoleak after endovascular repair of abdominal aortic aneurysm. *Journal of Vascular Surgery,* Vol.34, No.1, pp. 98-105, ISSN 0741-5214

Crawford, E. S., Saleh, S. A., Babb, J. W.,3rd, Glaeser, D. H., Vaccaro, P. S., & Silvers, A. (1981). Infrarenal abdominal aortic aneurysm: Factors influencing survival after operation performed over a 25-year period. *Annals of Surgery,* Vol.193, No.6, pp. 699-709, ISSN 0003-4932

Cuypers, P. W., Laheij, R. J., & Buth, J. (2000). Which factors increase the risk of conversion to open surgery following endovascular abdominal aortic aneurysm repair? The EUROSTAR collaborators. *European Journal of Vascular and Endovascular Surgery,* Vol.20, No.2, pp. 183-189, ISSN 1078-5884

Dattilo, J. B., Brewster, D. C., Fan, C. M., Geller, S. C., Cambria, R. P., Lamuraglia, G. M., et al. (2002). Clinical failures of endovascular abdominal aortic aneurysm repair: Incidence, causes, and management. *Journal of Vascular Surgery,* Vol.35, No.6, pp. 1137-1144, ISSN 0741-5214

Dillavou, E. D., Muluk, S. C., & Makaroun, M. S. (2006). Improving aneurysm-related outcomes: Nationwide benefits of endovascular repair. *Journal of Vascular Surgery,* Vol.43, No.3, pp. 446-452, ISSN 0741-5214

Finlayson, S. R., Birkmeyer, J. D., Fillinger, M. F., & Cronenwett, J. L. (1999). Should endovascular surgery lower the threshold for repair of abdominal aortic aneurysms? *Journal of Vascular Surgery,* Vol.29, No.6, pp. 973-985, ISSN 0741-5214

Giles, K. A., Landon, B. E., Cotterill, P., O'Malley, A. J., Pomposelli, F. B., & Schermerhorn, M. L. (2011). Thirty-day mortality and late survival with reinterventions and readmissions after open and endovascular aortic aneurysm repair in Medicare beneficiaries. *Journal of Vascular Surgery,* Vol.53, No.1, pp.6-13, ISSN 0741-5214

Gilling-Smith, G. L., Martin, J., Sudhindran, S., Gould, D. A., McWilliams, R. G., Bakran, A., et al. (2000). Freedom from endoleak after endovascular aneurysm repair does not equal treatment success. *European Journal of Vascular and Endovascular Surgery,* Vol.19, No.4, pp. 421-425, ISSN 1078-5884

Goodney, P. P., Tavris, D., Lucas, F. L., Gross, T., Fisher, E. S., & Finlayson, S. R. (2010). Causes of late mortality after endovascular and open surgical repair of infrarenal abdominal aortic aneurysms. *Journal of Vascular Surgery,* Vol.51, No.6, pp. 1340-1347, ISSN 0741-5214

Halak, M., McDonnell, C. O., Muhlmann, M. D., & Baker, S. R. (2007). Open surgical treatment of aneurysmal sac expansion following endovascular abdominal aneurysm repair: Solution for an unresolved clinical dilemma. *Vascular,* Vol.15, No.4, pp. 201-204, ISSN 1708-5381

Hallett, J. W.,Jr, Marshall, D. M., Petterson, T. M., Gray, D. T., Bower, T. C., Cherry, K. J.,Jr, et al. (1997). Graft-related complications after abdominal aortic aneurysm repair: Reassurance from a 36-year population-based experience. *Journal of Vascular Surgery,* Vol.25, No.2, pp.277-84; discussion pp. 285-286, ISSN 0741-5214

Harris, P., Brennan, J., Martin, J., Gould, D., Bakran, A., Gilling-Smith, G., et al. (1999). Longitudinal aneurysm shrinkage following endovascular aortic aneurysm repair: A source of intermediate and late complications. *Journal of Endovascular Surgery,* Vol.6 No.1, pp. 11-16, ISSN 1074-6218

Harris, P. L., Vallabhaneni, S. R., Desgranges, P., Becquemin, J. P., van Marrewijk, C., & Laheij, R. J. (2000). Incidence and risk factors of late rupture, conversion, and death after endovascular repair of infrarenal aortic aneurysms: The EUROSTAR experience. European collaborators on Stent/graft techniques for aortic aneurysm repair. *Journal of Vascular Surgery,* Vol.32, No.4, pp. 739-749, ISSN 0741-5214

Hobo, R., Buth, J., & EUROSTAR collaborators. (2006). Secondary interventions following endovascular abdominal aortic aneurysm repair using current endografts. A EUROSTAR report. *Journal of Vascular Surgery,* Vol.43, No.5, pp. 896-902, ISSN 0741-5214

Holzenbein, T. J., Kretschmer, G., Thurnher, S., Schoder, M., Aslim, E., Lammer, J., et al. (2001). Midterm durability of abdominal aortic aneurysm endograft repair: A word of caution. *Journal of Vascular Surgery,* Vol.33, No.2 (Suppl), pp. S46-54, ISSN 0741-5214

Johnston, K. W. (1994). Nonruptured abdominal aortic aneurysm: Six-year follow-up results from the multicenter prospective Canadian aneurysm study. Canadian society for vascular surgery aneurysm study group. *Journal of Vascular Surgery,* Vol.20, No.2, pp. 163-170, ISSN 0741-5214

Jones, J. E., Atkins, M. D., Brewster, D. C., Chung, T. K., Kwolek, C. J., LaMuraglia, G. M., et al. (2007). Persistent type 2 endoleak after endovascular repair of abdominal aortic aneurysm is associated with adverse late outcomes. *Journal of Vascular Surgery,* Vol.46, No.1, pp. 1-8, ISSN 0741-5214

Laheij, R. J., Buth, J., Harris, P. L., Moll, F. L., Stelter, W. J., & Verhoeven, E. L. (2000). Need for secondary interventions after endovascular repair of abdominal aortic aneurysms. intermediate-term follow-up results of a European collaborative registry (EUROSTAR). *The British Journal of Surgery,* Vol.87, No.12, pp. 1666-1673, ISSN 0007-1323

Makaroun, M., Zajko, A., Sugimoto, H., Eskandari, M., & Webster, M. (1999). Fate of endoleaks after endoluminal repair of abdominal aortic aneurysms with the EVT device. *European Journal of Vascular and Endovascular Surgery,* Vol.18, No.3, pp. 185-190, ISSN 1078-5884

Matsumura, J. S., & Moore, W. S. (1998). Clinical consequences of periprosthetic leak after endovascular repair of abdominal aortic aneurysm. endovascular technologies investigators. *Journal of Vascular Surgery,* Vol.27, No.4, pp. 606-613, ISSN 0741-5214

May, J., White, G. H., Waugh, R., Petrasek, P., Chaufour, X., Arulchelvam, M., et al. (2000). Life-table analysis of primary and assisted success following endoluminal repair of abdominal aortic aneurysms: The role of supplementary endovascular intervention in improving outcome. *European Journal of Vascular and Endovascular Surgery,* Vol.19, No.6, pp. 648-655, ISSN 1078-5884

May, J., White, G. H., Yu, W., Ly, C. N., Waugh, R., Stephen, M. S., et al. (1998). Concurrent comparison of endoluminal versus open repair in the treatment of abdominal aortic aneurysms: Analysis of 303 patients by life table method. *Journal of Vascular Surgery,* Vol.27, No.2, pp. 213-221, ISSN 0741-5214

May, J., White, G. H., Yu, W., Waugh, R., Stephen, M., Sieunarine, K., et al. (1997). Conversion from endoluminal to open repair of abdominal aortic aneurysms: A hazardous procedure. *European Journal of Vascular and Endovascular Surgery,* Vol.14, No.1, pp. 4-11, ISSN 1078-5884

Moore, W. S., Brewster, D. C., & Bernhard, V. M. (2001). Aorto-uni-iliac endograft for complex aortoiliac aneurysms compared with tube/bifurcation endografts: Results of the EVT/Guidant trials. *Journal of Vascular Surgery,* Vol.33, No.2 (Suppl), pp. S11-20, ISSN 0741-5214

Moore, W. S., Kashyap, V. S., Vescera, C. L., & Quinones-Baldrich, W. J. (1999). Abdominal aortic aneurysm: A 6-year comparison of endovascular versus transabdominal repair. *Annals of Surgery,* Vol.230, No.3, pp. 298-308, ISSN 0003-4932

Ouriel, K., Srivastava, S. D., Sarac, T. P., O'hara, P. J., Lyden, S. P., Greenberg, R. K., et al. (2003). Disparate outcome after endovascular treatment of small versus large abdominal aortic aneurysm. *Journal of Vascular Surgery,* Vol.37, No.6, pp. 1206-1212, ISSN 0741-5214

Peppelenbosch, N., Buth, J., Harris, P. L., van Marrewijk, C., Fransen, G., & EUROSTAR Collaborators. (2004). Diameter of abdominal aortic aneurysm and outcome of endovascular aneurysm repair: Does size matter? A report from EUROSTAR. *Journal of Vascular Surgery,* Vol.39, No.2, pp. 288-297, ISSN 0741-5214

Resch, T., Ivancev, K., Lindh, M., Nyman, U., Brunkwall, J., Malina, M., et al. (1998). Persistent collateral perfusion of abdominal aortic aneurysm after endovascular repair does not lead to progressive change in aneurysm diameter. *Journal of Vascular Surgery,* Vol.28, No.2, pp. 242-249, ISSN 0741-5214

Rutherford, R. B., & Krupski, W. C. (2004). Current status of open versus endovascular stent-graft repair of abdominal aortic aneurysm. *Journal of Vascular Surgery,* Vol.39, No.5, pp. 1129-1139, ISSN 0741-5214

Sampaio, S. M., Shin, S. H., Panneton, J. M., Andrews, J. C., Bower, T. C., Cherry, K. J., et al. (2009). Intraoperative endoleak during EVAR: Frequency, nature, and significance. *Vascular and Endovascular Surgery,* Vol.43, No.4, pp. 352-359, ISSN 1538-5744

Starnes, B. W., Andersen, C. A., Ronsivalle, J. A., Stockmaster, N. R., Mullenix, P. S., & Statler, J. D. (2006). Totally percutaneous aortic aneurysm repair: Experience and prudence. *Journal of Vascular Surgery,* Vol.43, No.2, pp. 270-276, ISSN 0741-5214

Steinmetz, E., Abello, N., Kretz, B., Gauthier, E., Bouchot, O., & Brenot, R. (2010). Analysis of outcome after using high-risk criteria selection to surgery versus endovascular repair in the modern era of abdominal aortic aneurysm treatment. *European Journal of Vascular and Endovascular Surgery,* Vol.39, No.4, pp. 403-409, ISSN 1078-5884

Steinmetz, E., Rubin, B. G., Sanchez, L. A., Choi, E. T., Geraghty, P. J., Baty, J., et al. (2004). Type II endoleak after endovascular abdominal aortic aneurysm repair: A conservative approach with selective intervention is safe and cost-effective. *Journal of Vascular Surgery,* Vol.39, No.2, pp. 306-313, ISSN 0741-5214

Timaran, C. H., Ohki, T., Veith, F. J., Lipsitz, E. C., Gargiulo, N. J.,3rd, Rhee, S. J., et al. (2005). Influence of type II endoleak volume on aneurysm wall pressure and distribution in an experimental model. *Journal of Vascular Surgery,* Vol.41, No.4, pp. 657-663, ISSN 0741-5214

Velazquez, O. C., Baum, R. A., Carpenter, J. P., Golden, M. A., Cohn, M., Pyeron, A., et al. (2000). Relationship between preoperative patency of the inferior mesenteric artery and subsequent occurrence of type II endoleak in patients undergoing endovascular repair of abdominal aortic aneurysms. *Journal of Vascular Surgery,* Vol.32, No.4, pp. 777-788, ISSN 0741-5214

Visser, J. J., Bosch, J. L., Hunink, M. G., van Dijk, L. C., Hendriks, J. M., Poldermans, D., et al. (2006). Endovascular repair versus open surgery in patients with ruptured abdominal aortic aneurysms: Clinical outcomes with 1-year follow-up. *Journal of Vascular Surgery,* Vol.44, No.6, pp. 1148-1155, ISSN 0741-5214

Zarins, C. K., Crabtree, T., Bloch, D. A., Arko, F. R., Ouriel, K., & White, R. A. (2006). Endovascular aneurysm repair at 5 years: Does aneurysm diameter predict outcome? *Journal of Vascular Surgery,* Vol.44, No.5, pp. 920-931, ISSN 0741-5214

Zarins, C. K., White, R. A., Hodgson, K. J., Schwarten, D., & Fogarty, T. J. (2000). Endoleak as a predictor of outcome after endovascular aneurysm repair: AneuRx multicenter clinical trial. *Journal of Vascular Surgery,* Vol.32, No.1, pp. 90-107, ISSN 0741-5214

Zarins, C. K., White, R. A., Schwarten, D., Kinney, E., Diethrich, E. B., Hodgson, K. J., et al. (1999). AneuRx stent graft versus open surgical repair of abdominal aortic aneurysms: Multicenter prospective clinical trial. *Journal of Vascular Surgery,* Vol.29, No.2, pp. 292-305; discussion pp. 306-308, ISSN 0741-5214

Zeebregts, C. J., Geelkerken, R. H., van der Palen, J., Huisman, A. B., de Smit, P., & van Det, R. J. (2004). Outcome of abdominal aortic aneurysm repair in the era of endovascular treatment. *The British Journal of Surgery,* Vol.91 No.5, pp. 563-568, ISSN 0741-5214

10

12-year Experience with the Endologix Powerlink^R Device in Endovascular Repair of Abdominal Aortic Aneurysms

Ziheng Wu[1], Lefeng Qu[2], Dieter Raithel[3] and Konstantinos Xiromeritis[3]
[1]Department of Vascular Surgery, First Affiliated Hospital, College of Medicine, Zhejiang University, Hangzhou
[2]Department of Vascular Surgery, Changhai Hospital Affiliated to the Second Military Medical University
[3]Department of Vascular and Endovascular Surgery, Nuremberg Southern Hospital,
[1,2]China
[3]Germany

1. Introduction

Since Parodi reported the first successful endovascular aneurysm repair procedure in 1991, this procedure has gained wide acceptance for the treatment of abdominal aortic aneurysms in the past two decades. This minimally invasive approach has been proven effective and safe in the treatment of abdominal aortic aneurysm patients with lower early morbidity and mortality rates compared to open surgery repair. Meanwhile, dozens of endografts have been designed for endovascular aneurysm repair, and most of them are now still undergoing modification and improvement. Although these devices have been improved over time, secondary procedures are required in up to 27% of patients following endovascular aneurysm repair. Complications of stent-graft migration, endoleaks, stent rupture/fracture, aortic neck dilatation and development of other aortoiliac aneurysms mandate lifelong patient follow-up.

Among these complications the most prevalent and concerning complications are distal migration (defined by the Society for Vascular Surgery as device movement of greater than 10 mm or lesser device movement necessitating secondary intervention) and Type I endoleak, putting the patients under an increasing risk of aneurysm rupture. Migration has a reported incidence of up to 45%, and has been shown in biomechanical analyses to be the result of both persistent downward flow upon the stent-graft bifurcation (affecting neck fixation), and transverse forces, resulting in device lateral movement (affecting neck fixation, component stability, and iliac fixation). Type I endoleak is closely associated with migration, and is certainly the most significant predictor of aneurysm increase, risk of rupture, and need for secondary intervention or open conversion repair.

Therefore, the most favorable design of endovascular aneurysm repair endograft should theoretically support to counteract the downward force of pulsatile blood flow and possibly prevent distal migration. Now on the market most of the endovascular aneurysm repair endografts are modular devices and deployed from proximal to distal. The Endologix

(Irvine, CA, USA) Powerlink^R device is the only unibody endograft which is deployed at the aortic bifurcation ("anatomical fixation"). From our nearly 16 years experience of more than 1700 (ending in November 2009) endovascular aneurysm repair cases with 13 different endografts, we prefer the Powerlink^R unibody bifurcated device for this challenge. Ending in December 2008, 612 cases of endovascular aneurysm repair were performed using the Powerlink^R device in our single center, in 513 patients the devices were implanted "anatomically" from the aortoiliac bifurcation to the renal artery level with or without proximal cuff and/or additional Palmaz^R stent. We have published our outcomes with the Powerlink^R for abdominal aortic aneurysms in the last years. In one article, the results included the cases that deployed not "anatomically". The objective of this report is to summarize our 12-year experience of endovascular aneurysm repair for abdominal aortic aneurysm with the Powerlink^R stent-graft deployed "anatomically".

2. Methods

2.1 Patient sample

From February 1999 to December 2008, 612 patients with infrarenal abdominal aortic aneurysm were evaluated for endovascular aneurysm repair treatment with the Endologix Powerlink^R endograft in our center. Of this cohort in 513 patients the devices were implanted "anatomically" from the aortoiliac bifurcation to the renal artery level with or without proximal cuff and/or additional Palmaz^R stent. According to the American Society of Anesthesiologists' physical status classification there were 60.8% (312/513) cases in ASA III/IV stage. The follow-up imaging was performed at 1 month, 6 months and yearly thereafter. Computed tomography angiograms with a 2.5-mm slice thickness were routinely performed to determine endovascular aneurysm repair eligibility. Data of these 513 patients were retrospectively analyzed in the study. Of these 513 patients, a special analysis was also made of data from 117 cases with short and/or angulated necks (from February 1999 to December 2007) (Table 1).

	Short neck (11-15 mm)	Very short neck (< 10 mm)	Angulated neck (> 60°)
Number of cases	54	26	37
Mean age, years	72.2	73.1	72.7
Male	50 (93%)	23 (88%)	32 (86%)
Mean AAA diameter, cm	5.8	6.1	6.3
ASA class III/IV	44 (81%)	21 (81%)	31 (84%)

Table 1. Demographics and Patients Characteristics

2.2 Endologix Powerlink^R system

The Powerlink^R main body device is an unibody bifurcated endograft consisting of a fully supported, high density, low porosity expanded polytetrafluoroethylene (ePTFE) graft with an endoskeleton constructed as a single-wire, cobalt chromium alloy body with limbs. The graft is attached to the stent only at the proximal and distal ends using surgical suture, a feature that results in excellent resistance to stent fracture or fatigue. Accessory proximal extensions are constructed in like manner, with both infrarenal configurations and suprarenal PowerFit™ configurations available (Figure 1).

Accessory limb extensions in straight, stepped, flared, and tapered configurations are available to permit customization to patient anatomy as needed (Figure 2). Device availability permits the treatment of patients with proximal aortic neck diameters of 18 to 32 mm, and distal iliac seal zone diameters of 10 to 23 mm. The low profile 19 Fr delivery system introducer requires only one surgically exposed femoral artery for deployment. Unique to this device, contralateral access is obtained percutaneously (9Fr) through a pre-cannulated contralateral limb. These features enable use of the device in patients with one small or severely diseased iliac access vessel, where with available proximal fixation devices, this is not possible. The Powerlink^R design and access flexibility thus increase the number of patients that can be electively treated by endovascular aneurysm repair. Moreover, the use of the integrated introducer sheath for accessory delivery and deployment and ancillary device introduction reduces the need for exchanges, thereby minimizing the potential for vessel intimal injury (Figure 3).

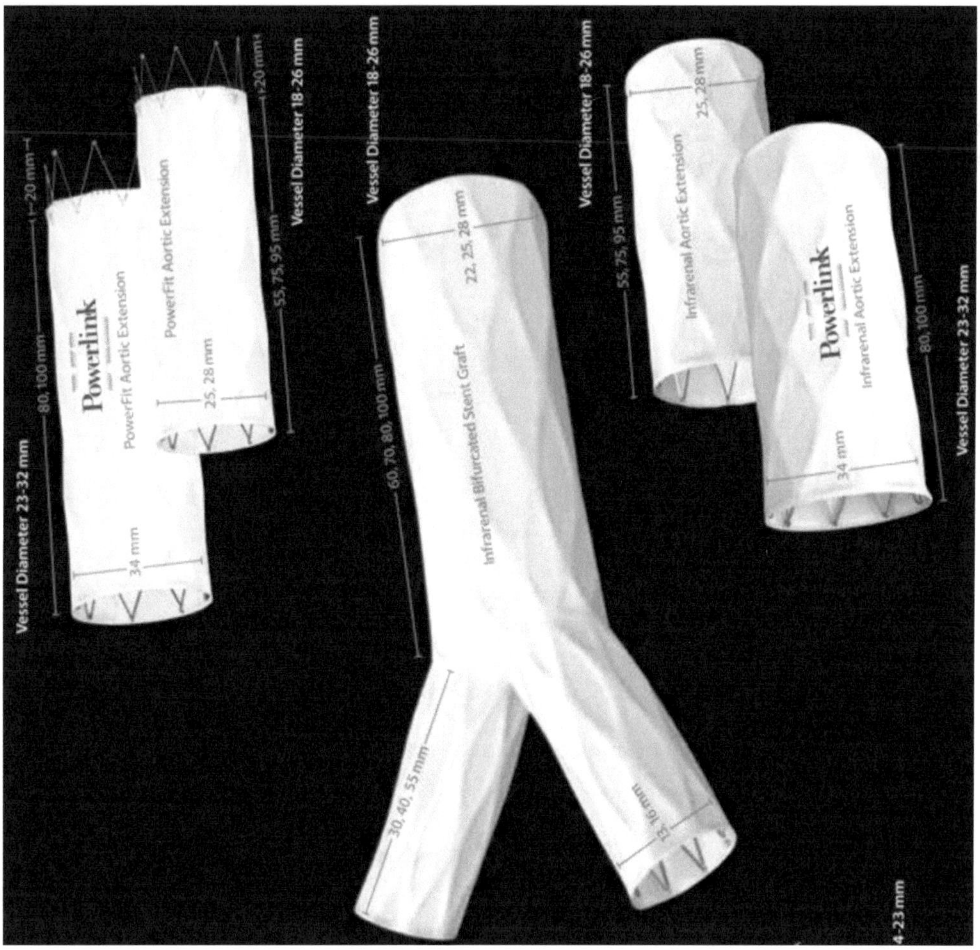

Fig. 1. Powerlink^R Endografts (Unibody bifurcated, PowerFit™)

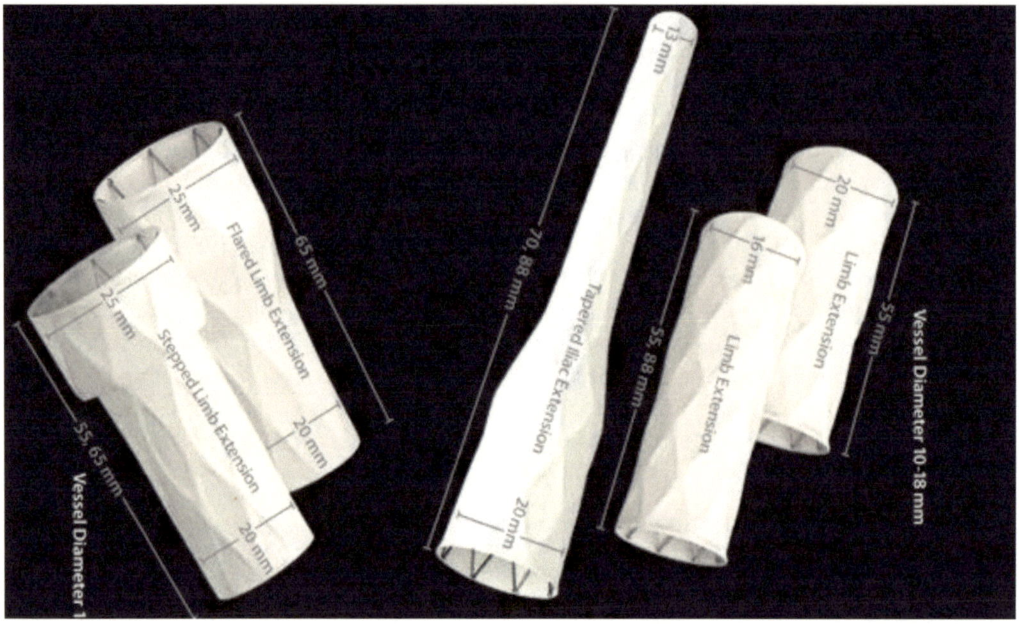

Fig. 2. Powerlink^{R} Endografts Accessory limb extensions (straight, tapered, flared and stepped extensions)

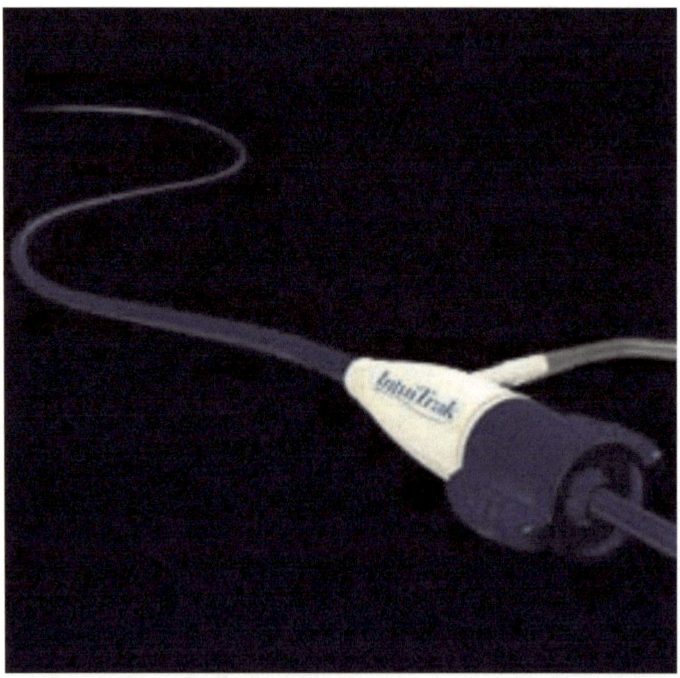

Fig. 3. IntuiTrak endovascular abdominal aortic aneurysm system (Flexible, low profile delivery system, anatomical fixation, Pre-cannulated 9F contralateral limb, Hydrophilic coated sheath, Simple and controlled deployment)

2.3 EVAR procedure with the Powerlink[R] system

Stent-graft selection is based on pre-operative and intra-operative measurements of aortic non-aneurysmal neck diameter, aortic length from the most caudal renal artery to the aortic bifurcation, and length from the aortic bifurcation to the hypogastric arteries. Procedures are performed in suitably equipped operating rooms or endovascular suites with operating room availability. Proper fluoroscopic imaging equipment and tools include a mobile C-arm, automated contrast injector, intraoperative angiography, and if preferred, intravascular ultrasound. Bifurcated and, as needed, proximal extension stent-graft models are chosen per established sizing algorithms, while achieving proximal seal and fully lining the infrarenal aorta. After angiography and aortic length verification with a marker catheter, the bifurcated stent graft delivery system contralateral guidewire is placed, and the integrated 19Fr introducer sheath is advanced over the stiff guidewire into the aorta. Under fluoroscopic visualization, the introducer sheath is retracted to expose the constrained bifurcated stent graft. The constrained device is then placed upon the aortoiliac bifurcation, after which the main body and each limb of the device are deployed using a simple yet metered control cord mechanism. This results in implantation of the device at the aortoiliac bifurcation (i.e., anatomical fixation). Based on the patient anatomy and intraoperative angiography, an accessory proximal extension is placed as needed to achieve adequate overlap with the bifurcated device and seal in the proximal neck (Figure 4). Limb extensions can similarly be placed as needed to accommodate patient anatomical needs. Balloon dilatation may be performed if desired.

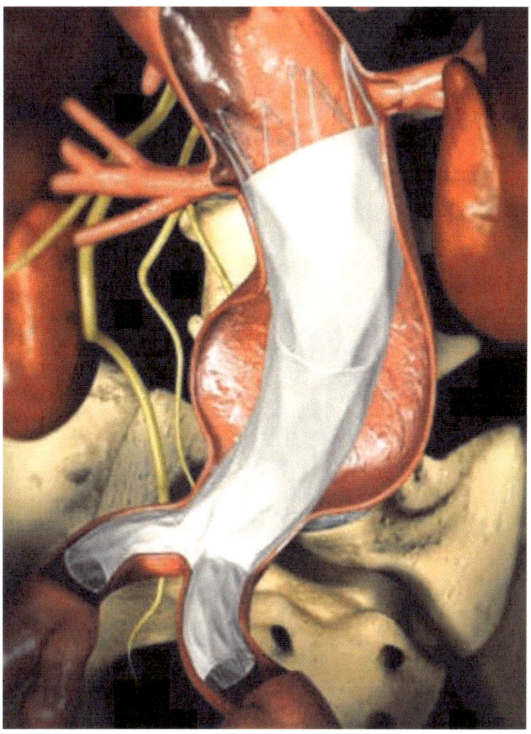

Fig. 4. Image of the Anatomically Fixed Powerlink[R] Implant. Full aortic relining and proximal seal are completed with the PowerFit™ proximal extension.

2.4 Palmaz^R stent and deployment procedure

Palmaz^R stents are inserted through a 14-F Check-Flo Performer introducer (Cook, Bloomington, IN, USA). The stent can be expanded to 14-25 mm correspondingly the length from 37.79-30.58 mm. The stent was advanced and deployed across the renal arteries and top of the graft with a MAXI LD PTA balloon dilation catheter (Cordis, Miami, FL, USA). We usually choose a P4014 Palmaz^R stent, a 25mm-diameter expandable balloon and a 45cm-long 14F sheath (Figure 5). The balloon had better be inflated one time whose surface is relatively coarse to prevent the stent from dislocation in the course of deployment. The Palmaz^R stent was asymmetrically hand-crimped on an expandable balloon that ensures that the proximal (cranial) aspect will expand first. A long sheath is placed distal to the target area. We regularly deploy the Palmaz^R stent with one third above the renal artery, since when we dilate the Palmaz^R stent, it shortens. Once the balloon and stent assembly is in position, the sheath is partially retracted to allow only the proximal (cranial) half of the balloon to expand, flaring the unsheathed proximal stent. The expanded proximal balloon prevents cranial stent migration. The sheath prevents distal (caudal) stent migration. Full retraction of the sheath allows the distal balloon and stent to expand, completing the stent deployment (Figure 6).

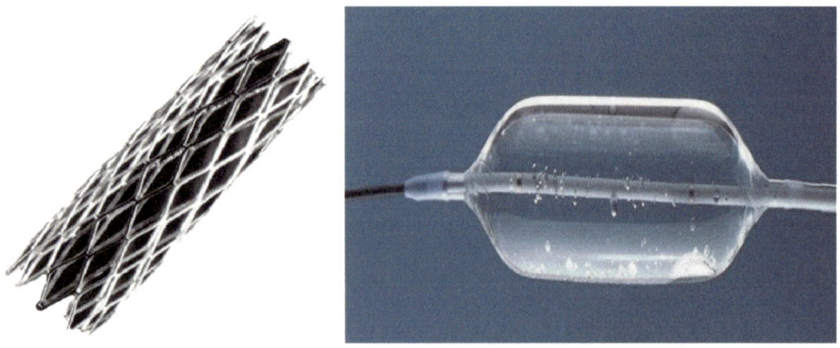

Fig. 5. A P4014 Palmaz^R stent and a MAXI LD PTA expandable balloon

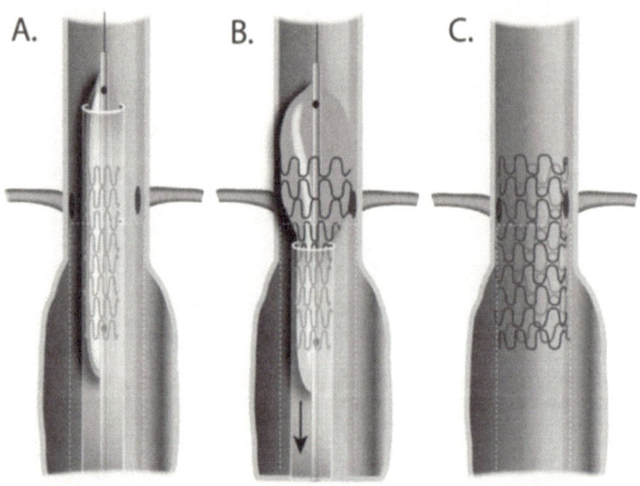

Fig. 6. Details of the deployment procedure of Palmaz^R stent. (A) The stent loaded off-center on the balloon is positioned at the intended area of deployment through the sheath under fluoroscopic guidance. (B) The sheath is partially retracted and the balloon is insufflated, deploying the proximal (cranial) portion of the stent. (C) Fully deployed stent.

2.5 Follow-up

All patients were evaluated before discharge; at 1 and 6 months; and annually thereafter to assess clinical symptoms, potential endoleaks, and aneurysm size. Computed tomography angiogram was performed at each visit; digital subtract angiography was used selectively in special cases, such as visible endoleak or aneurysm sac enlargement seen on computed tomography angiograms.

3. Results

This study cohort included 513 consecutive patients (mean age 72.9±8.0 years, male 461); the mean maximal aneurysm diameter was 54.6±8.9 mm. 86 (16.8%) cases underwent preliminary hypogastric embolisation in the presence of common iliac artery and/or hypogastric artery aneurysm or a too short common iliac artery. The technical success rate was 98.4% (505/513), emergent open conversion occurred in 8 cases (1.6%) because of delivery access problem. The proximal cuff was used in 61.0% (308/505), Palmaz^{R} stent in 20.6% (104/505), limb extension in 14.3% (72/505), retrograde iliac artery endarterectomy and femoral patchplasty in 27 (5.3%) cases, iliac-femoral graft interposition in two cases. Primary type Ia endoleak occurred in 20 cases (4.0%) and all were remedied intraoperatively by Palmaz^{R} stent or the endoleaks were considered so minimal that spontaneous vanish would be expected in close follow-up. 18 (3.5%) cases had type II endoleak and were under routine observation. Mean procedure time was 55±21 min. The 30-day mortality rate was 0.4% (2/513) (Table 2).

	Whole group	Short and/or angulated neck group
Case number	513	117
Range time	2/1999-12/2008	2/1999-12/2007
Technical success rate	98.4% (505/513)	97.4% (114/117)
Emergent conversion rate	1.6% (8/513)	2.6% (3/117)
Proximal cuff	61.0% (308/505)	100% (114/114)
Palmaz^{R} stent	20.6% (104/505)	72.8% (83/114)
Primary type Ia endoleak	4.0% (20/505)	5.3% (6/114)
Type II endoleak	3.5% (18/505)	4.4% (5/114)
30-day mortality rate	0.4% (2/513)	1.7% (2/117)

Table 2. Procedure details and perioperative complications

503 cases were followed up for mean 5.2 years (range, 2 months–9.5 years). Proximal type I endoleak existed in 6 cases (1.2%), all of them were primary type Ia endoleaks, 4 were revised with proximal cuff and/or Palmaz^{R} stent and 2 by selective open conversion. Type II endoleak existed in 22 cases (4.4%), limb occlusion rate was 1.0% (5/503), partial renal infarction occurred in 9 cases (1.8%) and selective open conversion rate was 1.6% (8/503). There were no aneurysms rupture, no device migration, no type III/IV endoleak and stent-graft rupture/fracture. A reduction in mean aneurysm sac diameters and volumes has been noted at every follow-up interval (Table 3).

Of the 117 patients with short and/or angulated neck, the technical success rate was 97.4% (114/117). Intraoperative complications included 3 (2.6%) emergent open conversions due to

delivery access problem, 6 (5.3%) primary type Ia endoleaks and 5 (4.4%) type II endoleaks. The 30-day mortality was 1.7% (2/117) (Table 2, 4).
The 2.6-year follow-up results showed 4 (3.6%) primary type Ia endoleaks, which were revised with proximal cuff and/or Palmaz^R stent. Limb occlusion occurred in 2 (1.8%) cases. There were no open conversion, no aneurysm rupture, no device migration, no type III/IV endoleaks and stent-graft rupture/fracture (Table 3, 5).

	Whole group	Short and/or angulated neck group
Case number	513	117
Follow-up case number	503	112
Follow-up mean period	5.2 years	2.6 years
Type Ia endoleak	1.2% (6/503)	3.6% (4/112)
Type II endoleak	4.4% (22/503)	2.7% (3/112)
Limb occlusion rate	1.0% (5/503)	1.8% (2/112)
Partial renal infarction	1.8% (9/503)	2.7% (3/112)
Selective conversion rate	1.6% (8/503)	0.0% (0/112)
Aneurysm rupture	0	0
Device migration	0	0
Type III/IV endoleak	0	0
Stent-graft rupture	0	0

Table 3. Intraoperative and postoperative results

	Short neck (n=54)	Very short neck (n=26)	Angulated neck (n=37)
Successful implantation	52 (96.3%)	26 (100%)	37 (97.3%)
Delivery access problem	2	0	1
One proximal cuff	50 (96.2%)	22 (84.6%)	29 (80.6%)
Two proximal cuffs	2 (3.8%)	4 (15.4%)	7 (19.4%)
Proximal Palmaz stent	42 (80.8%)	23 (88.5%)	18 (50.0%)
Limb extension	6 (11.5%)	3 (11.5%)	3 (8.3%)
Suprarenal fixation	48 (92.3%)	26 (100%)	33 (91.7%)
Infrarenal fixation	4 (7.7%)	0	3 (9.3%)
Retrograde iliac TEA	3 (5.8%)	1 (3.8%)	2 (5.6%)
Femoral patch/angioplasty	3 (5.8%)	2 (7.6%)	3 (8.3%)
Iliac-fem bypass	0	0	1
Proximal type I endoleak	3 (5.8%)	1 (3.8%)	2 (5.6%)
Type II	2 (3.8%)	1 (3.8%)	2 (5.6%)
Type III/IV	0	0	0

Table 4. Procedure details and intraoperative complications in the hostile neck anatomy group

	Short neck (n=54)	Very short neck (n=26)	Angulated neck (n=37)
Proximal type I endoleak	2 (3.8%)	1 (3.8%)	1 (2.8%)
Type II endoleak	2 (3.8%)	0	1 (2.8%)
Partial renal infarction	2 (3.8%)	0	1 (2.8%)
Distal migration	0	0	0
Stent kinking	0	0	0
Limb occlusion	1 (1.9%)	0	1 (2.8%)

Table 5. Mean 2.6 years follow-up results in hostile neck anatomy group

4. Discussions

The applicability of endovascular aneurysm repair in abdominal aortic aneurysms mainly depends on the aortoiliac anatomy and morphology. Among all the challenging factors limiting application of this minimally invasive technique, the infrarenal aortic aneurysm neck morphology is still the most important determinant. The infrarenal neck length and angulation are the first parameters we should consider in the indication for endovascular aneurysm repair. Some clinical studies have made it clear that abdominal aortic aneurysms with short and/or angulated necks for endovascular aneurysm repair have a high risk of stent-graft distal migration and proximal type I endoleak, which make up the exact criteria in challenging cases. In one EUROSTAR study, 5183 patients underwent endovascular aneurysm repair from October 1996 to January 2006. Incidence of stent-graft migration, proximal type I endoleak, proximal neck dilatation, secondary interventions, aneurysm rupture, and all-cause and aneurysm-related mortality were compared between patients with and without severe infrarenal neck angulation (> 60 degrees angle between the infrarenal aortic neck and the longitudinal axis of the aneurysm). In the short term (before discharge), stent-graft migration (OR 2.17, 95% CI 1.20 to 3.91, p=0.0105) and proximal type I endoleak (OR 2.32, 95% CI 1.60 to 3.37, p<0.0001) were observed more frequently in patients with severe infrarenal neck angulation. Over the long term, proximal type I endoleak (HR 1.80, 95% CI 1.25 to 2.58, p=0.0016), higher incidences of proximal neck dilatation (> or =4 mm) (HR 1.26, 95% CI 1.11 to 1.43, p=0.0004) and need for secondary interventions (HR 1.29, 95% CI 1.00 to 1.67, p=0.0488) were seen in the severe infrarenal neck angulation group. All-cause mortality, rupture of the aneurysm and aneurysm-related mortality were similar in patients with and without severe infrarenal neck angulation. In the subgroup of patients with an Excluder endograft, proximal endoleak at the completion angiogram (OR 4.49, 95% CI 1.31 to 15.32, p=0.0166) and long-term proximal neck dilatation (HR 1.67, 95% CI 1.20 to 2.33, p=0.0026) were more frequently observed in patients with severe infrarenal neck angulation.

The endovascular aneurysm repair mechanism is to construct an endoluminal exclusion channel inside the native aortoiliac artery to exclude the aneurysm from the dynamic blood flow to prevent rupture, and the endoluminal exclusion channel must be stable and sealed. But short necks are unable to provide sufficient proximal landing zone for secure fixation and seal; angulated necks are unable to provide proper anchoring adaptation for secure fixation and seal. Is there an optimal device to adapt to these challenging anatomies? Most of the authors and the currently available devices emphasize the proximal fixation with

bars/hooks/crimps and suprarenal fixation, but device distal migration is still unavoidable. Interestingly, all the currently available modular devices were designed to implant starting just below the renal arteries, which will result in hanging the device inside the aneurysm sac. From the dynamic mechanism, it is not stable, as the blood flow through the stent-graft acts as a displacing force, and the endograft is normally held in position by friction dependant on the radial force of the graft against the aortic wall and the contact surface between the graft material and the artery wall.
Completely contrary to these modular devices, the Powerlink^R one-piece long main body bifurcated stent-graft was designed to be implanted sitting on the native abdominal aortic bifurcation. We have termed this technique "Anatomical Fixation", which proved effective in eradicating distal migration. Mimicking construction of a building, the endoluminal exclusion channel can be built up to the renal artery level with an oversized long suprarenal proximal cuff. After endograft stability has been achieved, more attention should be paid to the proximal fixation and seal. A compulsory ballooning of the neck and the conjunction part was routinely carried out for better adaptation. Palmaz^R stent implantation depends on the angiogram outcome. We normally implant the Palmaz^R stent only if there is a high risk of proximal type I endoleak. A Palmaz^R stent is used in the neck to strengthen the radial fixation force and to adapt the graft to the aortic wall for better seal. Balloon-expandable Palmaz^R stent has been proven to provide better seal as well as fixation in treating hostile necks.
Qu et al reported their results of 612 eligible abdominal aortic aneurysm patients underwent endovascular aneurysm repair between 1999 and 2008 using the Powerlink^R System in our center. Of the 612 patients, 99 cases (16%) completed between 1999 and 2004 had the endograft deployed from the renal artery downward. The remaining 513 cases (84%) completed afterwards had the bifurcated stent-graft deployed onto the native aortoiliac bifurcation. Among the 513 cases, 146 cases (28%) were deemed as challenging anatomy with short and/or angulated neck. Technical success was achieved in 98.5% of patients (603/612). Intraoperative emergent open conversion occurred in 9 patients, 8 of which were due to delivery access problems and 1 due to rupture. 3 deaths and 2 limb occlusions were encountered perioperatively. During the follow-up (mean: 5.2 years; maximum: 9.5 years), 1 rupture and 7 migrations occurred, all of which were in patients in whom the device was fixed at the level of the renal arteries. The rates of late selective open conversion in the renal fixation and anatomical fixation groups were 4.0% and 1.9%, respectively. Likewise, the cumulative rates of proximal type I endoleak in the groups of renal fixation and anatomical fixation were 5.0% and 1.2%, respectively. Remarkably, no stent fracture, graft disruption and type III/type IV endoleaks were observed in any patient. Harlin et al also reported the new results of 44 consecutive eligible patients enrolled in eight US sites between 2006 and 2008. Each patient underwent a Powerlink^R infrarenal bifurcated stent-graft with anatomical fixation onto the native aortoiliac bifurcation and a suprarenal proximal cuff to achieve proximal sealing. Challenging infrarenal aortic neck anatomy was present in 93% of patients. Technical success rate was 100%. No aneurysm-related deaths, open conversions, migrations, or type III/IV endoleaks were observed. The majority of endoleaks (80%) observed during follow up were type II. The primary clinical success rate was 93%. Two secondary endovascular procedures were performed for type Ia or type Ib endoleak, and one surgical intervention was performed for resolution of limb occlusion. Significant reduction in sac diameter has been observed to up to 2 years. Between September 2005 and June 2008, a prospective, multicenter, pivotal US Food and Drug Administration trial of the Powerlink XL System for endovascular aneurysm repair was conducted at 13 centers. A total of 78 patients presenting with abdominal aortic aneurysm

and an infrarenal aortic neck up to 32 mm in diameter received the bifurcated stent-graft with anatomical fixation onto the native aortoiliac bifurcation and proximal sealing with a Powerlink XL infrarenal proximal extension stent-graft. Challenging infrarenal aortic neck anatomy was present in 85% of patients. Technical success was achieved in 98.7% of patients, with one patient requiring femoral-femoral bypass intraoperatively. Aneurysm exclusion was achieved in 100% of patients. At the one-month CT scan, the independent core lab identified a Type II endoleak in 13 patients, Type Ib and Type II endoleaks in one patient, and unknown endoleak in three patients. At 30 days, there were no deaths, open conversions, ruptures, or migrations. Through one year follow-up, Type II endoleak predominated (9/10 patients with endoleak), with one proximal Type I endoleak and no Type III/IV; no conversions, ruptures, or migrations have been observed. The one-year all-cause mortality rate was 6.4%, with 100% freedom from aneurysm-related mortality. Secondary procedures were performed within one year in five patients (6.4%) for treatment of proximal Type I endoleak (n = 2), proximal Type I/Type II endoleak (n = 1), and distal Type I endoleak (n = 2). Reduced or stable aneurysm sac diameter at one year was observed in 96% of patients. All these results suggest that anatomical fixation at the native aortic bifurcation can provide secure fixation for cases with hostile proximal aortic necks.
Short-term results suggested the use of the prophylactic adjunctive balloon-expandable Palmaz^{R} stents may decrease the incidence of secondary interventions related to challenging neck anatomy when used as an adjunctive measure with endovascular aneurysm repair. Cox et al reviewed their experience of endovascular aneurysm repair with use of the Palmaz^{R} stents in patients with hostile neck anatomy and type I endoleaks. Of 140 patients who underwent endovascular aneurysm repair between 2000 and 2004, they reviewed data of 19 patients in whom they used the proximal balloon-expandable stents. Palmaz^{R} stents were deployed in the proximal graft with transrenal extension. AneuRx (18/19) and Zenith (1/19) endografts were used in all of the patients. Of the 19 patients, 15 had the prophylactic stent placement for known hostile neck anatomy and 4 patients had stent placement for type I endoleak. Assisted primary technical success was achieved in all patients. Three patients had maldeployment of the endograft or proximal stent requiring additional endovascular interventions at the time of surgery. No endografts were deployed too low requiring stent placement. Procedure-related complications occurred in 2 of 19 patients. These included 1 operative death secondary to pneumonia and 1 patient who developed progressive renal failure. Short-term clinical success was achieved in 17 of 19 patients. Two patients required secondary interventions, 1 due to device migration with secondary conversion to open repair, and an endoleak, which, on angiogram, was a large type II endoleak successfully treated with coiling of the inferior mesenteric artery. One patient was observed to have a type II endoleak with no associated aneurysm enlargement. Another retrospective review was made of 250 consecutive abdominal aortic aneurysm cases with hostile necks that underwent commercially available endograft treatment adjunctive with the Palmaz^{R} stent in Arizona heart institute and Nuremberg south hospital from September 2005 to November 2009. The primary technical success rate was 83.6% (209/250). The mean time of follow-up was 23.4 months; the overall clinical success rate was 95.2% (238/250). The overall conversion rate was 2.4% (6/250) due to large proximal type I endoleak and sac enlargement. There was no neck dilation or graft migration. These results showed deployment of the Palmaz^{R} stent in hostile necks has proved to be easy, effective and safe.
At the beginning, most of the abdominal aortic aneurysm cases in our center were performed according to the publicly accepted anatomical criteria for endovascular aneurysm repair. With

accumulation of experience, the indication of endovascular aneurysm repair has been widely broadened. Abiding by the above philosophy, approximately 90%-95% of infrarenal abdominal aortic aneurysms in our unit can be treated with endovascular aneurysm repair, and we are treating more and more challenging cases (such as short neck, angulated neck, thrombus-affiliated neck, calcified neck and surface-irregular neck, et al) in this way.

In the whole group, with a mean 5.2-year long-term follow-up, the type Ia endoleak rate was only 1.2% (6/503). Even in the short and/or angulated neck group with mean 2.6-year mid-term follow-up, the proximal type I endoleak rate was 3.6% (4/112), without open conversion and distal migration. Our results have strongly demonstrated that the Endologix Powerlink^{R} endograft with "anatomical fixation" is very effective to prevent migration and type Ia endoleak for abdominal aortic aneurysms with challenging neck anatomy.

After building upon the foundation of the bifurcated endograft, a suprarenal proximal cuff with a long overlapping segment inside the bifurcated main body endograft is built up to the renal artery level. In our whole group, proximal long cuff was used in 61.0% (308/505) cases, and in the hostile neck group, all the patients had the proximal long cuff. This long cuff is not only used for prevention of type III endoleak but also useful for stretching the angulated segment of the infrarenal aorta, namely remodeling and straightening the proximal angulated neck. 20.6% (104/505) and 72.8% (83/114) patients had proximal Palmaz^{R} stents in the whole group and the hostile neck group, respectively, resulting in further remodeling of the infrarenal aorta with more contact area for better fixation and seal (Figure 7).

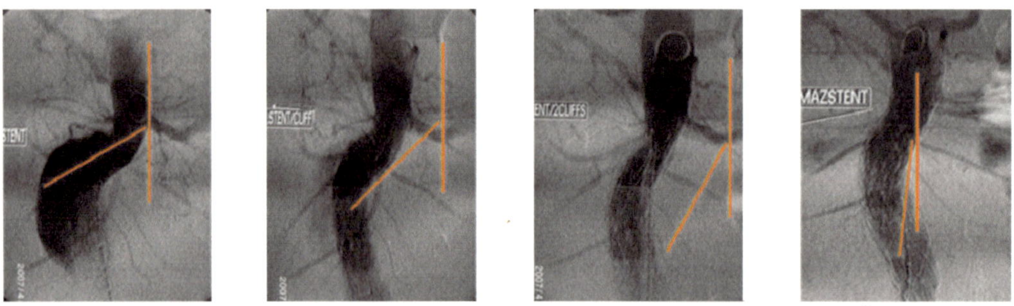

Fig. 7. Angiography-pictures after deployment of the Powerlink^{R} bifurcated main body stent, the first PowerFit^{TM} proximal cuff, the second PowerFit^{TM} proximal cuff, the Palmaz^{R} stent in turn

Regarding the device size choice, the Powerlink^{R} unibody bifurcated stent-graft is different from the modular devices. The distance from the lowest renal artery to the abdominal aortic bifurcation, and the distance from the aortic bifurcation to the hypogastric artery are important parameters for the size choice. Graft length is determined by the lengths of the native abdominal aorta and the common iliac artery. Graft diameter is determined by oversizing the endograft by 10-20% in excess of the measured neck diameter. Due to the several standard sizes of the main body, proximal cuff and limb extension, this system proved simple and easy for size selection. The most commonly used main body size in our unit is 25 mm in neck diameter, 10 cm in main body length, 16 mm in limb diameter, and 5.5 cm in limb length. The most commonly used suprarenal proximal cuff is 28 mm in diameter and 75 mm or 95 mm in length.

Common iliac aneurysm and/or hypogastric artery aneurysm or a too short common iliac artery can prevent safe and successful anchoring of the distal end of the limb of the stent. Some studies reported that common iliac artery aneurysms exist in about 20% to 30% of patients with abdominal aortic aneurysms who were examined for endovascular aneurysm repair. In our study, the applicability of endovascular aneurysm repair was increased by 16.8% (86/513) after preliminary hypogastric aneurysm embolization. Therefore, preliminary embolization of hypogastric artery with additional extension of the graft to the external iliac artery may expand the indication of endovascular aneurysm repair. But we all know that hypogastric artery embolization will cause pelvic ischemic complications such as buttock claudication, sexual dysfunction and other pelvic ischemia symptoms (e.g., gluteal necrosis, spinal cord ischemia, rectosigmoid ischemia, or limb ischemia). In our center, a retrospective review was conducted of all 101 consecutive patients (91 men; mean age 73.4 ± 8.7 years) who underwent preliminary embolization of 133 hypogastric arteries about 4 to 6 weeks prior to endovascular aneurysm repair from January 2005 to August 2009. Fourteen patients with 19 hypogastric arteries were treated using coils, while 87 patients were treated with Amplatzer Vascular Plugs in 114 hypogastric arteries. In the coil group, complete occlusion was achieved in 16 (84.2%) of 19 procedures. There were no acute pelvic ischemic symptoms after hypogastric artery embolization or endovascular aneurysm repair. Five (35.7%) patients had buttock claudication and 2 (16.7%) of 12 men experienced new erectile dysfunction after embolization. At a mean 42.2-month follow-up (range 14-58), 3 (21.4%) patients had a type II endoleak via retrograde flow in the hypogastric artery without aneurysm growth and were under observation. In the Amplatzer Vascular Plugs group, all 114 hypogastric arteries in 87 patients were successfully occluded; there was no device dislodgment or limb ischemia observed. Buttock claudication and new sexual dysfunction developed in 12 (13.8%) patients and 4 (5.1%) of 79 men after the procedure, respectively. During a mean 26.4-month follow-up (range 4-54), 2 (2.3%) patients developed distal type I endoleaks after endovascular aneurysm repair, but angiography confirmed that neither of the endoleaks was related to the vessel embolized with the Amplatzer Vascular Plugs. Comparing the outcomes of the treatment groups, the Amplatzer Vascular Plugs was placed with fewer intraoperative complications (p=0.013) and more complete occlusion (p=0.01) than coil embolization. The rate of buttock claudication was lower in the Amplatzer Vascular Plugs group (p=0.042). Our clinical researches showed that hypogastric aneurysm embolization prior to endovascular aneurysm repair is safe and effective. The Amplatzer^R Vascular Plug affords easier and more precise placement and provides more complete occlusion, with fewer intraoperative and postoperative ischemic complications than coil embolization.

For proximal type I endoleak, balloon angioplasty is first recommended in our experience. If it does not work, a Palmaz^R stent in the aneurysm neck is able to cure the endoleak. There were 20 cases and 6 cases of primary proximal type I endoleaks in the whole group and the short and/or angulated neck group after balloon angioplasty, respectively. But after the deployment of the palmaz^R stent, all of them were remedied or minimal that spontaneous vanish was expected by operators in the follow-up. During the mid-term or long-term follow-up, only 6 and 4 primary proximal type I endoleak still existed in the two groups. If there is still some space between the renal artery and the top of the stent-graft, a suprarenal proximal cuff with or without Palmaz^R stent can achieve a good result. Only 2 cases in the whole group underwent selective open conversion, the other 4 were all remedied by endovascular re-intervention.

Delivery access problems were the main reasons for emergent open conversion. In our study, all of the intraoperative emergent open conversion occurred because of the delivery access problems. But with the accumulation of our experience, for most stenotic iliac

arteries, pre-dilatation with an 8 mm or 10 mm angioplasty balloon can usually solve the problem. If not, we preferred retrograde iliac artery endarterectomy with Moll Ring cutter.
9 (1.8%) cases in the whole group suffered from partial renal infarction found on computed tomography scan, but the renal function was not impaired. Though all these 9 cases had suprarenal fixation, a controlled study from two pivotal US Food and Drug Administration trials using the Powerlink^R bifurcated stent-graft revealed that suprarenal fixation does not lead to a significant increase in acute renal events, renal impairment, or alteration in blood pressure compared with infrarenal fixation. During the trials, 283 patients underwent endovascular aneurysm repair with the Powerlink^R bifurcated stent-graft. A comparison of preoperative, perioperative (1 ~ 7 days), and postoperative (>7 days) alterations in serum creatinine, creatinine clearance and blood pressure was done. Renal adverse events were determined by computed tomography scan and clinical chart review and included renal infarction, renal artery stenosis (either progressive or requiring renal stent placement) and renal artery occlusion. Both suprarenal fixation and infrarenal fixation groups showed a significant increase in serum creatinine and a decrease in creatinine clearance over time. No significant difference in serum creatinine or creatinine clearance existed between groups during any time period. There were no differences in postoperative renal impairment (infrarenal, 10.2%; suprarenal, 7.6%, P = 0.634), the need for hemodialysis (infrarenal, 0.7%; suprarenal, 0%, P = 1.00), systolic and diastolic blood pressure during subsequent follow-up between treatment groups. There was no significant difference in the number of renal adverse events detected by computed tomography between the infrarenal fixation (10, 6.8%) group and the suprarenal fixation (3, 3.8%) group (P = 0.550).
Proximal fixation devices artificially elevate the aortoiliac bifurcation, requiring contralateral limb cannulation some distance from the patient's native aortoiliac bifurcation. In the case of a narrow distal aorta, bi-lobe or saccular aneurysms, such maneuvers can be challenging or unachievable. An example of this is highlighted in a recent report regarding a newer device, where the distal aortic diameter averaged 33mm in enrolled patients, more than 50% increased over that of patients enrolled in the Powerlink^R anatomical fixation trials. Even with this large distal aortic diameter, intraoperative limb stenosis requiring stenting occurred in 11% of patients, with intervention within 30 days for limb occlusion or thrombosis performed in 2.2% of patients, leading the authors to suggest prophylactic intraoperative limb stenting. It is not known if the long-term rate of limb kinking/occlusion will be similar to the 4.3% rate reported for other currently available devices. Interestingly, endografts with fully supported limbs (e.g., Excluder, Powerlink^R) appear to have greater resistance to intraoperative stenosis and kinking and the lowest reported rates of limb kinking or occlusion with long-term follow-up (1.7%, 1.2%). Because the Powerlink^R device includes a pre-cannulated contralateral limb requiring only 9Fr percutaneous access, anatomical fixation implantation eliminates the cannulation problem.
In a multinational registry analysis of patients presenting with coronary artery disease, cerebrovascular disease, or peripheral arterial disease, patients with abdominal aortic aneurysms were found to have a three-fold increased incidence of peripheral artery disease than those without abdominal aortic aneurysms. One cannot deny that preserving the native aortoiliac bifurcation after endovascular aneurysm repair to enable future peripheral interventions is an important consideration. The anatomically fixed Powerlink^R device relining the abdominal aorta offers the opportunity for such subsequent peripheral interventions post-endovascular aneurysm repair.
The complexity of abdominal aortic aneurysm is commonly characterized based on location and involvement of visceral vessels. Infrarenal aneurysms generally involve the infrarenal

aorta and may involve the aortoiliac vasculature. A subset of infrarenal aneurysms extend up to the level of but do not involve the renal arteries (juxtarenal aneurysms) or extend further to involve one or both of the renal arteries (pararenal aneurysms). As noted previously, a substantial proportion of infrarenal aneurysms are not suitable for endovascular aneurysm repair due to unfavorable proximal neck anatomy (e.g., severely angulated, dilated, short, or encroaching on or involving the renal arteries). In regulatory studies of infrarenal endovascular aneurysm repair, patients were carefully selected to ensure neck length and angulation requirements were met in order to optimize outcomes. Shorter length or greater angulation has been reported since the original trials to increase the risk of migration and Type Ia endoleak and associated with need for intervention. Owing to the increased risk of renal complications, mesenteric ischemia and other complications following open repair of juxtarenal or pararenal aneurysms compared to infrarenal aneurysms, researchers have sought to extend a totally endovascular technique to repair these aneurysms. In this treatment, it is essential to maintain the patency of the renal arteries and other visceral vessels. Up to now, only homemade or customized fenestrated stent-grafts with the use of commercially available uncovered or covered vascular stents have been used for the repair of juxtarenal aneurysms. The key limitation to this approach is the need to customize the design and manufacture of each stent-graft to a particular patient anatomy. This requires a lengthy period of time for planning, manufacture, and delivery of the device, and is very costly. As a result, physicians have begun to seek other options, such as hybrid debranching techniques or chimney techniques. However, these options remain suboptimal. The concept of an off the shelf alternative to customization has been postulated; however this has yet to be realized. More recently, an off-the-shelf fenestrated stent-graft system has been developed based on the Powerlink^R stent-graft. Integral to this system is the bifurcated stent-graft, anatomically fixed at the aortoiliac bifurcation, a fenestrated proximal extension with proprietary design, and compatible covered renal stents. All devices are constructed from cobalt chromium alloy for exceptional durability, and have a high density ePTFE covering. Initial estimates suggest this system will be applicable to 80% or more of patients with juxtarenal or pararenal aneurysm, without need for customization. Initial clinical experience will be available by the end of this year. Multicenter clinical trials are expected to commence in 2011, and if successful, would significantly increase the numbers of patients who could be treated endovascularly, would significantly reduce the time from diagnosis to treatment, and would represent significant improvement in cost effectiveness over the currently available options.

The field of endovascular aneurysm repair for abdominal aortic aneurysm has matured in recent years and is progressing into ever more challenging anatomy than treated in early trials. The problems of distal migration or endoleak remain, particularly in the more challenging anatomies. Clearly utilization of the native aortoiliac bifurcation as a strong foundation on which to place the Powerlink^R bifurcated stent-graft followed by achievement of proximal seal with an aortic extension if needed is a simple yet elegant way of mitigating the risk of migration and endograft destabilization. The emergence of anatomical fixation with the availability of a well designed off the shelf proximal extension and visceral branch grafts, starting clinical evaluation at this time, has strong potential to not only address a significant unmet clinical need, but to address global demands for cost-effective options for these patients. Furthermore, the prospective clinical validation of a totally percutaneous approach to endovascular aneurysm repair will serve to advance this technique and its use in properly selected patients. Other proximal fixation devices are in development or available in some regions that feature lower profile delivery systems and enhanced proximal fixation attachment mechanisms. A novel sac anchoring endovascular prosthesis (the Nellix device) is in final stages of regulatory review in Europe. This technology obliterates the aneurysm sac with a polymer-filled endobag and paving endoframe lumens. Although it has the potential to significantly reduce or eliminate the incidence of any endoleak, and thus reduce the surveillance necessary with other endovascular prostheses. Broader and longer term study will be necessary to validate this fully.

The next horizon yet to be addressed is the thoracic aorta, particularly the ascending aorta, where no adequate endovascular options yet exist. Although in final proprietary development at this time, a novel endografting approach utilizing a thoracic anatomical fixation technique with in situ fenestration and branch preservation is on the future horizon.

5. Conclusions

Our experience demonstrated that building up the endovascular exclusion system in the abdominal aortic aneurysms using the unibody Powerlink^R device with proximal cuff and/or additional Palmaz^R stent showed a satisfactory long-term outcome, even proved safe and effective in treating abdominal aortic aneurysms with short and/or angulated neck. With this intuitive approach, stent graft migration and its related potential complications are virtually eliminated. However, prospective longer follow-up in multicenter randomized controlled larger series are necessary to confirm these encouraging outcomes.

6. References

Armon, MP; Wenham, PW. & Whitaker, SC. (1998). Common iliac artery aneurysms in patients with abdominal aortic aneurysms. *Eur J Vasc Endovasc Surg,* Vol. 15, No. 3, (March 1998), pp. 255-257, ISSN 1078-5884

Alterman, DM. & Stevens, SL. (2008). The Excluder aortic endograft. *Perspect Vasc Surg Endovasc Ther.* Vol. 20, No. 2, (June 2008), pp. 136-148, ISSN 1531-0035

AbuRahma, AF; Campbell, J. & Stone, PA. (2009). The correlation of aortic neck length to early and late outcomes in endovascular aneurysm repair patients. *J Vasc Surg,* Vol. 50, No. 4, (October 2009), pp. 738-748, ISSN 0741-5214

Baumgartner, I; Hirsch, AT. & Abola, MT. (2008). Cardiovascular risk profile and outcome of patients with abdominal aortic aneurysm in out-patients with atherothrombosis: data from the reduction of atherothrombosis for continued health (REACH) registry. *J Vasc Surg,* Vol. 48, No. 4, (October 2008), pp. 808-814, ISSN 0741-5214

Brinster, CJ; Fairman, RM. & Woo, EY. (2011). Late open conversion and explantation of abdominal aortic stent grafts. *J Vasc Surg,* Epub ahead of print, (February 2011), ISSN 0741-5214

Cox, DE; Jacobs, DL. & Motaganahalli, RL. (2006). Outcomes of endovascular AAA repair in patients with hostile neck anatomy using adjunctive balloon-expandable stents. *Vasc Endovasc Surg,* Vol. 40, No. 1, (January-February 2006), pp. 35-40, ISSN 1538-5744

Cochennec, F; Becquemin, JP. & Desgranges, P. (2007). Limb graft occlusion following EVAR: clinical pattern, outcomes and predictive factors of occurrence. *Eur J Vasc Endovasc Surg,* Vol. 34, No. 1, (June 2007), pp. 59-65, ISSN 1078-5884

Chaikof, EL; Brewster, DC. & Dalman, RL. (2009). The care of patients with an abdominal aortic aneurysm: The Society for Vascular Surgery practice guideline. *J Vasc Surg,* Vol. 50, No. 4 Suppl, (October 2009), pp. S2-49, ISSN 0741-5214

Carpenter, JP; Garcia, MJ. & Harlin, SA. (2010). Contemporary results of Endovascular repair of abdominal aortic aneurysms: effect of anatomical fixation on outcomes. *J Endovasc Ther,* Vol. 17, No. 2, (April 2010), pp. 153-162, ISSN 1526-6028

Dillavou, ED; Muluk, SC. & Rhee, RY. (2003). Does hostile neck anatomy preclude successful endovascular aortic aneurysm repair? *J Vasc Surg,* Vol. 38, No. 4, (October 2003), pp. 657-663, ISSN 0741-5214

Donayre, CD; Zarins, CK. & Krievins, DK. (2011). Initial clinical experience with a sac-anchoring endoprosthesis for aortic aneurysm repair. *J Vasc Surg,* Vol. 53, No. 3, (March 2011), pp. 574-582, ISSN 0741-5214

Fulton, JJ; Farber, MA. & Marston, WA. (2005). Endovascular stent-graft repair of pararenal and type IV thoracoabdominal aortic aneurysms with adjunctive visceral reconstruction. *J Vasc Surg,* Vol. 41, No. 2, (February 2005), pp. 191-198, ISSN 0741-5214

Greenhalgh, RM; Brown, LC. & Kwong, GP. (2004). Comparison of endovascular aneurysm repair with open repair in patients with abdominal aortic aneurysm (EVAR trial 1), 30-day operative mortality results: randomized controlled trial. *Lancet,* Vol.364, No. 9437, (September 2004), pp. 843-848, ISSN 0140-6736

Henretta, JP; Karch, LA. & Hodgson, KJ. (1999). Special iliac artery considerations during aneurysm endografting. *Am J Surg,* Vol. 178, No. 3, (September 1999), pp. 212-218, ISSN 0002-9610

Hobo, R; Buth, J. & Eurostar collaborators. (2006). Secondary interventions following endovascular abdominal aortic aneurysm repair using current endografts. A EUROSTAR report. *J Vasc Surg,* Vol. 43, No. 5, (May 2006), pp. 896-902, ISSN 0741-5214

Hobo, R; Kievit, J. & Leurs, LJ. (2007). Influence of severe infrarenal aortic neck angulation on complications at the proximal neck following endovascular AAA repair: a Eurostar study. *J Endovasc Ther,* Vol. 14, No. 1, (February 2007), pp. 1-11, ISSN 1526-6028

Harlin, SA; Beasley, RE. & Feldman, RL. (2010). Endovascular abdominal aortic aneurysm repair using an anatomical fixation technique and concomitant suprarenal orientation: results of a prospective, multicenter trial. *Ann Vasc Surg,* Vol. 24, No. 7, (October 2010), pp. 921-929, ISSN 0890-5096

Jordan, WD Jr; Moore, WM Jr. & Melton, JG. (2009). Secure fixation following EVAR with the Powerlink XL System in wide aortic necks: results of a prospective, multicenter trial. *J Vasc Surg,* Vol. 50, No. 5, (November 2009), pp. 979-986, ISSN 0741-5214

Lee, ES. & Zarins, CK. (2004). Endograft migration: incidence, causes, and clinical significance. *Perspect Vasc and Endovasc Surg,* Vol. 16, No. 3, (September 2004), pp. 187-191, ISSN 1531-0035

Li, Z. & Kleinstreuer, C. (2006). Analysis of biomechanical factors affecting stent-graft migration in an abdominal aortic aneurysm model. *J Biomechanics,* Vol. 39, No. 12, (September 2005), pp. 2264-2273, ISSN 0021-9290

Leurs, LJ; Kievit J. & Dagnelie, PC. (2006). Influence of infrarenal neck length on outcome of endovascular abdominal aortic aneurysm repair. *J Endovasc Ther,* Vol. 13, No. 5, (October 2006), pp. 640-648, ISSN 1526-6028

Mehta, M; Sternbach, Y. & Taggert, JB. (2010). Long-term outcomes of secondary procedures after endovascular aneurysm repair. *J Vasc Surg,* Vol. 52, No. 6, (December 2010), pp. 1442-1449, ISSN 0741-5214

Nordon, IM; Hinchcliffe, RJ. & Manning, B. (2010). Toward an "off-the-shelf" fenestrated endograft for management of short-necked abdominal aortic aneurysms: an analysis of current graft morphological diversity. *J Endovasc Ther,* Vol. 17, No. 1, (February 2010), pp. 78-85, ISSN 1526-6028

Parodi, JC.; Palmaz, JC. & Barone, HD. (1991). Transfemoral intraluminal graft implantation for abdominal aortic aneurysms. *Ann Vasc Surg,* Vol.6, No. 4, (November 1991), pp. 491-499, ISSN 0890-5096

Prinssen, M; Verhoeven, EL. & Buth, J. (2004). A randomized trial comparing conventional and endovascular repair of abdominal aortic aneurysms. *N Engl J Med,* Vol.351, No. 16, (October 2004), pp. 1607-1618, ISSN 0028-4793

Parmer, SS. & Carpenter, JP. (2006). Endovascular aneurysm repair with suprarenal vs infrarenal fixation: a study of renal effects. *J Vasc Surg,* Vol. 43, No. 1, (January 2006), pp. 19-25, ISSN 0741-5214

Peterson, BG; Matsumura, JS. & Brewster, DC. (2007). Five-year report of a multicenter controlled clinical trial of open versus endovascular treatment of abdominal aortic aneurysms. *J Vasc Surg,* Vol. 45, No. 5, (May 2007), pp. 885-890, ISSN 0741-5214

Qu, LF; Hetzel, G. & Raithel, D. (2007). Seven years' single center experience of Powerlink unibody bifurcated endograft for endovascular aortic aneurysm repair. *J Cardiovasc Surg (Torino),* Vol. 48, No. 1, (February 2007), pp. 13-19, ISSN 0021-9509

Qu, L. & Raithel, D. (2008) Experience with the Endologix Powerlink endograft in endovascular repair of abdominal aortic aneurysms with short and angulated necks. *Perspect Vasc Surg Endovasc Ther.* Vol. 20, No. 2, (June 2008), pp. 158-166, ISSN 1531-0035

Qu, L. & Raithel, D. (2009) From clinical trials to clinical practice: 612 cases treated with the Powerlink stent-graft for endovascular repair of AAA. *J Cardiovasc Surg (Torino),* Vol. 50, No. 2, (April 2009), pp. 131-137, ISSN 0021-9509

Raithel, D; Qu, Lefeng. & Hetzel, G. (2006). A new concept in EVAR, In: *Endovascular Today,* May 2006, Available from
http://www.bmctoday.net/evtoday/2006/05/article.asp?f=EVT0506_08.html

Raithel, D. (2011). Endovascular Abdominal Aortic Aneurysm Repair: An Overview of the Anatomical Fixation Technique and Associated Outcomes with the Powerlink[R] Device. *J Interv Cardiol,* Epub ahead of print, (April 2011), ISSN 0896-4327

Stanley, BM; Semmens, JB. & Mai, Q. (2001) Evaluation of patient selection guidelines for endoluminal AA A repair with the Zenith stent-graft: the Australasian experience. *J Endovasc Ther,* Vol. 8, No. 5, (October 2001), pp. 457-464, ISSN 1526-6028

Schermerhorn, M; O'Malley, J. & Jhaveri, A. (2008). Endovascular vs. open repair of abdominal aortic aneurysms in the Medicare population. *N Engl J Med,* Vol.358, No. 5, (January 2008), pp. 464-474, ISSN 0028-4793

Torsello, G; Troisi, N. & Tessarek, J. (2010). Endovascular aortic aneurysm repair with the Endurant stent graft: early and 1-year results from a European multicenter trial. *J Vasc Interv Radiol,* Vol. 21, No. 1, (January 2010), pp. 73-80, ISSN 1051-0443

Wu, Z; Qu, L. & Ramaiah, V. (2011). Controversies and Updates in Vascular Surgery, Edizioni minerva medica, ISBN 13: 978-88-7711-701-4, TORINO, ITALY

Wu, Z; Raithel, D. & Ritter, W. (2011). Preliminary embolization of the hypogastric artery to expand the applicability of endovascular aneurysm repair. *J Endovasc Ther,* Vol. 18, No. 1, (February 2011), pp. 114-120, ISSN 1526-6028

11

Ruptured Abdominal Aortic Aneurysms

Antonello M.
Department of Cardiac, Thoracic and Vascular Sciences,
Vascular and Endovascular Surgery Section, University of Padua,
Italy

1. Introduction

Abdominal aortic aneurysm (AAA) rupture (RAAA) is defined as bleeding outside the adventitia of a dilated aortic wall. Ruptures are classified as free when they flow into the peritoneal cavity causing massive blood loss, usually associated with a high mortality rate, and as retroperitoneal which are characterized by minor blood loss since retroperitoneal tissues contain the hematoma. In a minority of cases AAAs rupture into the intestinal tract (frequently in the last portion of the duodenum) creating an aortic enteric fistula or into the cava vein. Differentiation between symptomatic and ruptured aneurysm is essential. Like patients with RAAA, individuals with symptomatic AAAs may present with a variable symptomatology ranging from mild tenderness to severe pain, but there is no blood outside the aortic wall at computed tomography angiography (CTA) or intraoperatively (Fig. 1).

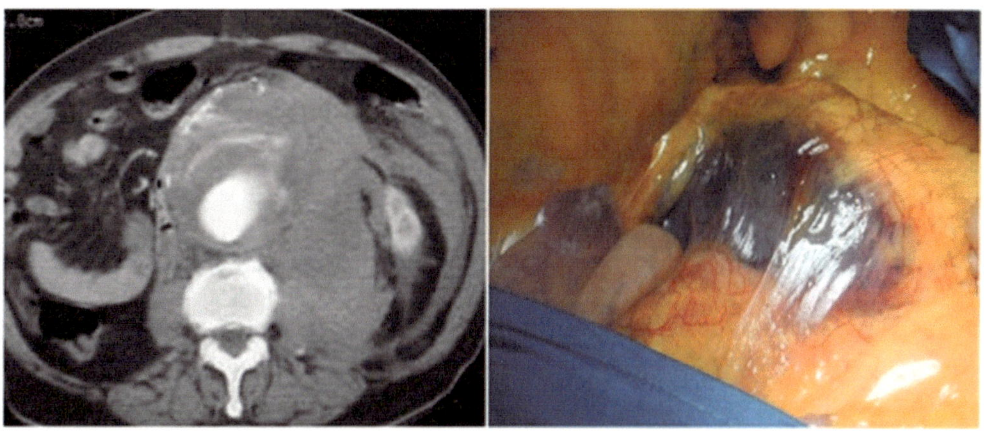

Fig. 1. Preoperative angio-CT showing a RAAA (panel A), and the intraoperative finding (panel B).

Pain is related to the aneurysm itself as a consequence of an acute expansion of the wall, intraluminal hemorrhage or bleeding into the thrombus, or it can be caused by other factors: cholecystitis, diverticulitis, pancreatitis. Patients who undergo elective AAA repair have the best prognosis, followed by patients with symptomatic aneurysms, who do not have hypotension, followed by patients with RAAA. The second of these must not be included in data concerning RAAA as they would artificially improve the outcome results.

The incidence of RAAA ranges between 5.6 and 17.5 per 100,000 person-years in the Western Hemisphere (Moll et al., 2006).

2. Diagnosis, transfer and preoperative care

The mortality rate associated with RAAA is especially high during transfer to the emergency room (ER) or other emergency settings and later in the operating theatre (OT). Most ruptures occur outside of the hospital and the time between onset of symptoms and arrival at the OT has been found to be critical in determining the final outcome. Funds have been provided by national and regional health organizations to plan specialized pre-hospital management and transportation, including the use of helicopters.

RAAA should be suspected in all patients over 50 complaining of abdominal or back pain, hypotension, and presenting with a pulsatile mass (the classic triad presentation). The mass may be obscured in patients with a large abdominal circumference. An episode of syncope can be indicative of orthostatic hypotension. An emergency Doppler ultrasound (DUS) should be performed to confirm the diagnosis in those patients. The patient should be transferred to the nearest high-volume hospital where an expert vascular/endovascular surgical team is available. Patients needing elective and RAAA repair whose surgeons have high annual procedure volumes are more likely to survive after surgery. A volume-outcome relationship has already been demonstrated for elective AAA repair as well as for other operations (Cho et al., 2008; Heikkinen et al., 2002; Dueck et al., 2004). It is unclear if surgeons with high annual procedure volumes become more expert and therefore produce superior outcomes or if better surgeons producing superior outcomes garner more referrals and thus become high-volume surgeons. Vascular surgeons, in any case, have better outcomes than general surgeons. RAAA patients of high-volume surgeons trained in vascular surgery have an adjusted 30-day mortality rate of 40.5%, compared with 43.9% for all other surgeons, with an absolute risk difference of 3.4%. Although the absolute difference in adjusted 30-day survival between high-volume vascular surgeons (3.5%) and all other surgeons (5.0%) was smaller for elective repairs, the number of elective operations is higher with respect to the number of RAAA repairs (Cho et al., 2008; Harris et al., 1991).

The statistics concerning surgeon volume and mortality suggest that it may be beneficial to regionalize RAAA repair to high-volume vascular surgeons. But the argument can also be made that regionalization can lengthen the time between the onset of symptoms and surgery while patients are being transferred from one hospital to another. Informed policy decisions concerning regionalization cannot be made until the time effect is compared with the benefit of being operated on by high-volume vascular surgeons. Patients may, however, prefer to undergo surgery closer to home, and this could nullify the small survival advantage for elective AAA repair.

This controversy seems to have been partially resolved by Endovascular Ruptured Aneurysm Repair (EVRAR). In a recent study by McPhee et al. who analyzed data gathered in the USA between 2001-2006, EVRAR was found to be independently associated with a lower postoperative mortality risk than was open surgical repair (odds risk 1.56), with the highest advantage found in high-volume centers for elective EVAR (McPhee et al., 2009).

When a RAAA is suspected a blood sample should be taken for analysis and cross matched (a minimum 8 units of blood cells and 4 units of blood plasma should be prepared) and a large intravenous access and a Foley catheter should be placed simultaneously.

Optimal management guidelines for preoperative crystalloid infusion in patients with severe hypotension have not been established. Aggressive resuscitation during which large quantities of fluids are administered can elevate systolic blood pressure (SBP) causing rupture of the temporary aortic seal that forms leading to further blood loss and worsening of hypotension (Johansen et al., 1991). The optimal strategy, termed permissive hypotension, seems to be providing minimal fluid infusion and the pharmacological resuscitation necessary to maintain consciousness with a SBP of about 80 mm Hg (50-90mm Hg) (Crawford 1991; Alric et al., 2003). When possible, red blood cells should always be used during resuscitation. There are no randomized trials comparing different types of resuscitation for RAAA. In a series of patients presenting with severe hypotension (SBP<90 mm Hg) survival was improved in those who received minimal fluid infusion and in whom permissive hypotension was maintained until they arrived in the OT (Bickell et al., 1994).

An emergency ultrasound examination should be performed by an expert operator to confirm the diagnosis once the patient has arrived in the ER and, if the patient is hemodynamically stable (consciousness and SBP >90 mmHg), a CTA should subsequently be performed to examine the aneurysm anatomy, to identify the rupture site, to plan aortic cross-clamping (supra or infra-renal), and to analyze the feasibility of endovascular repair. The unstable patient (unconsciousness and SBP<90 mmHg) should be taken directly to the OT (Fig. 2).

3. Open RAAA repair

Once in the OT, the patient must be quickly prepared and draped so that the operation can begin after induction of anesthesia that can itself cause severe hypotension if curare is used. An intra-arterial line to monitor blood pressure, a central vein catheter, and a nasogastric tube should be placed.

Conventional open surgical repair (OR), involving surgical exposure of the aorta and replacement of the aneurysm with a synthetic tube graft if possible, is the most common treatment for AAA. Its advantages include shorter operating times and limited overall systemic physiologic insult. A small (2-3 cm) iliac aneurysm or a moderate stenosis can be repaired at a later date. Systemic heparinization, which reduces bleeding complications, can be avoided although retrograde iliac flushing and injection of a heparinized flush solution into the iliac arteries is necessary to remove any soft clots and to reduce distal thrombosis. Once RAAA repair has been completed and before the aorta has been unclamped, which is always associated with significant hypotension, the anesthesiologist must verify that appropriate fluids are being administrated and that pressor agents and bicarbonate are prepared for use if required. Once the repair has been performed in about 25-30% of cases the abdomen cannot be closed without significant tension from a swollen bowel or a massive retroperitoneal hematoma or both that could lead to postoperative abdominal compartment syndrome secondary to an increase in intra-abdominal pressure. To avoid that complication an early or delayed closure of the abdomen using a non-absorbable mesh covered with polyurethane is indicated rather than a decompressive laparotomy, as it seems to reduce graft infection and multiple organ failure development (Rasmussen et al., 2002). Open AAA repair is a complex, major operation with high morbidity and mortality due to the combined effects of surgical exposure, hemorrhage, and aortic clamping which may induce lower torso ischaemia-reperfusion injury.

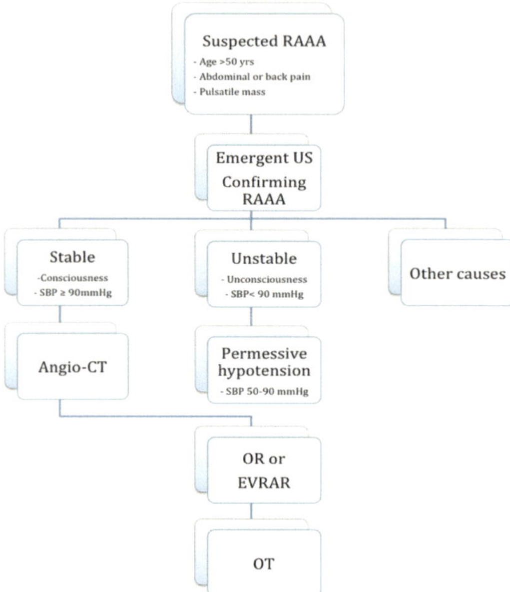

Fig. 2. Flow-chart showing a simplified protocol for the management of RAAA. *(OR: open repair, OT: operating theatre).*

4. Operative strategies for RAAA

The main goal of surgery to repair RAAA is to obtain a safe, rapid, and effective proximal cross-clamping of the aorta to interrupt hemorrhage. Different intraoperative approaches and strategies with regard to surgical and anesthetic aspects can be used to obtain aortic control and to improve the postoperative outcome.

4.1 The transperitoneal approach

The most common open approach is the transperitoneal one through a midline abdominal incision. Most surgeons prefer this technique because they are more confident with it and because it provides wide exposure of the infrarenal as well of the suprarenal aorta. It is possible, in fact, to rapidly dissect the infradiaphragmatic aorta and to cross-clamp the aorta at this point. To gain aortic control the left lobe of the liver must then be retracted to the right and the gastrohepathic omentum is opened allowing entry into the lesser sac. A nasogastric tube is usually used to identify the esophagus, which is retracted to the left. It is then possible to expose the aorta between the diaphragmatic crura, which is dissected with an electrocautery to facilitate a rapid, safe clamp placement. Once aortic control is obtained the clamp on the subdiaphragmatic aorta should be placed on the infrarenal neck if possible. The supraceliac aortic cross-clamping must be as short as possible to reduce visceral and renal ischemia. Some surgeons prefer to perform supraceliac aortic cross-clamping routinely to control hemorrhage readily and to avoid damage to the left renal vein and/or the gonadic veins which may take place during an infrarenal neck dissection when there is a large hematoma in that area. Some concerns have been voiced with regard to this method because supraceliac cross-clamping can worsen the visceral and renal ischemia induced by hemorrhagic shock, which in turn could contribute to often fatal multisystem organ failure.[32]

4.1.1 The left retroperitoneal approach

Some surgeons prefer the left retroperitoneal approach to the abdominal aorta because of the advantages that it offers with respect to the standard transabdominal access. It has, in fact, been associated with less severe intraoperative hypothermia, fluid loss, lower postoperative ventilatory deficit, and a shorter period of paralytic ileus (Chang et al. 1990). This exposure is, moreover, considered the approach of choice for patients with a so-called "hostile abdomen", those who have undergone multiple intraabdominal procedures or pelvic irradiation. It can also be useful in obese patients and in cases of horseshoe kidney (Wahlgren et al., 2007).

The approach provides wide access to the infradiaphragmatic aorta as a 10th intercostal incision is used allowing rapid control of the supraceliac aorta before the aneurysm is exposed through the hematoma. Some surgeons in fact, advocate its routine use for RAAA repair. A retrospective analysis (Chang et al., 1990) on RAAA treated via a retroperitoneal extended approach (10th intercostal incision, 25 pts) as opposed to a standard transperitoneal procedure (38 pts) revealed that there was a lower 30-day mortality (12% vs 34.%; $p<0.05$), less need for ventilatory support in the OT, and a shorter duration of paralytic ileus when the former was used. But a prospective randomized study (Cambria et al., 1990) analyzing the transperitoneal approach (59 pts) as compared to the retroperitoneal procedure (54 pts) reported finding no advantage to the former.

Some concerns have been voiced with regard to this approach and especially concerning the difficulty in controlling the right renal artery, and, if the aneurysm is large, exposure of the right iliac artery could be technically demanding. It is important then that the surgeon be familiar with a procedure which, at best, is difficult. The retroperitoneal approach may, moreover, be contraindicated in patients undergoing active cardiac massage for resuscitation or with a questionable diagnosis.

4.1.1.1 Balloon occlusion

According to some surgeons safe aortic control can be attained using an aortic occlusion balloon (AOB) placed in the visceral aorta under fluoroscopic guidance enabling laparotomy while avoiding the risk of rupturing the aneurysm and causing massive hemorrhage. Lieutenant Colonel Carl W. Huges first introduced the technique to repair traumatic rupture of the abdominal aorta in 1950 during the Korean war (Arthis et al., 2006). Many advancements have been made since then especially during the last decade. Newer techniques and materials are now used to obtain aortic control using a compliant AOB (Assar et al., 2009). The most common approach is to insert the AOB through a percutaneous transfemoral access using a 11 to 16 F sheath placed in the suprarenal or pararenal aorta over a stiff guidewire (Arthurs et al., 2006; Malina et al., 2005; Mayer et al., 2009). A compliant AOB is then passed through the sheath and inflated proximal to the RAAA. The sheath is advanced to support the inflated balloon from below to avoid distal dislocation. The sheath should be fixed firmly to prevent any displacement that can occur if blood pressure rises. The entire procedure should be performed under fluoroscopic guidance, but when this is unavailable confirmation of occlusion is generally associated to the loss of a palpable femoral pulse and an increase in blood pressure.

A transbrachial approach has also been described for RAAA (Matsuda et al., 2003). In 1964 Heimbecker first described remote transaxillary aortic control using AOB in RAAA (Heimbecker 1964). The advantages of transbrachial or axillary AOB placement is that the AOB inflated at the infrarenal aorta level does not interrupt the blood supply to the celiac, supramesenteric, and renal arteries. Important concerns have, however, been advanced with regard to this approach, and, in fact, it does seem to present some disadvantages. This technique may, in fact, involve a cutdown procedure to access the brachial artery and at times this may require a second operating team and dissection of the median nerve, potentially increasing the time for AOB placement. Most AOBs are large, bare, stiff, and difficult to pass in a blind fashion across the arch of the aorta. Oblique imaging may be necessary to traverse the arch into the descending thoracic aorta, while placement of a large sheath in the brachial artery may cause additional ischemic complications in the upper extremity.

Risks associated with AOB, the most catastrophic of which being that of provoking a free rupture in a contained RAAA, need be considered. A wire or catheter could feasibly exit through the site of the aortic rupture or the weakened aortic wall aggravating hemorrhage. Transfemoral AOB should then always be performed under fluoroscopic guidance to avoid this complication. Another potential obstacle could be percutaneously locating the common femoral artery in a hypotensive patient. Low et al (1986) reported a 58% success rate in the percutaneous cannulation of the common femoral artery to place an AOB in cases of traumatic exsanguinating hemorrhage. When the attempt fails, a femoral cutdown procedure is required and ultrasound-guided access techniques may be useful. The risk of visceral, spinal cord, and lower extremity ischemia in an already moribund patient is associated to any technique of proximal control depending on the extent of the preexisting shock and collateral flow. Aortic occlusion times vary and some surgeons limit balloon inflation time to 10 minutes with a variable period of deflation for reperfusion (Assar et al., 2009) because intermittent aortic occlusion is better tolerated. This technique can also be applied to gain control of the iliac arteries once the aneurismal sac is opened to avoid iliac vein lesions if there is a large hematoma.

4.1.1.2 Intraoperative Auto Transfusion (IAT) and red cell salvage

IAT is a method of blood conservation that reduces the need for allogeneic blood transfusions during AAA surgery (Alric et al., 2003; Takagi H et al., 2007). In a systematic review including 2 small randomized controlled trials, Alvarez et al (2004) did not find evidence that IAT decreases exposure to allogeneic blood transfusions (ABT) during infrarenal AAA surgery. Since the time that review was written, the results of two large randomized controlled trials have been published. In a recent meta-analysis of randomized controlled trials published before 2007, Takagi et al reported that IAT reduces the risk of ABT in elective AAA surgery, and its use has been recommended even for RAA (Markovic et al., 2009). Once IAT becomes routine in all AAA surgeries and all operators have become familiar with it, its use may become commonplace during RAAA repair protocols.

IAT has obvious advantages as blood volume and normothermia are maintained because of the rapidity with which blood is salvaged and returned to the patient. Two basic blood salvage and replacement methods are possible: washed and unwashed (whole blood) autotransfusion. Cell washing devices can theoretically remove potentially toxic byproducts of injured red blood cells, such as activated clotting proteins and activated complement, but they also eliminate beneficial blood components such as platelets and clotting proteins. Although heparin is added by the autotransfusion system, it is removed when the blood is washed by an autotransfusion device. Unwashed autotransfusions return not only platelets and proteins but also unwanted free hemoglobin and activated coagulation factors known to increase the frequency of transfusion-related coagulopathy or nephropathy and its use has thus been entirely abandoned. Dilutional coagulopathy is considered the major adverse event related to the use of cell washing systems. Administration of fresh frozen plasma and platelets is recommended when more than 8 units of autologous blood have been returned (Marty-Ane et al., 1995). IAT is particularly useful in the treatment of massive hemorrhage during which rapid reinfusion of large volumes of blood can be lifesaving and it is most effective when the salvage and reinfusion of shed blood can be accomplished at flow rates compatible with the degree of hemorrhage. Postoperative coagulation disorders and hypothermia-induced coagulopathies are prevented to a large extent by autotransfusion which returns warmer blood products (Marty-Ane et al., 1995).

4.1.1.2.1 Renal function

The incidence (ranging between 26 and 42%) of renal failure after RAAA is remarkably high. Of patients with renal failure, 11-40% require postoperative dialysis with an associated mortality rate of 76-89% (Harris et al., 1991; Magee et al., 1992). Impairment in renal function has been associated with suprarenal cross-clamping, duration of cross clamping >30 minutes, preexisting conditions of renal dysfunction (serum creatinine > 2 mg/dl), shock, and age over 80 (Bonventre 2007; Nicholson et al., 1996). The etiology of renal dysfunction is multifactorial and many who develop it have sustained major insult to other organs. Ischaemic renal injury affects the tubules at the level of the outer medullar, which primarily include the thick ascending loop of Henle and the S3 portion of the proximal convoluted tubule. Tubular cell death is now considered characterized by both necrosis and apoptosis. Necrosis results from profound cellular adenosine triphosphate (ATP) depletion and is characterized by a sequence of events that begins with loss of cell polarity and of the epithelial brush border, followed by the loss of the integrity of tight junctions and the appearance of integrins such as intercellular adhesion molecule 1 on the cell surface. These interact with leukocyte adhesion molecules to mediate an inflammatory response with the release of cytotoxic mediators. Cells then slough into the tubular lumen and further impair already compromised filtrate flow. Tubular cell apoptosis is also triggered by ischaemia through as yet uncharacterized mechanisms, also resulting in cell loss, but there is no inflammatory component, and the resultant apoptotic bodies are phagocytosed by macrophages or surviving epithelial cells. Apoptosis is also observed in the recovery phase during epithelial proliferation and probably has a role in restoring a normal tubular structure. Clinically, the initial observation is that of a loss of urinary concentrating ability as the medullary gradient dissipates, followed by a decline in urine output as tubules become obstructed and denuded (Bonventre 2007).

Some intraoperative strategies concerning anesthetic and surgical aspects can be utilized to protect the renal parenchyma. Use of mannitol, an osmotic diuretic and the earliest pharmacological agent utilized to protect renal function following vascular surgery, continues to be controversial. In a randomized controlled study, Nicholson et al reported that it reduces renal injury following infrarenal AAA, but in a recent review Hersey et al. (2008) concluded that there is no evidence that mannitol preserves renal function during aortic surgery. Mannitol infusion, nevertheless, is the most commonly used method to protect renal parenchyma from ischemic damage and from ischemic-reperfusion injury. Its use has been shown to protect renal function during elective surgery when suprarenal aortic cross-clamping does not exceed 60 minutes (Deriu et al., 2001). The dose commonly used is a bolus of 25 mg IV administered before or immediately after aortic cross-clamping. Mannitol seems to increase tubular fluid volume through its osmotic effect and by reducing tubular cell swelling and hence resistance to flow. Since it is a hydroxyl radical scavenger, it is effective in an ischaemia-reperfusion injury setting (Hersey & Poullis 2008).

Another pharmacological therapy that can be begun before or during supraceliac aortic cross-clamping is fenoldopam mesylate, a dopamine-1 agonist receptor which improves plasmatic renal blood flow to the cortex and medullary regions. The dose used to obtain renal effects is 0.05/0.003 µg per kilogram per minute, is well below that usually needed to lower systemic blood pressure (Halpenny et al., 2002; Gilbert et al., 2001). There is no data on its usefulness during RAAA surgery, but those effects on renal function noted during aortic surgery probably could presumably apply to RAAA as well.

Other drugs such as dopamine, dopexamine, calcium channel antagonists and natriuretic peptide have been proposed, but their use is still limited and further studies are needed.

Several intra-operative surgical strategies are applicable to protect renal tissue from prolonged cross-clamping ischemia. Many surgeons utilise the local cooling of the kidneys to protect the tissue from protracted cross-clamping ischemia by cyclic or continuous perfusion of renal arteries with cold solutions (Ringer's lactate or saline) (Allen et al., 1993; Kashyap et al., 1997). Ice slushes can be applied to the kidney surface to further ensure hypothermia, if exposure is retroperitoneal. But hypothermia of the renal parenchyma remains a problem when the kidney remains *in situ*, and the results found using this method are controversial with regard to the prevention of post-operative renal failure (Allen et al., 1993). In the light of our research studies and preliminary clinical reports, we utilize short-term kidney arterial blood reperfusion whenever clamping ischemia exceeds 30 min.

Reperfusion is achieved by re-establishing pulsatile normothermic blood flow either through the repaired renal artery or, in the majority of operative procedures, through the Pruitt–Inahara shunt (500-50-9F. Ideas for MedicineTM, Cryo-Life® Comp, St. Petersburg, FL, U.S.A.).

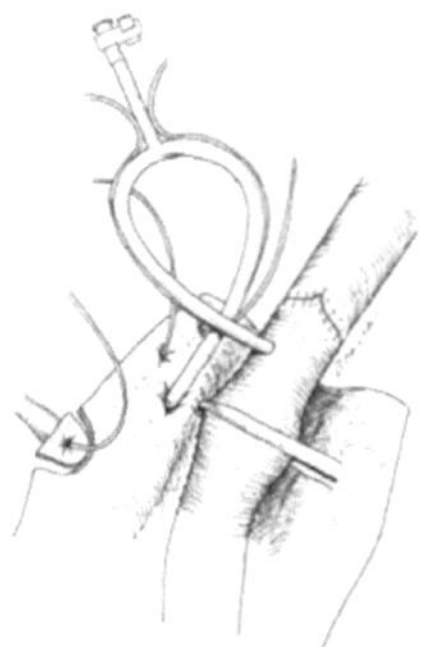

Fig. 3. The temporary renal reperfusion is achieved by re-establishing pulsatile normothermic blood flow through a Pruitt–Inahara shunt (500-50-9F. Ideas for MedicineTM, Cryo-Life® Comp, St. Petersburg, FL, U.S.A.) when the procedure requires more than 30 min of renal artery cross clamping. The proximal end of the shunt is inserted into the tubegraft and its distal end into the renal artery. After 3 min of blood the aorta and the renal artery are clamped, the shunt is promptly removed and the renal artery reconstruction completed. The reperfusion is repeated every 30 min if necessary.

This technique can protect renal parenchyma from prolonged clamping ischemia (up to 100 min) (Deriu et al., 2001).

5. Postoperative complications

The most frequent complications after surgery for RAAA are listed in Table 1.

	Incidence	Associated mortality
Postoperative bleeding	12-14%	-
Colonic ischemia	3-13%	73-100%
Respiratory failure	26-47%	34-68%
Renal dysfunction	26-42%	-
Postoperative dialysis	3-18%	76-89%
Myocardial infarction	14-24%	19-66%
Major arrhythmia	19-23%	40-48%
Congestive heart failure	18-21%	39-42%
Multisystem organ failure	59-66%	65-71%
Paraplegia and paraparesis	1.1-2.3%	45-53%

Table 1. Major postoperative complications following open repair for RAAA.

Uncontrollable haemorrhage during RAAA repair is a major cause of perioperative mortality (Davies et al., 1993; Milne et al., 1994). Patients with coagulopathic haemorrhage must undergo timely administration of fresh frozen plasma, platelets, cryoprecipitate and antifibrinolytic agents. But in patients arriving in the OT with signs of severe haemorrhagic shock, these measures may be insufficient to restore normal haemostatic function in the face of persistent hypoperfusion, acidosis and hypothermia by the end of the operation. In this clinical situation, intra-abdominal packing is recommended to control further bleeding, to optimize organ perfusion, and to correct metabolic disturbances in the intensive therapy unit (van Herwaarden et al., 2001). Concerns have been advanced with regard to this technique and the possibility of secondary intra-abdominal infective complications noted in 13% in an early postoperative period and in 18% in a later phase and as a result the technique is not commonly used in open RAAA repair (Johnston 1994).

Colon ischemia can develop as a single mucosal lesion or as necrosis involving the full-thickness of the colon with or without perforation. Several factors are thought to be responsible for colonic ischemia: severe hypotension, preoperative inferior mesenteric artery (IMA) patency, the presence of a collateral supply from the superior mesenteric, and the site of hematoma. The patency of at least one hypogastric artery is generally considered acceptable to ensure adequate intestinal perfusion. After RAAA repair the colon must be carefully inspected and in case of doubt the IMA should be reimplanted and/or the hypogastric arteries should be inspected by ultrasound examination to verify their patency. If colonic ischemia is suspected during the postoperative period, a colonscopy should be performed as it is considered diagnostic, and colon resection, associated with a high mortality rate (50%), may be necessary (Harris et al., 1991; Johnston 1994).

Myocardial infarction, associated with an high mortality rate (20-65%), develops as a result of excessive cardiac workload due to blood loss, aggressive resuscitation efforts, clamping and declamping in patients often with pre-existing history of ischemic coronary artery disease %).[61] Rapid diagnosis and treatment of this fatal complication is imperative.

Multiple-organ failure (MOF) is the major cause of death in the intensive care unit after successful RAAA repair.[62] Some factors such as suprarenal aortic cross-clamping and longer operative duration of aortic clamping seem to be involved in its development (Bauer et al., 1993). Infection and shock are the two most common clinical predisposing factors and processes such as severe tissue injury or pancreatitis that induce a major inflammatory response seem to be capable of initiating a cascade of events that culminates in MOF (Deitch 1992; Haveman et al., 2008). Regardless of the cause, MOF generally follows a predictable course, beginning with the lungs and followed by hepatic, intestinal, and renal failure, in that order. Hematologic and myocardial failure are usually later manifestations of MOF, while the onset of alterations involving central nervous system alterations can occur either early or late. This classical sequential pattern of organ failure can be modified, however, by pre-existing disease or by a precipitating clinical event. Renal failure, for example, may precede hepatic or even pulmonary failure in subjects with intrinsic renal disease or in patients who have sustained prolonged periods of shock, while hepatic or myocardial failure may be an early or even the initial manifestation of this syndrome in a patient with cirrhosis or myocardial damage. These clinical exceptions illustrate the biologic principle that, although systemic responses are similar in patients developing MOF, the exact sequence of organ failure can be influenced by the individual's acute disease processes or physiologic reserve (Deitch 1992).

One hypothesis concerning the development of MOF after RAAA surgery is based on the "two hit" theory: the rupture and repair of an AAA is a combination of two ischemic-reperfusion injuries (Lindsay et al., 1999). The first ischemic event is hemorrhagic shock, which sets off an inflammatory response, followed by resuscitation causing the first reperfusion injury. The second ischemic event is aortic cross-clamping followed by the aortic declamping causing the second reperfusion injury.

This theory supports the microcirculatory hypothesis of MOF according to which organ injury is related to ischemia or vascular endothelial injury. In the macrophage hypothesis, instead, prolonged activation of macrophages results in excessive production, surface expression, and liberation of cytokines and other products, which through a cascade effect involving humoral and cellular effector systems exert deleterious local and systemic effects. The former hypothesis includes several distinct but to some extent overlapping potential mechanisms of injury, including inadequate tissue and cellular oxygen delivery, the ischemia-reperfusion phenomenon, and tissue injury due to endothelial-leukocyte interactions (Reilly et al., 1991; Granger et al., 1988). There are, thus, many points in which the microcirculatory and macrophage hypotheses of organ failure overlap and interact (Deitch 1992; Pober & Cotran, 1990). Clinical and experimental observations have in fact clearly demonstrated that systemic inflammation adversely affects the microcirculation, while ischemia can exaggerate the host's inflammatory response to subsequent stimuli by activating neutrophils and priming macrophages (Deitch 1992).

Prognosis appears to be directly related to both the number of organs that fail and the length of time the patient is in organ failure, but our ability to predict outcome in individual cases is not so precise as to supersede clinical judgment in determining when further treatment is futile.

The first cause of death in the surgical intensive care unit is MOF, and the best treatment is prevention. In spite of the development of new-generation antibiotics and ever more sophisticated techniques of organ support, our ability to save patients once MOF has set in has not appreciably improved over the last two decades (Deitch 1992). New therapeutic strategies aiming to prevent and/or limit the development of the physiologic abnormalities inducing organ failure are needed to improve survival in these patients.

6. Results after RAAA repair

The mortality rate of RAAA remains exceedingly high; in fact with the exception of only a few series (Crawford 1991, Lawrie et al., 1980), it ranges between 30 and more than 70% in most reports (Mureebe et al., 2008; Bown et al., 2002; Johansen et al., 1991; Bauer et al., 1993). If these statistics include patients who died at home or during transportation to the hospital, the mortality rate approaches 90% (Dueck et al., 2004). Poor survival rates have been reported throughout the last few decades despite advancements in specialized pre-hospital management and transportation, rapid emergency diagnostic evaluation and aneurysm repair by high-volume vascular surgery teams, and sophisticated post-operative intensive care units (Darling et al., 1996; Bown et al., 2002; Alric et al., 2003; Bauer et al., 1993; Dueck et al., 2004; Antonello et al., 2009).

In the light of high mortality rates and high hospital costs, some attempts have been made to identify pre-operative variables that might be used to select patients for surgery (Antonello et al., 2009; Boyle et al., 2003; Calderwood et al., 2004; Tambyraja et al., 2008a, 2008b). While this approach may be justified in our cost-effective age, its ethical and legal implications need to be pondered. The decision to deny operative treatment to a patient with a RAAA can be made only on an individual basis and can be justified only in those cases characterized by poor quality of life due to a precarious general clinical status or mental condition. Variables and scoring systems (Tab. 2), have recently been developed to identify patients with a prohibitive operative risk for RAAA repair.

Among these, the Glasgow Aneurysm Score (GAS) seems to be the most simple and accurate in identifying those patients unfit for emergency repair surgery (Antonello et al., 2007; Korhonen et al., 2004). Sufficient data are still lacking in the literature with regard to these systems, GAS included, and large prospective studies are certainly warranted.

The best approach to RAAA remains, in any case, prevention. DUS screening programs for AAA in men over 65 have recently been attempted to reduce mortality (Scott et al., 1995, 2002; Lindholt et al.). The rationale behind these programs is that ultrasound is a valid, fast, safe method to detect AAAs, with an estimated sensitivity and specificity of 98 and 99%, respectively, and that perioperative mortality for elective AAA is lower than 5% in most centers (Lindholt et al., 1999). The Multicenter Aneurysm Screening Study (MASS) results published in 2002 in the Lancet journal showed that ultrasound screening performed over a 29 month period in men between 65 and 74 reduced the AAA mortality risk by 42% (Ashton et al., 2002). Two other reviews on this topic were later published by Cochrane (Cosford et al., 2007) and Lindholt et al. who confirmed these findings and reported a significant mid-term reduction in AAA-related and overall mortality after 3-5 yrs, data that has been verified by long-term analysis. There is, instead, insufficient evidence demonstrating usefulness in women. While ultrasound screening is relatively inexpensive, further analysis is needed, and all the latest findings concerning this subject must be examined carefully whenever health care administrators are considering population-based screening programs.

	Odds ratio (95%CI)
Age >80 year	1.5-3
Female sex	1.5-2
Hypotension < 80mmhg	2.5-3.5
Renal impairment	2-3.5
Pulmonary disease	1.5-2.2
Haemoglobin <8 g/l	1.8-2
Hematocrit <30%	1.8-2.5
Diabetes	1.3-1.8
Coronary artery disease	1.7-2.2
Suprarenal cross clamping	1.8-2.5
	Area under the roc curve (95% CI)
Hardman Index	0.69
GAS°	0.64
ERAS§	0.72
Possum	0.69

* Physiological and Operative Score for Enumeration of mortality and Morbidity
° Glasgow Aneurysm Score
§ Edinburgh ruptured aneurysm score

Table 2. Principle risk factors and Scoring Systems developed to predict survival after open repair for RAAA.

7. Quality of life after RAAA

The long-term impact on quality of life after AAA repair is debatable. Health, of course, cannot be defined simply as the absence of disease and infirmity, but implies physical, mental, and social well-being. Traditional outcome measures with regard to vascular surgery, such as graft patency and complication rates, are certainly important. These measures tend, nevertheless, to reflect a technical point of view towards the procedure rather than concern for the impact that the event has had on the patient as a whole. Measuring quality of life (QL) before and after surgery is one way to evaluate the patient's perception of health and well-being. In extreme situations, a technically successful operation might leave a patient significantly debilitated by morbidity associated with the surgery. This seems to be a very real possibility, in fact, for survivors of AAA repair, given the high operative morbidity and mortality rates. The most frequently used questionnaires are the Rosser index (Korhonen et al., 2003; Joseph et al., 2002) (a measure of physical disability and psychological distress) and the Medical Outcomes Study Short Form-36 Health Survey (McDaniel et al., 2000; Reemtsma & Morgan, 1997; Chetter et al., 1997) (Sf-36; a generic QL measurement tool) promoted by the American Society for Vascular Surgery and validated for use in patients with vascular disease.

In studies utilizing the Rosser index, not widely validated for vascular patients, a significant reduction was found in the level of functional capacity in the RAAA group with respect to

patients who underwent elective repair (Magee et al., 1992; Hennessy et al., 1998). Biases emerged in these reports as the studies were small and the patients were not matched for comorbidities, so it is difficult to ascertain if the populations (elective vs emergency) were similar.
Larger studies with matched populations (elective vs emergency) were performed using the SF-36 by Tambyraja et al. (2005) and Hill et al. (2007) who reported that there were no significant differences in QL in the two groups. These studies also suggested that long-term RAAA survivors had the same QL as those who underwent open elective repair surgery.

8. Endovascular repair

Endovascular aortic repair is a new catheter-based, imaging guided procedure that has the potential to redefine the traditional approach to the treatment of AAA. Since it was first described by Parodi in 1991 (Parodi et al., 1991), its role in RAAA repair continues to be debated. In fact, while most published data drawn from non-randomised studies (Mayer et al., 2009) suggest that EVRAR is feasible in selected patients and in institutions specialized in endovascular techniques, the only published randomized control study by Hinchliffe et al. (2002) showed no benefit in terms of mortality or complications. But since that trial included symptomatic but non-ruptured AAA patients it is difficult to interpret these results. Long-term findings are needed to assess if EVRAR effectively treats endoleaks, prevents late ruptures, and ensures stent-graft integrity. The potential advantages of EVRAR with respect to open repair, such as reduced blood loss, less need for transfusions, and shorter stays in the ICU seem to be due to a decreased physiological insult. As EVRAR obviates the need for laparotomy, direct surgical exposure, handling of abdominal contents, and aorto-iliac clamping, it is an attractive alternative and potentially helpful in reducing the mortality rate of RAAA (Ten Bosh et al., 2010; Harkin et al., 2007; Sadat et al., 2008; Dillon et al., 2007).
Different strategies are employed to treat RAAA using endovascular therapy.
Proximal aortic control during EVRAR is obtained using a balloon placed in the visceral aorta via the brachial or the femoral accesses. The use of a balloon occlusion device is however associated to the risk of renal and splanchnic ischemia and distal embolization does not prevent on-going blood loss from ilio-femoral arteries.
The most common procedure is aorto-unifemoral graft. The advantage of this method is that the aneurysm is quickly excluded from the circulation since introduction and deployment is rapid, and the contralateral gate does not need to be engaged as opposed to the bifurcated endograft which can be time consuming in some situations. Stent grafts may offer wider applicability but can be used only when unilateral iliac anatomy is suitable, but a femoro-femoral crossover is nevertheless required (Fig. 4).
Thanks to the recent diffusion of the endovascular technique most RAAAs are treated using aorta-bi-iliac endografting, and no differences in outcomes have been found in the two types of endografts (Moll et al., 2011).
Abdominal compartment syndrome is a major cause of death after EVRAR and increases short-term mortality up to 5 times compared to that in patients with normal intra-abdominal pressure. All EVRAR patients should be monitored for this syndrome by frequent bladder pressure readings and open surgery must be considered when bladder pressure rises over 20 mm Hg (Djavani et al., 2011). The major concerns regarding

endovascular treatment in emergency situations are the patient's hemodynamic condition and time delays during the preoperative work up. The Montefiore RAAA Management Protocol (Harkin et al., 2007) seems to provide solutions and foresees using the endovascular approach in all patients with presumed ruptured aortoiliac aneurysms. Recent studies on EVRAR outline the procedure's many benefits observed in selected groups of patients with an anatomical suitability for EVAR, commonly reported at 60% (range 18-83%) (Ten Bosh et al., 2010, 2011). In those cases there was a reduction in the mortality rate, in the length of time spent in intensive care, and in the total time spent in the hospital traditionally associated with open repair. But due to heterogeneity and biases these results should be interpreted with caution (Sadat et al., 2008; Dillon et al., 2007). Large multicenter randomized controlled trials will establish the efficacy of EVRAR.

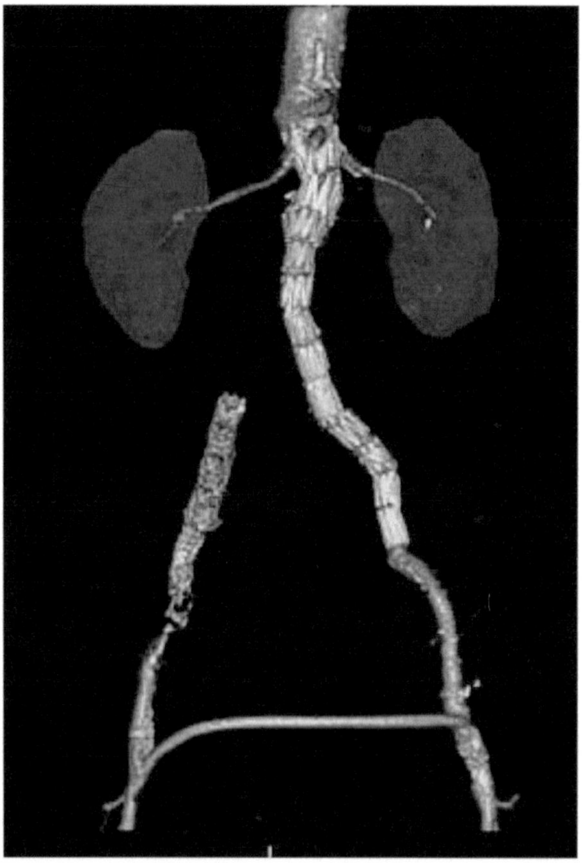

Fig. 4. Post-operative angio-CT showing an aorto-unifemoral endograft with a femoro-femoral cross-over performed for a RAAA

A pilot study recently outlined the difficulty in carrying out that kind of study (Hinchliffe et al., 2006). Some of the problems included: obtaining informed consent from patients with hemodynamic instability, inclusion of patients unsuitable for EVAR as well as traditional repair, immediate availability of CTA instrumentation, expert endovascular teams, and endograft devices.

9. Conclusions

Despite an increase in the volume of patients undergoing elective AAA repair over recent decades, the number of patients with RAAA has not fallen significantly (Johansson et al., 1994; Acosta et al., 2006; Wanhainen et al., 2008). Although the surgical mortality rate for elective AAA repair has steadily improved due to advancements in operative techniques and perioperative care and has fallen to less than 2% in specialized centres and 5% in less-specialized hospitals, the mortality rate of RAAA has not significantly changed over the past three decades and still ranges between 30 and 70% according to recent reports (Heller et al., 2000; Marty-Ane et al., 1995; Mureebe et al., 2008; Cho et al., 2008; Darling et al., 1996). The high mortality seems to be related to a combination of hemorrhagic shock and lower torso ischaemia followed by reperfusion injury despite successful revascularization (Harris et al., 1991; Bown et al., 2002)

Given the poor outcomes after open RAAA repair and in the light of lower perioperative morbidity and mortality after EVAR, some centers have adopted EVAR protocols for RAAA repair. Excellent results have been reported by those centers where the mortality rate has fallen to as low as 30%(Ten Bosch et al., 2010; Visser et al., 2007). But despite these results this technique cannot be offered to all patients with RAAA due to anatomic considerations (short neck, poor iliac access) and it has been estimated that only about 60% are anatomically suitable. (Visser et al., 2007; Ten Bosch et al., 2010, 2011) Additional factors reducing the applicability of EVRAR are institutional limitations, such as the lack of trained endovascular surgeons and/or endovascular equipment. But beyond the inherent difficulties and limitations connected to its use, EVRAR seems to present very important benefits confirming its usefulness and value as a modern surgical option for RAAA repair (Veith et al., 2003).

10. Acknowledgment

The author would like to thanks Linda Inverso for her help in preparing the manuscript and S. Bonvini for his wonderful illustration.

11. References

Acosta S, Ogren M, Bengtsson H, Bergqvist D, Lindblad B, Zdanowski Z. Increasing incidence of ruptured abdominal aortic aneurysm: a population-based study. *J Vasc Surg.* 2006; 44: 237-243.

Adam DJ, Fitridge RA, Raptis S. Intra-abdominal packing for uncontrollable haemorrhage during ruptured abdominal aortic aneurysm repair. *Eur J Vasc Endovasc Surg.* 2005; 30: 516-519.

Allen BT, Anderson CB, Rubin BG, Flye MW, Baumann DS, Sicard GA. Preservation of renal function in juxtarenal and suprarenal abdominal aortic aneurysm repair. *J Vasc Surg.* 1993; 17: 948-58; discussion 958-9.

Alvarez GG, Fergusson DA, Neilipovitz DT, Hebert PC. Cell salvage does not minimize perioperative allogeneic blood transfusion in abdominal vascular surgery: a systematic review. *Can J Anaesth.* 2004; 51: 425-431.

Alric P, Ryckwaert F, Picot MC, Branchereau P, Colson P, Mary H, Marty-Ane C. Ruptured aneurysm of the infrarenal abdominal aorta: impact of age and postoperative complications on mortality. *Ann Vasc Surg.* 2003; 17: 277-283.

Antonello M, Lepidi S, Kechagias A, Frigatti P, Tripepi A, Biancari F, Deriu GP, Grego F. Glasgow aneurysm score predicts the outcome after emergency open repair of symptomatic, unruptured abdominal aortic aneurysms. *Eur J Vasc Endovasc Surg.* 2007; 33: 272-276.

Antonello M, Frigatti P, Maturi C, Lepidi S, Noventa F, Pittoni G, Deriu GP, Grego F. Open repair for ruptured abdominal aortic aneurysm: is it possible to predict survival? *Ann Vasc Surg.* 2009; 23: 159-166.

Arthurs Z, Starnes B, See C, Andersen C. Clamp before you cut: Proximal control of ruptured abdominal aortic aneurysms using endovascular balloon occlusion--Case reports. *Vasc Endovascular Surg.* 2006; 40: 149-155.

Ashton HA, Buxton MJ, Day NE, Kim LG, Marteau TM, Scott RA, Thompson SG, Walker NM, Multicentre Aneurysm Screening Study Group. The Multicentre Aneurysm Screening Study (MASS) into the effect of abdominal aortic aneurysm screening on mortality in men: a randomised controlled trial. *Lancet.* 2002; 360: 1531-1539.

Assar AN, Zarins CK. Endovascular proximal control of ruptured abdominal aortic aneurysms: the internal aortic clamp. *J Cardiovasc Surg (Torino).* 2009; .

Bauer EP, Redaelli C, von Segesser LK, Turina MI. Ruptured abdominal aortic aneurysms: predictors for early complications and death. *Surgery.* 1993; 114: 31-35.

Bickell WH, Wall MJ,Jr, Pepe PE, Martin RR, Ginger VF, Allen MK, Mattox KL. Immediate versus delayed fluid resuscitation for hypotensive patients with penetrating torso injuries. *N Engl J Med.* 1994; 331: 1105-1109.

Boyle JR, Gibbs PJ, King D, Shearman CP, Raptis S, Phillips MJ. Predicting outcome in ruptured abdominal aortic aneurysm: a prospective study of 100 consecutive cases. *Eur J Vasc Endovasc Surg.* 2003; 26: 607-611.

Bonventre JV. Pathophysiology of acute kidney injury: roles of potential inhibitors of inflammation. *Contrib Nephrol.* 2007; 156: 39-46.

Bown MJ, Nicholson ML, Bell PR, Sayers RD. Cytokines and inflammatory pathways in the pathogenesis of multiple organ failure following abdominal aortic aneurysm repair. *Eur J Vasc Endovasc Surg.* 2001; 22: 485-495.

Bown MJ, Sutton AJ, Bell PR, Sayers RD. A meta-analysis of 50 years of ruptured abdominal aortic aneurysm repair. *Br J Surg.* 2002; 89: 714-730.

Calderwood R, Halka T, Haji-Michael P, Welch M. Ruptured abdominal aortic aneurysm. Is it possible to predict outcome? *Int Angiol.* 2004; 23: 47-53.

Cambria RP, Brewster DC, Abbott WM, Freehan M, Megerman J, LaMuraglia G, Wilson R, Wilson D, Teplick R, Davison JK. Transperitoneal versus retroperitoneal approach for aortic reconstruction: a randomized prospective study. *J Vasc Surg.* 1990; 11: 314-24; discussion 324-5.

Crawford ES. Ruptured abdominal aortic aneurysm. *J Vasc Surg.* 1991; 13: 348-350.

Chang BB, Shah DM, Paty PS, Kaufman JL, Leather RP. Can the retroperitoneal approach be used for ruptured abdominal aortic aneurysms? *J Vasc Surg.* 1990; 11: 326-330.

Chetter IC, Spark JI, Dolan P, Scott DJ, Kester RC. Quality of life analysis in patients with lower limb ischaemia: suggestions for European standardisation. *Eur J Vasc Endovasc Surg.* 1997; 13: 597-604.

Cho JS, Kim JY, Rhee RY, Gupta N, Marone LK, Dillavou ED, Makaroun MS. Contemporary results of open repair of ruptured abdominal aortoiliac aneurysms: effect of surgeon volume on mortality. *J Vasc Surg.* 2008; 48: 10-7.

Cosford PA, Leng GC. Screening for abdominal aortic aneurysm. *Cochrane Database Syst Rev.* 2007; (2): CD002945.

Darling RC,3rd, Cordero JA,Jr, Chang BB, Shah DM, Paty PS, Lloyd WE, Leather RP. Advances in the surgical repair of ruptured abdominal aortic aneurysms. *Cardiovasc Surg.* 1996; 4: 720-723.

Davies MJ, Murphy WG, Murie JA, Elton RA, Bell K, Gillon JG, Jenkins AM, Ruckley CV. Preoperative coagulopathy in ruptured abdominal aortic aneurysm predicts poor outcome. *Br J Surg.* 1993; 80: 974-976.

Deitch EA. Multiple organ failure. Pathophysiology and potential future therapy. *Ann Surg.* 1992; 216: 117-134.

Deriu GP, Grego F, Lepidi S, Antonello M, Milite D, Zaramella M, Damiani N. Short-term arterial blood reperfusion of normothermic kidney in renal artery and abdominal aorta reconstructive surgery. *Eur J Vasc Endovasc Surg.* 2001; 21: 314-319.

Djavani Gidlund K, Wanhainen A, Bjorck M. Intra-abdominal Hypertension and Abdominal Compartment Syndrome after Endovascular Repair of Ruptured Abdominal Aortic Aneurysm. *Eur J Vasc Endovasc Surg.* 2011.

Dillon M, Cardwell C, Blair PH, Ellis P, Kee F, Harkin DW. Endovascular treatment for ruptured abdominal aortic aneurysm. *Cochrane Database Syst Rev.* 2007; (1): CD005261.

Dueck AD, Kucey DS, Johnston KW, Alter D, Laupacis A. Survival after ruptured abdominal aortic aneurysm: effect of patient, surgeon, and hospital factors. *J Vasc Surg.* 2004; 39: 1253-1260.

Dueck AD, Kucey DS, Johnston KW, Alter D, Laupacis A. Long-term survival and temporal trends in patient and surgeon factors after elective and ruptured abdominal aortic aneurysm surgery. *J Vasc Surg.* 2004; 39: 1261-1267.

Gilbert TB, Hasnain JU, Flinn WR, Lilly MP, Benjamin ME. Fenoldopam infusion associated with preserving renal function after aortic cross-clamping for aneurysm repair. *J Cardiovasc Pharmacol Ther.* 2001; 6: 31-36.

Granger DN. Role of xanthine oxidase and granulocytes in ischemia-reperfusion injury. *Am J Physiol.* 1988; 255: H1269-75.

Halpenny M, Rushe C, Breen P, Cunningham AJ, Boucher-Hayes D, Shorten GD. The effects of fenoldopam on renal function in patients undergoing elective aortic surgery. *Eur J Anaesthesiol.* 2002; 19: 32-39.

Harkin DW, Dillon M, Blair PH, Ellis PK, Kee F. Endovascular ruptured abdominal aortic aneurysm repair (EVRAR): a systematic review. *Eur J Vasc Endovasc Surg.* 2007; 34: 673-681.

Harris LM, Faggioli GL, Fiedler R, Curl GR, Ricotta JJ. Ruptured abdominal aortic aneurysms: factors affecting mortality rates. *J Vasc Surg.* 1991; 14: 812-8; discussion 819-20.

Haveman JW, Zeebregts CJ, Verhoeven EL, van den Berg P, van den Dungen JJ, Zwaveling JH, Nijsten MW. Changes in laboratory values and their relationship with time after rupture of an abdominal aortic aneurysm. *Surg Today.* 2008; 38: 1091-1101.

Heimbecker RO. An Aortic Tampon for Emergency Control of Ruptured Abdominal Aneurysm. *Can Med Assoc J.* 1964; 91: 1024-1025.

Heikkinen M, Salenius JP, Auvinen O. Ruptured abdominal aortic aneurysm in a well-defined geographic area. *J Vasc Surg.* 2002; 36: 291-296.

Heller JA, Weinberg A, Arons R, Krishnasastry KV, Lyon RT, Deitch JS, Schulick AH, Bush HL,Jr, Kent KC. Two decades of abdominal aortic aneurysm repair: have we made any progress? *J Vasc Surg.* 2000; 32: 1091-1100.

Hennessy A, Barry MC, McGee H, O'Boyle C, Hayes DB, Grace PA. Quality of life following repair of ruptured and elective abdominal aortic aneurysms. *Eur J Surg.* 1998; 164: 673-677.

Hersey P, Poullis M. Does the administration of mannitol prevent renal failure in open abdominal aortic aneurysm surgery? *Interact Cardiovasc Thorac Surg.* 2008; 7: 906-909.

Hill AB, Palerme LP, Brandys T, Lewis R, Steinmetz OK. Health-related quality of life in survivors of open ruptured abdominal aortic aneurysm repair: a matched, controlled cohort study. *J Vasc Surg.* 2007; 46: 223-229.

Hinchliffe RJ, Bruijstens L, MacSweeney ST, Braithwaite BD. A randomised trial of endovascular and open surgery for ruptured abdominal aortic aneurysm - results of a pilot study and lessons learned for future studies. *Eur J Vasc Endovasc Surg.* 2006; 32: 506-13; discussion 514-5.

Johansen K, Kohler TR, Nicholls SC, Zierler RE, Clowes AW, Kazmers A. Ruptured abdominal aortic aneurysm: the Harborview experience. *J Vasc Surg.* 1991; 13: 240-5; discussion 245-7.

Johansson G, Swedenborg J. Little impact of elective surgery on the incidence and mortality of ruptured aortic aneurysms. *Eur J Vasc Surg.* 1994; 8: 489-493.

Johnston KW. Ruptured abdominal aortic aneurysm: six-year follow-up results of a multicenter prospective study. Canadian Society for Vascular Surgery Aneurysm Study Group. *J Vasc Surg.* 1994; 19: 888-900.

Joseph AY, Fisher JB, Toedter LJ, Balshi JD, Granson MA, Meir-Levi D. Ruptured abdominal aortic aneurysm and quality of life. *Vasc Endovascular Surg.* 2002; 36: 65-70.

Kashyap VS, Cambria RP, Davison JK, L'Italien GJ. Renal failure after thoracoabdominal aortic surgery. *J Vasc Surg.* 1997; 26: 949-55; discussion 955-7.

Korhonen SJ, Kantonen I, Pettila V, Keranen J, Salo JA, Lepantalo M. Long-term survival and health-related quality of life of patients with ruptured abdominal aortic aneurysm. *Eur J Vasc Endovasc Surg.* 2003; 25: 350-353.

Korhonen SJ, Ylonen K, Biancari F, Heikkinen M, Salenius JP, Lepantalo M, Finnvasc Study Group. Glasgow Aneurysm Score as a predictor of immediate outcome after surgery for ruptured abdominal aortic aneurysm. *Br J Surg.* 2004; 91: 1449-1452.

Lawrie GM, Crawford ES, Morris GC,Jr, Howell JF. Progress in the treatment of ruptured abdominal aortic aneurysm. *World J Surg.* 1980; 4: 653-658.

Lindholt JS, Vammen S, Juul S, Henneberg EW, Fasting H. The validity of ultrasonographic scanning as screening method for abdominal aortic aneurysm. *Eur J Vasc Endovasc Surg.* 1999; 17: 472-475.

Lindholt JS, Norman P. Screening for abdominal aortic aneurysm reduces overall mortality in men. A meta-analysis of the mid- and long-term effects of screening for abdominal aortic aneurysms. *Eur J Vasc Endovasc Surg.* 2008; 36: 167-171.

Lindsay TF, Luo XP, Lehotay DC, Rubin BB, Anderson M, Walker PM, Romaschin AD. Ruptured abdominal aortic aneurysm, a "two-hit" ischemia/reperfusion injury: evidence from an analysis of oxidative products. *J Vasc Surg.* 1999; 30: 219-228.

Low RB, Longmore W, Rubinstein R, Flores L, Wolvek S. Preliminary report on the use of the Percluder occluding aortic balloon in human beings. *Ann Emerg Med.* 1986; 15: 1466-1469.

Magee TR, Scott DJ, Dunkley A, St Johnston J, Campbell WB, Baird RN, Horrocks M. Quality of life following surgery for abdominal aortic aneurysm. *Br J Surg.* 1992; 79: 1014-1016.

Malina M, Veith F, Ivancev K, Sonesson B. Balloon occlusion of the aorta during endovascular repair of ruptured abdominal aortic aneurysm. *J Endovasc Ther.* 2005; 12: 556-559.

Markovic M, Davidovic L, Savic N, Sindjelic R, Ille T, Dragas M. Intraoperative Cell Salvage versus Allogeneic Transfusion during Abdominal Aortic Surgery: Clinical and Financial Outcomes. *Vascular.* 2009; 17: 83-92.

Mayer D, Pfammatter T, Rancic Z, Hechelhammer L, Wilhelm M, Veith FJ, Lachat M. 10 Years of Emergency Endovascular Aneurysm Repair for Ruptured Abdominal Aortoiliac Aneurysms: Lessons Learned. *Ann Surg.* 2009; 249: 510-515.

Marty-Ane CH, Alric P, Picot MC, Picard E, Colson P, Mary H. Ruptured abdominal aortic aneurysm: influence of intraoperative management on surgical outcome. *J Vasc Surg.* 1995; 22: 780-786.

Matsuda H, Tanaka Y, Hino Y, Matsukawa R, Ozaki N, Okada K, Tsukube T, Tsuji Y, Okita Y. Transbrachial arterial insertion of aortic occlusion balloon catheter in patients with shock from ruptured abdominal aortic aneurysm. *J Vasc Surg.* 2003; 38: 1293-1296.

McDaniel MD, Nehler MR, Santilli SM, Hiatt WR, Regensteiner JG, Goldstone J, McCarthy WJ, White JV. Extended outcome assessment in the care of vascular diseases: revising the paradigm for the 21st century. Ad Hoc Committee to Study Outcomes Assessment, Society for Vascular Surgery/International Society for Cardiovascular Surgery, North American Chapter. *J Vasc Surg.* 2000; 32: 1239-1250.

McPhee J, Eslami MH, Arous EJ, Messina LM, Schanzer A. Endovascular treatment of ruptured abdominal aortic aneurysms in the United States (2001-2006): a significant survival benefit over open repair is independently associated with increased institutional volume. *J Vasc Surg.* 2009; 49: 817-826.

Milne AA, Murphy WG, Bradbury AW, Ruckley CV. Postoperative haemorrhage following aortic aneurysm repair. *Eur J Vasc Surg.* 1994; 8: 622-626.

Moll FL, Powell JT, Fraedrich G, Verzini F, Haulon S, Waltham M, van Herwaarden JA, Holt PJ, van Keulen JW, Rantner B, Schlosser FJ, Setacci F, Ricco JB, European Society for Vascular Surgery. Management of abdominal aortic aneurysms clinical practice guidelines of the European society for vascular surgery. *Eur J Vasc Endovasc Surg.* 2011; 41 Suppl 1: S1-S58.

Mureebe L, Egorova N, Giacovelli JK, Gelijns A, Kent KC, McKinsey JF. National trends in the repair of ruptured abdominal aortic aneurysms. *J Vasc Surg.* 2008; 48: 1101-1107.

Nicholson ML, Baker DM, Hopkinson BR, Wenham PW. Randomized controlled trial of the effect of mannitol on renal reperfusion injury during aortic aneurysm surgery. *Br J Surg.* 1996; 83: 1230-1233.

Parodi JC, Palmaz JC, Barone HD. Transfemoral intraluminal graft implantation for abdominal aortic aneurysms. *Ann Vasc Surg.* 1991; 5: 491-499.

Pober JS, Cotran RS. The role of endothelial cells in inflammation. *Transplantation.* 1990; 50: 537-544.

Rasmussen TE, Hallett JW,Jr, Noel AA, Jenkins G, Bower TC, Cherry KJ,Jr, Panneton JM, Gloviczki P. Early abdominal closure with mesh reduces multiple organ failure after ruptured abdominal aortic aneurysm repair: guidelines from a 10-year case-control study. *J Vasc Surg.* 2002; 35: 246-253.

Reemtsma K, Morgan M. Outcomes assessment: a primer. *Bull Am Coll Surg.* 1997; 82: 34-39.

Reilly PM, Schiller HJ, Bulkley GB. Pharmacologic approach to tissue injury mediated by free radicals and other reactive oxygen metabolites. *Am J Surg.* 1991; 161: 488-503.

Sadat U, Boyle JR, Walsh SR, Tang T, Varty K, Hayes PD. Endovascular vs open repair of acute abdominal aortic aneurysms--a systematic review and meta-analysis. *J Vasc Surg.* 2008; 48: 227-236.

Scott RA, Wilson NM, Ashton HA, Kay DN. Influence of screening on the incidence of ruptured abdominal aortic aneurysm: 5-year results of a randomized controlled study. *Br J Surg.* 1995; 82: 1066-1070.

Scott RA, Bridgewater SG, Ashton HA. Randomized clinical trial of screening for abdominal aortic aneurysm in women. *Br J Surg.* 2002; 89: 283-285.

Takagi H, Sekino S, Kato T, Matsuno Y, Umemoto T. Intraoperative autotransfusion in abdominal aortic aneurysm surgery: meta-analysis of randomized controlled trials. *Arch Surg.* 2007; 142: 1098-1101.

Tambyraja AL, Fraser SC, Murie JA, Chalmers RT. Functional outcome after open repair of ruptured abdominal aortic aneurysm. *J Vasc Surg.* 2005; 41: 758-761.

Tambyraja AL, Murie JA, Chalmers RT. Prediction of outcome after abdominal aortic aneurysm rupture. *J Vasc Surg.* 2008; 47: 222-230.

Tambyraja AL, Lee AJ, Murie JA, Chalmers RT. Prognostic scoring in ruptured abdominal aortic aneurysm: a prospective evaluation. *J Vasc Surg.* 2008; 47: 282-286.

Ten Bosch JA, Teijink JA, Willigendael EM, Prins MH. Endovascular aneurysm repair is superior to open surgery for ruptured abdominal aortic aneurysms in EVAR-suitable patients. *J Vasc Surg.* 2010; 52: 13-18.

Ten Bosch JA, Willigendael EM, van Sambeek MR, de Loos ER, Prins MH, Teijink JA. EVAR Suitability is not a Predictor for Early and Midterm Mortality after Open Ruptured AAA repair. *Eur J Vasc Endovasc Surg.* 2011; .

van Herwaarden JA, van Vroonhoven TJ. Abdominal packing for surgically uncontrollable hemorrhage in ruptured abdominal aortic aneurysm repair. *J Vasc Surg.* 2001; 33: 195-196.

Veith FJ, Ohki T, Lipsitz EC, Suggs WD, Cynamon J. Treatment of ruptured abdominal aneurysms with stent grafts: a new gold standard? *Semin Vasc Surg.* 2003; 16: 171-175.

Visser JJ, van Sambeek MR, Hamza TH, Hunink MG, Bosch JL. Ruptured abdominal aortic aneurysms: endovascular repair versus open surgery--systematic review. *Radiology.* 2007; 245: 122-129.

Wahlgren CM, Piano G, Desai T, Shaalan W, Bassiouny H. Transperitoneal versus retroperitoneal suprarenal cross-clamping for repair of abdominal aortic aneurysm with a hostile infrarenal aortic neck. *Ann Vasc Surg.* 2007; 21: 687-694.

Wanhainen A, Bylund N, Bjorck M. Outcome after abdominal aortic aneurysm repair in Sweden 1994-2005. *Br J Surg.* 2008; 95: 564-570.

12

Endovascular Repair of the Ruptured Aneurysm

Jane Cross, Peter Harris and Toby Richards
University College Hospital,
United Kingdom

1. Introduction

Despite advances in the management of ruptured abdominal aortic aneurysms (RAAA), the mortality remains high. Approximately 6,000 men per year die from RAAA in England and Wales, accounting for 2% of deaths(1). In 2009 the UK National Vascular Database reported approximately 17% of aneurysms treated were ruptured, with an open mortality of 38%(2). The significant operative mortality for open repairs may reflect an irrecoverable physiological insult at the time of operation. Avoidance of laparotomy, retroperitoneal dissection and aortic cross clamping make endovascular techniques appealing for this high risk patient cohort.

Over the last decade, Endovascular Aneurysm Repair (EVAR) has become an established alternative to open surgery for the management of elective Abdominal Aortic Aneurysms (AAA). EVAR confers reduced early mortality(3), shorter operating time, fewer post-operative complications, reduced blood transfusion requirements, shorter ITU and hospital stay(4).

EVAR for RAAA was first reported in 1994(5). Currently its use is limited to specialist centres in the UK. The VASCUNET(6) multi-national database in 2008 reported 7466 RAAA of which 6468 were managed by open repair and only 478 by EVAR. The open mortality rate was 33% compared to 15% for EVAR. However, current published data for REVAR are subject to selection bias and the benefit of REVAR is unclear(7). EVAR is likely to be offered to stable patients or high surgical risk patients(8) and unstable patients are likely to have an open repair. Protocols and standard operating procedures are often reported incompletely or not at all making interpretation of results difficult. A pilot RCT was terminated early(9) due to slow recruitment at a single site and an over optimistic power calculation, and the evidence from single centre reports, systematic reviews and population based studies is weak.

This chapter outlines the patient selection, operative parameters, and post operative complications together with an evidence review for REVAR.

2. Patient selection

Indications for REVAR are variable between institutions. REVAR is used to treat all anatomically suitable RAAA in some centres, whereas its use is confined to haemodynamically stable patients in others; definitions of haemodynamic stability also vary(10). There are still many centres in the UK without a dedicated REVAR team and REVAR may not be routinely offered out of hours.

2.1 Haemodynamic parameters

Selection bias of previous studies suggested that REVAR was suitable only for stable patients. Hypotensive patients were considered unsuitable because of potential delays in obtaining a CT scan. However this has recently been challenged by the concept of "permissive hypotension" and hypotension is now not considered to preclude the use of EVAR.
Animal models of uncontrolled haemorrhage showed increased bleeding(11) and decreased survival when systolic blood pressure alone was the goal of resuscitation. In theory, increased fluid resuscitation leads to increased arterial and venous pressure, dilution of clotting factors and decreased blood viscosity. Permissive hypotension is the restrictive use of fluid therapy(12) to maintain SBP below normal physiological parameters with the aim of minimising blood loss prior to definitive intervention. Fluid input is titrated to maintain brain/vital organ perfusion. Whilst some authors advocate a SBP > 80mmHg to avoid cardiac, splanchnic, renal and brain ischaemia(13), others allow the SBP to fall to 50mmHg or less without fluid administration as long as the patient is moving and talking(14).

2.2 Anatomical criteria

Most centres require preoperative contrast enhanced CT to assess anatomical suitability for EVAR. Approximately 50% of patients presenting as an emergency are thought to be anatomically suitable for EVAR(15-16). Although, there is variability in the rapid availability of CT scans, pre procedural CT scans do not appear to significantly delay treatment or have an impact on outcome(9, 17) and the majority of patients who reach hospital with RAAA are stable enough to undergo a CT(18) prior to intervention. Newer "Hybrid" operating/angio suites often incorporate a CT scanner. This may decrease the delay between presentation and procedure commencement by reducing transfer time.

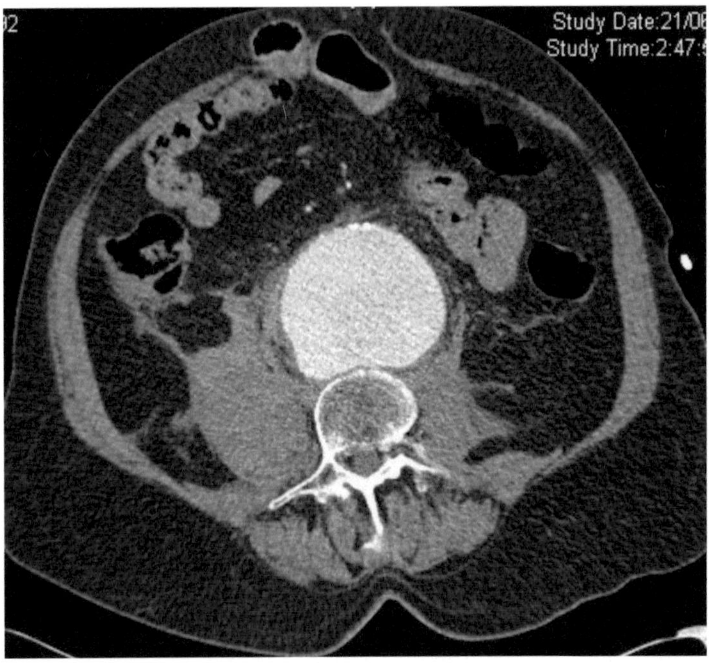

Fig. 1. A. CT scan of a contained ruptured AAA

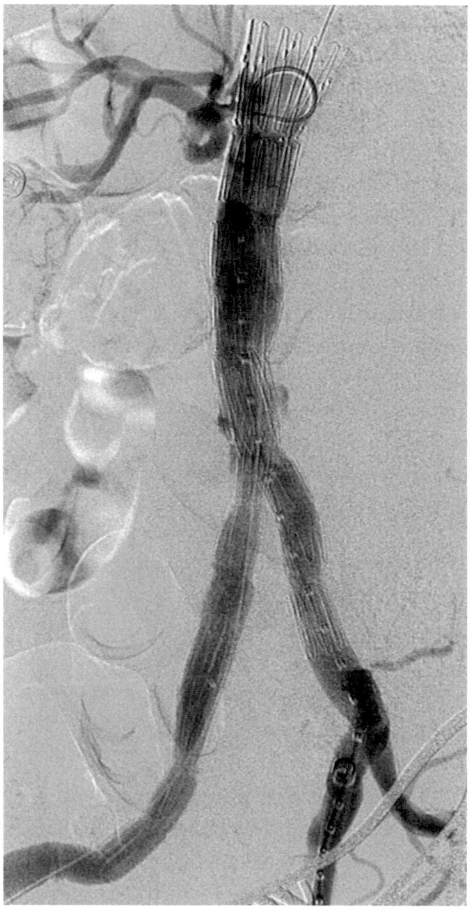

Fig. 1. B. The same patient following successful REVAR with a bifurcated graft. Note the right common iliac artery was aneurysmal necessitating coverage of the right internal iliac artery.

In unstable patients, CT may be avoided by performing intra-operative fluoroscopy to directly evaluate aneurysm morphology(10, 19). Graft sizing measurements are taken using calibrated catheters. However, this does not accurately show thrombus or atheroma lining the graft landing zones and was only able to predict the correct size of the graft in 60% of patients in an elective series.

RAAA usually present at a larger size with more adverse anatomical features than asymptomatic AAA(20). Data shows a significant increase in graft (procedural) related mortality in patients with adverse anatomy(8). In such cases open repair may be the preferred option. Although eligibility criteria are the same as those used for elective EVAR, the primary objective is survival and not long term durability of the device and it may be appropriate to consider less stringent anatomical criteria in patients with ruptured AAA(21-22). There is evidence that successful procedures can occur in the presence of adverse morphology. Alsac et al included neck angulation to 90° and reported EVAR to be suitable in 59% of cases(23), Moore advocated graft placement in necks of less than 10mm in length with the use of ancillary bare metal stenting of the pararenal neck(24). Metha et al accepted

necks as short as 5mm(21). Others have suggested electively covering the renal arteries in the emergency setting(22) a scenario that was fatal in the cases in this case series.
Another option for an unsuitable neck is to design and manufacture a fenestrated stent graft out of a commercially available device(25). However, it takes time to prepare the graft and some of the materials needed for construction e.g. fenestration markers are not routinely available. This is clearly not an option in the haemodynamically unstable patient. With the development of "off the shelf" fenestrated stent grafts, emergency fenestrated EVAR may become a more common future development.
Newer techniques such as "chimney" or "snorkel" procedures (fig 2) have been successfully reported for REVAR(25-26). This uses a technique of parallel stents for branching arteries and allows proximal placement of an endograft in the setting of a very short neck (2-3mm). Flow is secured to the branch arteries by inserting the renal artery stents simultaneous to the deployment of the aortic stent graft; this increases the number of short necked aneurysms that can be treated dramatically. This technique has also been used as a bail out option following inadvertent coverage of the renal arteries by converting to immediate laparotomy and retrogradely cannulating the renal arteries.

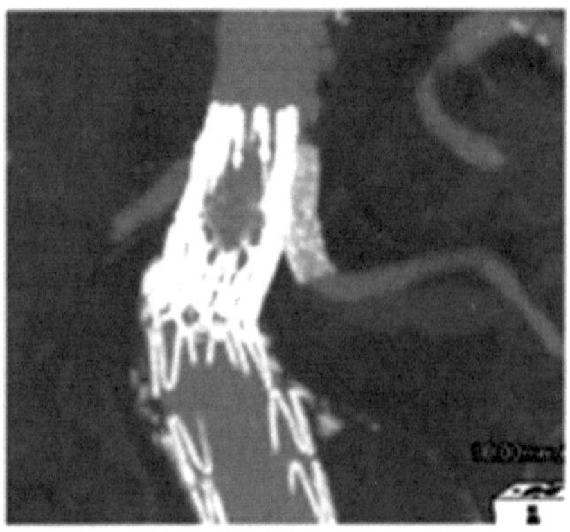

Fig. 2. CT showing a snorkel graft.

3. Procedure details

3.1 Theatre set up

Emergency EVAR should be undertaken in centres experienced and familiar with EVAR, where a multidisciplinary training programme and a pan-departmental protocol for the management of emergency EVAR can be effectively established. No individual factor leads to increased complications of emergency surgery, small errors often as a result of lack of familiarity, can compound to disrupt the normal planned sequential steps involved in graft placement. A dedicated REVAR team should therefore be available at all times with cross-departmental multidisciplinary training and rehearsal(21, 24).
Centres should have access to an endovascular suite with good quality imaging. A "Hybrid suite" is an ideal scenario and allows easy conversion to open surgery if necessary. Experience with adjunctive procedures and availability of different endograft options may facilitate EVAR in adverse anatomy(21, 27). Good imaging is vital for complex and /or ancillary procedures, cannulation and stenting of the renal arteries in case of pararenal top stent EVAR placement, placement of top cuff extension pieces, coiling of the internal iliac

artery for limb extension and potentially in the future for the use of iliac bifurcation devices or preloaded fenestrated devices.
In America EVAR has steadily increased for ruptured AAA. However, a reduction in mortality following REVAR was only seen in larger high volume centres. Lesperance et al showed a mortality of 21% in teaching hospitals compared to 55% at non-teaching hospitals(28). Other studies have also shown improved survival in experienced high volume centres(10) (26 v 46% mortality for REVAR(29)). Further, a 22.5% absolute risk reduction in mortality was seen after implementation of a structured protocol for management of RAAA and the use of an algorithm favouring endovascular repair(30). It is likely that the management of REVAR will be centralised to major regional vascular centres for optimal outcome.

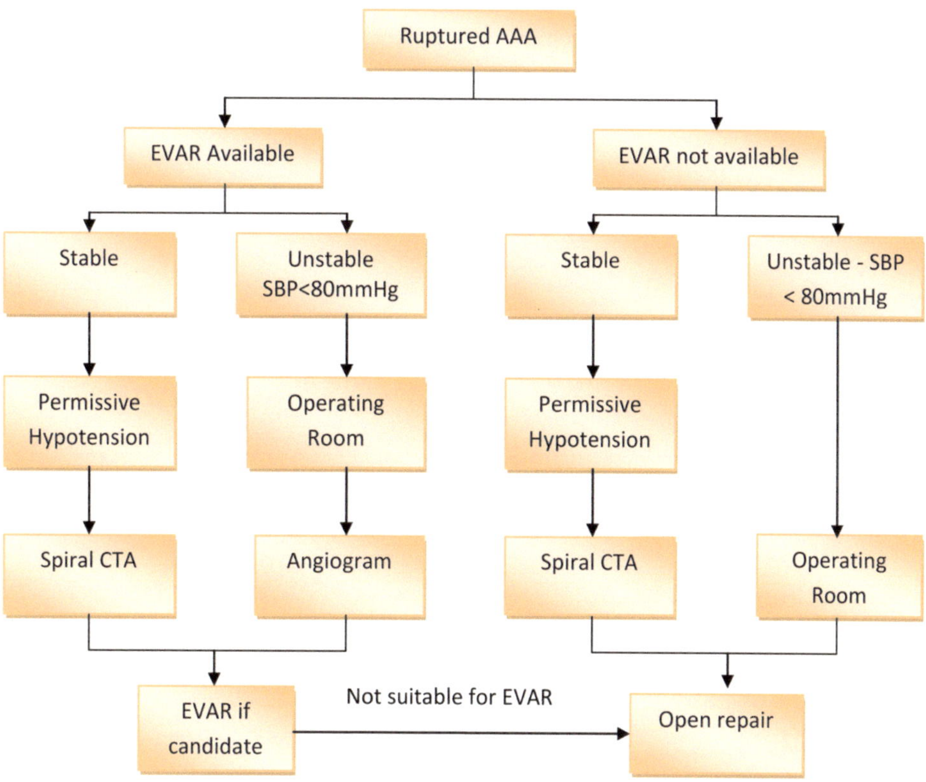

Fig. 3. An algorithm used by a centre in Canada(24).

3.2 Anaesthesia

REVAR may be performed under general anaesthesia, epidural or local anaesthesia with sedation(31). Induction of general anaesthesia inhibits the sympathetic vascular tone thereby inducing acute haemodynamic changes. It can also cause loss of abdominal muscle tone which may precipitate a free rupture from a previous aortic tamponade. REVAR under local anaesthetic is therefore often the preferred method and may improve patient outcome(32). Inadequate analgesia however may lead to restlessness and conversion to GA may be required. Although bifurcated grafts may be completed under local anaesthetic, AUI stent grafts require conversion to GA for the femoro-femoral bypass graft.

3.3 Haemorrhage control

Most patients who reach hospital with RAAA are stable and among those patients that reach hospital alive, around 90% of the deaths take place more than 2 hours after arrival(18). In the majority of cases swift deployment of the endograft results in successful haemorrhage control(13). However, patients with life threatening haemodynamic instability require immediate proximal occlusion of the aorta to control bleeding. This can be rapidly established by inflation of a compliant latex balloon placed via either the brachial or femoral routes to provide temporary haemostasis prior to definitive aneurysm exclusion(14).

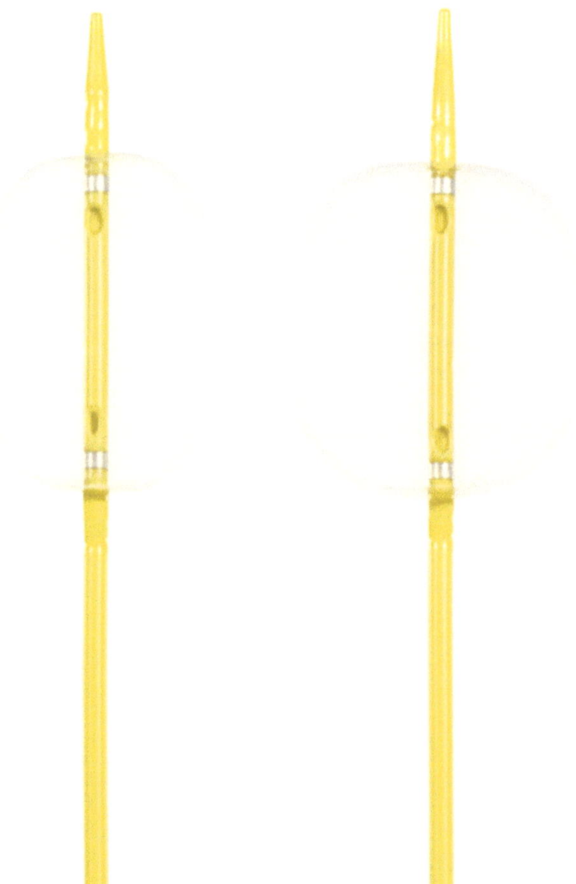

Fig. 4. Aortic occlusion balloon

A brachial approach may prevent distal migration of the balloon and allow transfemoral insertion of the stent graft with the aortic balloon still inflated. However, percutaneous brachial/axillary puncture is difficult in a shocked patient and surgical cut down is time consuming. Descending aortic catheterisation from the right arm is associated with the risk of cerebral emboli and the left sided approach may interfere with positioning of the C-arm fluoroscope.

Percutaneous femoral puncture may be easier in the hypotensive patient(33). The descending aorta is catheterised and a sheath inserted into the supra-/para renal aorta. The balloon is passed through the sheath and inflated. The sheath is advanced to support the inflated balloon from below and avoid distal dislocation when the blood pressure rises. The aortic stent graft is inserted from the contralateral groin via a stiff wire running outside the inflated balloon. The sheath that supports the balloon must also protrude above the stent graft to allow withdrawal of the balloon into the sheath after the endograft has been released; otherwise it is impossible to retrieve the balloon past the deployed stent graft. Conventional iodinated contrast may poorly delineate the aortic branches due to arrest of the blood flow. CO2 angiography is a useful adjunct(33). The balloon itself may occlude the renal arteries and should be cranially repositioned if the renal arteries cannot be identified. A second aortic balloon is inflated inside the main body of the stent graft as soon as the main body has been deployed and the primary balloon and supporting sheath are removed. This minimises visceral branch ischaemia.

Complications of aortic occlusion balloons include renal and splanchnic ischaemia and embolisation(34). The majority of patients do not require an occlusion balloon and the balloon should only be used in life threatening haemorrhage. The indications for aortic balloon control vary between centres and it may be used in approximately 18-23% of patients(10).

3.4 Graft configuration

Both bifurcated and aortouni-iliac(AUI) devices can be successfully used. A recent survey found that approximately 75% of grafts used are modular and 25% are unibody(10). Although AUI devices require a GA for the subsequent femoro-femoral crossover, they can be used to exclude contralateral common iliac aneurysms, are quick and easy to deploy(35) and may produce faster haemorrhage control. An appropriate inventory of suitable grafts and accessories must be stocked and available for procedural and unexpected contingencies.

4. Morbidity and mortality

Current evidence suggests that REVAR may be of benefit in the reduction of peri-operative morbidity and mortality as compared with open repair, in particular for haemodynamically stable patients. Single centres have reported small series with a mortality for REVAR of 15.6-24%(23, 36-37) and two multi-centre studies reported similar results of 26-45%(29, 38) mortality. In a systematic review of 22 studies REVAR was associated with reduced mortality (odds ratio 0.624)(39) and a further review showed a pooled mortality of 21%(40). However a randomised controlled trial failed to demonstrate a benefit with a mortality rate of 53% for both open repair and REVAR.

REVAR may be associated with lower postoperative physiological complications, reduced ITU and hospital stay compared to open repair(29, 39). REVAR is associated with an increased mortality (OR 7.2) in high surgical risk patients(41) compared to REVAR in low risk patients and may not be the "easier option" for high risk patients. These results should be used to influence the consent process for such patients.

4.1 Visceral ischaemia

The incidence of ischaemic colitis in elective EVAR is around 1%(42). The cause is multi-factorial and includes interruption of the inferior mesenteric artery, microembolisation, hypoperfusion, abdominal compartment syndrome and interruption of the hypogastric arteries. REVAR patients are likely to be more susceptible and the incidence of colonic ischaemia may be as high as 20%(43). This may be proportional to the level of pre-operative hypotension(44). Although previous reports suggest that it is safe to cover one or even both internal iliac arteries in the elective setting(45-46), reports of colonic ischaemia have followed an occlusion of at least one internal iliac artery.

4.2 Compartment syndrome

Abdominal compartment syndrome is an important cause of multi organ failure and occurs in around 10 -12% of patients(10, 47). Some centres routinely measure the bladder pressure and open the abdomen in the absence of organ failure(32, 48). Other centres only perform laparostomies in the presence of deteriorating BP, lung and renal function(14, 49). The intra-abdominal pressure may be increased secondary to the retroperitoneal haematoma in REVAR patients and surgical decompression is occasionally needed. Successful outcome depends on early recognition, early conservative treatment to reduce intra-abdominal hypertension (diuretics, colloids and neuromuscular blockade) and decompression if abdominal compartment syndrome develops.

4.3 Endoleak

Although late technical failures are more likely with inaccurate graft placement, difficult anatomy in the emergency setting may mean acceptance of a potentially inadequate repair. It may be better to return the patient to theatre once stabilised in the post operative period, prior to discharge to improve the seal zone.
It is likely that the incidence of type 1 endoleak is higher for REAVR than elective EVAR. However, these are poorly reported and the true incidence is unclear. Most REVAR series are small with short term follow up only, making meaningful data extraction difficult. However published series have shown a type I endoleak rate of 11.7 - 15.7% and a type II rate of around 25%(13, 32) for REVAR. A type 1 endoleak in a RAAA is a potential cause of ongoing haemorrhage and should be treated urgently.

5. Future trials

Three randomised controlled trials are currently underway, the Dutch AJAX trial, the French ECAR trial and the UK IMPROVE Trial.

5.1 The AJAX trial

The Amsterdam Acute Aneurysm Trial(50) is a multi-centre randomised controlled trial. Stable, anatomically suitable patients are randomised to either open repair or REVAR. The primary endpoint is 30 day mortality and severe morbidity and the secondary endpoints are quality of life and cost effectiveness. Started in 2004, the trial was based on an initial recruitment of just 80 patients. No significant difference was seen and recruitment has therefore been extended twice and is still ongoing.

5.2 ECAR trial

The Endovasculaire vs Chirurgie dans les Anevrysmes Rompus is a multi centre randomised controlled trial(51). All consecutive patients with ruptured aorto-iliac aneurysms who are haemodynamically stable (SBP>80), and have favourable anatomy are included. The primary outcome is 30 day mortality. Secondary outcomes are cardiovascular, pulmonary, gastrointestinal, renal and neurological morbidity, time in ITU and volume of blood transfused. All stable patients undergo CT scan and patients who are anatomically suitable are randomised to open repair or EVAR. The study started in 2008 and aims to recruit around 160 patients.

5.3 IMPROVE trial

The UK based Immediate Management of the Patient with Rupture: Open Versus Endovascular Repair (IMPROVE)(52) is a multi-centre international randomized controlled trial currently underway. This study differs from the previous two because it recruits "all comers". Patients with a clinical diagnosis of RAAA are randomized to either immediate CT scan and endovascular repair whenever anatomically suitable, or to open repair with CT scan being optional. The protocol of permissive hypotension is incorporated. Recruitment started in October 2009 and it is anticipated 600 patients will be required to show a 14% survival benefit for EVAR. The trial addresses whether the anticipated reduced mortality and morbidity associated with EVAR is offset by the relatively greater ease of access and speed to conventional surgery.

6. Conclusion

The use of EVAR is feasible in patients who present with a ruptured or acutely symptomatic AAA. Current evidence is weak and has likely inclusion bias; however published mortality rates are lower for REVAR than for open repair. Patient selection for REVAR varies between centres but the concept of "permissive hypotension" has increased the patient cohort undergoing REVAR. Mortality rates are lower in high volume centres; this may reflect experience in centres familiar with emergency EVAR, experience with adjunctive procedures, establishing control in heamodynamically unstable patients by supra renal aortic occlusion balloon placement, and the use of large balloon mounted stents to reinforce a short or angulated neck. Availability of different endograft options may facilitate EVAR for adverse anatomy and access to an endovascular suite with good quality imaging is undeniably beneficial. REVAR may also be associated with lower postoperative physiological complications, reduced ITU and hospital stay compared to open repair. However further studies are needed to produce concrete evidence. Current international multi-centre trials are underway to determine the benefit.

7. References

[1] Earnshaw JJ, Shaw E, Whyman MR, Poskitt KR, Heather BP. Screening for abdominal aortic aneurysms in men. BMJ. 2004 May 8;328(7448):1122-4.
[2] Lees S. The National Vascular Database Report 2009. 2009.
[3] Endovascular aneurysm repair versus open repair in patients with abdominal aortic aneurysm (EVAR trial 1): randomised controlled trial. Lancet. 2005 Jun 25-Jul 1;365(9478):2179-86.
[4] Prinssen M, Verhoeven EL, Buth J, Cuypers PW, van Sambeek MR, Balm R, et al. A randomized trial comparing conventional and endovascular repair of abdominal aortic aneurysms. N Engl J Med. 2004 Oct 14;351(16):1607-18.
[5] Yusuf SW, Whitaker SC, Chuter TA, Wenham PW, Hopkinson BR. Emergency endovascular repair of leaking aortic aneurysm. Lancet. 1994 Dec 10;344(8937):1645.
[6] Gibbons. The European Society for Vascular Surgery Second Vascular Surgery Database Report. 2008.

[7] Dillon M, Cardwell C, Blair PH, Ellis P, Kee F, Harkin DW. Endovascular treatment for ruptured abdominal aortic aneurysm. Cochrane Database Syst Rev. 2007(1):CD005261.
[8] Richards T, Goode SD, Hinchliffe R, Altaf N, Macsweeney S, Braithwaite B. The importance of anatomical suitability and fitness for the outcome of endovascular repair of ruptured abdominal aortic aneurysm. Eur J Vasc Endovasc Surg. 2009 Sep;38(3):285-90.
[9] Hinchliffe RJ, Bruijstens L, MacSweeney ST, Braithwaite BD. A randomised trial of endovascular and open surgery for ruptured abdominal aortic aneurysm - results of a pilot study and lessons learned for future studies. Eur J Vasc Endovasc Surg. 2006 Nov;32(5):506-13; discussion 14-5.
[10] Veith FJ, Lachat M, Mayer D, Malina M, Holst J, Mehta M, et al. Collected world and single center experience with endovascular treatment of ruptured abdominal aortic aneurysms. Ann Surg. 2009 Nov;250(5):818-24.
[11] Holmes JF, Sakles JC, Lewis G, Wisner DH. Effects of delaying fluid resuscitation on an injury to the systemic arterial vasculature. Acad Emerg Med. 2002 Apr;9(4):267-74.
[12] van der Vliet JA, van Aalst DL, Schultze Kool LJ, Wever JJ, Blankensteijn JD. Hypotensive hemostatis (permissive hypotension) for ruptured abdominal aortic aneurysm: are we really in control? Vascular. 2007 Jul-Aug;15(4):197-200.
[13] Alsac JM, Kobeiter H, Becquemin JP, Desgranges P. Endovascular repair for ruptured AAA: a literature review. Acta Chir Belg. 2005 Apr;105(2):134-9.
[14] Veith FJ, Ohki T. Endovascular approaches to ruptured infrarenal aorto-iliac aneurysms. J Cardiovasc Surg (Torino). 2002 Jun;43(3):369-78.
[15] Rose DF, Davidson IR, Hinchliffe RJ, Whitaker SC, Gregson RH, MacSweeney ST, et al. Anatomical suitability of ruptured abdominal aortic aneurysms for endovascular repair. J Endovasc Ther. 2003 Jun;10(3):453-7.
[16] Hoornweg LL, Wisselink W, Vahl A, Balm R. The Amsterdam Acute Aneurysm Trial: suitability and application rate for endovascular repair of ruptured abdominal aortic aneurysms. Eur J Vasc Endovasc Surg. 2007 Jun;33(6):679-83.
[17] Boyle JR, Gibbs PJ, Kruger A, Shearman CP, Raptis S, Phillips MJ. Existing delays following the presentation of ruptured abdominal aortic aneurysm allow sufficient time to assess patients for endovascular repair. Eur J Vasc Endovasc Surg. 2005 May;29(5):505-9.
[18] Lloyd GM, Bown MJ, Norwood MG, Deb R, Fishwick G, Bell PR, et al. Feasibility of preoperative computer tomography in patients with ruptured abdominal aortic aneurysm: a time-to-death study in patients without operation. J Vasc Surg. 2004 Apr;39(4):788-91.
[19] Peppelenbosch N, Zannetti S, Barbieri B, Buth J. Endograft treatment in ruptured abdominal aortic aneurysms using the Talent AUI stentgraft system. Design of a feasibility study. Eur J Vasc Endovasc Surg. 2004 Apr;27(4):366-71.
[20] Szilagyi DE, Smith RF, DeRusso FJ, Elliott JP, Sherrin FW. Contribution of abdominal aortic aneurysmectomy to prolongation of life. Ann Surg. 1966 Oct;164(4):678-99.
[21] Mehta M, Taggert J, Darling RC, 3rd, Chang BB, Kreienberg PB, Paty PS, et al. Establishing a protocol for endovascular treatment of ruptured abdominal aortic aneurysms: outcomes of a prospective analysis. J Vasc Surg. 2006 Jul;44(1):1-8; discussion
[22] Lee RW, Rhodes JM, Singh MJ, Davies MG, Wolford HY, Diachun C, et al. Is there a selection bias in applying endovascular aneurysm repair for rupture? Ann Vasc Surg. 2008 Mar;22(2):215-20.

[23] Alsac JM, Desgranges P, Kobeiter H, Becquemin JP. Emergency endovascular repair for ruptured abdominal aortic aneurysms: feasibility and comparison of early results with conventional open repair. Eur J Vasc Endovasc Surg. 2005 Dec;30(6):632-9.
[24] Moore R, Nutley M, Cina CS, Motamedi M, Faris P, Abuznadah W. Improved survival after introduction of an emergency endovascular therapy protocol for ruptured abdominal aortic aneurysms. J Vasc Surg. 2007 Mar;45(3):443-50.
[25] Resch T. Proportion of Ruptured AAAs Suitable for EVAR in view of Chimney and Homemade Fenestrated Endografts. www.veithsymposiumorg/pdf/vei/2624pdf.
[26] Schlosser FJ, Aruny JE, Freiburg CB, Mojibian HR, Sumpio BE, Muhs BE. The chimney procedure is an emergently available endovascular solution for visceral aortic aneurysm rupture. J Vasc Surg. 2011 Jan 26.
[27] Albertini JN, Perdikides T, Soong CV, Hinchliffe RJ, Trojanowska M, Yusuf SW. Endovascular repair of abdominal aortic aneurysms in patients with severe angulation of the proximal neck using a flexible stent-graft: European Multicenter Experience. J Cardiovasc Surg (Torino). 2006 Jun;47(3):245-50.
[28] Lesperance K, Andersen C, Singh N, Starnes B, Martin MJ. Expanding use of emergency endovascular repair for ruptured abdominal aortic aneurysms: disparities in outcomes from a nationwide perspective. J Vasc Surg. 2008 Jun;47(6):1165-70; discussion 70-1.
[29] Greco G, Egorova N, Anderson PL, Gelijns A, Moskowitz A, Nowygrod R, et al. Outcomes of endovascular treatment of ruptured abdominal aortic aneurysms. J Vasc Surg. 2006 Mar;43(3):453-9.
[30] Starnes BW, Quiroga E, Hutter C, Tran NT, Hatsukami T, Meissner M, et al. Management of ruptured abdominal aortic aneurysm in the endovascular era. J Vasc Surg. 2010 Jan;51(1):9-17; discussion -8.
[31] Lachat ML, Pfammatter T, Witzke HJ, Bettex D, Kunzli A, Wolfensberger U, et al. Endovascular repair with bifurcated stent-grafts under local anaesthesia to improve outcome of ruptured aortoiliac aneurysms. Eur J Vasc Endovasc Surg. 2002 Jun;23(6):528-36.
[32] Mayer D, Pfammatter T, Rancic Z, Hechelhammer L, Wilhelm M, Veith FJ, et al. 10 years of emergency endovascular aneurysm repair for ruptured abdominal aortoiliac aneurysms: lessons learned. Ann Surg. 2009 Mar;249(3):510-5.
[33] Malina M, Veith F, Ivancev K, Sonesson B. Balloon occlusion of the aorta during endovascular repair of ruptured abdominal aortic aneurysm. J Endovasc Ther. 2005 Oct;12(5):556-9.
[34] Low RB, Longmore W, Rubinstein R, Flores L, Wolvek S. Preliminary report on the use of the Percluder occluding aortic balloon in human beings. Ann Emerg Med. 1986 Dec;15(12):1466-9.
[35] Chuter TA, Faruqi RM, Reilly LM, Kerlan RK, Sawhney R, Wall SD, et al. Aortomonoiliac endovascular grafting combined with femorofemoral bypass: an acceptable compromise or a preferred solution? Semin Vasc Surg. 1999 Sep;12(3):176-81.
[36] Kubin K, Sodeck GH, Teufelsbauer H, Nowatschka B, Kretschmer G, Lammer J, et al. Endovascular therapy of ruptured abdominal aortic aneurysm: mid- and long-term results. Cardiovasc Intervent Radiol. 2008 May-Jun;31(3):496-503.
[37] Chagpar RB, Harris JR, Lawlor DK, DeRose G, Forbes TL. Early mortality following endovascular versus open repair of ruptured abdominal aortic aneurysms. Vasc Endovascular Surg. 2010 Nov;44(8):645-9.
[38] Peppelenbosch N, Geelkerken RH, Soong C, Cao P, Steinmetz OK, Teijink JA, et al. Endograft treatment of ruptured abdominal aortic aneurysms using the Talent

aortouniiliac system: an international multicenter study. J Vasc Surg. 2006 Jun;43(6):1111-23; discussion 23.

[39] Sadat U, Boyle JR, Walsh SR, Tang T, Varty K, Hayes PD. Endovascular vs open repair of acute abdominal aortic aneurysms--a systematic review and meta-analysis. J Vasc Surg. 2008 Jul;48(1):227-36.

[40] Mastracci TM, Garrido-Olivares L, Cina CS, Clase CM. Endovascular repair of ruptured abdominal aortic aneurysms: a systematic review and meta-analysis. J Vasc Surg. 2008 Jan;47(1):214-21.

[41] Jordan WD, Alcocer F, Wirthlin DJ, Westfall AO, Whitley D. Abdominal aortic aneurysms in "high-risk" surgical patients: comparison of open and endovascular repair. Ann Surg. 2003 May;237(5):623-9; discussion 9-30.

[42] Miller A, Marotta M, Scordi-Bello I, Tammaro Y, Marin M, Divino C. Ischemic colitis after endovascular aortoiliac aneurysm repair: a 10-year retrospective study. Arch Surg. 2009 Oct;144(10):900-3.

[43] Champagne BJ, Lee EC, Valerian B, Mulhotra N, Mehta M. Incidence of colonic ischemia after repair of ruptured abdominal aortic aneurysm with endograft. J Am Coll Surg. 2007 Apr;204(4):597-602.

[44] Bast TJ, van der Biezen JJ, Scherpenisse J, Eikelboom BC. Ischaemic disease of the colon and rectum after surgery for abdominal aortic aneurysm: a prospective study of the incidence and risk factors. Eur J Vasc Surg. 1990 Jun;4(3):253-7.

[45] Mehta M, Veith FJ, Ohki T, Cynamon J, Goldstein K, Suggs WD, et al. Unilateral and bilateral hypogastric artery interruption during aortoiliac aneurysm repair in 154 patients: a relatively innocuous procedure. J Vasc Surg. 2001 Feb;33(2 Suppl):S27-32.

[46] Wolpert LM, Dittrich KP, Hallisey MJ, Allmendinger PP, Gallagher JJ, Heydt K, et al. Hypogastric artery embolization in endovascular abdominal aortic aneurysm repair. J Vasc Surg. 2001 Jun;33(6):1193-8.

[47] Djavani Gidlund K, Wanhainen A, Bjorck M. Intra-abdominal Hypertension and Abdominal Compartment Syndrome after Endovascular Repair of Ruptured Abdominal Aortic Aneurysm. Eur J Vasc Endovasc Surg. 2011 Mar 14.

[48] Hechelhammer L, Lachat ML, Wildermuth S, Bettex D, Mayer D, Pfammatter T. Midterm outcome of endovascular repair of ruptured abdominal aortic aneurysms. J Vasc Surg. 2005 May;41(5):752-7.

[49] Mehta M, Darling RC, 3rd, Roddy SP, Fecteau S, Ozsvath KJ, Kreienberg PB, et al. Factors associated with abdominal compartment syndrome complicating endovascular repair of ruptured abdominal aortic aneurysms. J Vasc Surg. 2005 Dec;42(6):1047-51.

[50] Amsterdam Acute Aneurysm trial: background, design, and methods. Vascular. 2006 May-Jun;14(3):130-5.

[51] Desgranges P, Kobeiter H, Castier Y, Senechal M, Majewski M, Krimi A. The Endovasculaire vs Chirurgie dans les Anevrysmes Rompus PROTOCOL trial update. J Vasc Surg. 2010 Jan;51(1):267-70.

[52] Powell JT, Thompson SG, Thompson MM, Grieve R, Nicholson AA, Ashleigh R, et al. The Immediate Management of the Patient with Rupture: Open Versus Endovascular repair (IMPROVE) aneurysm trial--ISRCTN 48334791 IMPROVE trialists. Acta Chir Belg. 2009 Nov-Dec;109(6):678-80.

Late Complications Following Aortic Aneurysm Repair

Michiel L.P. van Zeeland and Lijckle van der Laan
Department of Vascular Surgery, Amphia Hospital
The Netherlands

1. Introduction

Abdominal aortic aneurysm affects 5-10 % of men and 1,3% of women (Cosworth & Leng, 2007). Current treatment of aortic aneurysm is going through rapid changes. The first successful open repair with a homograft was performed in 1951 (Dubost et al. 1952). Initially, the aneurysm wall was completely removed which could lead to major complications. Creech modified the technique and combined repair with a graft with aneurysmorhapphy which simplified the technique and improved results (Creech, 1966). Late complications after open surgical repair are infrequent but also poorly monitored. It is generally assumed that if patients have survived this major surgical procedure, few complications occur. Endovascular aneurysm repair (EVAR) is gaining popularity since the mid-nineties (Parodi et al., 1991). Despite major technical improvements in endografts, follow-up is essential after endovascular repair. Recent studies reported up to 40% of aneurysms growing after EVAR, even in recent years (2004-2008) (Schanzer et al., 2011). These growing aneurysms pose the vascular surgeon for new clinical problems which sometimes require unorthodox interventions. An overview of late complications of both open and endovascular abdominal aortic aneurysm repair is given along with specific solutions from the literature and our own experience. Table 1 summarizes the late complications and estimated incidence form the literature.

Common late complications after aortic aneurysm repair			Estimated Incidence
Open repair	Graft related	Anastomotic aneurysm	1-10%
		Graft occlusion	<1%
		Infection	0.2-2%
		Aortoenteric fistula	0.3-2.5%
	Non-graft related	Incisional herniae	30-90%
		Small bowel obstruction	Unknown *
		Sexual dysfunction	Up to 80%
		Buttock claudication	Unknown
EVAR**	Graft related	Infection	1-3%
		Migration, kinking, occlusion	1-14%
		Rupture	1-9%

*Single Study showed 2.6% (Siporin et al., 1993), **Endovascular Aneurysm Repair.

Table 1. Late complications after aneurysm repair

2. Late complications after open aneurysm repair

2.1 Graft related complications

Late complications after successful AAA repair are infrequent. Anastomotic aneurysms are infrequent in the literature (1-10%), but this might be an underestimation due to a lack of follow-up. Repair can be performed open or endovascular. Infectious complications are also rare after open AAA repair. An infected aortic prosthesis represents one of the most difficult challenges for the vascular surgeon today. Diagnosis is usually obvious but occasionally unclear even after extensive clinical and radiological investigations. Mortality and amputation rates continue to be high. Various treatment options will be discussed, from definitive surgical repair to a non-operative approach comprised of drainage and long term antibiotic treatment. Our own unpublished data on non-operative management will be presented. Aortoduodenal fistulae can present with hemorrhage or as an infected prosthesis. Treatment is also extremely challenging for the vascular surgeon with high mortality rates. Graft thrombosis is infrequent and usually caused by coexistent iliac occlusive disease.

2.1.1 Anastomotic aneurysm

2.1.1.1 Incidence of anastomotic aneurysm

Plate et al published on of the earliest reports on late complications (Plate et al., 1985). A study of over 1000 AAA patients with 6 year follow-up showed anastomotic aneurysms but no fistula. Forty-nine true, 14 anastomotic, and five dissecting aneurysms were detected in 59 patients 5 years after the initial aneurysm repair. These aneurysms were located in the thoracic (24), thoracoabdominal (five), or abdominal aorta (11), and in the iliac (six), femoral (17), popliteal (four), and renal arteries (one). Only one of 26 patients presenting with a rupture of one of these secondary aneurysms survived. There was a significant association between preoperative hypertension and recurrent aneurysm. The authors suggest that subsequent vascular disease, including recurrent aneurysms and graft complications, cause significant late morbidity and mortality after repair of abdominal aortic aneurysm. They suggest that careful follow-up and adequate control of hypertension may allow reduction in morbidity and an improvement in late survival. Hertzer et al. reported much less graft-related complications(0.4%) with 5-year follow-up, although only clinically evident (as opposed to computed tomography scan-detected) events were considered (Hertzer et al., 2002). Conrad et al. described a cohort of 540 open non-ruptured AAA repairs (Conrad et al.,2007). 152 Of them had follow-up CT scans which revealed 13 graft-related complications identified in 11 patients, including 7 anastomotic pseudoaneurysms (4 proximal and 3 distal). Three of the four proximal and two of the three distal cases underwent open operative repair. The remaining two were observed because of concomitant co morbidities. Hallett reported a 9.4% graft-related complication rate (mostly anastomotic pseudoaneurysms) after open AAA repair at an average follow-up of 5.8 years with late surveillance imaging on most patients (Hallett et al., 1997). Finally, Biancari et al. report of a 15.4% late graft-related complication rate with a median follow-up of 8 years (Biancari et al., 2002). This is significantly worse than the previous reports and may be related to the inclusion of ruptured AAA repairs. Edwards et al. set out to examine late follow-up of aortic surgery (Edwards et al., 1992). They performed ultrasonography of 111 patients and discovered eleven paraanastomotic aneurysms, including 7 pseudoaneurysms and 4 true aneurysms of the adjacent aorta. The majority were seen after 7 years.

2.1.1.2 Surgical management of anastomotic aneurysm

Surgical treatment of anastomotic pseudoaneurysm is a technically challenging procedure and requires dissection through previous scarred operative sites in patients who are likely to have more co morbidity than those with primary aortic surgery. As a result, mortality and morbidity rates of aortic redo surgery are higher than those associated with primary prosthetic reconstructions (van Herwaarden et al., 2004; Mulder et al., 1998; Treiman et al., 1988). Allen et al. reported an overall 73% major postoperative complication rate and an operative mortality rate of 21% in 29 patients who were treated for anastomotic aneurysms of the abdominal aorta (Allen et al., 1993). Endovascular treatment of anastomotic aneurysms after aortic surgery seems a promising technique. Small series have been published on the subject. Yuan et al. constructed endovascular grafts from PTFE sutured to Palmaz stents and treated 10 patients with 12 aneurysms. No mortality occurred and 1 wound hematoma was observed. After a mean of 16 months of follow-up, no graft related complications occurred. Van Herwaarden treated 14 patients with either anastomotic or iliac aneurysms after previous aortic repair, using commercially available stent grafts. Eleven patients recovered without sequelae and 3 patients required a second intervention (2 open and 1 endovascular) after 12 months follow-up (Van Herwaarden et al., 2004). The authors warned us for the placement of a tube endovascular graft in a normal graft body. For better columnar strength, bifurcated stents should be used.

Ruptured (para)anastomotic aneurysms are even more challenging for the vascular surgeon. The mortality rate of patients with ruptured (para)anastomotic aneurysm arriving in the hospital is very high. Endovascular repair has been described in a few cases (Syfrodas et al., 2008). Our group also described an already unresponsive patient in severe hemorrhagic shock who was treated with an aortic occlusion balloon for hemodynamic stabilization and subsequent stent placement to exclude a ruptured iliac aneurysm. The patient recovered uneventfully (Menke et al., 2010).

In conclusion, for (para)anastomotic aneurysms, endovascular treatment seems to have advantages over open repair with good mid-term results.

2.1.2 Graft occlusions

Large series mention few graft occlusions after open aneurysm repair. Hallett et al. reported 6 graft thromboses after 10 years of follow-up of 307 grafts (Hallett et al., 1997). One tube occluded, the others were bifurcated. Conrad et al. performed CT scanning of 152 of 540 open repairs. There were four graft limb occlusions in the bifurcated grafts that were treated with open thrombectomy and revision of the distal (femoral) anastomosis (Conrad et al., 2007). The Dutch Randomized Endovascular Aneurysm Repair (DREAM) trial followed 178 open and 173 EVAR cases and found a total of 3 occlusions after open repair and 12 after EVAR (De Bruin et al., 2011). The long term outcome of the EVAR 1 trial showed 22 graft thromboses in 1216 repairs, 2 after open and 20 after EVAR (Greenhalgh et al., 2010).

Treatment of graft thrombosis can be performed open or endovascular. Usually, stenosis of the distal anastomosis is the cause. Open repair and revision of the distal anastomosis is required in these cases. We recommend the use of a graft thrombectomy catheter. Intra-arterial thrombolysis is increasingly used in graft acute thrombosis with good results. Also, recent reports on ultrasound-accelerated thrombolysis are promising (Schrijver et al., 2011).

2.1.3 Graft infection and management

2.1.3.1 Incidence and diagnosis of graft infection

Aortic vascular graft infection is an infrequent complication of aortic surgery. Large series showed an incidence of 0.2-2% graft infections after open aortic surgery (Hallett et al., 1997; Hertzer et al., 2002). The DREAM trial reported no graft infections in open repair and 2 after EVAR (De Bruin et al., 2010). Conrad followed 540 aortic grafts and described two graft infections which were identified and treated with graft removal (Conrad et al., 2007). Diagnosis is suspected with, fever, elevated serum CRP and leukocyte count and fluid collections around the graft on CT scan, in the absence of other possible causes of fever. Confirmation of the diagnosis is through culture of a micro-organism from the area of the graft. In unclear cases, FDG-PET-CT has proven to be a useful tool in the work-up for diagnosis of aortic graft infection (Bruggink et al., 2010).

2.1.3.2 Microbiology of graft infection

It has been proposed to divide the spectrum of aortic graft infections into early and late presentations (Bandyk, 2002). Early infections usually present within the first 3 months after implantation and spread rapidly whereas late infections usually occur after this period and tend to be more confined with respect to extent of infection. Most commonly, both types are initiated during graft implantation via contamination from patient skin flora. Early <4 months graft infection generally is caused by S. aureus or Gram-negative bacteria and frequently originates from a failure of primary wound healing. The presence of hematoma, lymphatic fistula, and devitalized tissue increase the risk for graft infection and should be treated aggressively with wound exploration, debridement, and primary wound closure. The majority (>80%) of graft infections are diagnosed more than 4 months after graft implantation. These infections are most commonly with S. Epidermidis, which produce a low-grade infection with a polysaccharide biofilm (slime-like appearance). Other pathogens include Escherichia coli, Pseudomonas spp., Proteus, Salmonella and Klebsiella pneumoniae, Listeria Monocytogenes and Corynebacteriae (own unpublished data). These pathogens are most likely to have colonized the graft after implantation. Whenever possible, pathogen(s) should be identified before treatment, permitting bactericidal-level antibiotics to be administered pre- and postoperatively. If the infecting organism has not been isolated, broad-spectrum antibiotics should be given. When S. aureus or S. epidermidis is the most likely pathogen, parenteral therapy with a first- or second-generation cephalosporin and vancomycin are appropriate. Once operative cultures have isolated all infecting organisms, treatment should be modified based on antibiotic susceptibility testing of the recovered strains. No evidence is available on the duration of antibiotic administration after treatment by graft excision, but at least 4 weeks of systemic antibiotics is recommended in the literature. After in situ prosthetic replacement or prosthetic graft preservation procedures, long-term antibiotic therapy is recommended (parenteral antibiotics for 6 weeks, followed by oral antibiotics for to 6 months) (Bandyk, 2002) . On the other hand, our personal experience is that some patients require life-long antibiotics. We have encountered cases where on cessation of antibiotic treatment, fever returned and subsided again after restarting antibiotic treatment.

2.1.3.3 Surgical management of graft infection

Excision of the infected aortic prosthesis and extra-anatomic bypass grafting through a noninfected field has been the most common treatment for patients with aortic graft infection. Results of the use of this approach have gradually improved since its introduction by Blaisdell et al. in 1970, particularly after the observation of Reilly et al. that staged extra-anatomic bypass grafting followed by graft excision was associated with lower mortality and improved initial limb salvage (Blaisdell et al., 1970; Reilly et al., 1987). Seeger et al. reported a series of 36 cases with infected aortic prosthesis. Four patients (11%) died in the postoperative period, and two patients died during follow-up as a direct consequence of extra-anatomic bypass grafting and aortic graft removal (one died 7 months after extra-anatomic bypass graft failure, one died 36 months after aortic stump disruption). One additional patient died 72 months after failure of a subsequent aortic reconstruction, so that the overall treatment-related mortality was 19%, whereas overall survival by means of life table analysis was 56% at 5 years. No amputations were required in the postoperative period, but four patients (11%) required amputation during follow-up. 5 patients had some form of axillopopliteal reconstruction, 3 of which occluded within one year and all were occluded after 5 years. This group abandoned axillopopliteal reconstructions and performed in situ replacement if outflow problems existed (Seeger et al., 2000).

Aortic graft infection can also be treated with simultaneous aortic graft excision and in situ aortic graft replacement with a variety of new aortic grafts (an autogenous graft, a homograft or a new prosthetic graft). Clagett et al. and Nevelsteen et al. have reviewed the use of autogenous grafts constructed from deep femoral veins to treat 41 and 15 patients with infected aortic grafts. Postoperative mortality rates were 10% and 7%, respectively, in these studies, and early amputation rates were 5% and 7%. Furthermore, Clagett reported that primary and secondary graft patency rates at 5 years were 83% and 100%, 5-year limb salvage was 86%, and significant lower extremity edema was uncommon (Clagett et al., 1997; Nevelsteen et al., 1995). A Dutch group produced excellent results with spiralised great saphenous veins as an aortic replacement for and infected prosthesis (van Zitteren et al. 2011). They treated 5 patients and reported no deaths and no amputations after 13 months of follow up.

2.1.3.4 Non-operative management of graft infection in the compromised patient

In some cases, graft removal is not feasible because of poor clinical condition of the patient after emergency aneurysm repair, a hostile abdomen or severe co-morbidity. Different methods of preserving the infected graft have been attempted. We have described two patients with infected grafts, unfit for immediate graft removal. The first was treated only by specific antibiotic treatment and the second was treated with percutaneous drainage and antibiotic treatment aimed at the cultured microorganism. To date, both patients are alive. One is on life-long antibiotic therapy (own unpublished data, Figures 1 and 2).

Calligaro et al. reported a 20 year experience with nine patients unfit for graft explantation. Principles of treatment were percutaneous or operative drain placement into retroperitoneal abscess cavities and along the graft, with instillation of antibiotics three times daily, repeated debridement of infected groin wounds, and intravenous antibiotic therapy for at least 6 weeks. They concluded that partial or complete graft preservation combined with aggressive drainage and groin wound debridement is an acceptable option for treatment of infection involving an entire aortic graft in selected patients with prohibitive risks for total graft excision. This treatment may be compatible with long-term survival and protracted absence of signs or symptoms of infection (Calligaro et al., 2003).

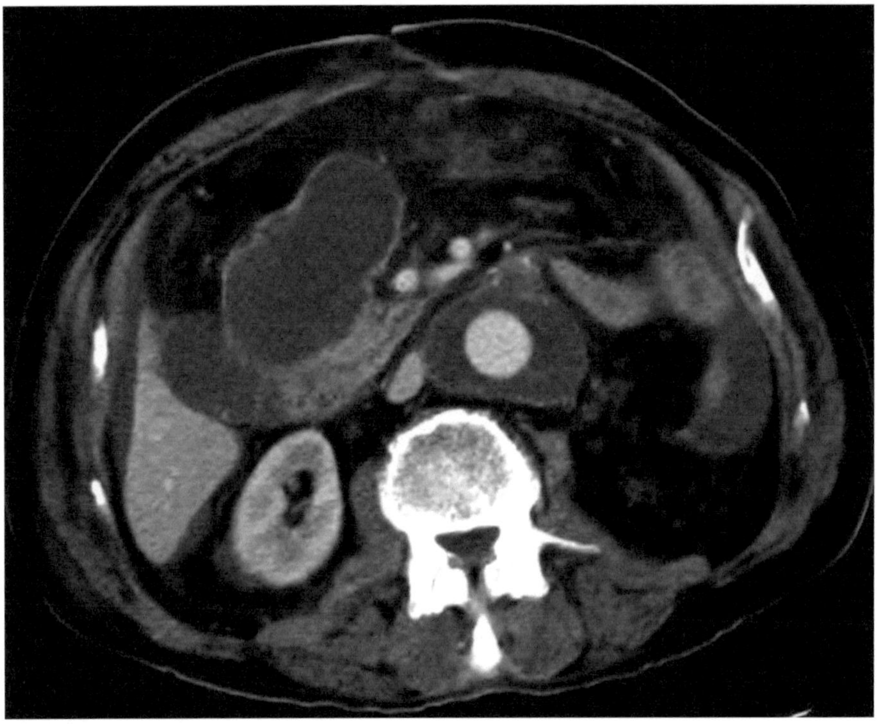

Fig. 1. Abdominal CT angiography shown an abscess and perigraft fluid.

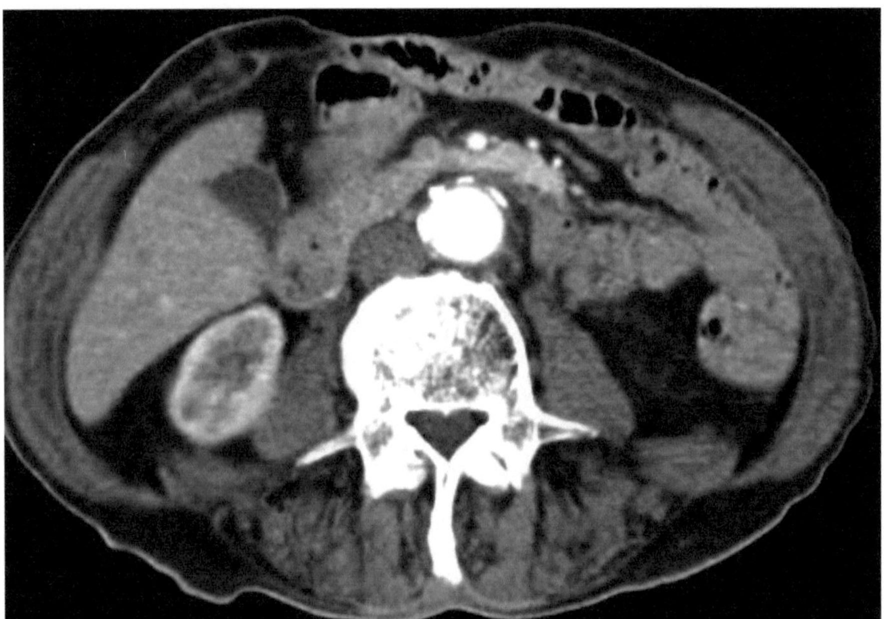

Fig. 2. Abdominal CT angiography after percutaneous drainage of abscess and 2 years of antibiotic treatment.

In conclusion, the treatment of the patient with an infected graft is a major challenge. The fitness of the patient is the most important factor in management, while virulence of the micro-organism is another factor . In young, fit patients, graft removal and in situ repair seems the most durable option. Extra-anatomic repair can be a less invasive procedure for the compromised patient. In severely compromised patients or those with a hostile abdomen, conservative management is feasible.

2.1.4 Aortoenteric fistula

Secondary aortoenteric fistulae complicate 0.3%-2.5% of all open aortic surgical procedures (Plate 1985, Bergquist 1987). On presentation, upper gastro-intestinal bleeding, hemorrhagic shock and fever may be present. Diagnosis is confirmed with gastroduodenoscopy and CT angiography. Despite prompt open repair, secondary aortoenteric fistula remains a very lethal condition with mortality rates up to 50% (Kakkos, 2011).

A small series buy Kuestner et al. described extra-anatomic bypass followed a few days thereafter by graft removal. Aortic stump blow out is a feared complication, and occurred in 9.1%. The major amputation rate was also 9.1%. Total mortality was as high as 27% (Keustner, 1993). Results are comparable with similar surgical management of infected prosthesis. Because of poor outcome, other attempts have been made to treat this complication. As with infected prosthesis, in situ repairs as described by Nevelsteen et al. and Clagett et al. have reasonable results.

Kakkos et al. recently published a comparison of open versus endovascular treatment of aortoenteric fistulae. Eight patients were treated with EVAR and 17 with open repair, of which 12 with extra-anatomical bypass and graft removal. There was a short term survival benefit after EVAR (0% mortality) and open repair (35% mortality). This difference had disappeared after two years because of excess recurrent disease in the EVAR group. The authors conclude that EVAR might be used in the future as a bridge to definitive repair (Kakkos et al., 2011)

2.2 Non-graft related complications

The magnitude of laparotomy related late complications has been poorly appreciated until recently. This is probably because of lack of proper follow-up. Nowadays, more attention has focused on non-vascular complications of open AAA repair. Giles et al. did an excellent survey on more than 40.000 Medicare beneficiaries after open repair or EVAR in the United States. Readmissions and reinterventions were 7.0 per 100 person-years after open repair. Laparotomy-related reinterventions had a considerably high 30-day mortality rate of 8.5% (Giles et al. 2011). This illustrates the major impact on health caused by laparotomy for open aortic repair.

2.2.1 Incisional hernia

Incisional hernia is an often underestimated complication after open abdominal aortic aneurysm repair

Incidences as high as 90% after midline laparotomy are reported in the literature after surgery for aneurysm (Fassiadis et al., 2005). This was with routine use of ultrasound and not all hernia demanded treatment. Others report lower incidence: 30% (Holland et al., 1996). The cause of high incidence of hernia after aneurysm surgery is thought to be a consequence of a connective tissue disorder. Transverse incisions have shown fewer hernias and may have the same exposure of the aorta (Fassiadis et al., 2005). A recent report from the UK showed the feasibility of a minilaparotomy for open aortic aneurysm repair (Hafez et al., 2011). They performed a 10 cm transverse supraumbilical laparotomy in 83 non-obese patients with AAA and reported a low mortality rate of 2.4% and only 2 incisional hernias. This excellent result is most likely a single surgeon experience. Besides that, the technique required 3 years to develop. A recent trial showed less incisional hernia with primary mesh closure of laparotomy after elective AAA repair (Bevis et al., 2010). In our experience, midline laparotomy is still the standard approach in open aneurysm repair. Especially in the setting of a vascular teaching hospital, we need maximum exposure of the aorta. Further research is required to determine the overall applicability of different techniques to minimize the morbidity of incisional hernia.

2.2.2 Small bowel obstruction

After laparotomy, incidence of small bowel obstruction (SBO) is estimated at 5-30%, depending on type of surgery. (Barmparas et al. 2010) After aortic surgery the literature is scarce and major trials do not report readmissions for SBO or reoperations. SBO in the immediate postoperative phase relatively infrequent after aortic surgery. An incidence of 2.6% is mentioned with a reoperation rate of 41%. (Siporin et al. 1993). De Bruin et al. described 2 immediate and 1 late bowel obstruction after open aneurysm repair (De Bruin et al., 2010). According to Crowson et al. the overall rate of gastrointestinal complications after infrarenal aortic aneurysm repair is 6.6%. In their series of 472 aortic aneurysm repairs, a small bowel obstruction developed after surgery in only two patients, caused by adherence to the aneurysmal sac and a deep tension suture having pierced the small bowel, respectively. (Crowson et al., 1984). More long-term data are not available for SBO after aortic surgery.

An unusual cause of SBO is duodenal obstruction, which has been described in the literature in case reports. This can be caused by the postoperative development of a retroperitoneal hematoma after aneurysm repair. (Tessier et al., 2003; Rijken & Butzelaer, 1996)

2.2.3 Sexual dysfunction

In the first edition of Rutherford's Vascular Surgery, the potential impact of aortic surgery on postoperative sexual function was not even mentioned. Nowadays, we recognize the importance of preserving blood flow to the internal iliac arteries and avoiding injury to the autonomic nerves flanking the aortoiliac bifurcation. Beyond these basic principles, however, we remain rather ignorant of the impact of vascular surgery on sexual function. Erectile dysfunction is frequently reported after open aneurysm repair, in tube and bifurcated grafts up to 83%. Obtaining meaningful data on this subject is difficult because of poor response rates to questionnaires (Lee et al., 2000). A prospective study from Netherlands showed that both EVAR and open elective AAA repair have an impact on sexual function in the early postoperative period but the recovery to the preoperative level was faster with EVAR than after OR (Prinssen et al., 2004).

2.2.4 Buttock claudication

Buttock claudication has been warned for when both internal iliacs are interrupted in open as well as endovascular aneurysm repair. A study by Mehta described the single center experience of 48 cases with both internal iliacs sacrificed during open repair or EVAR. Forty-one percent developed buttock claudication but after one year, only 14% still complained. The article describes high ligation of the internal iliac and preservation of side branches of external iliac and femoral vessels as well as systemic heparinisation as possible contributors to their good results in this controversial technique. (Mehta et al., 2004)

2.3 Long term survival

Survival after AAA repair is largely dependent on co morbidities. After open surgery, 6-year survival is approximately 70%. Not surprisingly, systemic complications of atherosclerosis cause most late deaths after AAA repair. Myocardial infarction, cerebrovascular events en other aneurysms are the major causes of death. Vascular complications account for two thirds of late deaths following aneurysm repair. Cancer is the second cause of late mortality (10-15%), followed by pulmonary disease. In 1985, Plate et al. followed up 1,112 patients who underwent abdominal aortic aneurysm repair. Follow-up, ranging from six to 12 years, was complete in 1,087 patients (97.7%). The most frequent cause of late deaths was coronary artery disease (45.6%) and significant morbidity related to the peripheral vascular system had developed in 94 patients, and led to 8.4% (48 patients) of all late deaths (Plate et al., 1985).

3. Late complications after endovascular aneurysm repair

With the start of endovascular repair, initiated with the fist report by Parodi in 1991, a new era of aneurysm repair had started (Parodi et al.,1991). The first randomized trials comparing endovascular with open aneurysm repair have not been published until 2004. Two recently published randomized trials comparing the effectiveness of open surgical and endovascular repair for the treatment of abdominal aortic aneurysms have demonstrated a significantly lower mortality rate for patients undergoing EVAR. However, the initial short-term survival advantage for patients undergoing EVAR was lost after long-term follow-up. A significant proportion of the late deaths of patients undergoing EVAR were due to aneurysm rupture. These concerning findings raise questions about the effectiveness and durability of EVAR to prevent death caused by abdominal aortic aneurysm rupture. (De Bruin et al., 2010; Greenhalgh et al., 2004)) Late aneurysm-related complications are more frequent after endovascular repair and pose the vascular surgeon for different challenges.

3.1 Infectious complications

Infectious complications are equally frequent after endovascular and open repair, and affects about 1-3% of patients. Management principles are similar to those of any infected prosthesis. However, the treatment depends on the patients' condition and the virulence of the micro-organism. Both open surgical repair with graft removal and non-operative treatment are feasible. Mortality remains very high.

3.1.2 Surgical technique of stent graft removal from the aorta

A specific problem of graft removal is the suprarenal fixation of stents at the renal arteries.
Our group reported a new method of removing an infected endoprosthesis from the abdominal aorta using a wire cutter. Three months after placement of an endovascular abdominal endoprosthesis for a ruptured aneurysm, the patient returned with an infection

of the aortic endoprosthesis. The endoprosthesis had been fixed with barbs and hooks above the renal arteries and was surgically explanted by using a wire cutter to cut the hooks. The bare suprarenal stent was left in place. The patient was discharged one month after stent removal, and was treated with oral antibiotics for another ten weeks. At one year follow-up the patient showed no clinical, biochemical, or radiological signs of infection. A Zenith endoprosthesis requires a dangerous procedure because the hooks of the bare stent are engaged into the supra-renal aorta. This case report documented a new technique to safely remove an infected endoprosthesis with the help of a wire cutter (Dolmans et al. 2009). Another group from the Netherlands described a different technique using the barrel of a syringe with the top end removed to slide over the endoprosthesis cranially to withdraw the hooks from the aortic wall (Koning et al. 2006).

3.2 Device related complications

3.2.1 Endoleak

Up to 23-36% patients require a reintervention after endovascular repair. This is most frequently because of an endoleak. Endoleak is defined as persistent blood flow outside the lumen of the endoluminal graft but within the aneurysm sac, as determined by an imaging study. Endoleaks will not be discussed here, as they are dealt with in another chapter.

3.2.2 Stent migration, kinking and occlusion

Long-term results of EVAR are now being published more and more. Long term results of randomised trials show 1-10% graft problems such as kinking, migration and occlusion after 6 years of follow up (De Bruin et al. 2010, Greenhalgh et al. 2010). A large study of secondary procedures after EVAR described 13.6 % migration and 7.4% limb occlusion (Mehta et al., 2010). Despite technical improvement in endovascular devices, device failures continue to occur in recent studies.

Waasdorp et al. studied the importance of iliac fixation to secure endograft fixation (Waasdorp et al. 2009). 154 Talent™ stent grafts were followed up with serial CT imaging. Proximal endograft migration occurred in 32 of 154 patients (21%) at a follow-up duration of 32; 13 migrations required treatment (8%). Migration was more frequent in patients treated with aorto-uniiliac devices than bifurcation devices. The migrator group had significantly shorter proximal and distal endograft fixation lengths. By multivariate regression analysis, proximal and distal endograft fixations were significant predictors for endograft migration at follow-up.

In our clinic we observed that in 66 Zenith® (COOK MEDICAL INC.,Bloomington, IN, USA) stentgrafts, nine out of 12 complications which required reintervention were due to problems with one of the leg extensions. This was the first study that clearly specified the percentage of problems with leg extensions in EVAR with one specific device (75%). We advise that during placement of a Zenith endovascular graft, extra attention should be paid to optimal placement of the leg extensions (Bindsbergen van et al., 2008).

3.2.3 Aneurysm rupture after EVAR

Rupture after EVAR is the ultimate failure of this treatment. Giles et al. reported 0.13 ruptures per 100 person-years after EVAR versus 0.01 after open repair (Giles et al., 2011). Mehta described 8.6% aneurysm rupture after EVAR with a mean follow up of 29 months (Mehta et al. 2010). Half of these ruptures were treated endovascular and half with open repair. Mortality was 7% vs. 25% respectively without statistical significance. Some have proposed that previous EVAR protects your patient from hemodynamic instability and improves survival in case of rupture. 30-day mortality was 28.5 % in previously treated patients and 38.7% in primary ruptures. This was not a significant difference (Coppi et al., 2009). Others claim the opposite: more mortality after previous EVAR. Kelso et al. reported 19% mortality and 9% excluding ruptures (Kelso et al., 2010). Recently, Schanzer reported an alarming increase in aneurysm size after EVAR in 40% of cases (Schanzer et al., 2011). This percentage increased in time during the study period (1999-2008). The authors suggested a liberalization of the instructions for use as a possible cause for this increase. Growing aneurysm diameter is sign of incomplete exclusion of the aneurysm and can therefore predict rupture.

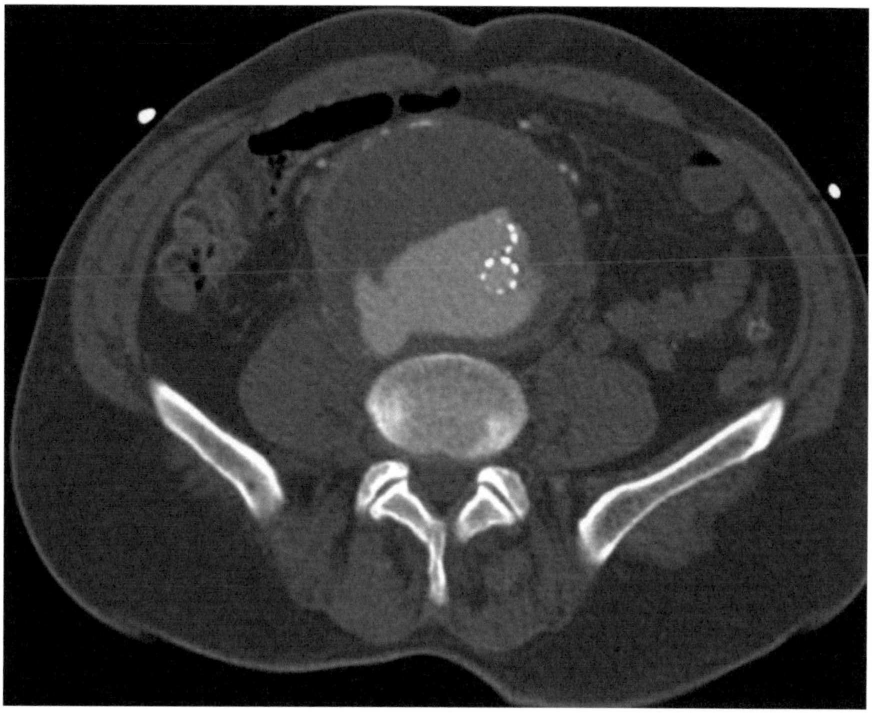

Fig. 3. A symptomatic aortic aneurysm 4 years after placement of uniiliac stent-graft for RAAA. Notice the type 3 endoleak as two parts of the graft are not connected.

In conclusion, EVAR is increasingly popular in current vascular practice, although questions keep rising on the durability of EVAR in the long term. In our practice EVAR will be first choice in most elective AAA patients with favorable anatomy. Young patients (<65 years) will be considered for open repair even with favorable EVAR anatomy. On the other hand, in vascular cripples with unfavorable anatomy, we do go outside de instructions for use of EVAR. Long term results of two European randomized trials have shown no benefit after 2 years and an increase in secondary procedures 4 years after EVAR (De Bruin et al. 2010, Greenhalgh et al., 2010). Therefore, the chances for the vascular surgeon of having to perform reoperative surgery on previously treated aneurysms, open or endovascular, will increase in the future.

3.3 Follow-up after endovascular repair

As shown in the previous paragraph, follow-up is necessary after endovascular aneurysm repair to detect complications before rupture. The optimal follow-up regimen is under debate in the literature, as little is known about how current endovascular grafts will perform in the future. Different imaging studies are being used. CT angiography is the gold standard, sometimes combined with plain abdominal x-ray. Because of increasing awareness of the disadvantages of CT scanning, other follow-up regimens are currently under study. Abdominal duplex ultrasound scanning (plain or contrast-enhanced), combined with plain abdominal x-ray are a reasonable alternative. Aneurysm size, endoleak type I and III can be detected with duplex. Despite its low positive predictive value, Manning et al. found duplex ultrasound to be a sensitive test for the detection of clinically significant endoleaks. Given concerns about cumulative radiation exposure and cost the authors see a future for ultrasound in follow-up of stable aneurysms after EVAR.

There is currently no consensus on the optimal follow up regimen. In our clinic, we still perform CT scanning combined with plain abdominal x-ray. In the future, duplex scanning may play a role in follow up.

4. Conclusion

This overview shows that late complications after open aortic aneurysm repair are an important health issue. Especially considering the fact that elective aneurysm repair is a procedure performed on asymptomatic patients. Late complications after open repair should not be underestimated, in light of the high mortality of re-interventions. Endovascular solutions for late complications of open repair such as pseudoaneurysm are promising. On the other hand, major concerns about the durability of EVAR appeared in recent studies. This indicates that there is still a role for open repair. However, we believe that endovascular repair will expand even more in the near future. With an ageing population and increasing rates of endovascular repair, the vascular surgeon will probably encounter more late endovascular complications. The challenge for the current vascular surgeon lies in the prevention and detection of these complications. Familiarity with both open and endovascular techniques give the future vascular surgeon the possibility to manage these complications adequately.

5. References

Allen, R., Schneider, J. & Longenecker, L. (1993). Paraanastomotic aneurysms of the abdominal aorta, *Journal of Vascular Surgery*. Vol. 18, No. 3, (September 1993), pp. 424-432

Bandyk, D. (2002). Antibiotics—Why so many and when should we use them? *Seminars in Vascular Surgery*, Vol. 15, No. 4, (December 2002), pp. 268-274

Barmparas, G., Branco, B. & Schnüriger, B. (2010). The Incidence and Risk Factors of Post-Laparotomy Adhesive Small Bowel Obstruction. *Journal of Gastrointestinal Surgery*, Vol.14, No. 10, (October 2010), pp. 1619-1628

Bergqvist, D., Alm, A. & Claes, G. (1987). Secondary aortoenteric fistulas - an analysis of 42 cases. *European Journal of Vascular Surgery*, Vol. 1, No. 1, (February 1987), pp. 11-18

Bevis P., Windhaber, R. & Lear, P. (2010). Randomized clinical trial of mesh *versus* sutured wound closure after open abdominal aortic aneurysm surgery. *British Journal of Surgery*, Vol. 97, No. 10, (October 2010), pp. 1497-1502

Biancari F., Ylonen, K. & Anttila, V. (2002). Durability of open repair of infrarenal abdominal aortic aneurysm: a 15-year follow-up study. *Journal of Vascular Surgery*, Vol. 35, No. 1, (January 2002), pp. 87-93

Bindsbergen van, L., Dolmans, D. & Van der Laan, L. (2008) Endovascular aneurysm repair with Zenith graft. Complications caused by leg extensions. *Journal of Cardiovascular Surgery (Torino)*, Vol. 49, No. 3, pp. 311-316

Blaisdell, F., Hall, A. & Lim, R. (1970). Aorto-iliac arterial substitution utilizing subcutaneous grafts. *Annals of surgery*, Vol. 172, No. 5, (November 1970), pp. 775-80.

Bruggink, J., Glaudemans, A. & Saleem, B. (2010). Accuracy of FDG-PET-CT in the diagnostic work-up of vascular prosthetic graft infection. *European Journal of Vascular and Endovascular Surgery*, Vol. 40 Pp. 348-354.

Calligaro, K., Veith, F. & Yuan, J. Intra-abdominal aortic graft infection: complete or partial graft preservation in patients at very high risk. *Journal of Vascular Surgery*, Vol. 38, No. 6, (December 2003), pp. 1199-1205

Chaikof, E., Blankensteijn J. & Harris, H. for the Ad Hoc Committee for Standardized Reporting Practices in Vascular Surgery of The Society for Vascular Surgery/American Association for Vascular Surgery. (2002). Reporting standards for endovascular aortic aneurysm repair. *Journal of Vascular Surgery*, Vol. 35, No. 5, (May 2002), pp. 148-60

Clagett, G., Valentine R. & Hagino R. (2007). Autogenous aortoiliac/femoral reconstruction from superficial femoral-popliteal veins: feasibility and durability. *Journal of Vascular Surgery*, Vol. 25, No. 2, (February 1997), pp. 255-270

Conrad, M., Crawford, R.& Pedraza, J. (2007). Long-term durability of open abdominal aortic aneurysm repair *Journal of Vascular Surgery*, Vol. 46, No. 4, (October 2007), pp. 669-675

Coppi, G., Gennai, S. & Saitta, G. (2009). Treatment of ruptured abdominal aortic aneurysm after endovascular abdominal aortic repair: A comparison with patients without prior treatment *Journal of Vascular Surgery*, Vol. 49, No. 3. (March 2009), pp. 582-588

Cosford, P. & Leng, G. (2007). Screening for abdominal aortic aneurysm. *Cochrane Database Systematic Review*, Vol. 18, No. 2, (April 2007), D002945

Creech O. (1966). Endo-aneurysmorrhaphy and treatment of aortic aneurysm. *Annals of Surgery* Vol. 164, No. 6, (December 1966), pp. 935-946

Crowson, M., Fielding, J. & Black, J. (1984). Acute gastrointestinal complications of infrarenal aortic aneurysm repair. *British Journal of Surgery*, Vol. 71, No. 11, (November 1984), pp. 825-828

De Bruin J., Baas, A. & Buth, J. (2010). Long-term outcome of open or endovascular repair of abdominal aortic aneurysm. *New England Journal of Medicine, Vol.* 362, No. 20, (May 2010) pp. 1881-1889

Dolmans D., Ho G. & Van Der Laan L. (2009). Surgical removal of an infected aortic endoprosthesis using a wire cutter. *Journal of Cardiovascular Surgery (Torino), Vol.* 50, No.3, (June 2009), pp. 411-414

Dubost C, Allary, M. & Oeconomos, N. (1952). Resection of an aneurysm of the abdominal aorta: reestablishment of the continuity by a preserved human arterial graft, with result after five months. *AMA Archives of Surgery,* Vol. 64, No. 3, (March 1952), pp. 405-8

Edwards, J., Teefey, S. & Zierler, R. (1992). Intraabdominal paraanastomotic aneurysms after aortic bypass grafting. *Journal of Vascular Surgery,* Vol. 15, No. 2, (February 1992), pp. 344-350

Greenhalgh, R., Brown, L. & Kwong, G. EVAR Trial Participants. (2004). Comparison of endovascular aneurysm repair with open repair in patients with abdominal aortic aneurysm (EVAR trial 1), 30-day operative mortality results: randomised controlled trial. *The Lancet,* Vol. 364, No. 9437, (September 2004), pp. 843-848

Greenhalgh, R., Brown, L. & Powell, J. The United Kingdom EVAR Trial Investigators. (2010). Endovascular versus open repair of abdominal aortic aneurysm. *The New England Journal of Medicine,* Vol. 362, No. 20 (May 2010), pp. 1863-1871

Fassiadis, N., Roidl, M. & Andrews, S. (2005). Randomized clinical trial of vertical or transverse laparotomy for abdominal aortic aneurysm repair. *British Journal Surgery,* Vol. 92, No. 10, (October 2005), pp. 1208-11

Giles, K., Landon, B & Cotterill, P. (2011). Thirty-day mortality and late survival with reinterventions and readmissions after open and endovascular aortic aneurysm repair in Medicare beneficiaries. *Journal of Vascular Surgery,* Vol. 53, No. 1, (January 2011), pp. 6-13

Sfyroeras, G., Lioupis G. & Bessias, N. (2008). Endovascular Treatment of a Ruptured Para-Anastomotic Aneurysm of the Abdominal Aorta. *Cardiovascular Intervention Radiology,* Vol. 31, Suppl. 2, (July 2008) pp. S79–S83

Hafez, H. Makhosini, M. & Abbassi-Ghaddi, N. (2011). Transverse minilaparotomy for open abdominal aortic aneurysm repair. *Journal of Vascular Surgery,* Vol. 53, No. 6, (June 2011), pp. 1514-1519

Hallett, J., Marshall, D. & Petterson T. (1997). Graft-related complications after abdominal aortic aneurysm repair: reassurance from a 36-year population-based experience. *Journal of Vascular Surgery,* Vol. 25, No. 2, (February 1997), pp. 277-284, discussion 285-286

Hertzer, N., Mascha, E. & Karafa, M. (2002). Open infrarenal abdominal aortic aneurysm repair: the Cleveland Clinic experience from 1989 to 1998. *Journal of Vascular Surgery,* Vol. 35, No. 6, (June 2002), pp. 1145-1154

Herwaarden van, J., Waasdorp, E. & Bendermacher, B. (2004). Endovascular Repair of Paraanastomotic Aneurysms after Previous Open Aortic Prosthetic Reconstruction. *Annals of Vascular Surgery,* Vol. 18, No. 3, (May 2004), pp. 280-286

Holland, A., Castleden, W. & Norman, P. (1996). Incisional hernias are more common in aneurysmal disease. *European Journal of Vascular and Endovascular Surgery,* Vol. 12, No. 2, (August 1996), pp. 196-200

Kakkos, S., Antoniadis, P. & Klonaris, C. (2011). Open or endovascular repair of aortoenteric fistulas? A multicentre comparative study. *European Journal of Vascular and Endovascular Surgery,* Vol. 41, No. 5, (May 2011), pp. 625-634

Kelso, R., Lyden, S. & Butler, B. (2009). Late conversion of aortic stent grafts. *Journal of Vascular Surgery,*Vol. 49, No. 3 (March 2009), pp. 589-595

Koning, O., Hinnen, J-W. & van Baalen, J. (2006). Technique for safe removal of an aortic endograft with suprarenal fixation. *Journal of Vascular Surgery* , Vol 43, No. 4, (April 2006), pp. 855-857

Kuestner, L., Reilly, L., & Jicha, D. (1995). Secondary aortoenteric fistula: contemporary outcome with use of extraanatomic bypass and infected graft excision. *Journal of Vascular Surgery*, Vol. 21, No. 2, (February 1995), pp. 184-195, discussion 195-196

Lee, E., Kor, D. & Kuskowski, M. (2000). Incidence of Erectile Dysfunction after Open Abdominal Aortic Aneurysm Repair, *Annals of Vascular Surgery,* Vol. 14, No. 1, (January 2000), pp. 13-19

Manning, B., O'Neill, S. & Haider, S. (2009). Duplex ultrasound in aneurysm surveillance following endovascular aneurysm repair: a comparison with computed tomography aortography. *Journal of Vascular Surgery*, Vol. 49, No. 1, (January 2009), pp. 60-65

Mehta, M., Veith, F., & Darling C. (2004). Effects of bilateral hypogastric artery interruption during endovascular and open aortoiliac aneurysm repair. Journal of Vascular Surgery, Vol. 40, No. 4, (October 2004), pp. 698-702

Mehta, M., Sternbach, Y. & Taggert, J. (2010). Long-term outcomes of secondary procedures after endovascular aneurysm repair. Journal of Vascular Surgery, Vol. 52, No. 6, (December 2010), pp. 1442-1448

Menke, V., Castenmiller, P. & Van der Laan, L. (2010). Stent Grafting a Ruptured Para-anastomotic Iliac Aneurysm. *Vascular and Endovascular Surgery,* Vol. 44, No. 6, (Augustus 2006), pp. 479-482

Mulder, E.; van Bockel, J. & Maas, J. (1998). Morbidity and mortality of reconstructive surgery of noninfected false aneurysms detected long after aortic prosthetic reconstruction. *Archives of Surgery, Vol.* 133, No. 1, pp. (January 1998), pp. 45-49

Mussa, F., Hedayati, N. & Zhou, W. (2007). Prevention and treatment of aortic graft infection. *Expert Review of Anti-Infective Therapy*, Vol. 5, No. 2, (April 2007), pp. 305-315

Nevelsteen, A., Lacroix, H. & Suy, R. (1995). Autogenous reconstruction with the lower extremity deep veins: an alternative treatment of prosthetic infection after reconstruction surgery for aortoiliac disease. *Journal of Vascular Surgery* Vol. 22, No. 2, (August 1995), pp. 129-34

Parodi, J., Palmaz, J. & Barone, H. (1991). Transfemoral intraluminal graft implantation for abdominal aortic aneurysm. *Annals of Vascular Surgery,* Vol. 5, No. 6, (November 1991), pp. 491-499

Prinssen, M., Buskens, E. & Nolthenius, R. (2004). Sexual dysfunction after conventional and endovascular

AAA repair: Results of the DREAM trial. *Journal of Endovascular Therapy,* Vol. 11, pp.613-20.

Prinssen, M., Verhoeven E. & Buth J. (2004). A randomized trial comparing conventional and endovascular repair of abdominal aortic aneurysms. *The New England Journal of Medicine*, Vol. 351, No. 16, (October 2004), pp. 1607-1618

Reilly, M., Stoney, R. & Goldstone, J. (1987). Improved management of aortic graft infection: the influence of operation sequence and staging. *Journal of Vascular Surgery*, Vol. 5, No. 3 (March 1987), pp. 421-431

Schanzer, A., Greenberg, R. & Hevelone, N. (2011). Predictors of abdominal aortic aneurysm sac enlargement after endovascular repair, *Circulation*, Vol. 123, (April 2011), E-pub ahead of print may 2011

Schrijver, A., Reijnen, M. & van Oostayen, J. (2011). Initial Results of Catheter-Directed Ultrasound-Accelerated Thrombolysis for Thromboembolic Obstructions of the

Aortofemoral Arteries: A Feasibility Study. *Cardiovascular Intervention Radiology*. (May 2011) [Epub ahead of print]

Seeger, J., Pretus, H.& Welborn, M. (2000). Long-term outcome after treatment of aortic graft infection with staged extraanatomic bypass grafting and aortic graft removal. *Journal of Vascular Surgery*; Vol. 32, No. 3, (September 2000), pp. 451-461

Siporin, K., Hiatt, K.& Treiman, R. (1993). Small bowel obstruction after abdominal aortic surgery. *The American Surgeon*, Vol. 59, No. 12, (December 1993), pp. 846-849

Tessier, D. & Brophy, C. (2003). Causes, diagnosis, and management of duodenal obstruction after aortic surgery. *Journal of Vascular Surgery*, Vol. 38, No. 1, (July 2003), pp. 186-189

Treiman, G., Weaver, F. & Cossman, D. (1988). Anastomotic false aneurysms of the abdominal aorta and the iliac arteries. *Journal of Vascular Surgery*, Vol. 8, No. 3, (September 1988), pp. 268-273

Waasdorp, E., de Vries, J. & Sterkenburg, A. (2009). The association between iliac fixation and proximal stent-graft migration during EVAR follow-up: mid-term results of 154 Talent devices, *European Journal of Vascular and Endovascular Surgery*, Vol. 37, No. 6, (June 2009), pp. 681-687

Yuan, J., Marin, M. & Veith, F. (2009). Endovascular grafts for noninfected aortoiliac anastomotic aneurysms (1997), *Journal of Vascular Surgery* ,Vol. 26, No. 2, (June 2009), pp. 210-221

Zitteren van, M,. Steenhoven van der, T. & Burger, D. (2011). Spiral vein reconstruction of the infected abdominal aorta using the greater saphenous vein: preliminary results of the Tilburg experience, *European Journal of Vascular and Endovascular Surgery*, Vol. 41, No. 5,(May 2011), pp. 637-646. URL: http://www.spiralvein.org

14

Abdominal Aortic Graft Infection

Dimitrios Tsapralis, Anestis Charalampopoulos and Andreas M. Lazaris
Attikon Teaching Hospital, University of Athens
Greece

1. Introduction

Despite the advances in operative techniques and perioperative management of patients suffering from abdominal aortic aneurysms (AAAs) or occlusive aorto-iliac disease, there are many early and late complications related to aortic graft insertion, either in open or endovascular approach, that every vascular surgeon should bear in mind. One of the most dreaded complication is the infection of prosthetic aortic grafts which continues to be problematic despite improvements in biomaterials and fabrication of prosthetics, refinements in implantation techniques, and better understanding of the pathogenesis of graft infections.
This article reviews the epidemiology, pathogenesis, diagnosis, and current state-of -the art management of prosthetic aortic graft infections.

1.1 Incidence and risk factors

The overall incidence of aortic graft infection has probably changed little in the past two decades despite an improved understanding of graft infections and more specified efforts at prevention (Perera et al., 2006). The true incidence of graft infections is difficult to establish and depends on how one defines the problem (graft infection or graft exposure in a nonhealing wound), the graft material (autogenous vein, Dacron, polytetrafluoroethylene [PTFE]), the duration of follow-up, and other factors (Chiesa et al., 2002; Perera et al., 2006). However, most recent series document an incidence ranging from just under 1% to as high as 6%, with an overall incidence of approximately 4% (Bisdas et al., 2010; FitzGerald et al., 2005). It is estimated that the cost of caring for a patient with an infected vascular graft currently averages $40,000 (Ali et al., 2009).
Both patient variables and technical factors predispose to the development of vascular graft infections. Patient factors include disease processes such as diabetes mellitus, obesity, uremia, malnutrition, and immunosuppressive states (Yeager et al., 1992). Ulceration or infection in an extremity distal to a graft and emergency procedures are also known to increase infectious risks (Perera et al., 2006). Wound healing complications, such as cellulitis, seroma, lymphocele, hematoma, or skin necrosis, further contribute to graft infections (Gutowski, 1998). Reoperation in the early postoperative period for thrombosis or bleeding is an additional predisposing factor. Special emphasis should be placed to the higher incidence of infection accompanied the implementation of aortofemoral bypass grafts compared to aortoiliac grafts, since the groin area is frequently contaminated and prone to wound complications (Yeager et al., 1992).

1.2 Pathogenesis

The vast majority of prosthetic aortic graft infections occur as a result of bacterial contamination of the perigraft space around the time of original graft placement. Under these circumstances, endogenous skin flora constitutes the causative organisms of such infections. Most patients who undergo arterial revascularization or aneurysm repair have significant numbers of mucin-producing coagulase-negative staphylococci on their skin, and at least 15% have methicillin-resistant (MRSA) strains preoperatively (Kieffer et al., 2001). Incomplete sterilization of instruments or grafts rarely does play a role in the incidence of aortic graft infections, but breaks in sterile technique, particularly during emergency procedures, are more common (Valentine, 2001). Graft seeding by bacteria from transected lymphatics in the presence of distal extremity infections may be important. Moreover, microorganisms from the native arterial thrombus or arteriosclerotic plaque may contaminate grafts. Careful culturing of the arterial wall during elective procedures demonstrates the presence of microorganisms in about 40% of specimens (Farkas et al., 1993; Hsu et al., 2004). Other studies suggest that aortic graft infections increase from 2% to approximately 10% if arterial wall cultures are positive, but some authors have concluded that bacteria in aneurysm contents is not linked to subsequent graft infections (Macbeth et al., 1984). Concomitant contaminated procedures increase the likelihood of prosthetic infection and should be avoided whenever possible. Lengthy procedures and those with larger blood loss are associated with higher infection rates (Yeager et al., 1992).

Irrespective of the origin or the type of offending microorganism, the pathogenetic mechanism of the ensuing infection represents a common denominator. During the early postoperative period, the fluid filled (blood, serum, lymph) perigraft environment is poorly perfused and relatively isolated from the natural host defenses (Chiesa et al., 2002). These poorly vascularized, perigraft fluid collections serve as a receprive medium for bacteria, enabling their survival and proliferation. Any early contamination of the perigraft space with even low numbers of bacteria, can lead to eventual prosthetic graft infection. Without early contamination, however, the prosthetic material becomes incorporated into surrounding, vascularized tissues, which functionally obliterates the perigraft space and, after several months, appears to render the graft more resistant to infection.

As described below in the section of clinical presentation, the prosthetic vascular graft infections are classified as early or late depending on presentation before or after four months from the time of surgical implantation. Even when considering the pathogenesis of late graft infections, the majority of them are caused by graft contamination at the time of implantation with indolent disease progression, in a manner identical to that mentioned previously in detail. Nevertheless, other mechanisms unique in this subgroup of patients with late presentation, comprise transient bacteremia and mechanical erosion of the graft into surrounding tissues (Kibria et al., 2010; Lazaris et al., 2009). Erosion into the urinary or gastrointestinal tracts or through the skin occurs in 1% to 3% of patients. Graft-enteric fistula complicates 0,6% to 2,3% of cases of aortic graft placement (Koshy et al., 2010). Transient bacteremia is presumed to be an occasional mechanism for late graft infections.

1.3 Microbiology

Staphylococcus species are the most common causative organism of aortic graft infections (Kaebnick et al., 1987; Sharp et al., 1994). This fact is consistent with our understanding that the pathogenesis of prosthetic graft infection is related to bacterial contamination at the time of graft placement. Staphylococcus epidermidis is the slow-growing, slim-producing organism classically causing late, indolent graft infection. The more virulent Staphylococcus aureus typically causes early graft infection and frequently is associated with overt signs of sepsis. It is estimated that Staphylococcus aureus accounts for approximately 25% to 50% of graft infections (FitzGerald et al., 2005). Methicillin-resistant (MRSA) strains of Staphylococcus aureus are increasingly common in early infections, and gram-negative bacilli, such as Enterobacter, Klebsiella, Escherichia coli, Proteus, and Pseudomonas, have also been slowly increasing in frequency (Kitamura et al., 2005).

For all organisms, bacterial adherence to the prosthetic graft is the initial event in the process of graft infection. Adherence is dependent on physical characteristics of the graft, such as pore size and surface are, and upon chemical properties, such as hydrophobicity (O'Brien & Colin, 1992). The production of an extracellular glycocalyx (mucin, slime) by staphylococci promotes adherence to biomaterials and provides protection against host defenses. This biofilm decreases antibiotic penetration and impairs phagocyte and antibody functions but will stimulate a chronic inflammatory process around an infected prosthesis. Organisms that produce a biofilm are more difficult to culture from an infected graft. Proteases produced by gram-negative organisms contribute to the higher rates of vessel wall necrosis, anastomotic disruption, and pseudoaneurysm formation with infectionfrom these bacteria (Kitamura et al., 2005; O'Brien & Colin, 1992). Finally, it is important for every vascular surgeon to bear in mind that, in contrast to primary aortic infections, Salmonella almost never is the causative organism for prosthetic graft infection.

1.4 Prevention

As indicated above, the preponderance of evidence suggests that in the majority of cases bacterial seeding of the conduit at the time of implantation leads the way to the development of postoperative graft infection whenever such an infection manifests. Based on this observation, it seems safe to conclude that careful observation of fundamental principles of patient management during that critical perioperative period can minimize the incidence of this detrimental complication. At first, prophylactic antibiotics should be administered intravenously before the skin incision. Although there is no compelling evidence that antibiotic use prevents frank infection, there is good evidence that the incidence of surgical site infection is reduced, and wound infection is an important contributor to graft infection in many cases (Kayser et al., 1978). The duration of antibiotic therapy postoperatively is controversial. Although there is no strong support for such policy, it is reasonable to continue antibiotics for 24 hours postoperatively (Barie & Eachempati, 2005). Because skin flora is an important source of graft contamination, the operative field should be widely cleansed with povidone-iodine solution, and ischemic or ulcerative lesions in the limbs should be isolated (Barie & Eachempati, 2005; Mangram et al., 1999). Lymphatics are another potential route of infection, and thus lymphatic tissue should be ligated and sharply divided. Last, the duration of hospitalization during the primary aortic graft insertion might interfere with the development of a graft infection at a later stage. Patients who are hospitalized for a prolonged time before operative intervention undergo an alteration in their microbial flora and may be at an increased risk of developing graft infection secondary to colonization with resistant organism (Angle et al, 2002)..

Thorough investigation has been centered for many years around the potential benefit of antibiotic-bonded Dacron and PTFE grafts to resist infection (O'Connor et al., 2006; Wilson,

2001). Most work has focused on rifampin-bonded grafts, which have been shown to elute the antibiotic at the implantation site for only a few days, possibly limiting their efficacy in this regard (Bandyk et al., 2001). Although there is some evidence that they are effective against Staphyococcus epidermidis and Staphylococcus aureus, they may have more limited efficacy against gram-negative organisms and MRSA Staphylococcus species.

1.5 Clinical presentation and classification

Patients with aortic prosthetic graft infection may present early (within 4 months) or late (after 4 months) following original graft placement (Orton et al., 2000). Szilagyi classified early infections of vascular prostheses into three grades according to the depth of wound involvement as assessed by clinical observation and wound exploration (Szilagyi et al., 1972). Grade I infections involve only the skin (celullitis); Grade II involve the subcutaneous tissue; and Grade III involve the prosthesis. Samson has modified the widely used classification system of extracavitary vascular graft infections established by Szilagyi (Samson, 1988). These modifications allow for more precise prognostication and directed treatment. Early graft infections, presented within the first 4 months after implantation, are typically caused by Staphylococcus aureus and gram-negative bacilli, and are accompanied by systemic signs of infection, including malaise, fever, and leukocytosis. Wound infections, anastomotic disruptions with bleeding, and tender groin masses are also common presenting signs (Valentine, 2001). Graft thrombosis, physical evidence of pseudoaneurysm, and distal embolization may also occur. Acute infection of intraabdominal aortic graft is rare but should be suspected when fever, leukocytosis, persistent adynamic ileus, and abdominal tenderness are present in the perioperative period without other evident etiologies.

Most aortic graft infections relate to aortobifemoral grafts and involve one or both the inguinal regions. In such cases the manifestation of infection is often obvious and consists in development of erythema overlying the graft, a palpable fluid collection, a draining sinus tract, or a pseudoaneurysm. The presence of any of the above signs revealed during physical examination should be assumed to be indicative of graft infection (Bandyk & Esses, 1994).

Conversely, the presentation of late-onset infections (presented after the first 4 months after implantation) tends to be subtle, without any specific signs or symptoms. Absence of fever is not uncommon. These patients are more likely to present with complications of aortic graft infection, such as pseudoaneurysm, sepsis or gastrointestinal bleeding as a result of erosion of the graft into the gastrointestinal tract, and hydronephrosis (Bandyk & Esses, 1994). Aortoenteric fistula may involve any segment of the large or small bowel, but the third and fourth portions of duodenum are the most common sites. In some instances, the anastomosis between the graft and the aorta remains intact, and erosion of the intact graft into the intestine causes mucosal bleeding. Alternatively, the anastomosis may communicate directly with the intestinal lumen, as a result of a pseudoaneurysm. A "herald bleed" from mucosal erosion usually precedes massive gastrointestinal bleeding from an established aortoenteric fistula (Montgomery & Wilson, 1996).

1.6 Diagnosis

The diagnosis of aortic graft infections is usually made on the ground of clinical findings, supported by radiological and microbiological investigations (FitzGerald et al., 2005). When a vascular surgeon raises the possibility of prosthetic graft infection, there are numerous modalities in his/her armamentarium that he/she has to recourse to in order to confirm or exclude that possibility. Unfortunately, under some circumstances, no laboratory or imaging modality can completely exclude the likelihood of aortic graft infection, and operative exploration is necessary to establish its diagnosis. In cases when signs of infection are evident in the inguinal region, duplex ultrasonography is often considered the best initial screening test. Features such as perigraft fluid or anastomotic pseudoaneurysm found at ultrasound, represent supportive evidence to the clinical suspicion. In addition, duplex ultrasound evaluates the patency of peripheral vessels of the afflicted extremity, playing a central role in drawing a potential surgical plan (Calligaro & Feith, 1991). It is of less benefit for diagnosis of intraabdominal graft infections due to the deep location of such grafts and the difficulty in discrimination of subtle findings.

Computed tomography (CT) scan is the most commonly performed study and the standard against which all other imaging modalities are compared (Mark et al., 1982). Both intravenous and oral contrast media are necessary to identify the graft lumen and the relationship of the prosthesis to adjacent structures (FitzGerald et al., 2005). CT scan has sensitivity more than 95% and specificity in the range of 85% when the criteria of perigraft fluid, perigraft soft tissue attenuation, ectopic gas, pseudoaneurysm, or focal bowel wall thickening are used (Balink & Reijnen, 2007). Importantly, CT scan provides an assessment of the entire graft in contrast to duplex ultrasound as mentioned before. In the early postoperative period, it may be difficult to distinguish graft infection from normal postoperative changes even with CT scan. Perigraft air is not common beyond 1 week after operation, but it is not pathognomonic of graft infection until 4-7 weeks after surgery (Qvarfordt et al., 1985; Soetevent et al., 2004). Similarly, perigraft fluid that persists beyond 4 months postoperatively is highly suspicious for the presence of infection (Qvarfordt et al., 1985). In the initial 4 months after surgery, perigraft fluid may be present without infection, and CT-guided aspiration may assist with definitive diagnosis when clinical circumstances raise such a possibility.

Magnetic resonance imaging (MRI) has a somewhat higher accuracy for diagnosis of intraabdominal graft infections than CT scan because of its superiority for discrimination of tissue planes, particularly in the retroperitoneum (Olofsson et al., 1988). Hence, it is quite sensitive in the detection of small amounts of perigraft fluid, but differentiation between gas in the perigraft space and calcifications in the native arterial wall may be difficult (FitzGerald et al., 2005). Owing to signal characteristics on T-1 and T-2 weighted images, MRI permits differentiation of perigraft fluid and inflammatory changes of surrounding structures from acute and chronic hematoma. However, MRI does not allow distinction between the various types of nonhemorrhagic fluid (infected vs. sterile) (Olofsson et al., 1988). Compared with CT, reconstruction of multiple tissue planes is more easily performed, and nephrotoxicity from intravenous agents may be avoided. In conclusion, because of its wide availability, lower cost, and high sensitivity and specificity, CT scan should be considered the standard reference among imaging modalities for the diagnosis of aortic graft infection. Even when graft infection manifests in the groin and documented with the use of duplex ultrasound, it is imperative to complement the work-up of the patient with CT in order to stage accurately the extent of infection and plan the surgical or conservative management.

Radioisotope scans with labeled leukocytes or immunoglobulin (indium or gallium) may confirm the presence of infection and outline its extent. Indium is considered more accurate than gallium due to higher background levels caused by nonspecific intestinal uptake of gallium (Mark et al, 1985). Accuracy rates for indium-labeled leukocyte scans are reported to be 90% to 100% in most studies, but both false-positive and false-negative results may occur. False-positive studies are more common in the first 3-4 months postoperatively, when there is normal inflammation in perigraft region. Correlation of positive findings with anatomic results from CT or MRI scans is useful to minimize false-positive scans. Several modifications of radioisotopic labeling techniques have been used and claimed to supplant CT scan as the first line in the diagnosis of aortic graft infections, but none have achieved this goal despite their promising initial results (Delgado et al., 1999; Mark et al., 1985; Palestro et al., 2001).

Compared with other anatomic imaging studies, arteriography is of limited value for the diagnosis of vascular graft infections because of false-negative results when native vessels are not involved in the infectious process. Arteriography is of assistance when planning reoperation for aortic graft infection because of its assessment of proximal and distal circulations and characterization of graft anastomosis. However, CT angiography or MR angiography have been predominated over arteriography, even in operation planning.

Sinography may demonstrate communication with the prosthetic graft and, thus, definitely confirms the diagnosis. However, a negative study does not preclude the presence of infection.

Gastrointestinal endoscopy should be considered in any patient with a possible gastrointestinal bleeding source after aortic bypass grafting. Endoscopists should be aware that aortoenteric fistula most often occurs in the distal portions of duodenum. The absence of bleeding from other gastrointestinal (GI) sources should prompt a high level of suspicion for the presence of an aortoenteric fistula, even if there is not clear visualization of the graft or ulceration in the duodenum. When other GI sources of bleeding are excluded, surgical exploration and inspection of the duodenum and aortic graft may be the only method to confirm or exclude aortoenteric fistula before the hemodynamic decompensation of the patient takes place.

Apart from imaging modalities, blood cultures have an integral part in the evaluation of such patients, as they guide the antibiotic coverage, either in the form of preoperative preparation of the patient, or in the context of conservative management with preservation of the infected graft.

1.7 Treatment

1.7.1 Goals

In dealing with an infected vascular aortic graft, the primary goal of treatment is to save life and limb. This can be achieved by initial and long-term eradication of the local and systemic septic process and maintenance of normal arterial perfusion to involved tissues. Secondary goals are to minimize morbidity, to restore normal function, and to maintain long-term function without the need for repeated intervention or amputation.

1.7.2 Principles of management

Bunt (Bunt, 2001) has elegantly described 4 principles of management for vascular graft infections. First, excision of the graft as a foreign body potentiating infection. Second, wide and complete debridement of devitalized and infected tissue to provide a clean wound in which healing can occur. Third, establishment of vascular flow to the distal bed. Fourth, institution of intensive and prolonged antibiotic coverage to reduce sepsis and prevent secondary graft infection.

The gold standard for treatment of an infected prosthetic aortic graft remains explantation of the graft and reperfusion of the area by placement of a new graft through an extra-anatomic uninfected route. However, recently it has been recognized that the bacterial characteristics of early versus late abdominal graft infections differ (early graft infections generally associated with more virulent organisms whereas late graft infections with less virulent organisms). Similarly to pathogen factors (type of microorganisms, virulence), the extent of graft infection, and antibiotic susceptibility guide appropriate operative selection. This has led to a plethora of alternative operative and antimicrobial strategies. Route of reconstruction (in situ versus extra-anatomic), timing and sequence of the procedures, type of bypass conduit, and manner of excision (partial versus complete) remain under controversy. Recently, endovascular options have been proposed, enriching the armamentarium of available treatment options, but also complicating the proper decision algorithm. The lack of sufficient Level I evidence data, allow occasionally an ad hoc choice of the proper treatment in each case (Perera et al., 2006).
With few exceptions, the treatment of aortic graft infection is surgical. Definitely, patient hemodynamic stability and antibiotic coverage are essential. Patients with hemodynamic instability secondary to hemorrhage from aortoenteric fistula or ruptured pseudoaneurysms require immediate resuscitation and operation. Limited efforts using the dogma of hypotensive haemostasis in order to stabilize the patient and allow further evaluation and planning may be appropriate. The patient's condition and ability to tolerate a definitive procedure as an emergency must be weighed against the option of a limited initial procedure and subsequent definitive management (staged operation).

1.7.2.1 Antibiotics

When prosthetic graft infection is suspected, empiric agents should be selected based on the presumed organism and expected sensitivities and initiated after appropriate cultures have been taken. For example, an early infection should be treated with agents active against methicillin-resistant staphylococci and gram-negative bacilli. Late infections that are presumed to be caused by coagulase negative staphylococci are treated with vancomycin, with or without rifampin (Perera et al., 2006). Antibiotics should be adjusted once the etiologic microorganism and its sensitivity have been identified. The length of antibiotic coverage is controversial, and recommendations are for a minimum of 2 to 4 weeks of parenteral antibiotics (Perera et al., 2006). Oral antibiotics are typically administered for an additional 1 to 6 months period, but some authors have recommended lifetime administration in cases when preservation of the potentially infected graft is warranted (Barrie & Eachempati, 2005).
There is no consensus on which agents are preferred for initial empiric therapy before adjustments can be made based on culture results. The British Society of Antimicrobial Chemotherapy (BSAC) Steering Group on the treatment of hospital infections has recommended treatment with cefuroxime and metronidazole, with or without amoxicillin, as suitable empirical therapy for early-onset prosthetic vascular graft infections. Ciprofloxacin and clindamycin should be considered as second line treatment in penicillin-allergic patients. However, as S. aureus is the organism most likely to be isolated in early-onset infections and, as methicillin resistance is increasingly common, empirical treatment should include a glycopeptides according to regional epidemiologic data (Darouiche, 1994). With regard to late-onset infections, guidelines recommend that antibiotic treatment be deferred until the infective etiology has been confirmed, except in the critically ill (.

1.7.2.2 Surgery

Succesful surgical treatment of aortic graft infection requires balancing strict adherence to the principles of managing the problem while trying to predict a patients' ability to withstand the proposed operation. Operative strategies include graft excision without revascularization, graft excision with extra-anatomic bypass procedures, and graft excision with in situ reconstruction using a prosthetic conduit, allograft, or autogenous tissue.

The extent of graft involvement should guide the extent and type of the operation, and, thus, should be scrutinized thoroughly. Limited infections may be treated by excision of the involved segment and preservation of the uninvolved, well-incorporated graft. Because graft infection may be more extensive at operation than indicated by preoperative studies, the surgeon should be prepared to change his/her plan according to the intraoperative findings.

As there is no evidence-based support for the efficacy, safety, and appropriateness of the graft salvage approach in the routine management of patients with aortic graft infections, and details of its outcomes come from case reports and series only, the explantation of the graft and vascular reconstruction is still considered the sine qua non for these patients to be cured. All of the reconstructive options are valid and appropriate depending upon patient characteristics, extent and virulence of infection, and severity of underlying vascular disease. It is a mistake to think that a single surgical approach is applicable to all patients with this condition. Knowing the pros and cons of each procedure, the vascular surgeon can tailor the surgical plan to the individualized requirements, and achieve the best outcome possible in each case.

1.7.3 Restoring perfusion in lower limbs

a. No revascularization

Graft excision without revascularization is associated with a 33-36% amputation rate and is rarely performed today (Bunt, 2001). It is usually reserved for patients with aortic graft infections with known thrombosed grafts but yet viable extremities. Often, the original indication for graft placement, as well as whether the graft was placed in an end-to-end or end-to-side manner is a crucial factor in determining the need for distal revascularization. The degree of limb ischemia and presence of collateral circulation are the most important aspects of selecting this option. For example, patients having grafts placed for occlusive disease with rest pain or tissue loss are more likely to need a bypass to restore blood to the distal bed. On the contrary, patients that had an aortic graft implantation for purely aneurysmal disease or claudication may not necessarily require a lower limbs revascularization procedure. Also, grafts having end-to-side configuration are more likely to have native collateral circulation still intact, thus being less likely to require a lower extremity revascularization.

b. Extra-anatomic bypass

Extra-anatomic bypass is a good option for the treatment of an infected aortic graft when groin infection is absent and lower extremity run-off is good. For instance, extra-anatomic bypass would be an excellent choice in a patient with an infected aortoiliac graft. The mortality and morbidity of this approach has decreased significantly since evidence supported preceding graft excision with extra-anatomic bypass rather than exploration and resection of the graft as the initial step. This reduces the duration of peripheral ischemia, operative blood loss, and attendant complications. One can stage the procedure by one or several days, especially in critically ill patients that require stabilization (Seeger et al., 2000). In the stable and good risk patient, we favor proceeding with graft excision under the same anesthetic, although there is only little evidence that the new extra-anatomic graft will experience thrombosis or become secondarily infected during the interval (Landry et al., 2000). Conversely, in patients who are bleeding the initial step should be exploration and removal of the infected graft.

In cases that involve groin infection due to prior aortofemoral bypass graft, the extra-anatomic reconstruction involves constructing the new femoral anastomosis to the profunda femoral artery (or superficial femoral artery) beyond the inguinal region through a lateral incision distal to the original femoral anastomosis. In these cases the PTFE axillofemoral graft is routed lateral to the anterior superior iliac spine circumventing the infected, original femoral incision. It should be emphasized that the aortic suture line, during aortic graft explantation, must be excised back to viable aortic tissue and oversewn in two layers with propylene suture, using omentum or prevertebral fascia to support the suture line. If necessary, one or both renal arteries may be sacrificed to obtain a satisfactory aortic stump closure, and splenorenal or hepatorenal bypass (or both) is carried out as needed. The periaortic tissue should be cultured and aggressively debrided.

The advantages of extra-anatomic bypass are that they may be physiologically less stressful to the patient, especially in the context of staged approach, they are technically straightforward, and there is minimal lower extremity ischemic time (Lehnert et al., 1993). The disadvantages consist in poor patency (about 60% at 5 years), especially in patients with multilevel occlusive disease, a 10% to 20% reinfection rate, that often proves fatal, the potential of aortic stump blow out, the high long-term amputation rate, estimated in the range of 30%, and the need for lifelong antithrombotic therapy (Lehnert et al., 1993; Mussa et al., 2007).Reinfection of extra-anatomic bypass following removal of an infected aortic prosthesis is a limb- and life-threatening problem about which little is known (Gordon et al., 1999). Thre are few options left other than to try to construct a new extra-anatomic bypass through uninfected tissues. This is usually not feasible, especially when distal, femoral anastomotic sites are involved with infection. Gorgon et al, has performed in situ femoral-popliteal vein reconstruction along with removal of the infected extra-anatomic bypass with satisfactory results (Gordon et al., 1999).

c. In-situ reconstruction

Because of persistent problems with durability and patency, as well as the other aforementioned complications, many authors have advocated the use of in situ reconstructions (Bandyk et al., 2001; Clagett et al., 1997; Noel et al., 2002). In situ arterial allografts were used extensively for infrarenal aortic replacement during the first decade of aortic surgery, but they were abandoned in the early 1960's due to difficulties in procurement and preservation, late degeneration, and availability of suitable aortic prosthetic grafts (DeBakey & Creech, 1954; Oudot & Beaconsfield, 1953). Allograft replacement, compared with the conventional method of graft excision and axillofemoral bypass, has the advantages of being expedient, associated with lower amputation rates (on the average 2%), and averting complications such as aortic stump blow out and reinfection or occlusion events (Verhelst et al., 2000). It also enables surgical reconstruction of hypogastric and deep femoral arteries, as indicated, thereby preventing the development of postoperative ischemic colitis or lower limb ischemia. However, mixed results have been reported regarding the efficacy of in situ replacement of infected aortic grafts with arterial homografts (Vogt et al., 1996). In one report, a 20% mortality was associated with this method of treatment (Speziale et al., 1997). Aortic allografts are also subject to long-term complications such as aneurysmal dilation, late allograft rupture, and thrombosis (Brown et al., 2009). Reinfection of allografts, although lower than in extra-anatomic bypass grafting, may also occur and usually proves fatal. Currently, aortic allografts are available only on a limited basis. Their shortage diminishes their use in situations where they may be most useful, namely in patients who are unstable, for example, those with actively bleeding aortoenteric fistula.

The same advantages and disadvantages accompany the use of antibiotic-treated prosthetic grafts. Their placement is expedient and technically straightforward, thus rendering them a reasonable option in critically ill, unstable patients. Moreover, they leave no aortic stump and are associated with relatively low amputation rate (Batt et al., 2003). We do not use in situ replacement with antibiotic-coated prosthetic grafts as the reported results are very poor, except in the replacement of one limb of an aortic graft infected with Staphylococcus epidermitis (Young et al., 1999). We have occasionally used such grafts in the initial temporizing treatment of aortoenteric fistula, thereby converting an unstable patient into a more stable with an infected aortic graft needing further treatment. Typically, the new prosthetic graft is soaked in rifampin, 60mg/ml, for 15 minutes before implantation (Walker et al., 1987). However, the reinfection rate is high and unpredictable, and patients must undergo lifelong antibiotic therapy.

d. Neo-aortoiliac bypass procedures

Because of the limitations of the other procedures, the use of in situ autogenous venous reconstruction technique, also termed neoaortoiliac system or NAIS procedure, has known great advocacy since its first description by Clagett in 1993 (Clagett et al., 1993). We should give credit to Erenfield who introduced first the concept of autogenous replacement of infected aortic grafts but it was Clagett' s introduction of the graft constructed of femoral popliteal veins that made the routine use of this method feasible. Early attempts that made use of greater saphenous vein grafts proved unsuccessful because the small caliber of the venous conduit resulted in low patency rates. Subsequent attempts using larger-caliber femoropopliteal (FPV) vein grafts, proved highly successful. FPV grafts have excellent long-term patency and are resistant to reinfection. Moreover, they are ideal conduits for patients with multilevel occlusive disease, in whom venous grafts would have better patency than prosthetic grafts. The 5-year patency rates for aortoiliac/aortofemoral reconstructions using FPV grafts range from 85% to 100% (Beck et al., 2008). According to the conventional method described by D'Addio and Clagett in 1993, the patient is prepared and draped from the nipples to the feet under general anesthesia (Clagett et al., 1993). A longitudinal incision along the course of the Sartorius muscle is used to expose an adequate length of the deep femoral and popliteal veins. The side branches are divided and ligated. Care is taken to preserve the profunda femoris vein in order to reduce the incidence of postoperative venous hypertension. The aortic graft is then exposed, either through a transperitoneal or retroperitoneal exposure and excised. Complete debridement of the aorta and surrounding tissues is performed. A sufficient length of deep vein is harvested. Reconstruction of the aortofemoral continuity is accomplished by either creating a bifurcated pantaloon graft, or by a unilateral aortofemoral graft, combined with an iliofemoral crossover graft.

A modification of the conventional NAIS procedure has been advocated by many authors in recent years. It is termed staged NAIS and refers to any aortoiliofemoral reconstruction using deep femoral popliteal veins in the treatment of aortic graft infections that is not completed in a single operation (Ali et al., 2008). At the initial operation, the deep veins are exposed, the side branches are divided and suture-ligated, and the incisions temporarily closed over closed-suction drains. The femoral veins are left in situ, so that flow is not interrupted. Overnight, sequential, compression devices are recommended, in addition to the use of low molecular weight heparin, as a prophylaxis against deep vein thrombosis.

The next day, the infected aortic graft is excised and the aortic reconstruction performed. In selected patients with graft occlusion and ischemia, the NAIS procedure may be further staged by performing unilateral revascularization of the most ischemic leg first, followed by revascularization of the contralateral limb at a later date.

Harvest of the deep vein is a critical part of the operation and has to be done meticulously. The staging of NAIS procedure, with harvesting the vein a day before definitive reconstruction, does not seem to cause any ill effects, and, in fact, may be beneficial in selected groups of patients (Modral et al., 2004). Especially in the presence of limb-threatening ischemia in conjunction with aortic graft infection, the advocates of the staged version, argue that deep femoral popiliteal vein mobilization may cause disruption of collaterals and precipitate acute ischemia. In such cases, the authors recommend that aortofemoral bypass be performed in the ischemic limb first, followed by femorofemoral bypass to the contralateral limb within 4 to 18 days later (Ali et al., 2008).

The advantages of autogenous femoroepopliteal vein replacement (NAIS) can be summarized as follows: a) superior long-term patency, limb salvage, b) minimal chance or reinfection, c) no aortic stump in the context of infected field, d) long-term antibiotic/antithrombotic therapy unnecessary (Lopera et al., 2008). Although reasonable limb salvage rates can be achieved using extra-anatomic bypass, achieving this goal requires careful follow up and multiple graft revisions or even new graft procedures. The advent of NAIS procedure has essentially obliterated the need for a secondary intervention in such fragile patients.

The main disadvantage is that the procedure is time consuming and technically demanding. The mean operating time is 8 hors and the lower extremity ischemic time is longer than that of patients undergoing the other procedures (Lopera et al., 2008). An additional disadvantage is the 20% incidence of short-term venous morbidity requiring leg fasciotomy (Modral et al., 2004).

A modification of the NAIS procedure with the use of the superficial femoral arteries as autologous neo-aortoiliac grafts have sporadically been reported in the literature as well (Dinis de Gama et al., 2004).

e. Conservative treatment

In an attempt to avoid submitting high-risk patients to a complex procedure with high morbidity and mortality, many authors have reported on a more conservative strategy, including aggressive local wound care with preservation of most, or all, of the involved graft (Calligaro et al., 2003). Although traditionally used in peripheral vascular graft infections, local care may also be carried out in selected patients with aortic graft infection. So, when clinical signs and preoperative imaging studies indicate that the infection is localized to the groin in a patient having undergone an aortofemoral bypass, drainage of all gross infection, extensive soft-tissue debridement, repetitive wound dressing changes, and the administration of antibiotics both topically and parenterally may effect sterilization of the wound and allow healing to occur by secondary intention. There have been few if any well-designed trials to study antimicrobial therapy as the main treatment of prosthetic aortic graft infection. Most studies are carried out by surgeons, and, as such, antibiotic therapy is mentioned as adjunct to surgical treatment. There is no evidence on which to decide the optimal duration of antibiotic administration (Perera et al., 2006). As mentioned above, this may vary from 2 weeks to one year, although a minimum of 4-6 weeks of intravenous therapy, followed by up to 6 months of oral therapy is commonly recommended (Nevelsteen et al., 1995). A small number of cases in which operation was deemed an unacceptably high risk to the patient have reported success with long-term suppressive treatment, including in some occasions lifelong antibiotic administration (Baddour, 2001; Roy & Grove, 2000).

A recent addition to our therapeutic armamentarium in managing infected aortic graft infection, when infection is suspected to be confined to one or both groins and the patient considered high risk to be submitted to operation, has been the use of a vacuum-assisted closure system (VAC). It has been reported that VAC therapy reduces the bacteria count in open wounds; removing excess fluid in the wound may stimulate lymphatic and blood flow and increase oxygen concentration, thereby killing bacteria (Dosluoglu et al., 2005). Further experience is necessary to evaluate the potential for VAC therapy to eradicate graft infections in the groin.

Although a trial of graft salvage is considered warranted in selected patients, as it avoids the morbidity inherent in excising the original graft and performing arterial ligation and repair in an infected field and obviates the necessity to perform an extra-anatomic bypass that is susceptible to recurrent thrombotic episodes, there are several disadvantages to this approach. A protracted period of hospitalization is required at considerable financial cost, and during this interval, the graft and patient are vulnerable to a number of complications such as anastomotic hemorrhage, thrombosis, and superinfection with more virulent organisms. A baseline CT scan is performed in these patients prior to discharge. This examination serves as a useful scan for comparison during routine follow-up or if patients develop additional septic or graft complications.

In the absence of evidence or consensus the treatment of aortic graft infection is often somewhat ad hoc and varies from center to center. As a conclusion of what previously described, two are the main criteria of choosing a plan of action. First the extent of graft infection, according to the Szilagyi and Samson criteria, and second, the microorganism cultured. Patients with limited graft infection (Samson 3, i.e. involving the body of the graft but not at an anastomosis) can be considered for graft salvage or route salvage (in situ reconstruction), with aggressive debridement with muscle transposition. On the contrary, graft salvage likely has limited application in advanced infection (Sampson 4 & 5, i.e. infection surrounding an exposed anastomosis with or without bacteremia). In these cases, the current literature suggests excision of the graft and it should be performed if tolerated. With regard to the microorganisms cultured, graft preservation or in situ reconstructions should be attempted when low virulence organisms are found, such as S. epidermidis. Methicillin resistant S. aureus and gram negative bacteria when met in graft infection should lead to graft explantation and extra-anatomical arterial reconstruction, unless when there is only minor graft involvement.

1.8 Endovascular stent graft infection

There has been no reason to believe that endovascular aortic stent grafts would be immune from septic complications, particularly because these procedures are increasingly being performed outside of the formal operating room and by nonsurgical vascular specialists. The infection rate of endovascular grafts implanted for abdominal aortic aneurysm disease is unclear, but Fiorani et al estimated a rate around 0,4% (Fiorani et al., 2003). Due to the minimal invasive nature of the procedure compared with the open counterpart, it is expected to be associated with lower septic complications.

The pathogenetic mechanisms of endograft infections consist mainly due to the following reasons:

1. Breaks in sterile technique during its implantation,
2. Superinfection during bacteremia from a variety of sources,
3. Severe intraperitoneal or retroperitoneal inflammation (i.e. rupture of hollow viscus, necrotizing pancreatitis),
4. Inoculation of bacteria during postoperative percutaneous interventions to manage various types of endoleaks (Hulin & Morris, 2007).
5. External injury of endograft (Lazaris et al., 2009).

The management of patients with infected aortic endografts must be based on the same fundamental principles as those analyzed above. The gold standard involves the explantation of the graft with subsequent reconstruction according to individualized parameters (Setacci et al., 2010). Some reports on the use of surgical or percutaneous placement of drains into the aneurysmal sac abscess contiguous to the graft in conjuction with irrigation of the perigraft area with antibiotic instilled through the drains and simultaneous systemic antibiotics administration, show promising results and have altered the approach to patients without signs of severe sepsis (Blanch et al., 2010; Pryluck et al., 2010).

1.9 Outcome

The perioperative mortality in patients with aortic prosthetic graft infection has improved over the past two decades. The conventional approach of graft removal and extra-anatomic reconstruction is associated with 12% mortality and 2% incidence of aortic stump infection/disruption (2). Three-year survival is estimated at 63% (Kitamura et al., 2005). Clearly, axillofemoral graft complications occur more frequently in patients with infected aortofemoral prosthetic grafts than in those with aortoiliac bypasses. This is specifically related to the technical challenge posed when attempting to avoid infection in the femoral region and simultaneously construct a durable prosthetic extra-anatomic bypass. On the other hand, the autogenous femoral vein graft is resistant to infection and appears to have a 2-year patency rate that exceeds 90% (Ali et al., 2008).

2. Conclusion

Aortic graft infections could be considered as the most dreadful complications that a vascular surgeon may encounter with. However, there are therapeutic options that can achieve remarkable results. Achieving the best result requires that the attending vascular surgeon takes advantage of the best features of each of the management plans available in his/her armamentarium. None of the approaches described here represents a perfect solution to the problem. What has become clear in recent years, however, is that although many patients with graft sepsis will continue to require graft explantation, an increasing number of autogenous and allograft options are available that offer the opportunity to maintain in-line anatomic arterial perfusion and preserve long-term limb viability.

3. References

Ali, A.; McLeod, N.; Klapatapu, V.; Moursi, M. & Eidt, J. (2008). Staging the neoaortoiliac system: feasibility and short-term outcomes. *Journal of Vascular Surgery,* Vol.48, No.5, (Nov), pp.1125-1131, ISSN 1097-6809

Angle, N. & Freischlag, J.A. (2002) Prosthetic graft infections. In: Vascular Surgery: A Comprehensive Review, ch. 38, ed.6, ed. By Moore WS. Philadelphia: WB Saunders, pp. 741-750

Baddour, L.M. (2001). Long-term suppressive antimicrobial therapy for intravascular device-related infections. *American Journal of the Medical Sciences,* Vol.322, No.4, (Oct), pp. 209-212, ISSN 0002-9629

Balink, H. & Reijnen, M.M. (2007). Diagnosis of abdominal aortic prosthesis infection with fdg-pet/ct. *Vascular & Endovascular Surgery,* Vol.41, No.5, (Oct-Nov), pp. 428-432, ISSN 1538-5744

Bandyk, D.F. & Esses, G.E. (1994). Prosthetic graft infection. *Surgical Clinics of North America,* Vol.74, No.3, (Jun), pp. 571-590, ISSN 0039-6109

Bandyk, D.F.; Novotney, M.L.; Johnson, B.L.; Back, M.R. & Roth, S.R. (2001). Use of rifampin-soaked gelatin-sealed polyester grafts for in situ treatment of primary aortic and vascular prosthetic infections. *Journal of Surgical Research,* Vol.95, No.1, (Jan), pp. 44-49, ISSN 0022-4804

Barie, P.S. & Eachempati, S.R. (2005). Surgical site infections. *Surgical Clinics of North America,* Vol.85, No.6, (Dec), pp. 1115-1135, viii-ix, ISSN 0039-6109

Batt, M.; Magne, J.L.; Alric, P.; Muzj, A.; Ruotolo, C.; Ljungstrom, K.G.; Garcia-Casas, R. & Simms, M. (2003). In situ revascularization with silver-coated polyester grafts to treat aortic infection: Early and midterm results. *Journal of Vascular Surgery,* Vol.38, No.5, (Nov), pp. 983-989, ISSN 0741-5214

Beck, A.W.; Murphy, E.H.; Hocking, J.A.; Timaran, C.H.; Arko, F.R. & Clagett, G.P. (2008). Aortic reconstruction with femoral-popliteal vein: Graft stenosis incidence, risk and reintervention. *Journal of Vascular Surgery,* Vol.47, No.1, (Jan), pp. 36-43; discussion 44, ISSN 0741-5214

Bisdas, T.; Bredt, M.; Pichlmaier, M.; Aper, T.; Wilhelmi, M.; Bisdas, S.; Haverich, A. & Teebken, O.E. (2010). Eight-year experience with cryopreserved arterial homografts for the in situ reconstruction of abdominal aortic infections. *Journal of Vascular Surgery,* Vol.52, No.2, (Aug), pp. 323-330, ISSN 1097-6809

Blanch, M.; Berjon, J.; Vila, R.; Simeon, J.M.; Romera, A.; Riera, S. & Cairols, M.A. (2010). The management of aortic stent-graft infection: Endograft removal versus conservative treatment. *Annals of Vascular Surgery,* Vol.24, No.4, (May), pp. 554 e551-555, ISSN 1615-5947

Brown, K.E.; Heyer, K.; Rodriguez, H.; Eskandari, M.K.; Pearce, W.H. & Morasch, M.D. (2009). Arterial reconstruction with cryopreserved human allografts in the setting of infection: A single-center experience with midterm follow-up. *Journal of Vascular Surgery,* Vol.49, No.3, (Mar), pp. 660-666, ISSN 1097-6809

Bunt, T.J. (2001). Vascular graft infections: An update. *Cardiovascular Surgery,* Vol.9, No.3, (Jun), pp. 225-233, ISSN 0967-2109

Calligaro, K.D. & Veith, F.J. (1991). Diagnosis and management of infected prosthetic aortic grafts. *Surgery*, Vol.110, No.5, (Nov), pp. 805-813, ISSN 0039-6060

Calligaro, K.D.; Veith, F.J.; Yuan, J.G.; Gargiulo, N.J. & Dougherty, M.J. (2003). Intra-abdominal aortic graft infection: Complete or partial graft preservation in patients at very high risk. *Journal of Vascular Surgery*, Vol.38, No.6, (Dec), pp. 1199-1205, ISSN 0741-5214

Chiesa, R.; Astore, D.; Frigerio, S.; Garriboli, L.; Piccolo, G.; Castellano, R.; Scalamogna, M.; Odero, A.; Pirrelli, S.; Biasi, G.; Mingazzini, P.; Biglioli, P.; Polvani, G.; Guarino, A.; Agrifoglio, G.; Tori, A. & Spina, G. (2002). Vascular prosthetic graft infection: Epidemiology, bacteriology, pathogenesis and treatment. *Acta Chirurgica Belgica*, Vol.102, No.4, (Aug), pp. 238-247, ISSN 0001-5458

Clagett, G.P.; Bowers, B.L.; Lopez-Viego, M.A.; Rossi, M.B.; Valentine, R.J.; Myers, S.I. & Chervu, A. (1993). Creation of a neo-aortoiliac system from lower extremity deep and superficial veins. *Annals of Surgery*, Vol.218, No.3, (Sep), pp. 239-248; discussion 248-239, ISSN 0003-4932

Clagett, G.P.; Valentine, R.J. & Hagino, R.T. (1997). Autogenous aortoiliac/femoral reconstruction from superficial femoral-popliteal veins: Feasibility and durability. *Journal of Vascular Surgery*, Vol.25, No.2, (Feb), pp. 255-266; discussion 267-270, ISSN 0741-5214

Darouiche, R.O. (2004). Treatment of infections associated with surgical implants. *New England Journal of Medicine*, Vol.350, No.14, (Apr 1), pp. 1422-1429, ISSN 1533-4406

Debakey, M.E.; Creech, O., Jr. & Cooley, D.A. (1954). Occlusive disease of the aorta and its treatment by resection and homograft replacement. *Annals of Surgery*, Vol.140, No.3, (Sep), pp. 290-310, ISSN 0003-4932

Delgado, M.; Prats, E.; Benito, J.L.; Abos, M.D.; Garcia-Lopez, F.; Tomas, A.; Razola, P.; Pina, J.I. & Banzo, J. (1999). [scintigraphy with 99mtc-hmpao labeled leukocytes and computed tomography in the diagnosis of vascular graft infection. A comparative study]. *Revista Espanola de Medicina Nuclear*, Vol.18, No.2, pp. 77-83, ISSN 0212-6982

Dinis da Gama, A.; Rosa, A.; Soares, M. & Moura, C. (2004). Use of autologous superficial femoral artery in surgery for aortic prosthesis infection. *Annals of Vascular Surgery*, Vol.18, No.5, (Sep), pp. 593-596, ISSN 0890-5096

Dosluoglu, H.H.; Schimpf, D.K.; Schultz, R. & Cherr, G.S. (2005). Preservation of infected and exposed vascular grafts using vacuum assisted closure without muscle flap coverage. *Journal of Vascular Surgery*, Vol.42, No.5, (Nov), pp. 989-992, ISSN 0741-5214

Farkas, J.C.; Fichelle, J.M.; Laurian, C.; Jean-Baptiste, A.; Gigou, F.; Marzelle, J.; Goldstein, F.W. & Cormier, J.M. (1993). Long-term follow-up of positive cultures in 500 abdominal aortic aneurysms. *Archives of Surgery*, Vol.128, No.3, (Mar), pp. 284-288, ISSN 0004-0010

Fiorani, P.; Speziale, F.; Calisti, A.; Misuraca, M.; Zaccagnini, D.; Rizzo, L. & Giannoni, M.F. (2003). Endovascular graft infection: Preliminary results of an international enquiry. *J Endovasc Ther*, Vol.10, No.5, (Oct), pp. 919-927, ISSN 1526-6028

FitzGerald, S.F.; Kelly, C. & Humphreys, H. (2005). Diagnosis and treatment of prosthetic aortic graft infections: Confusion and inconsistency in the absence of evidence or consensus. *Journal of Antimicrobial Chemotherapy*, Vol.56, No.6, (Dec), pp. 996-999, ISSN 0305-7453

Gordon, L.L.; Hagino, R.T.; Jackson, M.R.; Modrall, J.G.; Valentine, R.J. & Clagett, G.P. (1999). Complex aortofemoral prosthetic infections: The role of autogenous superficial femoropopliteal vein reconstruction. *Archives of Surgery*, Vol.134, No.6, (Jun), pp. 615-620; discussion 620-611, ISSN 0004-0010

Gutowski, P. (1998). [aortoiliac graft infection as a diagnostic and treatment problem]. *Annales Academiae Medicae Stetinensis*, Vol.Suppl 41, pp. 1-72, ISSN 1427-440X

Hsu, R.B.; Chen, R.J.; Wang, S.S. & Chu, S.H. (2004). Infected aortic aneurysms: Clinical outcome and risk factor analysis. *Journal of Vascular Surgery*, Vol.40, No.1, (Jul), pp. 30-35, ISSN 0741-5214

Hulin, S.J. & Morris, G.E. (2007). Aortic endograft infection: Open surgical management with endograft preservation. *European Journal of Vascular and Endovascular Surgery*, Vol.34, No.2, (Aug), pp. 191-193, ISSN 1078-5884

Kaebnick, H.W.; Bandyk, D.F.; Bergamini, T.W. & Towne, J.B. (1987). The microbiology of explanted vascular prostheses. *Surgery*, Vol.102, No.4, (Oct), pp. 756-762, ISSN 0039-6060

Kaiser, A.B.; Clayson, K.R.; Mulherin, J.L., Jr.; Roach, A.C.; Allen, T.R.; Edwards, W.H. & Dale, W.A. (1978). Antibiotic prophylaxis in vascular surgery. *Annals of Surgery*, Vol.188, No.3, (Sep), pp. 283-289, ISSN 0003-4932

Kibria, R.; Rao, P.K. & Siva, S. (2010). Secondary aortoenteric fistula presenting with recurrent episodes of sepsis. *Southern Medical Journal*, Vol.103, No.6, (Jun), pp. 594-595, ISSN 1541-8243

Kieffer, E.; Sabatier, J.; Plissonnier, D. & Knosalla, C. (2001). Prosthetic graft infection after descending thoracic/ thoracoabdominal aortic aneurysmectomy: Management with in situ arterial allografts. *Journal of Vascular Surgery*, Vol.33, No.4, (Apr), pp. 671-678, ISSN 0741-5214

Kitamura, T.; Morota, T.; Motomura, N.; Ono, M.; Shibata, K.; Ueno, K.; Kotsuka, Y. & Takamoto, S. (2005). Management of infected grafts and aneurysms of the aorta. *Annals of Vascular Surgery*, Vol.19, No.3, (May), pp. 335-342, ISSN 0890-5096

Koshy, A.K.; Simon, E.G. & Keshava, S.N. (2010). Education and imaging. Gastrointestinal: Aortoenteric fistula. *Journal of Gastroenterology and Hepatology*, Vol.25, No.5, (May), pp. 1014, ISSN 1440-1746

Landry, G.J.; Moneta, G.L.; Taylor, L.M., Jr. & Porter, J.M. (2000). Axillobifemoral bypass. *Annals of Vascular Surgery*, Vol.14, No.3, (May), pp. 296-305, ISSN 0890-5096

Lazaris, A.M.; Tsapralis, D.; Patapis, P.; Mproutzos, E.; Tzathas, H.; Kakisis, J.D. & Vasdekis, S.N. (2009). Aortoiliac endograft-enteric fistula due to an ingested toothpick. *Journal of Vascular Surgery*, Vol.50, No.3, (Sep), pp. 640-643, ISSN 1097-6809

Lehnert, T.; Gruber, H.P.; Maeder, N. & Allenberg, J.R. (1993). Management of primary aortic graft infection by extra-anatomic bypass reconstruction. *European Journal of Vascular Surgery*, Vol.7, No.3, (May), pp. 301-307, ISSN 0950-821X

Lopera, J.E.; Trimmer, C.K.; Josephs, S.; Dolmatch, B.; Valentine, R.J. & Clagett, G.P. (2008). Neoaortoiliac reconstructions using femoropopliteal veins: Mdct angiography findings. *AJR. American Journal of Roentgenology*, Vol.191, No.2, (Aug), pp. 569-577, ISSN 1546-3141

Macbeth, G.A.; Rubin, J.R.; McIntyre, K.E., Jr.; Goldstone, J. & Malone, J.M. (1984). The relevance of arterial wall microbiology to the treatment of prosthetic graft infections: Graft infection vs. Arterial infection. *Journal of Vascular Surgery*, Vol.1, No.6, (Nov), pp. 750-756, ISSN 0741-5214

Mangram, A.J.; Horan, T.C.; Pearson, M.L.; Silver, L.C. & Jarvis, W.R. (1999). Guideline for prevention of surgical site infection, 1999. Hospital infection control practices advisory committee. *Infection Control and Hospital Epidemiology*, Vol.20, No.4, (Apr), pp. 250-278; quiz 279-280, ISSN 0899-823X

Mark, A.; Moss, A.A.; Lusby, R. & Kaiser, J.A. (1982). Ct evaluation of complications of abdominal aortic surgery. *Radiology*, Vol.145, No.2, (Nov), pp. 409-414, ISSN 0033-8419

Mark, A.S.; McCarthy, S.M.; Moss, A.A. & Price, D. (1985). Detection of abdominal aortic graft infection: Comparison of ct and in-labeled white blood cell scans. *AJR. American Journal of Roentgenology*, Vol.144, No.2, (Feb), pp. 315-318, ISSN 0361-803X

Modrall, J.G.; Sadjadi, J.; Ali, A.T.; Anthony, T.; Welborn, M.B., 3rd; Valentine, R.J.; Hynan, L.S. & Clagett, G.P. (2004). Deep vein harvest: Predicting need for fasciotomy. *Journal of Vascular Surgery*, Vol.39, No.2, (Feb), pp. 387-394, ISSN 0741-5214

Montgomery, R.S. & Wilson, S.E. (1996). The surgical management of aortoenteric fistulas. *Surgical Clinics of North America*, Vol.76, No.5, (Oct), pp. 1147-1157, ISSN 0039-6109

Mussa, F.F.; Hedayati, N.; Zhou, W.; El-Sayed, H.F.; Kougias, P.; Darouiche, R.O. & Lin, P.H. (2007). Prevention and treatment of aortic graft infection. *Expert Rev Anti Infect Ther*, Vol.5, No.2, (Apr), pp. 305-315, ISSN 1744-8336

Nevelsteen, A.; Lacroix, H. & Suy, R. (1995). Autogenous reconstruction with the lower extremity deep veins: An alternative treatment of prosthetic infection after reconstructive surgery for aortoiliac disease. *Journal of Vascular Surgery*, Vol.22, No.2, (Aug), pp. 129-134, ISSN 0741-5214

Noel, A.A.; Gloviczki, P.; Cherry, K.J., Jr.; Safi, H.; Goldstone, J.; Morasch, M.D. & Johansen, K.H. (2002). Abdominal aortic reconstruction in infected fields: Early results of the united states cryopreserved aortic allograft registry. *Journal of Vascular Surgery*, Vol.35, No.5, (May), pp. 847-852, ISSN 0741-5214

O'Brien, T. & Collin, J. (1992). Prosthetic vascular graft infection. *British Journal of Surgery*, Vol.79, No.12, (Dec), pp. 1262-1267, ISSN 0007-1323

O'Connor, S.; Andrew, P.; Batt, M. & Becquemin, J.P. (2006). A systematic review and meta-analysis of treatments for aortic graft infection. *Journal of Vascular Surgery*, Vol.44, No.1, (Jul), pp. 38-45, ISSN 0741-5214

Olofsson, P.A.; Auffermann, W.; Higgins, C.B.; Rabahie, G.N.; Tavares, N. & Stoney, R.J. (1988). Diagnosis of prosthetic aortic graft infection by magnetic resonance imaging. *Journal of Vascular Surgery*, Vol.8, No.2, (Aug), pp. 99-105, ISSN 0741-5214

Orton, D.F.; LeVeen, R.F.; Saigh, J.A.; Culp, W.C.; Fidler, J.L.; Lynch, T.J.; Goertzen, T.C. & McCowan, T.C. (2000). Aortic prosthetic graft infections: Radiologic manifestations and implications for management. *Radiographics*, Vol.20, No.4, (Jul-Aug), pp. 977-993, ISSN 0271-5333

Oudot, J. & Beaconsfield, P. (1953). Thrombosis of the aortic bifurcation treated by resection and homograft replacement; report of five cases. *AMA Arch Surg*, Vol.66, No.3, (Mar), pp. 365-374, ISSN 0096-6908

Palestro, C.J.; Weiland, F.L.; Seabold, J.E.; Valdivia, S.; Tomas, M.B.; Moyer, B.R.; Baran, Y.M.; Lister-James, J. & Dean, R.T. (2001). Localizing infection with a technetium-99m-labeled peptide: Initial results. *Nuclear Medicine Communications*, Vol.22, No.6, (Jun), pp. 695-701, ISSN 0143-3636

Perera, G.B.; Fujitani, R.M. & Kubaska S.M. (2006). Aortic graft infection: Update on Management and Treatment Options. *Vasc Endovascular Surg*, Vol.40, No.1, (Jan), pp. 1-10, ISSN 1538-5744

Pryluck, D.S.; Kovacs, S.; Maldonado, T.S.; Jacobowitz, G.R.; Adelman, M.A.; Charles, H.C. & Clark, T.W. (2010). Percutaneous drainage of aortic aneurysm sac abscesses following endovascular aneurysm repair. *Vasc Endovascular Surg*, Vol.44, No.8, (Nov), pp. 701-707, ISSN 1938-9116

Qvarfordt, P.G.; Reilly, L.M.; Mark, A.S.; Goldstone, J.; Wall, S.D.; Ehrenfeld, W.K. & Stoney, R.J. (1985). Computerized tomographic assessment of graft incorporation after aortic reconstruction. *American Journal of Surgery*, Vol.150, No.2, (Aug), pp. 227-231, ISSN 0002-9610

Roy, D. & Grove, D.I. (2000). Efficacy of long-term antibiotic suppressive therapy in proven or suspected infected abdominal aortic grafts. *Journal of Infection*, Vol.40, No.2, (Mar), pp. 184-204, ISSN 0163-4453

Samson, R.H.; Veith, F.J.; Janko, G.S.; Gupta, S.K. & Scher, L.A. (1988). A modified classification and approach to the management of infections involving peripheral arterial prosthetic grafts. *Journal of Vascular Surgery*, Vol.8, No.2, (Aug), pp. 147-153, ISSN 0741-5214

Seeger, J.M.; Pretus, H.A.; Welborn, M.B.; Ozaki, C.K.; Flynn, T.C. & Huber, T.S. (2000). Long-term outcome after treatment of aortic graft infection with staged extra-anatomic bypass grafting and aortic graft removal. *Journal of Vascular Surgery*, Vol.32, No.3, (Sep), pp. 451-459; discussion 460-451, ISSN 0741-5214

Setacci, C.; De Donato, G.; Setacci, F.; Chisci, E.; Perulli, A.; Galzerano, G. & Siringano, P. (2010). Management of abdominal endograft infection. *Journal of Cardiovascular Surgery*, Vol.51, No.1, (Feb), pp. 33-41, ISSN 0021-9509

Sharp, W.J.; Hoballah, J.J.; Mohan, C.R.; Kresowik, T.F.; Martinasevic, M.; Chalmers, R.T. & Corson, J.D. (1994). The management of the infected aortic prosthesis: A current decade of experience. *Journal of Vascular Surgery*, Vol.19, No.5, (May), pp. 844-850, ISSN 0741-5214

Soetevent, C.; Klemm, P.L.; Stalenhoef, A.F. & Bredie, S.J. (2004). Vascular graft infection in aortoiliac and aortofemoral bypass surgery: Clinical presentation, diagnostic strategies and results of surgical treatment. *Netherlands Journal of Medicine*, Vol.62, No.11, (Dec), pp. 446-452, ISSN 0300-2977

Speziale, F.; Rizzo, L.; Sbarigia, E.; Giannoni, M.F.; Massucci, M.; Maraglino, C.; Santoro, E. & Fiorani, P. (1997). Bacterial and clinical criteria relating to the outcome of patients undergoing in situ replacement of infected abdominal aortic grafts. *European Journal of Vascular and Endovascular Surgery*, Vol.13, No.2, (Feb), pp. 127-133, ISSN 1078-5884

Szilagyi, D.E.; Smith, R.F.; Elliott, J.P. & Vrandecic, M.P. (1972). Infection in arterial reconstruction with synthetic grafts. *Annals of Surgery*, Vol.176, No.3, (Sep), pp. 321-333, ISSN 0003-4932

Valentine, R.J. (2001). Diagnosis and management of aortic graft infection. *Seminars in Vascular Surgery*, Vol.14, No.4, (Dec), pp. 292-301, ISSN 0895-7967

Verhelst, R.; Lacroix, V.; Vraux, H.; Lavigne, J.P.; Vandamme, H.; Limet, R.; Nevelsteen, A.; Bellens, B.; Vasseur, M.A.; Wozniak, B. & Goffin, Y. (2000). Use of cryopreserved arterial homografts for management of infected prosthetic grafts: A multicentric study. *Annals of Vascular Surgery*, Vol.14, No.6, (Nov), pp. 602-607, ISSN 0890-5096

Vogt, P.R.; von Segesser, L.K.; Goffin, Y.; Niederhauser, U.; Genoni, M.; Kunzli, A.; Lachat, M. & Turina, M.I. (1996). Eradication of aortic infections with the use of cryopreserved arterial homografts. *Annals of Thoracic Surgery*, Vol.62, No.3, (Sep), pp. 640-645, ISSN 0003-4975

Walker, W.E.; Cooley, D.A.; Duncan, J.M.; Hallman, G.L., Jr.; Ott, D.A. & Reul, G.J. (1987). The management of aortoduodenal fistula by in situ replacement of the infected abdominal aortic graft. *Annals of Surgery*, Vol.205, No.6, (Jun), pp. 727-732, ISSN 0003-4932

Wilson, S.E. (2001). New alternatives in management of the infected vascular prosthesis. *Surg Infect (Larchmt)*, Vol.2, No.2, (Summer), pp. 171-175; discussion 175-177, ISSN 1096-2964

Yeager, R.A. & Porter, J.M. (1992). Arterial and prosthetic graft infection. *Annals of Vascular Surgery*, Vol.6, No.5, (Sep), pp. 485-491, ISSN 0890-5096

Young, R.M.; Cherry, K.J., Jr.; Davis, P.M.; Gloviczki, P.; Bower, T.C.; Panneton, J.M. & Hallett, J.W., Jr. (1999). The results of in situ prosthetic replacement for infected aortic grafts. *American Journal of Surgery*, Vol.178, No.2, (Aug), pp. 136-140, ISSN 0002-9610

15

Gastrointestinal Complications of Abdominal Aortic Aneurysms

Emmeline Nugent and Paul Neary
National Surgical Training Centre, Royal College of Surgeons in Ireland
Ireland

1. Introduction

Although the gastrointestinal complications that occur secondary to repair of an aortic abdominal aneurysm (AAA) are uncommon they are associated with a significant increase in patient morbidity and mortality and therefore they warrant discussion. The gastrointestinal complications that we plan to review in detail in this chapter are ischaemic colitis, abdominal compartment syndrome, secondary aorto-enteric fistula, chylous ascites and ileus. We are also going to briefly discuss peptic ulcer disease, acute cholecystitis and acute pancreatitis and their relationship with AAA surgery.

Throughout the chapter we describe the incidence, aetiology, pathology, associated risk factors, diagnosis and management for each potential gastrointestinal complication in an evidence based manner.

Over the last two decades a new technique, endovascular surgery (EVAR), has been introduced as an alternative option for the management of an abdominal aortic aneurysm. The traditional approach, open repair, has long been regarded as a durable, effective procedure that is associated with a low rate of rupture with long-term follow up. However, the evolution of endovascular surgery has promised benefits when compared to the traditional approach. The advantages of the endovascular approach include a faster recovery time post-operatively and a reduction in the morbidity and mortality rates that occur with this condition. It also allows elderly patients and patients with co-morbidities that previously would have been considered unfit for surgery to undergo aneurysm repair in a safe manner. As part of our review of gastrointestinal complications following AAA repair, in this chapter we examine the impact, if any, that endovascular surgery has had on the type and frequency of these complications since its introduction.

2. Ischaemic colitis

2.1 Incidence

Ischaemic colitis is an infrequent but devastating complication following AAA repair. The intestinal mucosa is very sensitive to ischaemia and a sufficient reduction in blood flow can lead to this damaging condition. In ischaemic colitis it is only the mucosa of the bowel that is injured, the full thickness of the bowel wall remains unharmed.

The incidence of ischaemic colitis post open and elective repair of AAA is 1-3% (Van et al, 2000). The incidence following EVAR is similar. However the risk of ischaemic colitis increases to 10% in cases of open repair of a ruptured AAA. If routine post-operative colonoscopy is performed to screen for this condition the rate of detection dramatically rises to 9% for elective repair and has been reported to be found in up to 60% of patients following surgery for a ruptured aneurysm (Chen et al, 1996).

2.2 Aetiology

Any reduction in blood flow to the bowel wall mucosa can result in ischaemic colitis. With surgery for an AAA a reduction in blood flow can occur secondary to a reduction in circulating blood volume which can result, for example, due to blood loss or in a state of low cardiac output. Vasoconstriction of the splanchnic circulation occurring as part of the physiological response of the body to shock or due to the administration of vasopressive medication also results in a reduction of blood flowing to the bowel mucosa. Occlusion of the inferior mesenteric artery (IMA) or the internal iliac artery can lead to a reduction in blood flow to the bowel wall. This can arise due to external compression that occurs during operative repair, for example trauma caused by retraction, the intentional occlusion of the IMA that is associated with EVAR, or due to thrombus formation, arthero-embolisation or a haematoma formation.

In endovascular repair it has been proposed that ischaemic colitis could be attributed to the dislodgement of debris from the sac of the aneurysm during wire and graft manipulation. It has been suggested however, that the EVAR approach may reduce the severity of ischaemic colitis but there is currently a lack of conclusive data to support this (Elmarsay et al, 2000). Certainly a recent study has shown that there is at the very least no significant difference in the rates of ischaemic colitis following the open and EVAR approach (Bosch et al, 2010).

2.3 Pathology

During the fasting state the gastrointestinal tract only receives 20% of the overall cardiac output. This increases to 35% post-prandially, and of this, the mucosa receives 70% of the blood supply. The colon differs from the small bowel structurally, a difference that accounts for its greater susceptibility to a reduced blood flow volume. Firstly the sub-mucosal vascular plexuses are much more extensive in the small bowel when compared to the large bowel and secondly the large bowel has no villi and therefore it has no counter-current mechanism. In the case of hypotension or with a low cardiac output the micro-vascular arcades are the ones to suffer as they are (i) the last to get blood and (ii) in cases of shock the physiological response is to shunt blood away from the splanchnic circulation. The splenic flexure in particular is vulnerable to ischaemia as it is part of the "watershed" area - this is the area of the colon where the superior mesenteric artery and IMA both supply but are reliant on collaterals to bridge the gaps in-between. Within a fifteen minute window a reduction in blood flow leading to ischaemia can demonstrate structural changes in the mucosa. After three hours mucosal sloughing will be evident and after six hours transmural necrosis will manifest.

There are two main factors that cause structural damage, (i) hypoxia, due to a reduction in blood flow and (ii) reperfusion injury.

There are three steps in the pathophysiological process leading to ischaemic colitis; fluid loss, reperfusion injury and vasoconstriction of the splanchnic vasculature.

1. Fluid Loss: The amount of fluid lost during aortic surgery is considerable. Animal experiments have demonstrated that up to a third of circulating fluid (plasma) may be

lost after superior mesenteric artery occlusion (Geroulakos & Cherry, 2002). With a reduction in blood flow, the injured bowel loses its absorptive function while the crypt cells are spared and continue to secrete. Intraluminal exudation causes a further reduction in blood volume and distension of the bowel wall. The bowel becomes oedematous and there is transudation of fluid into the peritoneal cavity. When the arterial flow is then restored and blood flow returns to the gastrointestinal tract reactionary haemorrhage can occur into the bowel lumen.

2. Reperfusion injury: Anaerobic metabolism and acidosis trigger an inflammatory cascade. The main damaging effects of activating this cascade are caused by the production of free radicals (superoxide, peroxide and hydroxyl). The colonic mucosa is rich in the enzyme xanthine dehydrogenase which results in the production of reactive oxygen species and free radicals. The release of these free radicals causes a release of cytokines and platelet activating factor, which in turn activate and stimulate the release of monocytes, neutrophils and endothelin 1 (ET-1), which is a potent vasoconstrictor. The activation of polymorphonuclear leukocytes causes a systemic inflammatory response. The final result is end organ damage affecting the respiratory system, the renal system and leading to bone marrow failure. Further massive losses of fluid volume could result from disseminated intravascular coagulation (DIC) and the widespread increase in vascular permeability that this can bring.
3. Splanchnic vasoconstriction: Vasoconstriction can persist following revascularisation rendering perfusion inadequate.

The ischaemic colon loses its barrier function rapidly leading to invasion by luminal bacteria and endotoxin absorption. This takes place over a period of at least 24 hours. The mucosa sloughs off into the lumen which causes peristalsis, diarrhoea and bleeding. In the most severe of cases it leads to portal pyaemia and death. Less severe cases result in multi-organ damage and failure.

Three progressive stages of ischemic colitis are described (i) Grade 1: transient mucosal ischaemia, (ii) Grade II: mucosal and muscularis involvement which may result in healing with fibrosis and stricture formation (iii) Grade III: transmural ischaemia and infarction which results in gangrene and perforation. The mortality rate reaches 90% in patients with bowel infarction.

When comparing open surgery to EVAR it is likely that there is a different pathophysiological pattern at play. In EVAR there is no manipulation of the bowel which reduces the risk of trauma. As a result abdominal hypertension and compartment syndrome as a cause of ischaemic colitis is unlikely. Reperfusion injury to the bowel is also unlikely as the period of time during the operation when the aorta is occluded is short. It had been thought that sacrificing the IMA may account for ischaemic colitis in endovascular repair. However, it is now believed that preserving IMA patency may not be as important as previously thought. With EVAR there is a risk of micro-embolisation due to dislodging the thrombus or the artheromatous plaque during wire and graft manipulation and placement.

2.4 Risk factors

There are a number of factors that have been established as associated with a greater chance of ischaemic colitis. They can be divided into pre, peri or intra and post-operative risk factors (table 1).

	Risk Factors
Pre-operative	Ruptured AAA
	Mean systolic blood pressure <80mmHg
	Length of time spent hypotensive
	High disease severity score
	Age
	Female
Peri or intra-operative	Blood loss >2000ml
	Operating time >4 hours
	Body temperature <35 degrees
	Length of time aorta is cross-clamped
	Hospital case volume
	Internal iliac artery ligation
	Aotobifemoral grafting
Post-operative	Renal impairment
	Neutrophilia
	Metabolic acidosis
	Ionotropic support
	Bloody diarrhoea

Table 1. Risk Factors for Ischaemic Colitis (Bjorck et al, 1996; Neary et al, 2007; Perry et al, 2008; Becquemin et al, 2008; Levison et al, 1999)

Patients undergoing emergency AAA repair or that develop shock peri-operatively are at the greatest risk of developing ischaemic colitis. Here the incidence increases from 1-3% to 30% (Levison et al, 1999).

The type of surgical approach has not been found to be an independent predictor of ischaemic colitis. This has been challenged in particular with respect to the patency of the IMA. IMA patency has been demonstrated not to be associated with an increased risk of ischaemic colitis (Senekowitsch et al, 2006). This has been shown in open surgery where routine re-implantation of the IMA was compared to no re-implantation and in EVAR where the IMA is routinely blocked off. To date the importance of hypogastric artery patency has not been established in both open and EVAR repair. However, it does seem that it is not emerging as a significant risk factor (Geraghty et al, 2004).

2.5 Diagnosis

Ischaemic colitis can be seen at the time of open AAA repair. When this occurs a colectomy may need to be performed and the overall outcome for the patient is generally poor.

The mean time to diagnosis ischaemic colitis post-operatively is 5.5 days. In patients where a bowel resection is required there is an overall mortality rate of 80-90%. The sigmoid colon is the most commonly affected segment of large bowel followed by the rectum.

Presenting features are often insidious and include diarrhoea which may or may not be bloody and abdominal pain out of keeping with the clinical signs. The diagnosis often requires a high index of suspicion with specific investigations to confirm it. A high index of suspicion should be had in patients with persistent hypotension post-operatively, an elevated lactate, creatinine, leucocytes and other signs that point towards sepsis.

Features to be aware of on plain abdominal x-ray are non-specific and include; fluid levels, toxic colon dilation, intramural air and free air due to perforation. In severe clinical cases intra-portal air may be present. A barium enema may demonstrate thumb-printing which is present as a result of mucosal oedema. CT (contrast enhanced computed tomography) or MRI scans in the early stages may be normal or may show non-specific signs such as mucosal thickening or oedema. As ischaemic colitis progresses, scanning typically demonstrates a circumferential symmetrical wall thickening with fold enlargement. It may be useful to consider looking at the visceral arteries with MRA.

Endoscopy demonstrates a diagnostic accuracy of 92% (Assadian et al, 2008). But a histological diagnosis is the gold standard. On endoscopy there may be blood visible in the bowel lumen. If there is a suspicion that the colon may be ischaemic biopsies should be taken, even if the mucosa appears normal. In mild cases of ischaemic colitis the mucosa appears pale with petechiae, whereas in severe colitis the mucosa appears blue or black in colour and there may be slough or ulceration. Histological features on biopsy include; hyalinization of the lamina propria, atrophic appearing micro-crypts, lamina propria haemorrhage, full thickness mucosal necrosis and a diffuse distribution of pseudomembranes.

In the acute phase there is necrosis of the superficial epithelium and haemorrhage into the lamina propria. The intestinal crypts are spared. This stage is reversible, but it may progress. In the organising phase there is ulceration and associated granulation tissue formation without the presence of marked inflammatory changes. Iron deposits can be found also. The healed phase demonstrates architectural distortion of the crypts and a transmural fibrosis. Another diagnostic approach is an exploratory laparotomy.

In the setting of ischaemia these patients are at risk of developing pseudomembranous colitis. This is further exacerbated by the administration of prophylactic antibiotics.

Although postoperative clinical assessment with physical examination and laboratory tests is unreliable in predicting ischemic colitis, several intra-operative methods have demonstrated a certain degree of promise. These include inferior mesenteric artery stump pressure measurements, trans-serosal tissue oxygen tension measurements (tPO2), laparoscopy, and tonometry. Pulse oximetry could be another potentially helpful tool to monitor the colon for evidence of ischaemia (Yilmaz et al, 1999). Of these assessments, selective ligation of the IMA on the basis of intraoperative bowel inspection, colonic mesenteric Doppler signals, and IMA stump pressure have been the most encouraging. However, these techniques detect intra-operative changes and they may not accurately reflect or predict subsequent ischemic events.

Colonoscopy remains the diagnostic procedure of choice for assessing ischemic colitis.

2.6 Management

Early detection and treatment of ischaemic colitis is very important. The condition if diagnosed in the initial stages can be reversed.

Conservative management of ischaemic colitis can be employed if the ischaemia is not transmural and there is no evidence of multi-organ damage, the patient is clinically stable and they have no signs of peritonitis. Grade I and II bowel ischaemia can be treated with antibiotic therapy, intravenous fluids, bowel rest, and surveillance colonoscopy. Grade III ischaemia warrants an immediate laparotomy in an effort to decrease the mortality associated with this condition (Champagne et al, 2004). At laparotomy the ischaemic segment should be resected with both bowel ends being brought out as stomas. Patients that require an immediate laparotomy and bowel resection do worse in terms of outcome and have a significantly higher mortality risk. Surveillance colonoscopy is very important in the early grades of ischaemia and should be carried out at regular intervals as the ischaemia may become more extensive at any stage.

Although ischaemic colitis may be subclinical and only discovered on colonoscopy and biopsy it is still a significant condition, because despite resolution of the ischaemia, the gut mucosal barrier will have been altered. This allows the passage of bacteria and endotoxins into the portal circulation thereby causing sepsis and multi-organ failure. The true incidence of ischaemic colitis is probably much higher than the clinically evident incidence (Welch et al, 1998). Welch and colleagues performed a study where they scoped patients post-operative AAA repair and they found a very high rate of asymptomatic ischaemic colitis (30%) (Welch et al, 1998).

The monitoring of intra-abdominal pressure post-operatively is justified as an increase in intra-abdominal hypertension is associated with colonic ischaemia (Djavani et al, 2009). This approach can therefore allow early detection and treatment of ischaemic colitis. Another preventative approach, the effectiveness of which remains debatable is the role of re-implanting the IMA (Mitchell & Valentine, 2002). Arguments against this technique include the increased risk of bleeding from the anastomosis, the technically demanding nature of this procedure, and the increase in intra-operative time that it is associated with.

Major cardiac, respiratory and renal complications are associated with ischaemic colitis (Becquemin et al, 2008). Therefore it is easy to understand the seriousness of this gastrointestinal complication following AAA repair. A further complication of ischaemic colitis that presents at a late stage is a stricture of the colon. A stricture typically presents with features of subacute obstruction.

Overall there has been no difference in mortality demonstrated for ischaemic colitis occurring following open repair or endovascular surgery.

3. Abdominal Compartment Syndrome

3.1 Incidence

Abdominal compartment syndrome (ACS) occurs when a fixed compartment, defined by myofascial elements, becomes subject to increased pressure, leading to ischemia and organ dysfunction. ACS is the worst potential outcome that can occur with an elevation in intra-abdominal pressure (IAP). It is thought to be the most common cause of intestinal hypoperfusion and it also has significance in the setting of AAA repair. The incidence of ACS has been reported to be approximately 5 -18% in patients that do not undergo IAP monitoring and this increases to >10% when IAP is monitored. The incidence seems to be similar irrespective of whether open or EVAR repair is performed (Bjork et al, 2008; Bosch et al, 2010). The incidence is significantly greater in patients following a ruptured AAA (30%) and the associated mortality in this case can be up to 70% (Maker et al, 2009; Mehta, 2010). The diagnosis of abdominal compartment syndrome post AAA repair is a recognised prognostic indicator and is associated with an overall mortality rate of greater than 50%.

3.2 Aetiology

In open repair of an AAA the most significant contributors to an elevation in intra-abdominal pressure and subsequent development of ACS are manipulation of the intestines and mesenteric retraction occurring as a routine part of surgery.

The aetiology of ACS following endovascular repair is somewhat different. Factors associated with intra-abdominal hypertension following endovascular surgery include; (i) a retroperitoneal hematoma resulting in a space occupying lesion, (ii) continuous bleeding from the lumbar and inferior mesenteric arteries into the disrupted aneurysm sac or surrounding retroperitoneal tissues; this may be exacerbated by the systemic inflammatory response and associated coagulopathy that occurs in patients, in particular, those that have undergone emergency repair due to rupture, and (iii) similarly the increase in microvascular permeability that can lead to visceral and soft tissue oedema following ruptured AAA (Mehta, 2010).

3.3 Pathology

ACS is classified (Grade I-IV) based on the level of intra-abdominal pressure (table 2). In the critically ill patient without an AAA repair a normal IAP is considered to be 5-7mmHg. Grade I and II, where the IAP is between 12 and 20mmHg, can lead to impairment of renal function. This is followed by progressive dysfunction of all other organ systems.

Grade	Intra-abdominal Pressure (mmHg)
I	12-15
II	16-20
III	21-25
IV	>25

Table 2. Grading of Intra-abdominal Pressure according to WSACS Guidelines

A raised IAP of 20mmHg or more results in a reduction in the venous return to the heart and a decreased cardiac output. An increase in abdominal pressure also reduces venous flow to the various intra-peritoneal organs. Overall the outcome is that there is a reduction in perfusion of the various visceral organs resulting in bowel ischaemia. Mild cases of ischaemic colitis create an increase in intestinal permeability but in extreme cases bowel infarction can result.

The risk of increased IAP and therefore ACS has been proposed to be less in cases of endovascular repair. Studies have shown that EVAR is associated with less of a rise in inflammatory markers post-operatively when compared to open repair, a factor that as a consequence reduces the risk of a raised IAP and ACS (Junnarkar et al, 2003).

3.4 Risk factors

Risk factors for the development of intra-abdominal hypertension are multiple and can be divided into pre-operative, peri- or intra-operative and post-operative risk factors (table 3).

Studies have demonstrated that on comparing emergency open repair of a ruptured AAA to EVAR for a ruptured AAA, that those patients having open surgery had a significantly higher IAP post-operatively (Maker et al, 2009).

	Risk Factors
Pre-operative	Ruptured AAA
	Systolic blood pressure <70mmHg (>20 minutes)
	Haemoglobin <8 g/dl
	Shock
Peri- or intra-operative	Volume of blood loss
	Transfusion (platelet/>6 units red packed cells)
	>5 litres of intra-venous fluid
	Temperature <35 degrees
	Aortic occlusion balloon
	Time aorta cross-clamped
	Elevated activated partial thromboplastin time
Post-operative	Length of ICU stay
	PEEP score
	SIRS score
	pH <7.3

Table 3. Risk Factors for Intra-abdominal Hypertension

3.5 Diagnosis

Intra-abdominal pressure typically is at the highest level within 48 hours post-operatively.
Using intra-vesical pressure to monitor for intra-abdominal hypertension is central to the diagnosis of IAP and ACS. Intra-vesical pressure directly corresponds to IAP making this an easy to use diagnostic modality. In monitoring pressure levels readings should be taken on an hourly basis. A standard Foley catheter is placed in the bladder and measurements are taken with volume priming of 25mls of normal saline in the supine position during end expiration. The mid-axillary line serves as the zero reference point. Other parameters that warrant monitoring include the hourly urine output, lactate dehydrogenase levels and other markers of metabolic acidosis and respiratory function.

3.6 Management

The management approach for IAP needs to be proactive because if left untreated it may progress to ACS. Once there is a suspicion that ACS may develop prompt and concise management of the condition is warranted.
Some studies have reported avoiding the use of anti-coagulants, such as systemic heparin, in particular after EVAR in an attempt to reduce and limit the on-going bleeding that can occur from collateral vessels as a result of this procedure (Mehta, 2010). The thought process behind this is that continuous bleeding from collateral vessels can lead to a rise in IAP post-operatively. Other factors to consider are care with fluid administration and a trial of neuromuscular blockade in patients with the milder grades of raised IAP as a conservative approach.
Prevention is better than cure, and there is variance in the importance given to IAP monitoring. Certain centres measure IAP both intra-operatively and post-operatively on an

hourly basis. With a raised IAP, regardless of the presence of other associated risk factors, there is a drive towards recommending that these patients undergo decompression laparotomy (Mehta, 2010). Other studies have examined the role of leaving the abdomen open as a routine prophylactic measure against ACS. The open abdomen technique post AAA repair to safeguard against ACS was first described by Fietsman (Fietsman et al, 1989). It has a particularly relevant role following open repair for a ruptured aneurysm. Recording an intra-operative abdominal pressure of 12mmHg or above is described as an indication for this (Mayer et al, 2009). Here, it has been shown that in cases of ruptured AAA there is a 30% reduction in mortality associated with ACS using this technique (Mayer et al, 2009).

Management of ACS involves a decompression laparotomy as a matter of urgency. With this there are a number of different options available for further management. One option is the use of a plastic bag (Bogota bag) and a conventional secondary dressing as a temporary closure measure. Another option for temporary closure is the use of a vacuum-assisted closure (VAC) system (V.A.C., KCI International Inc, Amstelveen, The Netherlands). The exact underlying pathophysiological manner in which vacuum assisted closure devices work is not completely understood. It has been demonstrated that vacuum-assisted closure devices do exert anti-microbial activity (Morykwas et al, 1997) and they also stimulate granulation tissue formation (Moisidis et al, 2004; Morykwas et al, 2001). The device is thought to prevent abdominal wall retraction and as a result adds stability to the abdominal wall. In addition a vacuum-assisted closure device drains the excess intra-peritoneal fluid faster than a Bogota bag and therefore results in a faster decrease in IAP. This assists the patient in their recovery process and it also allows earlier closure of the abdomen.

The decision on the type of temporary closure device to use is made based on factors such as the volume of the intra-abdominal organs protruding from the abdomen following decompression laparotomy and a worry that bowel ischaemia leading to necrosis may occur in the patient. The use of a simple sterile plastic drape or bag allows for direct visualisation of the bowel and other intra-abdominal contents and is a convenient manner of observing for impending bowel ischaemia in a patient where this is a significant concern. A Bogota bag serves the same purpose, however it also has extra reserve capacity in that it allows for further intra-abdominal swelling to take place without impacting on venous return to the heart and general visceral perfusion (Mayer et al, 2009). In cases where a simple plastic bag or drape or the Bogota bag has been employed these temporary closure devices can be changed to a VAC closure device or a zip device at a later stage. This is generally undertaken when the patient is clinically stable, their organ dysfunction is improving and their intra-abdominal pressure remains stable or is decreasing. In patients with a VAC or zip device a high level of monitoring of IAP is required to ensure that the patient doesn't deteriorate and develop ACS again (Mayer et al, 2009).

The use of temporary closure devices or a staged or delayed closure in general is associated with an increased risk of ventral hernias, incisional hernias and fistulas.

A situation may arise where eventual direct closure of the abdomen is not feasible. This can occur in patients with a prolonged history of unresolving ACS that may have been complicated with infection. The options available at this stage include; the formation of a bilateral anterior rectus abdominus sheath turnover flap (Kushimoto et al, 2007). However, in the vast majority of cases the abdomen can be closed successfully after a median of ten days post laparostomy.

A delay in managing ACS is associated with a high mortality. It is also closely linked with ischaemic colitis. This in itself in patients who require a delayed decompression laparotomy and mesh closure is reported at 40%, compared with 6% in patients with early mesh abdominal closure for open ruptured AAA repair.

4. Secondary Aorto-enteric Fistula

4.1 Incidence

Secondary aortoenteric fistula (SAF) is one of the most dreaded of aortic graft complications. The incidence of SAF has increased since the introduction of prosthetic graft materials. It was first described by Brock in 1953 after homograft aortic repair (Walker et al, 1986).
The incidence has been reported as being between 0.3 - 2.0% (Kuestner et al, 1995; Menawat et al, 1997). There is a very high rate of surgical mortality associated with this complication with rates of 25 - 90% reported (Kuestner et al, 1995; Menawat et al, 1997). Heberer is credited with the first successful repair of such a fistula in 1957 (Walker et al, 1986). Overall the outcome associated with this complication is generally poor. It does occur in the endovascular setting but to a lesser extent (Bergqvist et al, 2008).

4.2 Aetiology

With open repair of AAA the aetiology is attributed to the formation of a pseudoaneurysm at the graft anastomosis, subclinical graft infection or mechanical factors related to the graft.
In the case of EVAR the formation of a secondary fistula is related to mechanical stent failure, or, distortion or migration of the stent (Janne et al, 2000; Norgren et al, 1998). Endotension has also been described to play a role. It can cause pressure necrosis of the wall of the aneurysm and the small bowel. Endotension, accelerating pressure necrosis, can occur secondary to an undetected or a subclinical endoleak or secondary to the transmission of pressure through a sealed thrombus (Ueno et al, 2006).
SAF is a rarer occurrence after endovascular repair as the adventitia of the aorta remains undisturbed. With EVAR there is no suture line or anastomosis and it is at these points where a fistula typically is found following open surgery.

4.3 Pathology

Injury to the bowel during dissection allows for fibrous contact between the bowel wall and the graft. This can result in a repetitive synchronous pulse traumatic injury. Mechanical erosion of prosthetic material into adjacent bowel most commonly occurs due to the lack of interposed retroperitoneal tissue or it can be associated with the excessive pulsation of a redundantly placed graft (Armstrong et al, 2005). The presence of an underlying graft infection, for example, staph epidermidis biofilm infection, can also lead to inflammatory adhesions and erosion (Bandyk et al, 1984).
The classical position of a SAF is described as being between the proximal aortic graft and the fourth part of the duodenum.

4.4 Risk factors

Risk factors for the formation of an aortoenteric fistula include; ruptured AAA repair, haematoma associated with surgical repair, thrombosis and wound infection. Other associated factors are male gender, increasing age and having an inflammatory or mycotic aneurysm.

With EVAR the most common complications are; endoleak and a migrated or kinked stent graft (Haussegser et al, 1999). These complications in turn add to the risk of developing a fistula. Coil embolization of an endoleak has also been reported as causing fistulae (Bertges et al, 2003).

4.5 Diagnosis

There is often a delay between the presentation and diagnosis of a SAF. The average interval between symptoms and presentation has been reported to be 47 days (range 8 - 180 days) (Armstrong et al, 2005). This is due to most investigative tests being negative or inconclusive. It is therefore very important to have a high index of suspicion for this condition. A poorer outcome is associated with a delay in recognition, diagnosis and definitive management.

There are two main patterns of presentation; bleeding and infection. A high index of suspicion is particularly required if the patient presents with what is known as a herald gastrointestinal bleed. Patients can also present with chronic melena, hematemesis or weight loss. However the typical presentation is with a herald bleed followed by a period of stability and then massive exsanguination and cardiovascular collapse. Patients presenting with symptoms and signs of sepsis can have fever, weight loss, an elevated white blood cell count and c-reactive protein, and abdominal or back pain indicating a retroperitoneal abscess.

Investigations include endoscopy, angiography and contrast studies. Angiography may be negative and at most show a small nipple at the anastomosis. The sensitivity of OGD for diagnosing a secondary aortoenteric fistula is less than 25%. Signs to be aware of on OGD include; fresh blood in the distal duodenum (often a paediatric colonoscope is required to advance this far), and visualising the graft in the base of the duodenal ulcer. To optimise diagnosis from CT investigation a high resolution, spiral, thin slice (3-5 mm) should be performed. On CT examination findings include; an obvious direct communication, loss of retroperitoneal soft tissue interposed between the overlying bowel and the proximal aortic graft, perigraft air and oedema. In patients following endovascular repair it often presents as a re-expanding AAA with associated inflammatory changes around the abdominal aorta (Ueno et al, 2006).

SAF can present as a late complication. The median time from primary operation to presentation has been reported to be two years (Bergqvist et al, 2008). One third of these patients that present late with the condition have been treated for hypovoleamic shock at some stage prior to diagnosis. This again underlines the importance of having a high index of suspicion for this clinical complication.

4.6 Management

A number of different operative approaches in the management of this complication have been described. Laparotomy is often performed in an emergent situation with the aim being to control bleeding, repair the fistula site, look for the source of infection and to reconstruct the vasculature. Primary repair may be useful in an elderly patient where you don't wish to subject them to a prolonged period of ischaemia due to aortic cross clamping. But this course of action doesn't address the underlying potential problem of a subclinical graft infection.

Traditionally, the management of SAF has involved the creation of an extra-anatomic bypass, with total excision of the graft and over-sewing of the aortic stump (Kuestner et al,

1995). The main objective of this type of surgery is to reduce the risk of infection. The bypass is usually tunnelled through non infected remote tissue planes that are generally axillobifemoral. The procedure itself has associated risks. The mortality rate is high at greater than 40%. There is a risk of a stump blow out rate of 16% and graft loss rates at one year of approximately 60%. Other associated complications include limb loss, and pelvic ischemia. It has also been reported to be the approach associated with the lowest mortality; however, this may be due to confounding factors such as performing the procedure in patients that are relatively heamodynamically stable and with little co-morbidity (Bergqvist et al, 2008).

Endovascular grafting has been successfully reported as a less invasive approach (Suzuki et al, 2005; Schlensak et al, 2000; Chuter et al, 2000). Endovascular grafting has also been successfully used as a temporary measure to control life threatening gastrointestinal bleeding allowing patient stability to be achieved. Endovascular repair is of benefit when the clinical status of the patient or their co-morbidities precludes open surgical intervention. This approach does not solve the underlying problem of the communication tract however. There have been reports on the use of N-butylcyanoacrylate in attempting to obliterate the tract (Finch & Heathcock, 2002). In the setting of an infection it is obviously a questionable method.

Other options that have been reported in the literature are omental patching and homografts. It is queried that both these approaches may have a role in controlling for post-operative infection (Vogt & Turina, 1999; Montgomery & Wilson, 1996). Staged procedures and the more conservative in situ graft replacement with antibiotic coated grafts have also been reported (Kavanagh et al, 2006; Reilly et al, 1987; Kieffer et al, 2004; Walker et al, 1986). In situ repair and revascularisation are associated with better outcomes in comparison to extra-anatomic bypass.

Following operative intervention a course of broad spectrum antibiotics covering for enteric flora is required. This is required in particular after graft replacement. The placement of a feeding jejunostomy at the time of operation should also be considered (Chenu 2009).

The risk of secondary rupture of the abdominal aorta following treatment for an aorto-enteric fistula has been reported as being between 9 and 17% (Kuestner et al, 1995; Menawat et al, 1997; Bergqvist et al, 1996). These figures add to the significant overall mortality risk associated with this complication.

5. Chylous ascites

5.1 Incidence

Chylous ascites is an unusual postoperative complication that can lead to significant mechanical, nutritional, and immunologic consequences for the patient. It can present following AAA repair. The incidence of chylous ascites following AAA repair has been reported to be between 0.03 - 0.1% (Pabst et al, 1993). The true incidence of this complication however is unknown as knowledge of it has mainly relied on case reports of which there have been 40 published to date in the literature.

5.2 Aetiology

It is hypothesised that dissection around the proximal infra-renal abdominal aorta can cause traumatic damage to the intestinal lymphatics and their recipients; the left lateral-aortic lymph nodes and the cisterna chyli. It is thought that cross clamping of the aorta may also contribute to the traumatic damage of the lymphatic system.

5.3 Pathology

There is a significant variation in the anatomy of the lymphatic channels in the abdomen. This can make it difficult to identify with ease the cisterna chyli and the other lymphatic channels. Identifying the lymphatic channels is made more difficult in the fasting state as there is a minimal amount of lymphatic fluid circulating through them. As a result they are easily lacerated during dissection. This can lead to stasis, fibrosis and rupture of the lymphatic channel into the aneurysmal wall which in turn can lead to the formation of an internal lymphatic fistula between the cisterna chyli or other main lymphatic trunks and the peritoneal cavity. It has been demonstrated that a partial or lateral tear in the cisterna chyli is less likely to heal and more likely to result in chylous ascites when compared to a complete transection, as a complete transection is more likely to spontaneously retract and seal itself off (McKenna & Stevick, 1983).

5.4 Risk factors

Chylous ascites occurs in 81% of cases secondary to AAA repair. Risk factors include upper or extensive dissection of the retroperitoneal space, difficult dissection following rupture of an AAA, an inflammatory aneurysm and previous abdominal aortic surgery. The presence of a proximal obstruction to the drainage of lymph from the abdomen is also an associated risk factor.

5.5 Diagnosis

Chylous ascites typically presents two weeks after AAA repair (Olthof et al, 2008). The mean presentation has been found to be 18.4 days (Sanger et al, 1991, Bahner & Townsend, 1990).
The most common signs and symptoms at presentation are abdominal distension and ascites following resumption of oral diet. The presence of intra-peritoneal fluid is confirmed by abdominal CT or ultrasound. The definitive diagnosis requires paracentesis. This reveals a lypaemic, sterile fluid which is milky in colour. Analysis of the fluid sample should demonstrate an alkaline pH, a total protein level of greater than 3 g/dl, total fat content between 0.4 and 4.0 g/dl and a predominance of lymphocytes on differential white blood count. If the patient is mechanically ventilated the diagnosis should be suspected in the presence of gradually progressing abdominal hypertension.
Other characteristic clinical features include a low serum albumin and a profound decrease in absolute lymphocyte count secondary to sequestration of lymphocytes into the ascitic fluid.

5.6 Management

The mortality rate associated with this condition has been reported to be as high as 18.5% (Garrett et al, 1989). However the literature also reports resolution in 60% of cases.
The goal of management is to reduce lymphatic flow. This is achieved with therapeutic paracenetesis combined with either total parenteral nutrition (TPN) or a medium chain triglyceride rich diet. For the first 14 days the patient should be kept nil per mouth and they should receive TPN. This is followed by a diet high in medium chain triglycerides. When this is commenced the TPN is weaned gradually. Abdominal girth measurement can aid monitor patient progress.
Second line treatment consists of placement of a peritoneovenous shunt. The main concern associated with shunt placement is sepsis. Operative ligation of the damaged lymphatic channel is another option. When operative ligation is undertaken it is important to ensure that the exact lymphatic leak is identified. This is difficult if the lymph fluid is clear. The use

of dye or feeding the patient cream pre-operatively have both been reported as aiding this process (Uchinami et al, 2005). Both these interventions are usually reserved for patients where conservative management has failed. Successful laparoscopic repair of the damaged lymphatic system has also been reported (Uchinami et al, 2005). The benefit of this approach is that it doesn't require as invasive surgery as open ligation and it reduces the risk of sepsis associated with shunt placement. Overall chylous ascites typically settles with the appropriate management.

6. Ileus

6.1 Incidence

Post-operative ileus is the most common complication to occur following abdominal surgery of any description. It is a problem that is difficult to prevent and is without solution. In the case of abdominal aortic repair it is both the most frequent gastrointestinal complication and overall post-operative complication. It occurs in up to 10% of patients (Sicard et al, 1995). On the other end of the spectrum mechanical obstruction of the small bowel, in particular, the duodenum, after abdominal aortic surgery is rare. Major studies have demonstrated that of patients undergoing AAA repair, small bowel obstruction occurred in 2.9%, with greater than 40% requiring operative intervention (Siporin et al, 1993).

6.2 Aetiology

Intra-operative handling of the bowel, and tissue trauma are thought to be the main causes of post-operative ileus. The use of foreign materials for example gauze swabs, the formation of haematomas and aneurysmal sac seromas also contribute. Superior mesenteric artery syndrome, where the duodenum is compressed between the retroperitoneum and the superior mesenteric artery as a result of a retroperitoneal haematoma is associated with ileus. This can also progress to mechanical bowel obstruction if left untreated. Adhesions however, are the most common cause of mechanical bowel obstruction.

6.3 Pathology

Many studies suggest that ileus is the result of an inhibition of intestinal contractility (Smith et al, 1977). Other studies show continued but uncoordinated contractions (Dauchel et al, 1976). The jejunum has been shown to be the main area of small bowel affected by a change in the pattern of bowel contractility following AAA repair (Miedema et al, 2002).
Oedema of the bowel wall results in ileus. The bowel wall becomes oedematous secondary to dissection, manipulation trauma and direct handling of the small bowel intra-operatively. This in turn stimulates an inflammatory cascade which is thought to cause an increase in the sympathetic response to the gastrointestinal tract.
There are two approaches the surgeon can take in open repair of an AAA; transabdominal and retroperitoneal. The transabdominal approach has been reported to be associated with a greater percentage of prolonged ileus and bowel obstruction post-operatively (Kudo et al, 2004) when compared with the retroperitoneal approach.

6.4 Risk factors

Studies have demonstrated that the longer the operative time and the greater the volume of intra-operative blood loss the greater the correlation with post-operative ileus and specifically the delayed passage of flatus (Miedema et al, 2002). Other factors that have also been found to be associated with post-operative ileus include hypoalbuminea, hypoproteinaemia and the presence of additional gastro-intestinal pathologies such as pancreatitis post-operatively. The length of the abdominal skin incision for abdominal aortic aneurysm repair has been determined to impact on the presence of ileus and time to return to normal diet. Hiromatsu and colleagues established that those patients with a skin incision of less than 15cm had a significantly smaller incidence of ileus when compared to a group of patients that had a skin incision of greater than 20cm (Hiromatsu et al, 2007). Laparoscopic repair has also demonstrated a shorter period of ileus and a quicker return to diet when compared to open repair (Coggia et al, 2005).

6.5 Diagnosis

Postoperative ileus is classically characterized by impaired intestinal motility and transit, absence of the passage of flatus, diminished bowel sounds, abdominal distension and intestinal dilatation. A patient with ileus typically presents with abdominal pain, nausea, and vomiting. On examination the abdomen is often distended and tender. The signs and symptoms typically are present within 24-48 hours post-operatively or when the patient attempts a return to fluids and diet. It can also present up to two weeks post the procedure.

Imaging such as plain x-rays of the abdomen and contrast studies aid in determining the extent of the ileus or obstruction. In the case of a non-resolving ileus or a suspected bowel obstruction a CT scan allows the underlying cause to be determined. If on CT scanning a cause is not found then it is most likely an adhesion that is causing the problem (Tessier et al, 2003).

A prolonged post-operative ileus is a significant contributor to postoperative morbidity and mortality (Johnson, 1989). This is particularly true of non-ruptured AAA repair. The presence of post-operative ileus slows the patients return to normal function. It results in a delayed discharge and is associated with the risk of other morbidities.

6.6 Management

Initial management should be conservative and involves the placement of a nasogastric (NG) tube which is left on free drainage and intravenous hydration. The patient should remain nil per mouth until the symptoms settle and drainage from the NG is minimal.

Determining the underlying cause can aid in planning management. If a specific cause is known for example, a haematoma, this should be drained or treated to allow resolution of symptoms. Where the symptoms do not settle after a period of greater than two weeks, typically operative intervention is required. Often the procedure is adhesiolysis. This in turn however increases the risk of wound infection and dehiscence, general sepsis and fistula formation post-operatively.

Some surgeons place a NG tube at the time of surgery in an effort to reduce nausea and vomiting. This is not evidence based but more associated with traditional practice.

Studies have examined the use of novel bioresorbable materials made from chemically modified hyaluronate acid and carboxymethylcellulose. These materials form a physicochemical barrier to prevent adhesion between adjacent tissue surfaces for up to seven days after surgery (Kudo et al, 2004).

The vast majority of patients (>80%) that are managed conservatively settle within a two week window and do not require surgical intervention (Tessier et al, 2003). Patients that ultimately require surgical intervention do so after a median duration of ten days conservative management (Tessier et al, 2003).

7. Acute pancreatitis

7.1 Incidence

Acute pancreatitis is a rare but recognised complication of AAA surgery. The true incidence of this condition is unknown and has been reliant on the reporting of case series in the surgical literature. It has been stated that the incidence is approximately 0.7% in open repair (Hashimoto & Walsh, 1999). In the presence of diabetes the incidence increases to 5% (Ryan et al, 2002). There has only been one case report, which the authors are aware of, to date with EVAR (James et al, 2008). One of the factors affecting the under-reporting of this complication is the often associated lack of a rise in amylase levels that can be found in particular with severe cases of pancreatitis.

7.2 Aetiology

The aetiology of acute pancreatitis specifically following AAA repair is not clear. One proposed theory is that of micro-emboli entering the pancreatic circulation leading to ischemia of the pancreas post-operatively (James et al, 2008). Another proposed aetiology is whereby aortic cross clamping, especially at the level of the supra-renal aorta, can result in peri-operative trauma which in turn leads to trauma and an inflammatory response.

7.3 Pathology

The spectrum of acute pancreatitis that has been described following AAA repair has varied from mild pancreatitis to more severe cases that are associated with pancreatic necrosis and a high mortality rate. In greater than 75% of known cases the pancreatitis was mild and the patients experienced a full recovery. Those patients however, that develop severe pancreatitis have been reported in one review as having a 100% mortality (Hashimoto & Walsh, 1999). This was due to multi-organ dysfunction and pancreatic necrosis. Conversely, as a point of interest, abdominal aortic aneurysms have been diagnosed following acute pancreatitis. This phenomenon is thought to be related to the release of enzymes such as elastase that cause lysis of the elastic component of the arterial vessel wall.

7.4 Risk factors

There are two known associated risk factors; (i) emergency surgery following a ruptured AAA and (ii) having diabetes mellitus (Ryan et al, 2002).

7.5 Diagnosis

The diagnosis of acute pancreatitis post-operatively is frequently associated with a delay. A raised amylase level often is just seen in mild cases of pancreatitis. In more severe cases of acute pancreatitis the amylase level can remain normal. Severe cases are usually picked up after a period of unexplained sepsis in a clinically deteriorating patient (Hashimoto & Walsh, 1999). On average severe cases of acute pancreatitis are diagnosed approximately two weeks following the initial aortic aneurysm surgery. Therefore a high index of suspicion is required for this complication in patients that develop signs and symptoms of sepsis post-operatively. The diagnosis is made using CT imaging. Features seen on CT include; diffuse or segmental pancreatic enlargement, irregularity or heterogeneity and lobularity of the pancreas, and obliteration of the peri-pancreatic fat planes. CT also allows areas of pancreatic necrosis to be detected. The presence of necrosis significantly impacts on the prognosis for the patient and is associated with a high rate of mortality.

7.6 Management

The management of acute pancreatitis following AAA repair adheres to the general supportive treatment protocol of bowel rest and intravenous fluid therapy, analgesia and nutritional support. Close monitoring for sepsis and multi-organ failure is also of importance. Regular CT scanning should be employed to monitor for disease progression and to screen for pancreatic necrosis. Assessment of severity should be carried out using pre-defined criteria such as Ranson and APACGE II severity scores. This allows modification of management protocols and risk stratification.

The mortality rate has been reported as ranging from 40% to an absolute level of 100% in severe cases of acute pancreatitis (Hashimoto & Walsh, 1999). With respect to preventing the development of acute pancreatitis post-operatively one proposition has been to perform an incidental cholecystectomy in patients with known cholelithiasis at the time of AAA repair (Hashimoto & Walsh, 1999). However, this intervention may be somewhat excessive as overall, acute pancreatitis, is a rare gastrointestinal complication of AAA surgery.

8. Acute colecystitis

8.1 Incidence

The incidence of acute cholecystitis has been reported as varying between 0.3 - 18% (Cadot et al, 2002). Overall acute cholecystitis complicating AAA repair is accepted to be a rare event.

8.2 Aetiology

Cholesterol crystallisation occurs in association with atherosclerotic disease. Patients with an AAA often will have atherosclerosis and therefore are predisposed to cholesterol gallstones. Often these are asymptomatic and therefore undiagnosed pre AAA repair. Embolization of cholesterol crystals can lead to ischaemia of the gallbladder which in turn is a cause of cholecystitis. Low flow states, such as hypovolaemia, may also cause gallbladder wall ischaemia and therefore cholecystitis. Following AAA surgery patients may also be at risk of developing acalculus cholecystitis.

8.3 Pathology

Cholecystitis may occur secondary to the presence of gallstones which can obstruct the cystic duct or other parts of the biliary tree or it may occur in the absence of calculi (acalculus choleystitis). Acalculus cholecystitis is more commonly found in critically ill patients and has a higher morbidity and mortality rate associated with it when compared to gallstone disease. It is also associated with a higher incidence of gallbladder perforation and gangrene. In the setting of AAA surgery the main pathophysiological process is thought to be due to bile stasis and the increased lithogenicity of bile. AAA patients are more predisposed to acalculus cholecystitis because of increased bile viscosity due to dehydration and blood loss. In patients that have a prolonged recovery where there is a delay in the return to normal diet a decrease in cholecystokinin-induced gallbladder contractions may result leading to bile stasis and a risk of cholecystitis.

8.4 Risk factors

Male gender, increasing age, emergency surgery, post-operative sepsis and hypotension or hypovolaemia are risk factors for acalculus cholecystitis. The presence of gallstones pre-operatively is a risk factor for calculus acute cholecystitis.

8.5 Diagnosis

Patients classically complain of right upper quadrant pain, nausea, vomiting and fever and on examination have abdominal tenderness, deranged liver function tests and an elevated white blood cell count. Having a high index of suspicion for acalculus disease is important as this complication has a worse prognosis and requires a more aggressive approach to treatment. The imaging modality of choice is ultrasound scanning. Features of gallbladder disease include; thickening of the gallbladder wall (>3mm), the presence of stones and pericholecystitic fluid.

Acute acalculous cholecystitis is the most common postoperative biliary complication after aortic surgery. The diagnosis should be entertained in patients with signs of abdominal sepsis after aortic surgery, especially those with a complicated postoperative course. Even if acute acalculous cholecystitis is diagnosed with ease, mortality remains high (Hagino et al, 1997).

8.6 Management

Acute cholecystitis is managed with intravenous fluid therapy, antibiotics and analgesia. The definitive treatment involves either (i) removal of the gallstones through ERCP or surgical removal of the gallbladder or (ii) the performance of a percutaneous cholecystostomy, which may be the treatment method of choice in patients that are otherwise too ill for surgical intervention.

There are centres that recommend a pre procedure cholecystectomy in patients with known cholelithiasis. The reasoning for this is that symptomatic gallbladder disease post-operatively is a significant contributor to morbidity and mortality when it occurs in a patient post AAA repair (D'Angelo et al, 1999).

9. Peptic Ulcer Disease

9.1 Incidence

The incidence of peptic ulcer disease (PUD) directly related to AAA repair is rare to begin with (0.9%) and its incidence has been further reduced by the routine incorporation of proton pump inhibitors (PPI's) into the management protocols of patients following AAA surgery (Achouh et al, 2006). In the literature there is a paucity of information on peptic ulcer disease associated with AAA, with the majority of reports having being published before the new millennium.

9.2 Aetiology

PUD after AAA surgery is theorized to be associated with (i) a decrease in gastric mucosal blood flow and (ii) the consumptive coagulopathy that can occur due to blood loss and the systemic inflammatory response that results from an AAA (Konno et al, 1991). This is particularly true following emergency surgery for a ruptured aneurysm and in patients with underlying co-morbidities pre-operatively.

9.3 Pathology

It has been found that a reduction in blood flow to the gastric mucosa and a rise in the prostaglandin content of the gastric mucosa both contribute to the development of PUD post AAA repair (Konno et al, 1994).

9.4 Risk factors

Risk factors include; previously treated PUD, ruptured AAA repair, coagulopathy (such as thrombocytopenia, altered thromboplastin time, reduction in fibrinogen levels), the volume of blood lost and the presence of DIC or SIRS post-operatively.

9.5 Diagnosis

In a patient with suspected PUD an OGD should be performed allowing direct visualisation of the peptic ulcer. At OGD biopsies should be taken to test for H. Pylori bacteria. OGD also allows for complications of PUD such, as bleeding, to be effectively managed.

9.6 Management

Symptomatic PUD, where the patient complains of epigastric pain, reflux symptoms and nausea can be treated with a course of PPI's. If H. Pylori is found to be present the patient requires a course of triple therapy. Active bleeding from a peptic ulcer needs to be expediently managed. This can be done at endoscopy using the injection of adrenaline to control bleeding. Surgical intervention is nowadays rarely necessary.

In the era before the regular use of PPI's, PUD in the setting of AAA repair was associated with a significant mortality, with reports of a mortality rate up to 30% (Achouh et al, 2006). Thankfully, although PUD may complicate the post-operative recovery pathway of the patient its overall morbidity and mortality has been significantly reduced.

10. Conclusion

All of the gastrointestinal complications discussed in this chapter require us, as physicians, to have a high index of suspicion for and knowledge of, following repair of an AAA. Although some of the complications we have detailed are rare in incidence they impact significantly on patient outcome, morbidity and mortality. The key gastrointestinal complications to be aware of following AAA surgery are ischaemic colitis, abdominal compartment syndrome and ileus. The introduction of EVAR has had a positive impact on the rate of some gastrointestinal complications, in other cases it has led to different pathophysiological pathways. As our knowledge base relies on literature reports it remains as yet to be seen what the full impact of endovascular surgery will have on outcomes following AAA repair in both the elective and emergent setting.

11. References

Achouh PE, Madsen K, Miller CC 3rd, Estrera AL, Azizzadeh A, Dhareshwar J, Porat E & Safi HJ (2006). Gastrointestinal complications after descending thoracic and thoracoabdominal aortic repairs: a 14-year experience. *J Vasc Surg*. Vol. 44, No. 3, pp. 442-6.

Armstrong PA, Back MR, Wilson JS, Shames ML, Johnson BL, & Bandyk DF (2005). Improved outcomes in the recent management of secondary aortoenteric fistula. *J Vasc Surg*, Vol. 42, pp. 660-6.

Assadian A, Senekowitsch C, Assadian O, Hartleb H, & Hagmüller GW (2008). Diagnostic accuracy of sigmoidoscopy compared with histology for ischemic colitis after aortic aneurysm repair. *Vascular*. Vol. 16, No. 5, pp. 243-7.

Bahner Jr DR, & Townsend R (1990). Chylous ascites after ruptured abdominal aortic aneurysm. *Contemp Surg*, Vol. 36, pp. 37-9.

Bandyk DF, Berni GA, Thiele BL, & Towne JB (1984). Aortofemoral graft infection due to Staphylococcus Epidermidis. *Arch Surg*, Vol. 119, pp. 102-8.

Becquemin JP, Majewski M, Fermani N, Marzelle J, Desgrandes P, Allaire E, & Roudat-Thoraval F (2008). Colon ischemia following abdominal aortic aneurysm repair in the era of endovascular abdominal aortic repair. *J Vasc Surg*, Vol. 47, pp. 258-63.

Bergqvist D, Bjorkman H, Bolin T, Dalman P, Elfstrom J, Forsberg O, Johansen L, Karacagil S, Karlqvist PA, Lanne T, Plate G, Ribbe E, Spangen L, Stenbeck J, Thomsen M, Wiklund B, & Angquist KA (1996). Secondary aorto-enteric fistulae - changes from 1973 to 1993. *Eur J Vasc Endovasc Surg*, Vol, 11, pp. 425-8.

Bergqvist D, Björck M, & Nyman R (2008). Secondary aortoenteric fistula after endovascular aortic interventions: a systematic literature review. *J Vasc Interv Radiol*. Vol. 19, No. 2, Pt. 1, pp. 163-5.

Bertges DJ, Villella ER, & Makaroun MS (2003). Aortoenteric fistula due to endoleak coil embolization after endovascular AAA repair. *J Endovasc Ther*, Vol, 10, pp. 130-135.

Björck M, Wanhainen A, Djavani K, & Acosta S (2008). The clinical importance of monitoring intra-abdominal pressure after ruptured abdominal aortic aneurysm repair. *Scand J Surg*. Vol. 97, No. 2, pp. 183-90.

Björck M, Bergqvist D, & Troëng T (1996). Incidence and clinical presentation of bowel ischaemia after aortoiliac surgery--2930 operations from a population-based registry in Sweden. *Eur J Vasc Endovasc Surg*. Vol. 12, No. 2, pp. 139-44.

Bosch TJA, Teijink JA, Willigendael EM, & Prins MH (2010). Endovascular aneurysm repair is superior to open surgery for ruptured abdominal aortic aneurysms in EVAR-suitable patients. J Vasc Surg. Vol. 52, No. 1, pp. 13-8.

Cadot H, Addis MD, Faries PL, Carroccio A, Burks JA, Gravereaux EC, Morrissey NJ, Teodorescu V, Sparacino S, Hollier LH, & Marin ML (2002). Abdominal aortic aneurysmorrhaphy and cholelithiasis in the era of endovascular surgery. *Am Surg*, Vol. 68, No. 10, pp. 839-843.

Champagne BJ, Darling RC, Daneshmand M, Kreienberg PB, Lee EC, Mehta M, Roddy SP, Chang BB, Paty PS, Ozsvath KJ, & Shah DM (2004). Outcome of aggressive surveillance colonoscopy in ruptured abdominal aortic aneurysm. *J Vasc Surg*, Vol. 39, pp. 792-6.

Chen JC, Hildebrand HD, Salvian AJ, Taylor DC, Strandberg S, Myckatyn TM, & Hsiang YN (1996). Predictors of death in nonruptured and ruptured abdominal aortic aneurysms. *J Vasc Surg*, Vol. 24, pp. 614-20.

Chenu C, Marcheix B, Barcelo C, & Rousseau H (2009). Aorto-enteric Fistula After Endovascular Abdominal Aortic Aneurysm Repair: Case Report and Review. *Eur J Vasc Endovasc Surg*. Vol. 37, pp. 401-40.

Chuter TA, Lukaszewicz GC, Reilly LM, Kerlan RK, Faruqi R, Sawhney R, Wall SD, Canto C, LaBerge JM, Gordon RL, & Messina LM (2000). Endovascular repair of a presumed aortoenteric fistula: late failure due to recurrent infection. *J Endovasc Ther*. Vol. 7, pp. 240-4.

Coggia M, Javerliat I, Di Centa I, Alfonsi P, Colacchio G, Kitzis M, & Goeau-Brissonniere O (2005). Total laparoscopic versus conventional abdominal aortic aneurysm repair: A case-control study. *J Vasc Surg*. Vol. 42, No. 5, pp. 906-910.

D'Angelo AJ, Kline RG, Faust GR, & Cohen JR (1999). Cholecystectomy during abdominal aortic aneurysm repair in patients with gallstones. *Vasc Surg*. Vol. 33, No. 6, pp. 705-710.

Dauchel J, Schang JC, Kachelhoffer J, Eloy R, & Grenier JF (1976). Gastrointestinal and myoelectric activity during the postoperative period in man. *Digestion*, Vol. 14, pp. 293-303.

Djavani K, Wanhainen A, Valtysson J, & Bjorck M (2009). Colonic ischaemia and intra-abdominal hypertension following open repair of ruptured abdominal aortic aneurysm. *BJS*, Vol. 96, pp. 621–627.

Elmarasy NM, Soong CV, Walker SR, Macierewicz JA, Yusuf SW, Wenham PW, & Hopkinson BR (2000). Sigmoid ischemia and the inflammatory response following endovascular abdominal aortic aneurysm repair. *J Endovasc Ther*. Vol. 7, pp. 21-30.

Fietsam R Jr, Villalba M, Glover JL, & Clark K (1989). Intra-abdominal compartment syndrome as a complication of ruptured abdominal aortic aneurysm repair. *Am Surg*. Vol. 6, pp. 396-402.

Finch L, & Heathcock B (2002). Emergent treatment of a primary aorto-enteric fistula with N-butyl 2-cyanoacrylate and endovascular stent.*J Vasc Intery Radiol*. Vol. 13, pp. 841-843.

Garrett HE Jr, Richardson JW, Howard HS, & Garrett HE (1989). Retroperitoneal lymphocele after abdominal aortic surgery. *J Vasc Surg*, Vol. 10, pp. 245–53.

Geraghty PJ, Sanchez LA, Rubin BG, Choi ET, Flye MW, Curci JA, Thompson RW, & Sicard GA (2004). Overt ischemic colitis after endovascular repair of aortoiliac aneurysms. *J Vasc Surg*. Vol. 40, pp. 413-8.

Geroulakos G, & Cherry Jr KJ. (2002) *Diseases of the visceral circulation*. Chapter: Ischaemic Colitis. Pages: 193 - 207. Arnold Publishers. ISBN 0340807229(hb). Great Britain.

Hagino RT, Valentine RJ, & Clagett GP (1997). Acalculous cholecystitis after aortic reconstruction. *J Am Coll Surg*. Vol. 184, No. 3, pp. 245-248.

Hashimoto L, & Walsh RM (1999). Acute pancreatitis after aortic surgery. *Am Surg*. Vol. 65, No. 5, pp. 423-426.

Hausegger KA, Tiesenhausen K, Karaic R, Tauss J, & Koch G (1999). Aortoduodenal fistula: a late complication of intraluminal exclusion of an infrarenal aortic aneurysm. *J Vasc Interv Radiol*, Vol. 10, pp. 747-750.

Hiromatsu S, Egawa N, Hosokawa Y, Ishihara K, Yokokura H, Tanaka A, & Aoyagi S (2007). A shorter skin incision technique for the repair of infrarenal abdominal aortic aneurysms. *Surg Today*. Vol. 37, No. 2, pp. 97-102.

James AD, Anderson HJ, Edwards R, & Sandison AJ (2008). Pancreatitis as a Complication of Endovascular Aneurysm Repair. *Eur J Vasc Endovasc Surg*, Vol. 35, pp. 310-311.

Janne d'Othee B, Soula P, Otal P, Cahill M, Joffle F, Cerene A, & Rousseau H (2000). Aorto-duodenal fistula after endovascular stent graft of an abdominal aortic aneurysm. *J Vasc Surg*, Vol. 31, pp. 190–5.

Johnson KW (1989). Multicenter prospective study of non-ruptured abdominal aortic aneurysm. Part II. Variables predicting morbidity and mortality. *J Vasc Surg*, Vol. 9, pp. 437-47.

Junnarkar S, Lau LL, Edrees WK, Underwood D, Smye MG, Lee B, Hannon RJ, & Soong CV (2003). Cytokine activation and intestinal mucosal and renal dysfunction are reduced in endovascular AAA repair compared to surgery. *J Endovasc Ther*. Vol. 10, pp. 195-202.

Kavanagh DO, Dowdall JF, Younis F, Sheehan S, Mehigan D, & Barry MC (2006). Aorto-enteric fistula: changing management strategies. *Ir J Med Sc*. Vol. 175, No. 1, pp. 40-44.

Kieffer E, Gomes D, Chiche L, Fleron MH, Koskas F, & Bahnini A (2004). Allograft replacement for infrarenal aortic graft infection: early and late results in a 179 patients. *J Vasc Surg*, Vol. 39, pp. 1009-17.

Konno H, Kaneko H, Maruo Y, Tatuo T, Nobuhiko N, Nakamura S, & Baba S (1994). Prevention of gastric-ulcer or acute gastric-mucosal lesions accompanying bleeding after abdominal aortic-aneurysm surgery. *W J Surg*, Vol. 18, No. 6, pp. 944-947.

Konno H, Sakaguchi S, & Hachiya T (1991). Bleeding peptic-ulcer after abdominal aortic-aneurysm surgery. *Arch Surg*, Vol. 126, No. 7, pp. 894-897.

Kudo FA, Nishibe T, Miyazaki K, Murashita T, Nishibe M, & Yasuda K (2004). Use of Bioresorbable Membrane to Prevent Postoperative Small Bowel Obstruction in Transabdominal Aortic Aneurysm Surgery. *Surg Today*, Vol. 34, pp. 648–651.

Kuestner LM, Reilly LM, Jicha DL, Ehrenfeld WK, Goldstone J, & Stoney RJ (1995). Secondary aortoenteric fistula: contemporary outcome with use of extraanatomic bypass and infected graft excision. *J Vasc Surg*, Vol. 21, pp. 184-96.

Kushimoto S, Yamamoto Y, Aiboshi J, Ogawa F, Koido Y, Yoshida R, & Kawai M (2007). Usefulness of the bilateral anterior rectus abdominis sheath turnover flap method for early fascial closure in patients requiring open abdominal management. *World J Surg*, Vol. 1, pp. 2-8.

Levison JA, Halpern VJ, Kline RG, Faust GR, & Cohen JR (1999). Perioperative predictors of colonic ischemia after ruptured abdominal aortic aneurysm. *J Vasc Surg*, Vol. 1, pp. 40-5.

Makar RR, Badger SA, O'Donnell ME, Loan W, Lau LL, & Soong CV (2009). The effects of abdominal compartment hypertension after open and endovascular repair of a ruptured abdominal aortic aneurysm *J Vasc Surg*, Vol. 49, pp. 866-72.

Mayer D, Rancic Z, Meier C, Pfammatter T, Veith FJ, & Lachat M (2009). Open abdomen treatment following endovascular repair of ruptured abdominal aortic aneurysms. *Vasc Surg*, Vol. 50, pp. 1-7.

McKenna R, & Stevick CA (1983). Chylous ascites following aortic reconstruction. *Vasc Surg*, Vol. 17, pp. 143-9.

Mehta M (2010). Endovascular aneurysm repair for ruptured abdominal aortic aneurysm: The Albany Vascular Group approach. *J Vasc Surg*, Vol. 52, pp. 1706-12.

Menawat SS, Gloviczki P, Serry RD, Cherry KJ Jr, Bower TC, & Hallett JW Jr (1997). Management of aortic graft-enteric fistulae. *Eur J Vasc Endovasc Surg*, Vol. Suppl A, pp. 74-81.

Miedema BW, Schillie S, Simmons JW, Burgess SV, Liem T, & Silver D (2002). Small bowel motility and transit after aortic surgery. *J Vasc Surg*, Vol. 36, pp. 19-24.

Mitchell KM, & Valentine RJ (2002). Inferior mesenteric artery reimplantation does not guarantee colon viability in aortic surgery. *J Am Coll Surg*. Vol. 194, No. 2, pp. 151-5.

Moisidis E, Heath T, Boorer C, Ho K, & Deva AK (2004). A prospective, blinded, randomized, controlled clinical trial of topical negative pressure use in skin grafting. *Plast Reconstr Surg, Vol.* 4, pp. 917-22.

Montgomery RS, & Wilson SE (1996). The surgical management of aortoenteric fistulas. *Surg Clin North Am, Vol.* 76, pp. 1147-57.

Morykwas MJ, Argenta LC, Shelton-Brown EI, & McGuirt W (1997). Vacuum-assisted closure: a new method for wound control and treatment: animal studies and basic foundation. *Ann Plast Surg, Vol.* 6, pp. 553-62.

Morykwas MJ, Faler BJ, Pearce DJ, & Argenta LC (2001). Effects of varying levels of subatmospheric pressure on the rate of granulation tissue formation in experimental wounds in swine. *Ann Plast Surg*, Vol. 5, pp. 547-51.

Neary P, Hurson C, Briain DO, Brabazon A, Mehigan D, Keaveny TV, & Sheehan S (2007). Abdominal aortic aneurysm repair and colonic infarction: a risk factor appraisal. *Colorectal Disease*, Vol. 9, No. 2, pp. 166–172.

Norgren L, Jernby B, & Engellau L (1998). Aortoenteric fistula caused by a ruptured stent-graft: a case report. *J Endovasc Surg, Vol.* 5, pp. 269–72.

Olthof E, Blankensteijn JD, & Akkersdijk GJM (2008). Chyloperitoneum Following Abdominal Aortic Surgery. *Vasc*, Vol. 16, No. 5, pp. 258-262.

Pabst TS, McIntyre KE Jr, Jr., Schilling JD, Hunter GC, & Bernhard VM (1993). Management of Chyloperitoneum After Abdominal Aortic Surgery. *Am J Surg*, Vol. 66, pp. 194-199.

Perry RJT, Martin MJ, Eckert MJ, Sohn VY, & Steele SR (2008). Colonic ischemia complicating open vs endovascular abdominal aortic aneurysm repair. *J Vasc Surg*, Vol. 48, pp. 272-7.

Rayan SS, Hamadan AD, Campbell DR, Akbari CM, Hook SC, Skillman J, LoGerfo FW, & Pomposelli FB Jr (2002). Is diabetes a risk factor for patients undergoing open abdominal aortic aneurysm repair? *Vasc Endovascular Surg*, Vol. 36, No. 1, pp. 33-40.

Reilly LM, Stoney RJ, Goldstone J, & Ehrenfeld WK (1987). Improved management of aortic graft infection: the influence of operation sequence and staging. *J Vasc Surg*, Vol. 5, pp. 421-31.

Sanger R, Wilmshurst CC, & Clyne CAC (1999). Chylous ascites following aneurysm surgery. *Eur J Vasc Surg*, Vol. 5, pp. 689-92.

Schlensak C, Doenst T, Spillner G, Blum U, Geiger A, & Beyersdorf F (2000). Palliative treatment of a secondary aortoduodenal fistula by stent graft placement. *Thorac Cardiovsac Surg*, Vol. 48, pp. 41-2.

Senekowitsch C, Assadian A, Assadian O, Hartleb H, Ptakovsky H, & Hagmüller GW (2006). Replanting the inferior mesentery artery during infrarenal aortic aneurysm repair: Influence on postoperative colon ischemia. *J Vasc Surg*, Vol. 43, pp. 689-94.

Sicard GA, Reilly JM, Rubin BG, Thompson RW, Allen BT, Flye MW, Schechtman KB, Young-Beyer P, Weiss C, & Anderson CB (1995). Transabdominal versus retroperitoneal incision for abdominal aortic surgery: report of a prospective randomized trial. *J Vasc Surg*, Vol. 21, pp. 174-81.

Siporin K, Hiatt JR, & Treiman RL (1993). Small bowel obstruction after abdominal aortic surgery. *Am Surg*, Vol. 59, pp. 846-9.

Smith J, Kelly KA, & Weinshilboum RM (1977). Pathophysiology of postoperative ileus. *Arch Surg*, Vol. 112, pp. 203-9.

Suzuki S, Imoto K, Uchida K, Haskiyama N, & Takanashi Y (2005). Endovascular Repair of a Presumed Aortoduodenal Fistula. *Ann Thorac Cardiovasc Surg*, Vol. 11, pp. 424-8.

Tessier DJ, & Brophy CM (2003). Causes, diagnosis, and management of duodenal obstruction after aortic surgery. *J Vasc Surg*, Vol. 38, pp. 186-9.

Uchinami M, Morioka K, Doi K, Nakamura T, Yoshida M, & Tanaka K (2005). Retroperitoneal laparoscopic management of a lymphocele after abdominal aortic surgery: A case report. *J Vasc Surg*, Vol. 42, No. 3, pp. 552-555.

Ueno M, Iguro Y, Nagata T, & Sakata R (2006). Aortoenteric Fistula After Endovascular Stent Grafting for an Abdominal Aortic Aneurysm: Report of a Case. *Surg Today*. 2006; Vol. 36, pp. 546–548.

Van DH, Creemers E, & Limet R (2000). Ischemic colitis following aortoiliac surgery. *Acta Chir Belg*, Vol. 100, pp. 21-7.

Vogt PR, & Turina MI (1999). Management of infected aortic grafts: development of less invasive surgery using cryopreserved homografts. *Ann Thorac Surg*, Vol. 67, pp. 1986-9.

Walker WE, Cooley DA, Duncan JM, Hallman JL, Ott DA, & Reul GJ (1986). The management of aortoduodenal fistula by in situ replacement of the infected abdominal aortic graft. *Ann Surg*, Vol. 205, pp. 727-32.

Welch M, Baguneid MS, McMahon RF, Dodd PD, Fulford PE, Griffiths GD, & Walker MG (1998). Histological study of colonic ischaemia after aortic surgery. *Br J Surg*. Vol. 85, No. 8, pp. 1095-8.

Yilmaz EN, Vahl AC, van Rij G, Nauta SHM, Brom HLF, & Rauwerda JA (1999). Endoluminal pulse oximetry of the sigmoid colon and the monitoring of the colonic circulation. *Cardiovascular Surg*, Vol. 7, No. 7, pp. 7

16

The Importance of Venous and Renal Anomalies for Surgical Repair of Abdominal Aortic Aneurysms

Roberto Jiménez and Francisco Morant
Hospital General Universitario de Alicante
Spain

1. Introduction

The presence of venous and renal anomalies can create technical difficulties during aortoiliac surgery, and the patients are most likely to suffer severe bleeding, thus the surgeon must be alert to detect these anomalies and to treat them correctly to avoid severe injuries.

2. Classification

The most frequent anomalies than can complicate abdominal aortic aneurysms (AAA) repair are:

- Major venous anomalies:
  - Renal vein anomalies:
    - Retroaortic left renal vein type I or II.
    - Circumaortic left renal vein.
  - Inferior cava vein anomalies:
    - Left-sided inferior vena cava or cava vein transposition
    - Double inferior vena cava: type I, II or III, right double cava.
    - Marsupial cava or preaortic iliac venous confluence.
    - Preureteral inferior vena cava, retrocaval ureter or circumcaval ureter.
    - Inferior vena cava malposition, anterior or posterior.
    - Agenesis of inferior vena cava.
- Genitourinary anomalies:
  - Fusion anomalies:
    - Horseshoe kidney: frequently fusion of inferior poles, exceptionally fusion of superior polo with inferior polo, or fusion of both superior poles.
    - Pancake kidney, lump kidney or pelvic horseshoe kidney: fusion of both poles.
  - Position anomalies, renal ectopia:
    - Congenital pelvic kidneys:
      - Unilateral or bilateral pelvic kidneys.
      - Crossed kidney with fusion.
      - Crossed kidney without fusion.

Unilateral crossed kidney with contralateral agenesic kidney.
Bilaterally crossed kidneys.
Acquired pelvis kidneys (renal transplant).
Multiple renal arteries, veins or ureters.

3. Epidemiology

3.1 Major venous anomalies

Congenital venous abnormalities in the retroperitoneal space are relatively infrequent and, under normal circumstances, asymptomatic, but have clinical importance in aortoiliac surgery. These anomalies have a low prevalence, the type I retroaortic left renal vein (LRV), with an incidence of 0.3–0.9% joining the inferior vena cava (IVC) in orthotopic position; the type II LRV that joins the IVC lower, at L4–L5 has an incidence of 0.4–0.9%; circumaortic LRV (0.5–1.4%); duplication of IVC (0.2–3%) and left-sided IVC (0.2–0.5%) (Aljabri et al., 2001; Bass et al., 2000).
The prevalence of marsupial cava in humans cannot be predicted, but it is probably very rare because only sporadic cases are described in literature, and studies of inferior cava anomalies do not even cite.
Retrocaval ureter is reported to be in 0,06-0,017% of autopsy materials. The incidence is greater in males than in females, with a ratio of 2,8:1 (Uthappa et al., 2002).
Agenesis of the IVC has an incidence of 0.0005% to 1% in the general population (Simon et al., 2006).

3.2 Genitourinary anomalies

Horseshoe kidney is a renal fusion anomaly estimated to be present in 0,25-0,6% of the population. It is twice as common in males as in females, while abdominal aortic aneurysm (AAA) occurs in 2% of the elderly. Horseshoe kidney associated with AAA is rare: it is found in only 0.12% of the patients that undergo AAA repair (Eze, et al., 1998; Makita et al., 2009; Yamamoto et al., 2006).
The pancake kidney also called fused pelvic kidney, is rare respect to other forms of ectopia, and its incidence cannot be estimated from the literature (Eckes & Lawrence, 1997; Krohn et al., 1999).
The incidence of congenital pelvic kidney has been estimated to be in 0,3%, due to an absence of migration of metanephros, and is the most frequent kidney ectopia. Crossed renal ectopia is an uncommon genitourinary anomaly, detected in 1 of 7000 autopsies. (Krohn et al., 1999; Marone et al., 2008 ; Morales & Greenberg, 2009 ; Sebe et al., 2004 ; Yano et al., 2003).
The prevalence of abdominal aortic aneurysm in patients with renal transplant is 1.01 to 6.7%. *De novo* AAA develops in the transplant population in younger subjects and has faster enlargement, suggesting that haemodialysis length, hypertension, dyslipidaemia and steroid therapy may play a role (Kaskarelis et al., 2006; Lepäntalo et al., 1999).
Multiple renal arteries are relatively frequent (15 to 30%), the incidence of a single additional renal artery is 23,2% and is more common on the left side (27,6%) and in males (33,1%) (Natsis et al., 2010).

4. Anatomy and etiology

IVC results of a complex embryological process between the sixth and tenth weeks of gestation. Three pairs of primitive veins: postcardinal, subcardinal and supracardinal veins,

appear in this order and form the four segments of the adult IVC: hepatic, suprarenal, renal and infrarenal (Fig.1).
The postcardinal veins appear first on the posterior aspect of the embryo. These veins regress, except for the distal aspects which became the iliac bifurcation. The subcardinal veins then appear anterior and medial to the postcardinal veins. The right subcardinal vein remains to form the suprarenal inferior vena cava, while the left subcardinal vein completely regresses. Subsequently, the supracardinal veins appear dorsally to the subcardinal veins. The left supracardinal vein then regresses, and the right supracardinal vein forms the infrarenal inferior vena cava (Minniti & Procacci 2002).

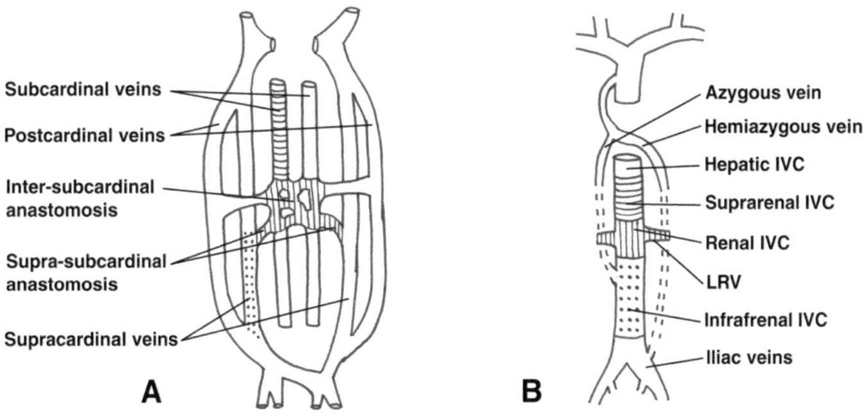

Fig. 1. Embryologic derivation of the inferior vena cava from 6-8 weeks of gestation (A) to the adult (B). IVC: inferior vena cava, LRV: left renal vein.

The most frequent anomalies are detected in the renal and infrarenal IVC, and there are some types of variants.

4.1 Retroaortic left renal vein

The vein crosses the aorta in posterior face instead of the anterior face like normally. There are two types (Karkos et al., 2001; Kraus et al., 2003):
In the *retroaortic LRV type I* the ventral preaortic limb of the renal venous collar is obliterated and the dorsal limb remains on the contrary of the normal evolution, joining the IVC in an orthotopic position at the level of the renal arteries (Fig. 2A).
In the *retroaortic LRV type II* the dorsal limb is detected in a lower position, at L4–L5, behind the aorta, and joins the IVC, gonadal or ascending lumbar veins (Fig. 2B).

4.2 Circumaortic left renal vein

In the circumaortic LRV, both the preaortic and retroaortic limb of the venous collar persists. There is a periaortic venous ring like in the embryonic state (Karkos et al., 2001) (Fig. 2C).

4.3 Transposition or left-sided inferior vena cava

Transposition or left-sided IVC develops from the persistence of the left instead of the right supracardinal vein, which occurs in the normal evolution. The left-sided infrarenal IVC typically joins the LRV, before it crosses the aorta to form a normal right-sided suprarenal IVC.

Probably it could be subclassified in *complete left-sided IVC*, if there is a preaortic trunk lying in front of the aorta and connected to the normal right suprarenal IVC (Fig. 3A) or *incomplete left-sided IVC* if this vein empties into the left renal vein (Fig. 3B). A complete transposition of the IVC to the left with hemiazygous continuation is extremely rare (Guray et al., 2004).

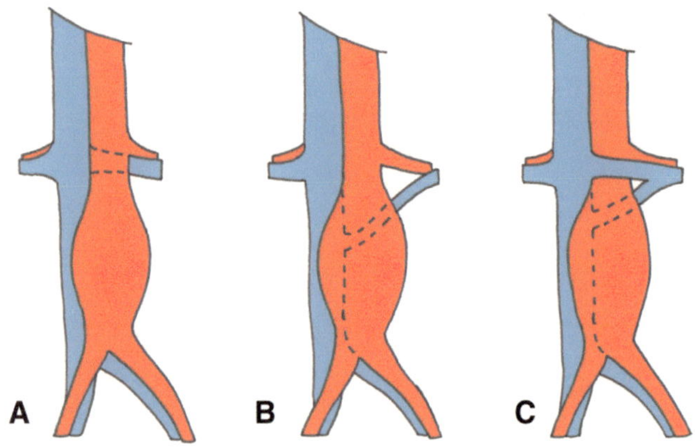

Fig. 2. Left renal vein anomalies. A, Retroaortic left renal vein type I. B, Retroaortic left renal vein type II. C, Circumaortic left renal vein

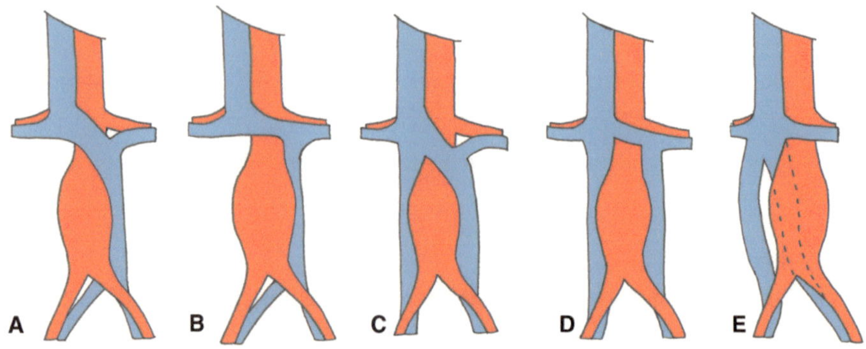

Fig. 3. Inferior vena cava (IVC) anomalies. A, Transposition or left-sided IVC. B, Left-sided IVC (incomplete). C, Duplication of the IVC. D, Double IVC (incomplete). E, Right-sided double IVC.

4.4 Double inferior vena cava

In the double IVC, both left and right supracardinal veins persist. The renal segment of the IVC develops from the right suprasubcardinal and postsubcardinal anastomoses, and the infrarenal segment develops from the right supracardinal vein. Persistence of both supracardinal veins results in duplication of the IVC. (Palit & Deb, 2002).

The left iliac vein ascends as duplicated left IVC and usually drains into the left renal vein, which then crosses anterior to the aorta and joins the right IVC in a normal fashion, *incomplete double IVC* (Fig. 3D) (Ng & Ng, 2009).

It is possible that the left IVC does not drains into the left renal vein, but after receiving the left renal vein it continues with a major preaortic trunk that travels obliquely and empties into the right IVC, *complete double IVC* (Fig. 3C). In contrast to the typical case of infrarenal duplication where the left IVC is quite smaller than the right IVC and empties into the left renal vein, there are several cases that involved the preaortic trunk, and the complete duplication of IVC could be subclassified into three types (Natsis et al., 2010):

Type I or major duplication: comprises two bilaterally symmetrical trunks and a preaortic trunk of the same caliber.

Type II or minor duplication: comprises two bilaterally symmetrical trunks, but smaller than the preaortic trunk.

Type III or asymmetric duplication: comprises small left IVC, larger right IVC and even larger preaortic trunk.

In the *right-sided double IVC* it is speculated that both of them are derived from the right supracardinal and subcardinal veins. Embryologically, the ventral vessel originates from the right subcardinal vein, whereas the dorsal vessel originates from the right supracardinal vein. (Sénécail et al., 2004 ; Nagashima et al., 2006 ; Ng & Ng, 2009).

In the double right IVC the left iliac vein crosses the midline behind or in front the aorta and ascends as double IVC, then joining at the renal level (Fig. 3E). There is a ventral-dorsal relationship between the two vessels. The right gonadal vein drains into the ventral vessel in majority of cases and into the IVC between the renal venous confluence and the confluence of the two vessels in other cases. (Nagashima et al., 2006; Tagliafico et al., 2007).

4.5 Marsupial cava or preaortic venous confluence

At fifth week embryo, three paired veins are roughly symmetrical (posterocardinal, supracardinal and sucardinal). At eighth week, a complex venous plexus appears in the lumbar region, with consolidation of various anastomoses between posterocardinal and supracardinal veins and with further development of circumumbilicous venous rings, which surround the future common iliac arteries on each side. By the tenth week, the ventral portion of the venous rings normally disappears. The persistence of a ventral anastomosis between interposterocardinal and supracardinal veins and the regression of the dorsal venous pathways gives rise to the preaortic common iliac veins confluence later on in fetal life (Natsis et al., 2003).

In this rare anomaly the normally right-sided inferior vena cava arise from an iliac vein confluence located anteriorly to the right common iliac artery and the aortic bifurcation rather than posteriorly (Fig. 4A) (Shindo et al., 1999).

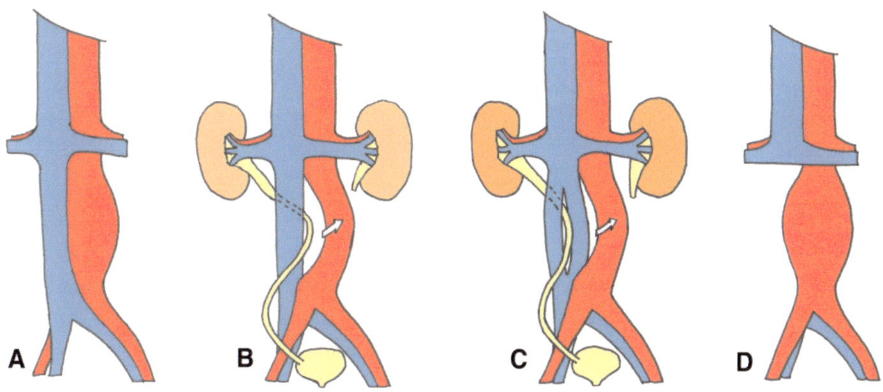

Fig. 4. Inferior vena cava (IVC) anomalies. A, Marsupial cava or preaortic venous confluence. B, Retrocaval ureter or pre-ureteric IVC. C, Transcaval ureter or periureteral venous ring. D Agenesis of infrarenal IVC.

Because such an anterior position of IVC is typical in most marsupials, as stated by McClure and Huntington in 1929, compared with the posterior position present in placental mammalians, it is used the term "marsupial cava" (Schiavetta et al., 1998).

4.6 Retrocaval ureter or circumcaval ureter

The embryological significance of the retrocaval ureter is, strictly speaking, an anomaly affecting the IVC and not the ureter. In embryology, the IVC normally develops from a plexus of fetal veins. The posterior cardinal and subcardinal veins lie ventrally, and the supracardinal veins lie dorsally. The left supracardinal veins and the lumbar portion of the right posterior cardinal vein atrophy and the subcardinal veins become the internal gonadal veins. A definitive right-sided IVC forms from the right supracardinal vein. If the postcardinal vein in the lumbar portion fails to atrophy and becomes the right-side IVC, the ureter is trapped dorsally to it. This occurs because the right postcardinal vein is positioned ventral to ureter in the definitive inferior vena cava, so the developing right ureter courses behind to the IVC.

Retrocaval ureter almost invariably involves the right side. In this uncommon venous anomaly the right ureter courses posterior to the IVC and partially encircles it. Right ureter's courses wings medially over pedicle of L3/4, passes behind the IVC, then exits anteriorly between IVC and aorta returning to its normal position, and produces varying degrees of proximal hydroureteronephrosis (Fig. 4B).

Bateson and Atkinson distinguished two types of retrocaval ureter according to the radiological appearance and site of ureteral narrowing (Uthappa et al., 2002; Shindo et al., 1999):

In type I (low loop), the ureter crosses behind the IVC at the level of the third lumbar vertebra and has a fish hook-shaped (S-shaped) deformity of the ureter. Marked hydronephrosis is seen in over 50% of patients.

In type II (high loop), the renal pelvis and upper ureter lie horizontally, and the retrocaval segment of the ureter is at the same level as the renal pelvis. The retrograde pyelogram shows a "sickle shape" of the involved ureter, generally with mild hydronephrosis. Type II is less common at around 10% of all cases.

Occasionally exits the *transcaval ureter or periureteral venous ring* and may cause ureteral obstruction (Fig. 4C) (Dillon, November 1991).

4.7 Inferior vena cava malposition, anterior or posterior

There has been described malposition of the inferior vena cava, anteriorly to an AAA or posterior at it. (Chauduri, 2011).

4.8 Agenesis of inferior vena cava

Agenesis of the IVC is often used to describe three different entities (Ruggeri el al., 2001):

- *Absence of the suprarenal IVC* results from failure to form the right subcardinal vein. The hepatic segment drains directly into the right atrium, and the blood from the infrarenal IVC returns to the heart through the azygos and hemiazygos veins.
- *Absence of the infrarenal IVC* with preservation of the suprarenal segment implies a failure of the development of the right supracardinal vein (Fig. 4D).
- *Absence of the entire IVC,* suggests that all three paired vein systems failed to develop properly.

4.9 Horseshoe kidney

The renal system is developed from three structures that follow in time: pronephros, mesonephros and metanephros. The embryologic kidneys ascend cranially and receive blood from multiple arteries of common iliac arteries and media sacra artery; the renal artery is formed later in the third month. If the migration does not happen it gives the pelvic kidney, and if a fusion occurs, gives the horseshoe kidney.

The normally separate left and right metanephric blastemas fuse prior to migration and rotation, resulting in a fused mass. During the development of the kidney, if the metannephric masses come into contact or fuse and their normal medial rotation is interrupted, the anomalous *horseshoe kidney* come about. The renal masses ascend in the abdomen; however, the renal isthmus that lies anterior to the aorta stops its cephalic migration at the level of the inferior mesenteric artery, giving an isthmus that lies over the distal aorta above the bifurcation.

There is a fusion at inferior poles of the kidneys at the midline in 90% of cases, with the majority of each kidney lying on its own side of the spine. The isthmus connecting the lower poles contains usually functional parenchyma but may be a fibrous band and is located anterior to the aorta and IVC and posterior to the inferior mesenteric artery. The renal pelvis is usually rotated anteriorly and ureters arise anteriorly or laterally, because the horseshoe kidney, similarly to the pelvic kidney cannot rotate (Fig. 5A).

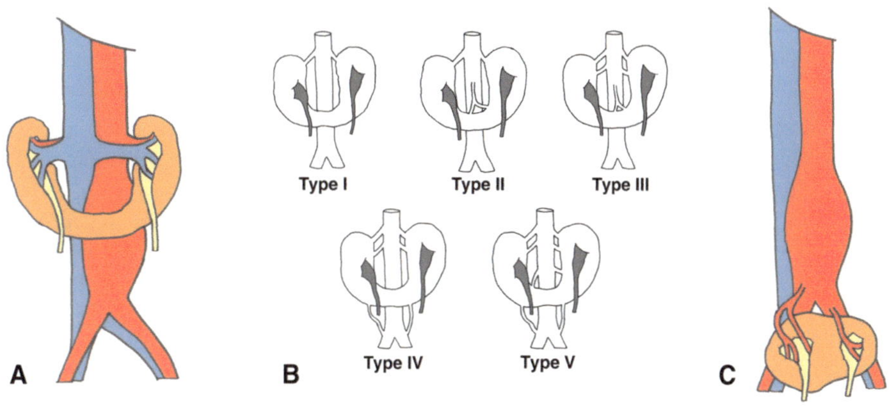

Fig. 5. Renal fusion anomalies. A, Horseshoe kidney. B, Vascularization of horseshoe kidney: type I, II, III, IV and V. C, Pancake kidney.

The blood supply to the horseshoe kidney can be quite variable, especially in the isthmus and lower poles. The abnormalities of blood supply have been reported in 60% to 74% of patients with horseshoe kidneys and frequently the isthmus and lower poles frequently have their own accessory renal artery from the aorta or iliac arteries. (Makita et al., 2009)

Different classifications exit for variable arterial blood supply in horseshoe kidney, like that proposed by Eisendrath (Fig. 5B) (Ruppert et al., 2004):

Type I: one renal artery for each side of the horseshoe kidney, 20% of cases.

Type II: one renal artery for each side with an aortic branch to the isthmus, 30%.

Type III: two arteries for each side and one renal isthmus artery, 15%.

Type IV: two arteries for each side with one or more arising from iliac arteries, including the isthmus branch, 15%.

Type V: multiple renal arteries originating from the aorta and mesenteric and iliac arteries, 20%.
Anatomically, the blood supply to the horseshoe kidney is controlled segmentally by the accessory arteries, and the collateral blood flow between the segments is minimum. The occurrence of the renal ischemia was as high as 74% and is recommended reconstructing the accessory artery whenever its diameter is 2 mm or more. (Makita et al., 2009).
The renal vein anatomy is normal, with two renal veins each from left and right portions of the horseshoe kidney draining into the cava in a standard position.

4.10 Pancake kidney or fused pelvic kidney

Although the embryologic development of pancake kidney has not been fully elucidated, it is thought that it arrests in the early stages of rotation and migration. The renal blastemas are completely fused at 4-8 week embryos, and consequently fails to migrate in a cephalic direction, leaving it in a pelvic location that is usually at or below the aortic bifurcation. (Eze et al., 1998).
As its name implies, there is complete fusion of renal parenchyma without the presence of an isthmus giving an irregularly lobulated kidney, which is nearly circular in outline. The kidney is normally located at the level of the aortic bifurcation and gives rise to two collecting systems from his anterior surface that join the bladder in the normal anatomic position. Various cases from literature report two, three or four renal arteries that supply the kidney from the aorta, the right or the left common iliac arteries. The only assumption one should make is that the renal blood supply will be variable in number and position of renal arteries and can often involve the distal aorta and iliac arteries. The venous drainage systems could be variable to the iliac vein and proximal vena cava (Fig. 5C). (Eze et al., 1998).

4.11 Congenital pelvic kidney

A pelvic kidney occurs when the blastema in the 5 to 7 week embryo inexplicably fails to ascend normally.
By definition, a pelvic kidney is located under a flat level between the two iliac crests. Left pelvic kidneys are more common than right ones. Adding variety to the anatomy is the fact that the pelvic kidney does not rotate medially, so its hilium is ventrally located. There is usually a normal short ureter entering the bladder on the ipsilateral side (Sebe et al., 2004).
It is possible to affirm than in pelvic position, the renal arteries are multiple in the most cases, much more frequent than in orthotopic position, where is evaluated a 30%. Whenever is a single renal artery (49% of cases), it origins systematically from the aortic bifurcation. When the renal arteries are double, in 40% cases, a branch is originated from aortic bifurcation, and the second branch can emanate from the ipsilateral or the contralateral common iliac artery or from internal iliac artery. In case of three or four arteries (11% of cases), a branch comes from aortic bifurcation and the others branches from iliac axis ipsi and contralateral. Rarely, blood supply is guaranteed by feeding arteries originating from inferior mesenteric arteries. In definitive, if there are multiple renal arteries (in more than 50% of cases), one of the branches origin systematically from aortic bifurcation, and the other branches comes from ipsilateral iliac axis and more rare from contralateral iliac axis. The venous vascularization of pelvic kidneys is never described. The pelvic renal veins are multiples and small caliber. They drain in the IVC and in ipsilateral common iliac vein (Fig. B) (Marone et al., 2008; Sebe et al., 2004).
The *single pelvic kidney* represents failure of ascend of the existing normal kidney beyond the true pelvis in combination with a congenital absence of the contralateral kidney (Morales & Greenberg 2005).

4.12 Acquired pelvis kidney (renal transplant)

The corpse kidney is situated in the pelvis, with anastomosis in iliac arteries and veins (Fig. 6C).

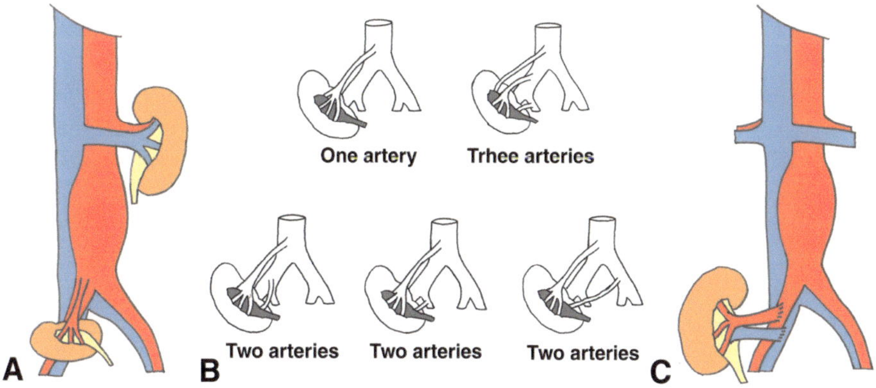

Fig. 6. Pelvic kidney. A, Congenital pelvic kidney. B, Vascularization of congenital pelvic kidney: one, two or three arteries. C, Acquired pelvic kidney (renal transplant).

4.13 Crossed renal ectopia

Causes may involve faulty development of the ureteric buds, vascular obstruction to the ascent of the kidneys, and environmental factors.

The ectopic kidney crosses the midline and lies contralateral to its normal position, and usually is fused to the normal kidney, so is called crossed fused ectopia. The ureter of the ectopic kidney crosses the midline to enter the bladder at its normal position. This type of kidney is most often malrotated (ventral helium) and situated below the normal kidney. The anomaly is more common in male patients, and frequently involves the left kidney.

The blood supply to the kidneys is from the aorta or the iliac arteries, and the number of renal arteries varies. Venous drainage may also be abnormal, but because venous structures are not involved in aortic surgery, there have been no reports regarding this. This anomaly can be classified into four types (Fig. 7): *Type A, crossed ectopia with fusion; type B, crossed ectopia without fusion; type C, solitary crossed ectopia; and type D, bilaterally crossed ectopia.* Type A is seen most frequently, and the other three types much less commonly. In this anomaly, the kidneys, including the nonectopic kidney, have an anomalous blood supply. (Yano et al., 2003)

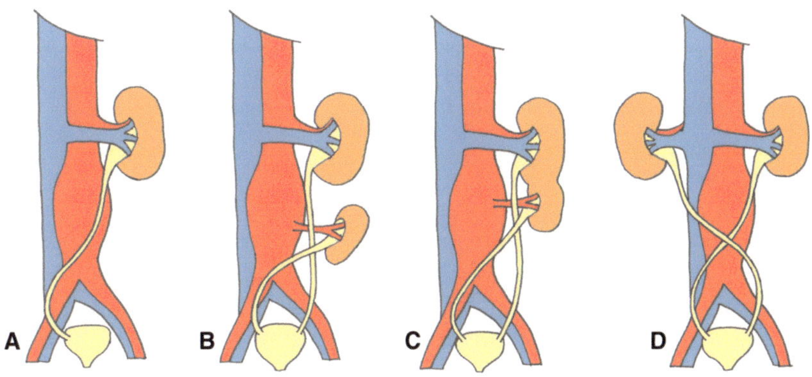

Fig. 7. Crossed renal ectopia. A, Solitary crossed kidney. B, Crossed kidney without or C, with fusion. D, Bilaterally crossed kidney.

4.14 Multiple renal arteries or renal veins

Renal arteries are derived from the embryonic mesonephric arteries. Regression of these arteries results in persistence of single mesonephric artery and formation of a single renal artery. Displasia of the mesonepric arteries gives rise to *multiple renal arteries* (Natsis et al., 2010).

Multiple renal veins are more frequent on the right side presumably due to the fact that the right postsubcardinal anastomosis does not regress, but participates in the formation of the renal segment of the IVC. As a consequence the dorsal renal vein may persist as well. On the contrary, the postsubcardinal anastomosis regresses on the left side and facilitates the regression of the left dorsal renal vein (Natsis et al., 2010).

The polar renal arteries are common, and usually of a small calibre, irrigating only a renal pole; double renal arteries is less frequent. Multiple renal veins can occur, but is less important because are not directly implied in aortic surgery.

5. Clinical

5.1 Major venous anomalies

These anomalies are asymptomatic usually. If there is a case with AAA ruptured into a *retraortic left renal vein* exit a clinical onset characterized by the unique syndrome: continuous abdominal bruit, abdominal and left flank pain with an associated pulsatile mass (Mansour triad) (Gabrielli et al., 2010).

Several cases report of thromboembolic events occurring in patient with *double IVC*. An increased incidence of thrombosis formation in double IVC has been seen, but the exact cause is unknown; some authors suggested than this may be related to the degree of narrowing of the vessel as it crosses the aorta. In patients who require IVC filter placement, separate filters are needed for both IVCs (Ng & Ng, 2009).

The *retrocaval ureter* or preureteral cava vein may give right flank pain, recurrent urinary tract infections, and microscopic or gross haematuria or hydronephrosis. There is a high incidence of calculi due to stasis. Hydronephrosis may be entirely silent without any symptoms, and the patients usually are in their third or fourth decades because of gradual development of hydronephrosis (Mahmood et al., 2005).

The i*nferior vena cava malpositions, anterior or posterior are* asymptomatic being a finding in the preoperative CT.

Recent reports confirm that *agenesis of the IVC* play a role as a strong predisposing factor for the development of deep venous thrombosis in young adults. An inadequate blood return through collaterals may increase the venous blood pressure in the veins of the legs, favoring venous stasis and subsequent deep venous thrombosis. (Schneider et al., 2002)

5.2 Genitourinary anomalies

Although about 1/3 of *horseshoe kidney* are asymptomatic, it can be complications like ureteropelvic junction obstruction with hydronephrosis, recurrent infections, recurrent calculus formation and increased incidence of Wilms tumors, transitional cell carcinoma and renal carcinoids.

The presence of a *pancake kidney* may predispose to recurrent urinary tract infection due to the short anomalous ureter that is prone to obstruction, but most of the reported cases are asymptomatic. (Eze et al., 1998).

In case of *pelvic kidney* there is a 32% of renovascular hypertension (Sebe et al., 2004)

6. Diagnostic

6.1 Major venous anomalies

Since computed tomography (CT) is routinely performed for the elective repair of AAA, usually these anatomical anomalies like *retroaortic LRV* (Fig. 8A y B), *circumaortic LRV* (Fig. 8C) and *left inferior vena cava* (Fig. 9A) are easily detected and the risk of the operation is minimized. CT has proven to be superior to ultrasound and phlebography for detecting IVC anomalies. Magnetic resonance imaging can be as effective as CT and avoids the risks of contrast nephropathy (Nishibe et al., 2004).

In emergency surgery for a ruptured AAA, diagnosed by ultrasound alone, venous anomalies may be injured during surgery resulting in serious bleeding. In case of a ruptured AAA a CT could be useful to detect venous and renal anomalies and to avoid severe injuries.

Radiologically, the presence of *double IVC* can be mistaken as a pathological lesion such as lymphadenopathy, or left periureteric dilatation. (Ng & Ng, 2009).

Characteristic computed tomography findings of *right double IVC* were a ventral-dorsal relationship between the two vessels and the unusual course of the left common iliac vein, passing ventral or dorsal to the aortic bifurcation or the right common iliac artery

The knowledge of variations like *marsupial cava* is especially important to surgeons, because it may cause problems in differential diagnosis from adenopathy.

The CT and the MRI are the most efficacious and least invasive method of confirm diagnosis of *retrocaval ureter*. Other entities that may produce medial deviation of the ureter include retroperitoneal fibrosis and retroperitoneal mass. (Uthappa et al., 2002).

Retrograde pyelogram or iv urogram may show marked dilatation of the right pelvicalyceal system and proximal ureter to the level of transverse process of L3 vertebra. In addition there is medial deviation of the ureter at the point of transition with the characteristic "S" shape. The distal few centimeters of the right ureter are of normal caliber.

Ultrasonography demonstrates the anatomy of the retrocaval ureter and is useful in follow-up patients for hydronephrosis, parenchymal atrophy, and nephrolithiasis. (Mahmood et al., 2005)

In *agenesis of the IVC* extensive collateral flow is observed, and the azygous and hemiazygous systems are particularly prominent; collaterals include the ascending lumbar veins, paravertebral venous plexus, and anterior abdominal wall veins.

The collateral circulation may simulate a paraspinal mass. The dilated azygous vein may be misinterpreted as a mediastinal mass on chest radiography, an the dilated collaterals in the abdomen could misinterpret as a enlarged pericaval lymph nodes in a CT abdominal, presumed a retroperitoneal lymphoma.

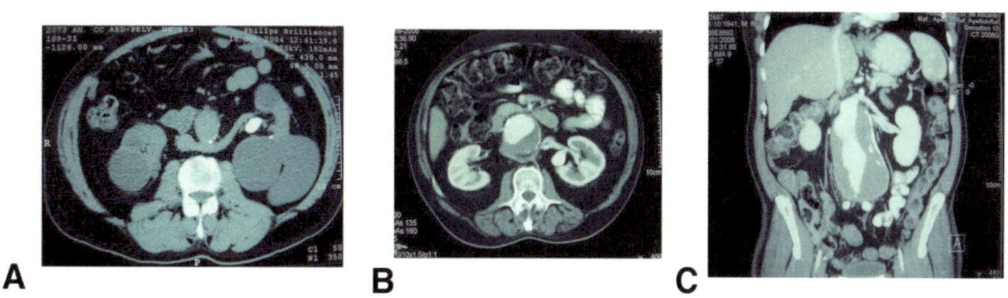

Fig. 8. Left renal vein (LRV) anomalies CT. A, Retroaortic left renal vein type I. B, Retroaortic LRV type II. C, Circumaortic LRV.

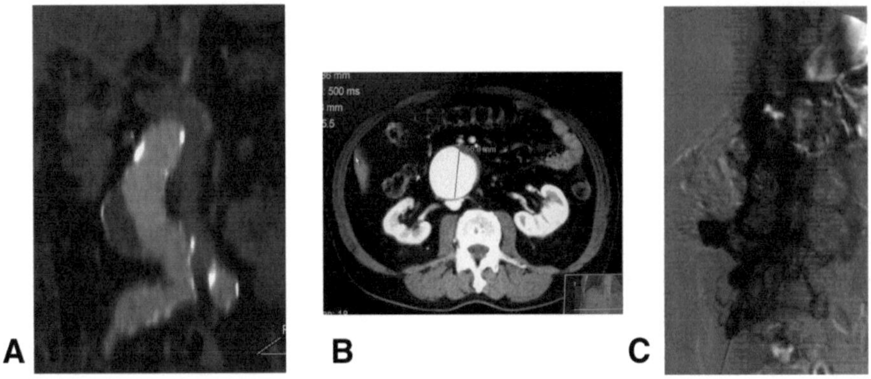

Fig. 9. Inferior vena cava (IVC) anomalies CT and arteriography. A, Left IVC. B, Posterior IVC. C, Agenesis of IVC.

6.2 Genitourinary anomalies

Preoperative knowledge of renal blood supply is of paramount importance to the vascular surgeon when working with anomalous kidneys. Abdominal aortic and iliac aneurysms are frequently repaired without routine preoperative angiographic examination; however, the presence of renal ectopia, often discovered by ultrasonographic or computed tomographic scanning, is a specific indication for preoperative angiographic examination.

With helical CT, adequate preoperative diagnosis of abdominal aortic aneurysm accompanied by *horseshoe kidney*, as well as determination of the arteries supplying the horseshoe kidney, are now easy. Such anatomy is important in determining the operative approach and procedure (Fig. 10A) (Makita et al., 2009; Yammamoto et al., 2006).

Renal scintigraphic scanning may also demonstrate whether the isthmus contains functioning tissue.

Computed tomography and magnetic resonance angiography allow providing information about both aortoiliac aneurysm anatomy and *pelvic kidney* (Fig 10B) feeding arteries and veins. Conventional intraarterial angiography is an invasive procedure but allows studying the renal artery anatomy with the highest sensitivity, identifying even small branches or accessory renal arteries that may be misdiagnosed with other techniques. Current technologies in the more recent angio-CT and angio-RM have significantly improved specifity and sensibility of these methods. In particular, the number and anatomical layout of the renal arteries should be established in advance of surgery, so that a surgical strategy for renal protection and arterial reimplantation can be formed. CT after the operation can disclose areas of renal infarction, suggesting that at least one renal artery originating from the aneurysm had been divided during the operation (Bui et al., 2007).

Duplex ultrasonography provide hemodynamic information such as alterations of peak systolic velocity that can occur in cases of severe kinking or dislocation of congenital pelvic kidney renal arteries in cases of huge associated aorto-iliac aneurysms.

Retrograde pyelography may provide further information about the path of the ureters and preoperative placement of ureteral catheter can enable the identification of an anomalous ureter.

There is renovascular hypertension in some cases, until 32%, but is difficult to diagnose in this cases with captopril isotopic gammagraphy. In hypertensive patients, preoperative base-line and captopril radionuclide renographic study may reveal the renovascular nature of the hypertension. It is possible that preoperatively hypertensive patients had postoperative captopril-renogram and serum creatinine levels returned to normal and were discharged without blood pressure medication (Hanif et al., 2005, Marone et al., 2008).

In *crossed renal ectopia* retrograde pyelography may provide further information about the path of ureters. Because arteries not identified at preoperative arteriography are occasionally found at surgery, too much confidence should not be placed on preoperative evaluation. To minimize the risk for complications, it also could be placed a ureteral catheter for intraoperative identification (Yano et al., 2003).

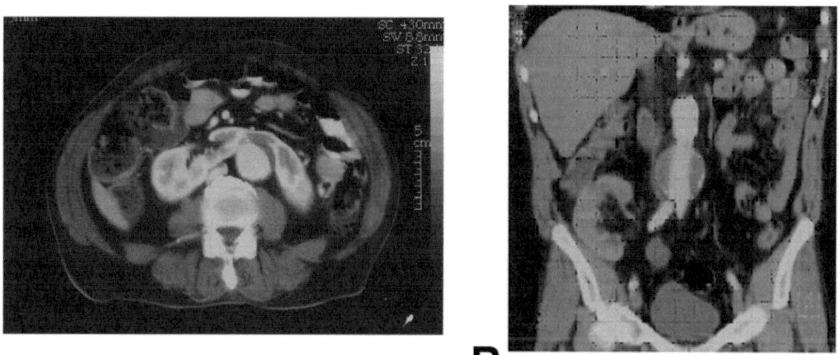

A B

Fig. 10. Genitourinary anomalies. A, Horseshoe kidney. B, Renal transplant.

7. Treatment

7.1 Retroaortic left renal vein

Exposure of the proximal aorta and performing the proximal graft anastomosis is the major technical problem associated with anomalies of the renal vein or IVC; an adequate control of the aneurysm neck can be achieved through a midline transperitoneal approach minimizing the retroaortic dissection and avoiding to encircle the aorta. Unlike other authors, we do not believe a left retroperitoneal approach is necessary. Clamping the aorta is feasible above or below a retroaortic LRV type I. (Shindo et al., 2000).

During the control of the patient's lumbar arteries from within the open sac of the aneurysm, there is a risk of damage especially in the case of retroaortic LRV type II. The vein can be damaged with the posterior stitches, resulting in severe bleeding or in the formation of a graft- LRV fistula. To avoid this, whenever possible, is better applying lumbar artery clips outside the AAA with visual control.

Sometimes it is necessary to ligate the normal LRV to control aneurysm's neck. Whenever LRV ligating is necessary, it should be performed close to the IVC in order to preserve the gonadal and adrenal veins that normally empty into the LRV, and thus maintain the left venous renal draining.

There has been described ruptured AAA with fistula to the retroaortic left renal vein, resolved with open surgery. Furthermore, the proximity of the arteriovenous fistula to the renal arteries increased the risk of endoleak type I because it influenced the sealing and fixation zone of the stent graft even more. (Gabrielli et al., 2010).

7.2 Left-sided inferior vena cava

Some authors prefer a left retroperitoneal approach in case of a left-sided IVC, which may be safer when preparing the perirenal aorta. A transperitoneal approach with division of the aberrant IVC as it crosses the aorta with subsequent anastomosis also has been suggested. Nevertheless, an adequate control of the aneurysmal neck can be achieved through a midline transperitoneal approach with sufficient cava mobilization (Fig. 11). There has been described an AAA with horseshoe kidney and left-sided inferior vena cava, resolved with open surgery (Evers et al., 2007; Giglia & Thompson 2004; Radermecker et al., 2008).

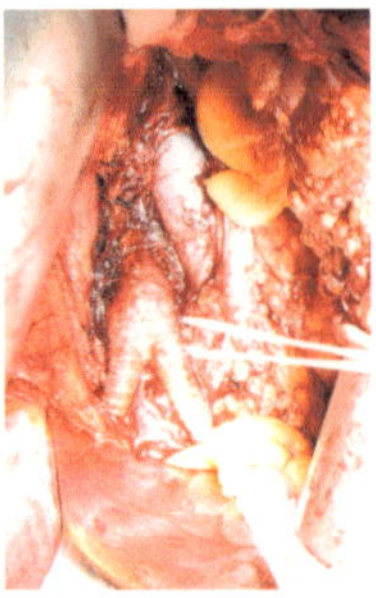

Fig. 11. Surgery image, left inferior vena cava and aortobifemoral bypass.

7.3 Double inferior vena cava

It has been suggested that the transperitoneal approach rather than retroperitoneal one should be adopted for patients with an abdominal aortic aneurysm and concomitant double IVC (Ng & Ng 2009). (Nagashima et al., 2006).

7.4 Marsupial cava or preaortic venous confluence

During elective surgery for AAA, the presence of this rare anomaly can be managed with little additional risk through the use of a long midline incision and transperitoneal route. With a careful blunt dissection of the right common iliac artery bifurcation, it is possible to gain distal control without mobilizing the caval confluence, which results strictly adherent to aorta. On the contrary, this anomaly is very troublesome if the distal aorta and right common iliac artery are approached retroperitoneally from the patient's right side (Schiavetta et al., 1998).

During emergency surgery, the priority of gaining quick control of the aorta and the iliac arteries through the retroperitoneal hematoma may lead to injury to major venous structures, excessive hemorrhage, and subsequent death. The inflammatory AAA poses another problem since an abdominal vein could be buried in the fibrosis, the preoperative mapping is important.

7.5 Retrocaval ureter

The retrocaval ureter can be inadvertently injured or ligated during aortoiliac surgery. Therefore, it is useful to identify such anomaly preoperatively. Ureteral stent (double J) may be helpful for stenting and drainage avoiding urine leakage and urosepsis.

Conservative treatment is necessary to those patients who have mild hydronephrosis without obvious symptoms, infection, worsening renal function, or stone formation. Ureteroureteral reanastomosis anterior to the vena cava with resection of the retrocaval segment is the widely favorite standard treatment; this reanastomosis can be done without resection of the retrocaval segment Laparoscopic or retroperioneoscopic ureterolisis and reconstruction of retrocaval ureter become popular in recent years with satisfactory success rate (Nagraj et al., 2006; Li et al., 2010).

7.6 Inferior vena cava malposition, anterior or posterior

Again is important identify these alteration of normal position of the vena cava due to not injury it during aortic surgery. With careful technique it could not be a problem.

7.7 Agenesis of inferior vena cava

The agenesic or hipoplasic cava vein difficult AAA dissection due the big collaterals with risk of haemorrhage. In the postoperative period may led deep venous thrombosis.
Patients with these venous anomalies, inflammatory AAA as well as elderly patients are at particularly high risk and could be candidates for endovascular procedures.

7.8 Horseshoe kidney

Horseshoe kidneys pose more technical difficulties because they limit access to the distal aorta and besides they are usually supplied by multiple renal arteries arising from the aorta, the AAA itself, or the iliac arteries. Although the retroperitoneal approach is recommended, the majority of authors describe the transperitoneal approach for most routine cases involving horseshoe kidney and abdominal aortic aneurysm. A retroperitoneal approach can need an adjunctive right iliac incision to facilitate clamping and manipulation of a right iliac aneurysm. The isthmus of the horseshoe kidney should not be divided unless it is thin and atrophic. Rather, the aortic graft usually can be tunneled beneath the kidney if the aorta is approached anteriorly. After resection of the isthmus, however, there are possibilities of hemorrhage, of formation of a hematoma in the retroperitoneum , or of vascular prosthesis infection associated with urine leakage (Makita et al., 2009; Yamamoto et al., 2006).
Cold perfusion is useful for renal preservation during temporary ischemia. Care must be taken, however, to revascularize the major arteries by reimplantation. Preoperative arteriography facilitates identification of these branches, but careful intraoperative dissection and inspection are required to avoid injury. Ligation of a small accessory artery diverging from an aneurysm did not affect postoperative renal functions. An accessory artery with a diameter of more than 2 mm requires reconstruction (Makita et al., 2009; Stroosma et al., 2001).
In the emergency setting the transperitoneal approach, less frequent re-anastomosis of renal arteries arising from the aneurysm, and more frequent separation of the renal isthmus were preferred to a retroperitoneal approach without separation of the isthmus, since the need for rapid vascular control lowered the threshold for division of the renal arteries and isthmus. (Stroosma et al., 2001).
In pluripathologic patients there are a high surgical risk and could be candidates for endovascular procedures. Endovascular aortic repair (EVAR) is feasible despite predictable technical difficulties (angulated neck, iliac aneurysm and occlusion) and the possibility or renal impairment. In patients with ruptured AAA and horseshoe kidney the EVAR treatment should be strongly considered (Chauduri, 2011; Saadi et al., 2008).
In presence of blood supply type I and II, according to Eisendrath, EVAR is preferable to open aneurysm repair in any patient in whom EVAR is technically feasible, if renal retention

values are normal. Non predominant accessory renal artery less than 3 mm in diameter providing the isthmus with blood can be covered without any problems. In the case of dominant accessory renal artery greater than 3 mm in diameter, we recommend diagnostic use of selective angiography to determine what proportion of the horseshoe kidney and how much parenchyma is supplied by the accessory renal artery. When a blood supply types III and IV exist, it must be decided on the basis of each case whether EVAR is feasible. In our view, type V cannot be repaired with EVAR (Galiñanes et al., 2011; Radermercker et al., 2004; Ruppert et al., 2004).

7.9 Pancake kidney

The presence of a large, relatively fixed renal mass impairs anterior transperitoneal access to the pelvic vessels, thus can be a successful repair via retroperitoneal procedures. The retroperitoneal approach, avoids the renal isthmus, collecting system, and venous anomalies. In addition, it provides direct access to the abdominal aorta, the hypogastric arteries, and its branches. The pancake kidney has no isthmus, and therefore dissection and retraction is the only means of exposure, with dissection of the kidney and gentle retraction the exposure was adequate without endangering the kidney, its blood supply and collecting system. Division of the parenchyma of the pancake kidney presents potential problems such as postoperative urinary leakage, renal vascular compromise, and eventual renal failure. If the aneurysm extends into the iliac arteries, aneurysmectomy poses a significant threat to renal salvage since complete mobilization of the pancake kidney is required with the attendant risk of vascular or parenchymal injury (Krohn et al., 1999).

Anomalous renal masses invariably have aberrant vasculature including abnormal venous drainage. Exanguinating hemorrhage can occur with inadverted venous injury, but this can be avoided by careful dissection around the pancake kidney. Renal blood must be preserved, as the sacrifice of any renal artery can result in renal necrosis and loss of renal function. In other cases, the renal arteries may arise from the aneurysm itself requiring reimplantation or bypass grafting or may be temporarily occluded to perform the aneurysm repair. The renal warm ischemia time and period of increased cardiac afterload were shortened by first performing the iliac artery anastomosis (Eze et al., 1998).

A variety of techniques are available that can be used to minimize the ischemic injury to the renal parenchyma:

Mannitol has been shown to be an affective scavenger of oxygen derived free radicals through its inhibition of thromboxane synthesis. It has been recommended as a standard precaution before aortic cross clamping in patient undergoing aneurysmectomy also with forced diuresis with furosemide. Low-dose dopamine has also been used for its renal protective effects. Dopamine is used intraoperatively and postoperatively to maximize renal vasodilatation. (Krohn et al., 1999)

The renal parenchyma can be preserved with the use of in situ cold perfusion (4°C) with lactated Ringer's or Collin's solution. To further diminish the effects of ischemia and reperfusion, selective renal perfusion techniques can also be used during aortic cross-clamping in specific cases, including the use of a variety of shunts and temporary bypass (Eckes & Lawrence, 1997).

7.10 Congenital pelvic kidney

In the majority of patients with a congenital pelvic kidney who underwent open repair developed significant, albeit largely transient, rises in creatinine value. Typically, this initial rise of creatinine levels is followed by a complete or near complete recovery which is consistent with that natural history of acute tubular necrosis (ATN). A preprocedure elevation of creatinine likely puts the patient at a higher risk for clinically apparent ATN postprocedure because of diminished functional renal reserve. (Bui et al., 2007).

In spite of all techniques for protection the pelvic kidney during aorta reconstruction ATN is common after surgery and tends to resolve within two weeks. Whether an episode of transient ATN shortens transplanted kidney life span is unknown, but we think is prudent to take reasonable steps to minimize ATN without adding complications to the procedure.

The risk factors currently associated with postoperative ATN include (1) the pelvic kidney constituting all functioning renal mass (congenital solitary pelvic kidney, renal transplant); (2) more than two anastomoses required to revascularize the kidney (e. g., reimplantation or bypass of the pelvic renal artery); (3) an elevated creatinine preoperatively; (4) poor collaterals such as occluded lumbars, inferior mesenteric artery, or internal iliac arteries or a measured aortic sac backpressure of <35 mm Hg; and (5) estimated aortic cross-clamp time for more than 50 min. (Bui et al., 2007).

Different mechanisms may plausibly be involved in renal function impairment, mainly related to malperfusion of congenital pelvic kidney such as aneurysm distal embolization, kinking of the renal artery, hemodynamic effects of abnormal pulsatility, and in the case of large lesions, due to depression of the renal parenchyma, renal veins, and the ureter and/or ureteropelvic junction. (Marone et al., 2008)

Renal function is more susceptible to ischemia in patients undergoing elective AAA repair who have transplanted kidneys than in patients with ectopic congenital pelvic kidneys. Except for patients with congenital solitary pelvic kidney, good results with congenital pelvic kidney should be expected as these patients had a normal kidney above the AAA that was not at risk of ischemic injury. Without the advantage of pre and postoperative nuclear renal isotope scans to assess excretion and flow, it is difficult to assess the degree of acute tubular necrosis in the congenital pelvic kidney in a patient with normal contralateral kidney.

Unlike a transplanted pelvic kidney, the congenital pelvic kidney may have a single renal artery, but their origin may be displaced to the distal aorta or even iliac arteries; or may has multiple renal arteries, one which may originate from the diseased distal aorta, requiring reimplantation. In cases of iliac aneurysm, it may be needed to reimplant the renal artery. If during aortic cross-clamping an ischemic discoloration of a segment of the kidney is observed that indicates the lack of a collateral vascular supply and the necessity of reimplanting the artery that supply that segment (Bui et al., 2007).

In case of renovascular hypertension refractory at treatment with an atrophic pelvic kidney it could be needed a nephrectomy for better hypertension control with less drugs (Sebe et al., 2004).

Because of the presence of congenital pelvic kidney, the renal function may be affected by intraoperative renal ischemia after aortic aneurysm repair and several methods of renal protection to prevent renal ischemic injury have been previously reported. These methods of renal preservation, also used during abdominal aneurysmectomy in renal transplant patients, can be divided in various groups: pharmacological systemic renal protection, in situ perfusion with hypothermic crystalloid solution, use of a temporary shunt and double proximal clamping technique, the use of perfusion with pump oxygenator or ex vivo perfusion are abandonee. In appropiate candidates, EVAR may be considered.

1. Systemic renal protection. The expansion of plasmatic volume with preoperatory hydration and the intraoperatory administration of furosemide and mannitol or dopamine to obtain forced diuresis before cross-clamping, reduce the risk of kidney loss, or acute tubular necrosis. These methods are safe and effective and can represent a good choice if associated to a fast aortic reconstruction.
2. In situ cooling techniques. To preserve renal function during supra-renal clamping for a longer time (60 to 90 min), it is possible to use selective infusions of bolus of cold (4°C) lactate Ringer's solution that can be repeated every 20 minutes or continuously infused to reduce the temperature of the kidney to 15-18°C. Some authors added 6-methylprednisolone and mannitol to this solution. Topical cooling kidney packing with ice slush is a complementary action in these cases. (Marone et al., 2008).
3. Temporary shunts. Temporary bypasses or shunts are performed from the axillary or subclavian artery or from the abdominal aorta above the aneurysm, or less frequently from the left atrial cavity or ascending aorta to the iliac or femoral vessels. A temporary extra-anatomic shunt maintains renal perfusion when conventional AAA repair is required. A shunt with partial extracorporeal circulation and pulsatile cold blood perfusion needs systemic anticoagulation; a shunt with centrifugal pump or a Gott shunt (heparin coated) does not need anticoagulation. However, all these procedures entail possible intimal arterial dissection or embolization and may increase the risk of haemorrhagic or infectious complications (Hanif et al., 2005; Maeda et al., 2009; Martin-Conejero et al., 2003).
4. Clamping and anastomoses techniques. The double proximal clamping technique, described by Lacombe offers a potential sufficient protection for medium time (less than 60 min) using backflow by lumbar, inferior mesenteric, and iliac arteries during completion of proximal aortic anastomosis. This technique involves completely dividing the aortic neck proximally between two clamps. The aortic back pressure after aortic cross-clamping is between 35 and 60 mm Hg, and experimentally, a renal blood flow under a low arterial pressure of only 25 mm Hg is adequate for organ survival (Lacombe , 1991, 2008)

Once the proximal anastomosis is complete, the sac can be opened and the distal anastomosis is performed while the pelvic kidney is perfused by retrograde flow from the ipsilateral internal and femoral arteries. The absence of a valid collateral circulation and the presence of a short proximal neck limit the use of this alternative. Some authors have pointed out that having two clamps together makes the proximal anastomosis more difficult. This technique has been modified by Hollis et al. to use a vascular stapler to avoid the distal clamp. The short proximal aortic neck may require placing the distal clamp across the proximal aneurysm sac. This compression of the sac could potentially lead to significant embolization. (Bui et al., 2007).

When using a bifurcated graft, performing the distal before the proximal anastomosis is another described technique for limiting clamp time. By taking the graft limb ipsilateral to the pelvic kidney and anastomosing it distal to the kidney on the external iliac artery, this anastomosis can be done without interrupting the normal aortoiliac flow to the pelvic kidney. Warm kidney ischemic time is then limited to the time it takes to do the proximal aortic anastomosis only.

5. Extracorporeal pump. Finally, another technical approach to this pathology is the renal perfusion using a femoral vein to femoral artery bypass using extracorporeal

oxygenation. This method offers a reliable protection but requires a perfusionist, a pump-oxygenation, and a groin incision for retrograde cannulation of the femoral artery and vein. The technique of *ex vivo* renal perfusion has been abandoned because of the risks of removing the transplant (Marone et al., 2008).

In suitable aneurysm candidates, the use of an endovascular graft can also be considered for treatment in patients with congenital pelvic kidneys. Endovascular repair obviates the need for renal protection as warm ischemic time is limited to ballooned graft placement. This is also especially attractive for high-risk patients with multiple comorbidities who otherwise may not tolerate open repair. Contrast load and excessive manipulation of the donor artery in renal allograft patients, however, need to be minimized in order to achieve optimal outcomes. However, there is a risk of vascular damage at the graft anastomotic site, so, if implant dislocation occurs, graft thrombosis may happen (Bui et al., 2007; Bertoni et al., 2010; Morales et al., 2009)

The decision to implant a bifurcated or an aorto-uni-iliac device depends on the anatomical characteristics of the aneurysm. The bifurcated stent graft maintains in-line flow to the renal transplant. The larger delivery system for the main body of the graft can be inserted *via* the contralateral iliac artery. On the other hand, the aorto-uni-iliac system has the potential disadvantages of an extra-anatomic approach, such as anastomotic stenosis, graft occlusion, and a small risk of crossover graft infection (Leon et al., 2009; Sadat et al., 2010).

In conclusion, to preserve renal function during open repair, various methods have been previously reported, but no procedure has been clearly considered the therapeutic gold standard. The congenital pelvic kidney is associated with a normal and functional contralateral kidney, so protective measures need not to be drastic. In our experience, the forced intraoperative diuresis with mannitol and furosemide and the main pelvic kidneys arteries selective perfusion with hypothermic lactate ringer solution, associated to a fast surgical technique, have proven to be safe and effective. (Marone et al., 2008).

7.11 Crossed renal ectopia

A ureteral stent can be placed preoperatively to prevent ureter intraoperative injury as a marker of the abnormal ureter. This shows that the ureter crosses the midline, and enters the bladder at its normal anatomic location. (Yano et al.,2003).

7.12 Acquired pelvic kidney (renal transplant)

The incidence of acute renal failure after aortic surgery in renal transplant patients has ranged from 1 to 8% in elective cases, and in patients with mild or moderate degree of renal dysfunction the morbidity rates are higher than in patients with normal renal function. Given the lack of collateralization of renal allograft, they are more susceptible to ischemic injury than congenital pelvic kidneys (Favi et al., 2005).

The aortic clamp during AAA repair may cause ischemia of the renal graft and diverse procedures have been performed to preserve the function of the transplanted organ. These methods are similar like described in congenital pelvic kidney. Successful surgical repair of AAA in patients with a transplanted kidney has been reported without any form of renal transplant protection, with judicious clamping and rapid anastomosis, although the warm ischemia time of the allograft should not take longer than 60 min. This option could be made difficult by the possibility of finding a very diseased calcific or malacious aortic wall due to dialysis and immunosuppressive therapy (Sckelly et al., 2002).

Standard open surgery without adjunctive shunts or bypasses remains a viable treatment option for these patients. Renal ischemia during aortic cross-clamping can be effectively reduced by cold graft perfusion and local hypothermia. In addition, the potential risk of atheromatous embolization to the transplanted kidney is less than for other temporary procedures of shunt or bypass. The endovascular technique may be used for patients who meet the anatomical criteria for endovascular repair and are at high risk for a conventional operation (Ailawadi et al., 2003; Khanmoradi et al., 2004; Karkos et al., 2006; Kokotsakis et al., 2009). The fever before EVAR in a kidney transplant patient is not always synonymous with infection; it may be a postimplantation syndrome. (Regidor et al., 2009).

It has been described an aortoiliac aneurysm resection and reconstruction with allograft together with simultaneous kidney transplantation as a one-stage procedure with good results. Also it has been described an aortic stent-graft explantation in a kidney transplant recipient (Hughes et al., 2009; Matia et al., 2008, 2009).

7.13 Multiple renal arteries

Accessory renal arteries can also be found during careful dissection of the aorta, usually arising more anteriorly than the normal lateral renal artery orifices. Those that are sufficiently large to supply distinct areas of renal parenchyma should be reimplanted onto the aortic graft if they arise from the AAA. This is facilitated by excising a surrounding collar (Carrel patch) of associated aortic wall along with the orifice.

8. Conclusion

Although uncommon, anatomical anomalies may lead to difficult situations and life-threatening bleeding. A preoperative CT is useful in the patients undergoing an AAA repair. Familiarity with these anomalies and safe operative technique is needed to avoid fatal complications. Endovascular techniques play an important role in AAA cases with venous and genitourinary anomalies if the patient has serious comorbidities and has adequate anatomical conditions in neck and iliac arteries.

9. Acknowledgment

To Carol, Celia and Miguel, for their patient and understanding.

10. References

Ailawadi G, Bedi A, Williams DM, Stanley JC & Upchurch GR. Endovascular treatment of aortic aneurysms in patients with renal transplants. *Journal of Vascular Surgery* Vol.37, No.3, (March 2003), pp. 693-6, ISSN 0741-5214.

Aljabri B, McDonald PS, Satin R, Stein LS, Obrand DI & Steinmetz OK. Incidence of major venous and renal anomalies relevant to aortoiliac surgery as demonstrated by computed tomography. *Annals of Vascular Surgery* Vol.15, No 6, (November 2001), pp. 615-618, ISSN 0890-5096.

Bass JE, Redwine MD, Kramer LA, Huynh PT & Harris JH. Spectrum of congenital anomalies of the inferior vena cava: cross-sectional imaging findings. *Radiographics* Vol.20, No.3, (May 2000), pp. 639-652, ISSN 0271-5333.

Bertoni HG, Girela G, Peirano M, Leguizamon JH, de la Vega A, Barone HD, Nutley M, Zhang Z, Douville Y & Guidoin R. A branched, balloon-deployable, aortomonoiliac stet-graft for treatment of AAA in a patient with a solitary intrapelvic kidney. *Journal Endovascular Therapy*, Vol.17, No.2, (April 2010), pp 261-5, ISSN 1526-6028.

Bui TD, Wilson SE, Gordon IL, Fujitani RM, Carson J & Montgomery RS. Renal function after elective infrarenal aortic aneurysm repair in patients with pelvic kidneys. *Annals of Vascular Surgery*, Vol.21, No.2, (March-April 2007), pp 143-148, ISSN 0890-5096.

Chaudhuri A. Exclusion of an infrarenal AAA with coincident horseshoe kidney and renovascular anomalies is feasible using a standard stent-graft. *European Journal of Vascular and Endovascular Surgery*, In press, available on line 25 February 2011, (Epub ahead of print), ISSN 1078-5884.

Dillon EH, Camputaro C. Nonobstructing periureteric venous ring: diagnosis with conventional and three-dimensional reconstruction CT. *American Journal of Roentgenology*, Vol.157, No. 5 (November 1991), pp 997-998. ISSN 0361-803X.

Evers DJ, Stoot JH & Breslau RJ, Symptomatic abdominal aortic aneurysm with inferior vena cava malposition. Acta Chirurgica Belgica, Vol.107, No.6, (November-December 2007), pp 693-4, ISSN 0001-5458.

Eckes D & Lawrence P. Bilateral iliac artery aneurysm and pancake kidney: a case report. *Journal of Vascular Surgery*, Vol.25, No.5, (May 1997), pp 927-30, ISSN 0741-5214.

Eze AR, White JV, Pathak AS & Grabowski MW. Pancake kidney: a renal anomaly complicating aortic reconstruction. *Annals of Vascular Surgery*, Vol.12, No.3, (May 1998), pp 278-281, ISSN 0890-5096.

Favi E, Citterio F, Tondolo V, Chirico A, Brescia A, Romagnoli J & Castagneto M. Abdominal aortic aneurysm in renal transplant recipients. *Transplantation Proceedings* Vol.37, No.6, (July-August 2005), pp. 2488-90, ISSN 0041-1345.

Gabrielli R, Rosati MS, Siani A & Marcucci G. Preoperative evaluation of retroperitoneal venous system anomalies during abdominal aortic aneurysm rupture. *Interactive Cardiovascular and Thoracic Surgery*, Vol.12, No.2, (February 2011), pp 278-80, ISSN 1569-9293.

Galiñanes EL, Quick J, Nichols WK, Ross CB, Faizer R & Morris ME. Horseshoe kidney and inflammatory abdominal aortic aneurysm. 2011, *Annals of Vascular Surgery*, in press, available on-line 27 January 2011, (Epub ahead of print), ISSN 0890-5096.

Giglia JS & Thompson JK. Repair of a thoracoabdominal aortic aneurysm in the presence of a left-sided inferior vena cava. *Journal of Vascular Surgery* Vol.40, No.1, (July 2004), pp. 161-163, ISSN 0741-5214.

Guray Y, Yelgec NS, Guray U, Ylmaz MB, Boyaci A & Korkmaz S. Left sided or transposed inferior vena cava ascending as hemiazygos vein and draining into the coronary sinus via persistent left superior vena cava: case report. *International Journal of Cardiology* Vol. 93, No.3-4, (February 2004), pp. 293-295, ISSN 0167-5273.

Hanif MA, Chandrasekar R & Blair SD. Pelvic kidney and aortoiliac aneurysm, a rare association, case report and literature review. *European Journal of Vascular and Endovascular Surgery*, Vol.30, No.5, (November 2005), pp 531-533, ISSN 1078-5884.

Hughes JD, Leon LR Jr & Goshima KR. Aortic stent-graft explantation in a kidney transplant recipient. *Annals of Vascular Surgery*, Vol.23, No.4, (July-August 2009), pp 535.e21-6, ISSN 0890-5096.

Karkos CD, Bruce IA, Thomson GJL & Lambert ME. Retroaortic left renal vein and its implications in abdominal aortic surgery. *Annals of Vascular Surgery* Vol.15, No.6, (November 2001), pp. 703-708, ISSN 0890-5096.

Karkos CD, McMahon G, Fishwick G, Lambert K, Bagga A & McCarthy MJ. Endovascular abdominal aortic aneurysm repair in the presence of a kidney transplant:

therapeutic considerations. *Cardiovascular and Interventional radiology* Vol.29, No.2, (March 2006), pp. 284-88, ISSN 0174-1551.

Kaskarelis IS, Koukoulaki M, Cappas I & Karkatzia F et al. Successful endovascular repair of ruptured abdominal aortic aneurysm in a renal transplant recipient. *Cardiovascular and interventional radiology* Vol.29, No.2, (April 2006), pp 279-283, ISSN 0174-1551.

Khanmoradi K, Brewster DC, Haddad FF & Cho SI. Endovascular repair of abdominal aortic aneurysm in a kidney transplant with 4-year follow-up. *Surgery* Vol.136, No.1, (July 2004), pp. 103, ISSN 1530-0358

Kokotsakis J, Kaskarelis I, Koukoulaki M, Athansasiou T, Skouteli E, Vougas V, Lioulias A & Drakopoulos S. Entire stent grafting of the thoracoabdominal aorta in a renal transplant recipient subsequent to extra-anatomical bypasses of the main abdominal vessels. *Annals of Thoracic Surgery*, Vol.87, No.2, (February 2009), pp 623-5, ISSN 0003-4975.

Kraus GJ & Goerzer HG. MR-angiographic diagnosis of an aberrant retroaortic left renal vein and review of the literature. *Clinical Imaging* Vol.27, No.2, (March-April 2003), pp. 132-134, ISSN 0899-7071.

Krohn DL, Sanchez LA, Wain RA & Veith FJ. Repair of bilateral common iliac artery aneurysms coexisting with a pelvic horseshoe kidney. *Annals of Vascular Surgery*, Vol.13, No.6, (November 1999), pp 625-628, ISSN 0741-5214.

Lacombe M. Aortoiliac surgery in renal transplant patients. *Journal of Vascular Surgery*, Vol.13, No.5, (May 1991), pp 712-718, ISSN 0741-5214.

Lacombe M. Surgical treatment of aortoiliac aneurysms in renal transplant patients. *Journal of Vascular Surgery*, Vol.48, No.2, (August 2008), pp 291-5, ISSN 0741-5214.

Leon LR, Glazer ES, Hughes JD, Bui TD, Psalms SB & Goshima KR. Aortoiliac aneurysm repair in kidney transplant recipients. *Vascular Endovascular Surgery*, Vol.43, No.1, (February-March 2009), pp 30-45, ISSN 1538-5744.

Lepäntalo M, Biancai F, Edgren J, Eklund B & Salmela K. Treatment options in the management of abdominal aortic aneurysm in patients with renal transplant. *European Journal of Vascular an Endovascular Surgery* Vol.18, No.2, (August 1999), pp. 176-8, ISSN 1078-5884.

Li HZ, Ma X, Qi L, Shi TP Wang BJ & Zhang X. Retroperitoneal laparoscopic ureteroureterostomy for retrocaval ureter: report of 10 cases and literature review. *Urology* Vol.76, No.4, (October 2010), pp 873-6, ISSN 0090-4295.

Maeda T, Watanabe N & Muraki S. Abdominal aortic aneurysm repair in a renal transplant recipient using a femoral v-a bypass. *Annals of Thoracic and Cardiovascular Surgery*, Vol.15, No.6, (December 2009), pp 415-417, ISSN 1341-1098.

Mahmood M, Tandon V, Dwivedi US & Singh PB. Retrocaval ureter: a rare entity in the spectrum of upper tract obstruction. *JK-practitioner* Vol.12, No.1, (January-March 2005), pp 24-25, ISSN 0971-8834.

Makita S, Yoshizaki T & Tabuchi N. A case of abdominal aortic aneurysm with horseshoe kidney. *Annals of Thoracic and Cardiovascular Surgery*, Vol.15, No.2, (April 2009), pp 15:129-132, ISSN 1341-1098.

Marone EM, Tshomba Y, Brioschi C, Calliari FM & Chiesa R. Aortoiliac aneurysm associated with congenital pelvis kidney: a short series of successful open repairs under hypothermic selective renal perfusion. *Journal of Vascular Surgery*, Vol.47, No.3, (March 2008), pp 638-44, ISSN 0741-5214.

Martin-Conejero A, Serrano-Hernando FJ, Reina-Gutierrez T, Rial-Horcajo R, Ponce-Cano AI & Blanco-Cañibano E. Surgery for aortoiliac aneurysm after kidney transplant. *Transplantations Proceedings*, Vol.35, No.8, (December 2003), pp 2953-7, ISSN 0041-1345.

Matia I, Adamec M, Varga M, Janousek L, Lipar K & Viklicky O. Aortoiliac reconstruction with allograft and kidney transplantation as one-stage procedure: long-term results. *European Journal of Vascular and Endovascular Surgery*, Vol.35, No.3, (March 2008), pp 353-7, ISSN 1078-5884.

Matia I, Pirk J, Lipar K & Adamec M. Successful surgical treatment of multilevel aortic aneurysms combined with renal transplantation. *Journal of Vascular Surgery*, Vol.50, No.1, (July 2009), pp 198-201, ISSN 0741-5214.

Minniti S & Procacci C. Congenital anomalies of the vena cava: embryological origin, imaging features and report of three new variants. *European Radiology* Vol.12, No.8, (August 2002), pp. 2040-2055, ISSN 0938-7994.

Morales JP & Greenberg RK. Customised stent graft for complex thoracoabdominal aneurysm associated with congenital pelvic kidney. *European Journal of Vascular and Endovascular Surgery*, Vol.37, No.5, (May 2009), pp 557-559, ISSN 1078-5884 .

Nagashima T, Lee j, Andoh K, Itoh T, Tanohata K, Arai M & Inoue T. Right double inferior vena cava: report of 5 cases and literature review. *Journal of Computer Assisted Tomography*, Vol.30, No.4, (July-August 2006), pp 642-5, ISSN 0363-8715.

Nagraj HK, Kishore TA & Nagalaskshmi S. Transperitoneal laparoscopic approach for retrocaval ureter. *Journal of Minimal Access Surgery*, Vol.2, No.2(April-June 2006), pp 81-82, ISSN 0972-9941.

Natsis K, Iordache G, Xepulias P & Tsikaras P. Preaortic iliac venous confluence. Marsupial vena cava. Case report. *Morphologie*, Vol.87, No.277, (June 2003), pp 21-23, ISSN 1286-0115.

Natsis K, Apostolidis S, Noussios G, Papathanasiou E, Kyriazidou A & Vyzas V. Duplication of the inferior vena cava: anatomy, embryology and classification proposal. *Anatomical Science International*, Vol.85, No.1, (March 2010), pp 56-60, ISSN 1447-6959.

Ng WT & Ng SSM. Double inferior vena cava: a report of three cases. *Singapore Medical Journal*, Vol.50, No.6, (Juny 2009), pp 211-13, ISSN 0037-5675.

Nishibe T, Sato M, Kondo Y, Kaneko K, Muto A, Hoshino R, Kobayashi Y, Yamashita M & Ando M. Abdominal aortic aneurysm with left-sided inferior vena cava. Report of a case. *International Angiology* Vol.23 No.4, (December 2004), pp. 400-402, ISSN 0392-9590.

Palit S & Deb S. A rare presentation of double inferior vena cava with anomalous pattern of azygos and hemiazygos venous system: a case report. *Journal of the Anatomical Society of India*, Vol.51, No.1, (June 2002), pp 65-67, ISSN 0021-9967.

Radermecker MA, Van Damme H, Kerzmann A, Creemers E & Limet R. Association of abdominal aortic aneurysm, horseshoe kidneys, and left-sided inferior vena cava: report of two cases. *Journal of Vascular Surgery*, Vol.47, No.3, (March 2008), pp 645-8, ISSN 0741-5214.

Regidor D, Ahijado FJ, Muñoz MA, Romero M, Roca A, Diaz-Tejeiro R, Leal I & Conde JL. Postimplantation syndrome in a kidney transplant patient: fever is not always synonymous with infection. *Transplantations Proceedings*, Vol.41, No.10, (December 2009), pp 4202-4, ISSN 0041-1345.

Ruggeri M, Tosetto A, Castaman G & Rodeghiero F. Congenital absence of the inferior vena cava: a rare risk factor for idiopathic deep vein thrombosis. *Lancet* Vol.357, No.9254, (February 10, 2001), pp. 441, ISSN 0140-6736.

Ruppert V, Umscheid T, Rieger J, Schmedt CG, Mussack T, Steckmeier B & Stelter WJ. Endovascular aneurysm repair: Treatment of choice for abdominal aortic aneurysm coincident with horseshoe kidney? Three case reports and review of literature. *Journal of Vascular Surgery*, Vol.40, No.2, (August 2004), pp 367-70, ISSN 0741-5214.

Saadi EK, Dussin LH, Moura L & Zago AJ. Endovascular repair of an abdominal aortic aneurysm in patient with horseshoe kidney: a case report. *Revista Brasileña de Cirugía Cardiovascular*, Vol.23, No.3, (July-September 2008), pp 425-428, ISSN 0102-7638.

Sadat U, Huguet EL & Varty K. Abdominal aortic aneurysm surgery in renal, cardiac and hepatic transplant recipients. *European Journal of Vascular and Endovascular Surgery*, Vol.40, No.4, (October 2010), pp 443-9, ISSN 1078-5884.

Schiavetta A, Cerruti R, Cantello C & Patrone P. Marsupial cava and ruptured abdominal aortic aneurysm. *Journal of Vascular* Surgery, Vol.28, No.4, (October 1998), pp 719-22, ISSN 0741-5214.

Schneider JG, Eynatten MV, Dugi KA, Duex M & Nawroth PP. Recurrent deep venous thrombosis caused by congenital interruption of the inferior vena cava and heterozygous factor V Leiden mutation. *Journal of Internal Medicine* Vol.252, No.3, (September 2002), pp. 276-280, ISSN 1365-2796.

Sebe P, Chemla E, Varkarakis J & Latrèmouille C. Variations anatomiques de la vascularisation des reins pelviens: à propos d'un cas et revue de la littérature. *Morphologie*, Vol.88, No.280, (April 2004), pp 24-26, ISSN 1286-0115.

Sénécail B, Josseaume T, Boeuf J, Hebert T, Waizi R & Nonent M. Right-sided duplication of the inferior vena cava. *Morphologie*, Vol.88, No.283, (December 2004), pp 183-7, ISSN 1286-0115.

Shindo S, Kobayashi M, Kaga S, Hurukawa H, Kubota K, Kojima A, Ijori K, Ishimoto T, Kamiya K & Tada Y. Retrocaval ureter and preaortic iliac venous confluence in a patient with an abdominal aortic aneurysm. *Surgical and Radiologic Anatomy*, Vol.21, No.2, (May 1999), pp 147-9, ISSN 0930-1038.

Shindo S, Kubota K, Kojima A, Iyori K, Ishimoto T, Kobayashi M, Kamiya K & Tada Y. Anomalies of inferior vena cava and left renal vein: risk in aortic surgery. *Annals of Vascular Surgery*, Vol.14, No.4, (November 2000), pp 393-6, ISSN 0890-5096.

Simon RW, Amann-Vesti BR, Pfammatter T & Koppensteiner R. Congenital absence ot the inferior vena cava: a rare risk factor for idiopathic deep-vein thrombosis. *Journal of vascular Surgery* Vol.44, No.2, (August 2006), pp. 416, ISSN 0741-5214.

Skelly CL, Farmer AM, Curi MA, Meyerson SL, Davidovitch RS, Woo DH & Schwartz LB. Aortic reconstruction in patients with functioning renal allograft. *Annals of Vascular Surgery* Vol.16, No.6, (November 2002), pp. 779-83, ISSN 0890-5096.

Stroosma OB, Koostra G & Schurink GW. Management of aortic aneurysm in the presence of a horseshoe kidney. *British Journal of Surgery*, Vol.88, No.4, (April 2001), pp 500-9 ISSN 1365-2168.

Tagliafico A, Capaccio E, Rosenberg I, Martinoli C & Derchi LE. Double right inferior vena cava associated with an anomalous venous ring encircling the right common iliac artery: report of a case with CT and US. *European Journal of Radiology Extra*, Vol.65, No.3, (December 2007), pp 111-115, ISSN 0720-048X.

Uthappa MC, Anthony D & Allen C. Retrocaval ureter: MR appearances. *The British Journal of Radiology*, Vol.75, No.890, (February 2002), pp 177-179, ISSN 0007-1285.

Yamamoto N, Mohri M, Kato G, Oki A & Tedoriya T. Isthmus of a horseshoe kidney overlying a ruptured abdominal aortic aneurysm: a case report. *Annals of Thoracic and Cardiovascular Surgery*, Vol.12, No.2, (April 2006), pp 149-51, ISSN 1341-1098.

Yano H, Konagai N, Maeda M, Itoh M, Kuwabara A, Kudou T & Ishimaru S. Abdominal aortic aneurysm associated with crossed renal ectopia without fusion: case report and literature review. *Journal of Vascular Surgery*, Vol.37, No.5, (May 2003), pp 1098-102, ISSN 0741-5214.

17

Isolated Iliac Artery Aneurysm

Shinichi Hiromatsu, Atsuhisa Tanaka and Kentarou Sawada
Kurume University School of Medicine
Japan

1. Introduction

Unlike abdominal and combined aortoiliac artery aneurysms, isolated iliac artery aneurysms (IIAAs) are uncommon. An isolated iliac artery aneurysm is defined as a twofold increase in the diameter of the iliac artery without a coexisting aneurysm at another location. IIAA was encountered infrequently in the past, comprising 0.9% to 4.7% of all intra-abdominal aneurysms according to a review of previous studies; however, in recent times, many asymptomatic IIAAs have been detected incidentally because of the widespread use of abdominal ultrasonography and computed tomography[1-3]. The frequency of IIAA compared to that of abdominal aortic aneurysm (AAA) ranges from 5.1% to 19.4%[4].

2. History

In 1817, Sir Astley Paston Cooper performed the first surgical ligation of the abdominal aorta proximal to the aneurysm for a traumatic external iliac artery (EIA) aneurysm in a 37-year-old man, but the man died 40 hours later[5,6]. In 1827, Valentine Molt performed the first successful ligation of the proximal iliac artery for a common iliac artery aneurysm (CIAA) in a 33-year-old farmer; 18 days later, he found that the aneurysm was nonpulsatile, and he removed the ligature percutaneously[7]. In 1912, Halsted[8] reported that only 5 of 15 (33.3%) patients who underwent iliac artery ligation for aneurysm survived the surgical procedure. In 1913, MacLaren[9] performed a successful ligation for a traumatic internal iliac aneurysm in a young woman. In 1923, more than a century after Cooper's first operation for IIAA, Rudolph Matas[10] performed the first successful proximal aortic ligation for a combined aortoiliac aneurysm in a young man with syphilis, who later died of tuberculosis.

3. Etiology and natural progression

The primary etiology is arteriosclerosis; however, IIAA also arises because of other predisposing conditions such as infection, dissection, fibromuscular dysplasia, trauma, and Marfan syndrome[11-13]. If arteriosclerosis causes an arterial bifurcation to become an obtuse rather than an acute angle, which is not morbid, the pulsation waves will be reflected more strongly[14]. This factor may account for the high incidence of abdominal aneurysm, and common and internal iliac artery aneurysms (iIAA's) may readily develop, because pulsation waves are generated very strongly at the common and internal iliac artery bifurcations owing to shortening of the distance to reflection of the pulse. However, because the EIA does not bifurcate before it becomes the common femoral artery, reflection of a pulsation wave does not readily occur, which may be the reason EIA aneurysms do not develop frequently. Furthermore, because the internal iliac artery branches off the common iliac artery after a short distance, the branch acts as a fulcrum, hindering the extension of an aneurysm along the long axis and expediting the expansion of the short axis diameter, which may facilitate rupture.

4. Incidence of aneurysm

We reviewed the cases of 183 men and 15 women in the literature[15-18], and our series consisted of 35 men and 6 women; which indicates male predominance. The mean age of the men and women in our series were 69.8 ± 10.8 years and 73 ± 7.9 years, respectively. IIAAs comprised 0.9% to 4.7% of all intra-abdominal aneurysms, as per the reports published before the last decade[1,2]. The frequency of IIAA compared to that of AAA was 5.1% to 19.4%, according to the reports published in the last decade, because improvements in diagnostic technology have increased detection of IIAAs[3,4]. Over the past 20 years, 41 patients with IIAA presented at the Kurume University School of Medicine. During the same period, 652 patients with AAA underwent surgery, including 52 patients with ruptured AAA (8%); therefore, the relative frequency of IIAA to that of AAA was 6.1% over a 20-year period at our hospital.

(Location of aneurysm) In the previous literature, 31 of 198 patients (15.7%) with IIAA had concurrent common and iIAA's, and the incidence was higher than the incidence in our series, which was 7.3% (3/41). The aneurysms were located in the common iliac artery in 31 patients and in the internal iliac artery in 7 (7.1%); EIA aneurysms were not observed. These findings are consistent with those of previous studies, which found that 57.1% (113/198) of IIAAs occurred in the common iliac artery, 26.3% (52/198) in the internal iliac artery, and 1.0% (2/198) in the EIA. CIAA was predominant in our series and in the series in the literature [1-4,15-18].

5. Frequency of rupture

Unlike abdominal aortic aneurysm, the natural progression of IIAA is not well defined. In the literature, the rate of rupture of an IIAA is high. Lowry and Kraft[1] reported that 75% of their patients presented with ruptured aneurysms. Similarly, Schuler and Flanigan reported that 51% of their patients had ruptured aneurysms. In an attempt to define the natural progression of these aneurysms, Schuler and Flanigan also reported the cases of 13 patients with untreated aneurysms. Nine of these patients (69%) died of aneurysm rupture after an average of just over 4 months after diagnosis[19]. In addition, the association between rupture and size is not defined. A threshold size of 3–4 cm was recommended in the era of open surgical repair, with its attendant increased morbidity[20]. In our series, the maximum diameter of the IIAAs was 3.2–13 cm (mean, 6.0 ± 1.9 cm). The diameter of the ruptured IIAAs was 5.0-13.0 cm (mean, 6.8 ± 2.1 cm), whereas that of nonruptured IIAAs was 3.2–7.5 cm (mean, 4.8 cm ± 1.1 cm). The diameter of the ruptured IIAAs was significantly greater than that of nonruptured IIAAs. Rupture occurred in 20 patients (48.8%). During the same period, 658 patients with AAA underwent surgery, of which 53 had ruptured aneurysms (8.1%). The frequency of ruptured IIAA was significantly higher than that of ruptured AAA.

The median maximum diameters of ruptured AAAs and ruptured IIAAs (measured at preoperative computed tomography [CT] scanning) were 7.2 ± 1.6 cm and 6.8 ± 2.1 cm, respectively.

6. Symptoms and diagnosis

IIAA may be masked by nonspecific signs and symptoms resulting from pressure on or erosion of adjacent structures, such as hydroureteronephrosis, hematuria, femoral or obturator neurological symptoms, and hemorrhagic stool[14,17,18], particularly in the absence of a pulsatile mass. If the physician, who encounters orthopedic, urologic, or lower abdominal symptoms, does not consider an aneurysm, the aneurysm may not be detected. Iliac aneurysms can be recognized early if the orthopedic surgeon, urologist, or gynecologist suspects this diagnosis; therefore, it is critical that they are aware of this disease. In the literature, IIAA could not be palpated as a pulsatile mass on abdominal examination in the case of 28 of 38 patients. IIAA is difficult to appreciate on an abdominal examination when a physician encounters a patient with lower abdominal pain. However, IIAAs could be palpated as pulsatile masses on rectal examination in 4 of 6 cases in previous studies[14-18,21-23]. Therefore, rectal examination is useful for the diagnosis of this aneurysm in a patient who complains of lower abdominal pain. In recent times, many asymptomatic IIAAs have been detected incidentally because of the widespread use of abdominal ultrasonography and three-dimensional CT.

7. Surgical indications and treatment strategies

The relative and absolute surgical indications for IIAA are minimum diameters of 3 and 4 cm, respectively. We present the treatment strategy for IIAA at our hospital. Most physicians recommend that patients with an IIAA of a diameter more than 3 cm, who are otherwise good surgical candidates, undergo elective repair[3]. We believe that IIAA has a great impact on the remainder of a patient's life because of a high incidence of rupture and fatality. The natural prognosis of IIAA is not clearly understood. However, patients with IIAA should undergo surgical repair if the patient is conscious, is not bedridden owing to a decrease in quality of life (QOL), and is not in the terminal stage of a malignant disease.

7.1 Surgical procedures

We recommend surgery, even in high-risk patients, because various procedures are available for IIAA treatment, depending on patient condition and aneurysm location. In addition, because commercial endografts have become widely available, we have offered endovascular iliac artery aneurysm repair (EVIAR) as an option to all anatomically appropriate patients with IIAAs of diameter more than 3–4 cm. The strategy for IIAA differs for CIAA and iIAA. Furthermore, each group has 2 categories, i.e., high risk and low risk, and the surgical procedure varies with patient suitability for EVIAR. The exclusion criteria for EVIAR were as follows: unfavorable anatomy (calcification, thrombus-lined aneurysm neck, bilateral common iliac aneurysms, excessive angulation, and iliac occlusive disease), a concomitant procedure, and surgeon preference.

7.1.1 The treatment strategies for CIAA

Figure 1 presents the treatment strategies for CIAA when anatomical characteristics exclude EVIAR. High-risk patients with an ipsilateral CIAA undergo thromboexclusion (TE) by coil or ligation of the proximal aneurysm neck, which necessitates femorofemoral bypass[21, 24], whereas those at lower risk are treated by aneurysmectomy with a bifurcated or local interposition prosthetic graft. For bilateral CIAAs, high-risk patients undergo TE with a bifurcated interposition prosthetic graft, whereas lower-risk patients are treated by aneurysmectomy with a bifurcated interposition prosthetic graft. When anatomical characteristics favor EVIAR, the treatment strategies for high-risk patients are the same as those for low-risk patients when EVIAR is used. Patients treated via an endovascular approach receive a unilateral iliac endograft if there is sufficient neck (usually 15 mm) present in the proximal common iliac artery. Otherwise, bifurcated aortoiliac stent grafts are used, which usually preserve at least 1 internal iliac artery. In all instances, the endograft limb is extended into the EIA landing zone (usually >20 mm). The ipsilateral internal iliac artery is addressed by covering the ostium with an endograft by coil embolization. Exclusion of the hypogastric artery by coil embolization and extension of the graft limb into the EIA are the most common.

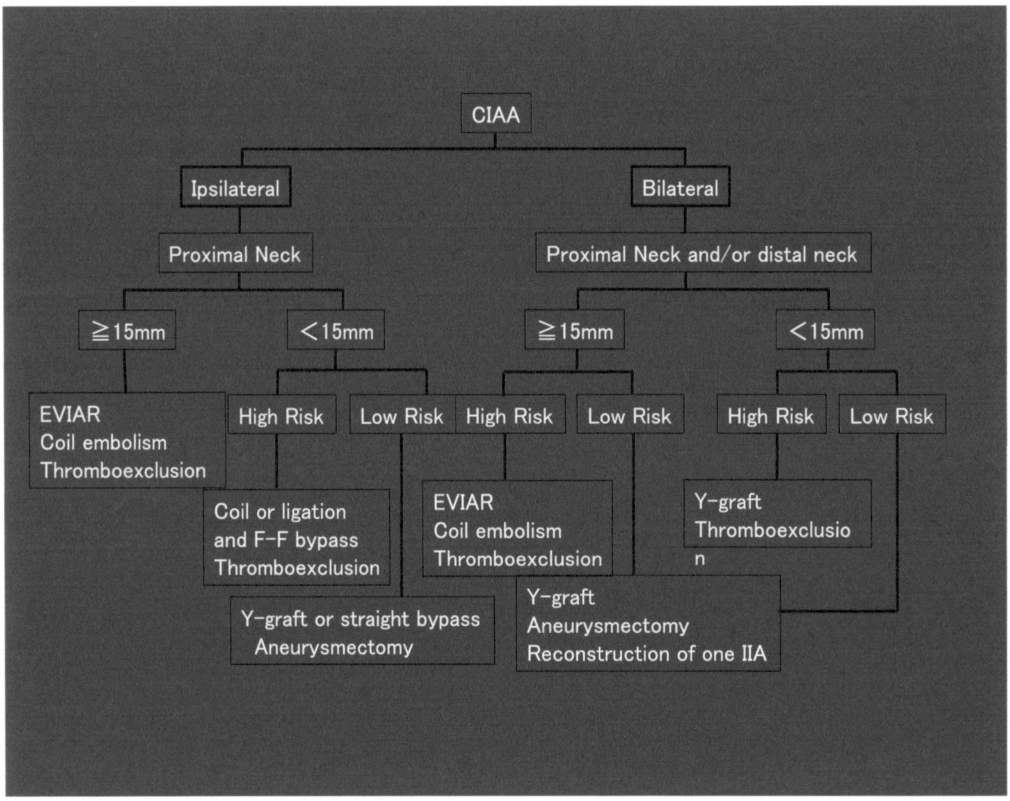

Fig. 1. The treatment strategies for CIAA

7.1.2 The treatment strategies for iIAA

Figure 2 illustrates the strategy for iIAA. High-risk patients with an ipsilateral iIAA undergo TE by coil or ligation of the proximal aneurysm neck, and those at lower risk are treated by endoaneurysmorrhaphy (EA) without reimplantation of the internal iliac artery. For bilateral iIAA, high-risk patients undergo TE by coil or ligation of the proximal aneurysm neck, whereas those at a low risk receive EA with a bifurcated interposition prosthetic graft. Both these procedures require unilateral reimplantation of an internal iliac artery.

When EVIAR is used, ipsilateral internal iliac artery aneurysm is coil-embolized, and the branches of the internal iliac artery are individually coil-embolized, if sufficient neck (usually 15 mm) is present in the proximal internal iliac artery. If the neck is short or absent in the proximal internal iliac artery, the proximal side is supported by a stent graft with extension into the EIA, and the branches are coil-embolized. In the case of bilateral internal iliac artery aneurysms, if the proximal aneurysm necks are <15 mm on both the sides, we recommend open surgery to preserve at least 1 internal iliac artery.

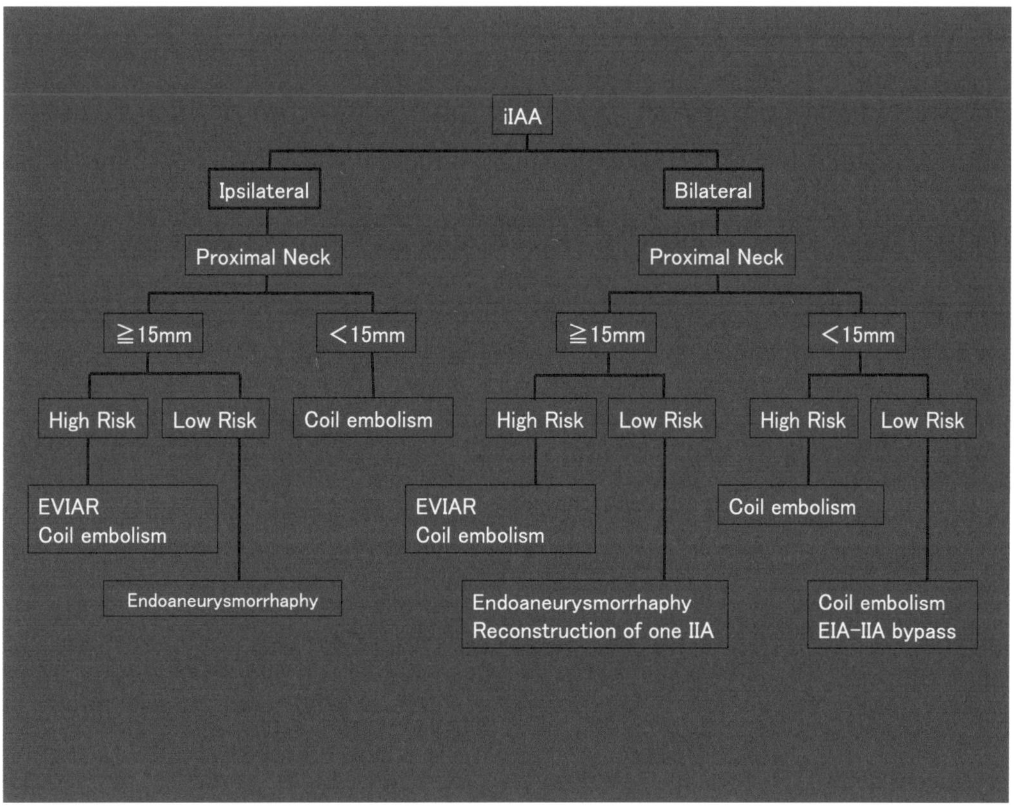

Fig. 2. The treatment strategies for iIAA

7.2 Other procedures

Recently, there has been considerable interest in percutaneous endovascular stent-graft repair of IIAA[20,25,26]. We have performed this procedure in 1 patient at our hospital, and the aneurysm was still reduced 5 years after the procedure without re-expansion. Casana et al. reported that endovascular repair of IIAA was initially successful in all the patients, although the median follow-up period was only 18 months[27]. However, Krupski et al. suggested that surgical repair might be more enduring and effective than percutaneous methods, because long-term results are still undetermined[20].

We believe that stent grafts will become the treatment of choice for IIAA in the future, assuming improvements in equipment and long-term results. When we perform EVIAR for CIAA at our department, we insert a tapered device from the abdominal aorta to the diseased EIA; on the other hand, for the contralateral iliac artery, we fenestrate a stent graft to maintain blood flow. Thus, the indications for EVIAR are as follows: (1) a unilateral common iliac artery aneurysm is present, (2) the aneurysm neck is ≥1 cm, (3) the diameter of the EIA into which the stent graft will be inserted is ≥8 mm, and (4) the contralateral internal iliac artery can be preserved. Patients who met all 4 of these criteria were included as subjects in the study. Further, recently we have been considering iIAA treatment with a stent graft, which involves the same surgical procedure for a stent graft for CIAA in addition to coil embolization of the iIAA.

8. Early and mid-term results

Several series have shown that 30-day mortality was 6%–7% for elective open procedures and 0% for elective EVIAR. However, 30-day mortality was 17%–50% for emergency open procedures and 33% for emergency EVIAR. The mid-term (36 months) primary graft patency rates in the open group and the EVIAR group were 100% and 95.6%–97%, respectively. In addition, the midterm (36 months) secondary intervention in the 2 groups was 0% and 11%–14%, respectively[28-33]. Endovascular repair for IIAA is safe and has similar intermediate-term outcomes to open repair. However, there are various procedures besides the placement of a bifurcated prosthetic graft for IIAA treatment[34]. Surgery should be performed immediately after IIAA diagnosis owing to the risk of rupture, even if patients are anatomically unsuitable for EVIAR. The IIAA treatment should be tailored to the patient's health status and the aneurysm anatomy.

9. Conclusion

Surgery should be performed immediately after IIAA diagnosis owing to the risk of rupture. We undertake surgical management even if the patient has a concomitant disease, because the treatment for IIAA can be performed with MIVS other than the placement of a bifurcated prosthetic graft. The IIAA treatment should be tailored to the patient's health status and the aneurysm anatomy.

10. References

[1] Lowry SF & Kraft RO. Isolated aneurysms of the iliac artery. Arch Surg 1978;113:1289–93.

[2] McCready RA. Isolated iliac artery aneurysms. Surgery 1983;93:688–93.

[3] Nachbur BH. Isolated iliac aneurysms. Eur J Vasc Surg 1991;5:375–81.
[4] Kasirajan V. Management of isolated common iliac artery aneurysms. Cardiovasc Surg 1998;6:171–7.
[5] Osler W. Remarks on arterio-venous aneurysm. Lancet 1915; 2:949.
[6] Cooper AP. Lectures on the principles and practice of surgery. 2nd ed. London: FC Westley; 1830. P. 153-76.
[7] Hager K. The illustrated history of surgery. New York: Bell Publishing; 1988.
[8] Halsted WS. The effect of ligature of the common iliac artery on the circulation and function of the lower extremitities. Trans Am Surg Assoc 1912; 30: 196-200.
[9] MacLaren A. Aneurysm of the internal iliac artery, probably following a severe instrumental delivery: operation and partial cure. Ann Surg 1913; 117:73-7.
[10] Matas R. Ligation of the abdominal aorta. Ann Surg 1925; 457: 457-62.
[11] Richardson JW, & Greenfield LJ, Natural history and management of iliac aneurysms. J Vasc Surg1998;8:165-71.
[12] Veith FJ, & Johnston KW. Endovascular treatment of abdominal aortic aneurysms: an innovation in evolution and under evaluation. J Vasc Surg 2002; 35: 183.
[13] Collin J, & Murie JA. Endovascular treatment of abdominal aortic aneurysm: a failed experiment. Br J Surg 2001; 88:1281-2.
[14] Lallemand RC. Role of the bifurcation in atheromatosis of the abdominal aorta. Surg Gynecol Obstet 1973; 137:987-90.
[15] Minato N. Isolated iliac artery aneurysm and its management. Cardiovasc Surg 1994; 2: 489-94.
[16] Shindo S. Inflammatory solitary iliac artery aneurysms: a report of two cases. Cardiovasc Surg 2001; 9:615-9.
[17] Katoh J. Rupture of anisolated internal iliac artery aneurysm into the rectum: report of a case. Surg Today 1995; 25:554-6.
[18] Katagiri M, & Kasuya S. Surgery for an isolated aneurysm of the internal iliac artery. Report of three cases. J Cardiovasc Surg (Trino) 1990; 31:118-20.
[19] Schuler JJ, & Flanigan DP: Iliac artery aneurysms. In Bergan J, YaoJST, editors: Diagnosis and treatment. New York, 1982, Grune and Strarron, pp 469-85.
[20] Krupski WC. Contemporary management of isolated iliac aneurysms. J Vasc Surg 1998;28:1–13.
[21] Boules TN. Endovascular management of isolated iliac artery aneurysms. J Vasc Surg 2006;44:29–37.
[22] Reuter SR, & Carson SN. Thrombosis of common iliac artery aneurysm by selective embolization and extraanatomic bypass. AJR 1980;134:1248–50.
[23] Matsumoto K. Surgical and endovascular procedures for treating isolatediliac artery aneurysms: ten-year experience. World J Surg 2004;28:797–800.
[24] Sahgal A. Diameter changes in isolated iliac artery aneurysms 1 to 6 years after endovascular graft repair. J Vasc Surg 2001;33:289–95.
[25] Chuter TA. Branched stent-grafts for endovascular repair of aortic andiliac aneurysms. Tech Vasc Interv Radiol 2005;8:56–60.
[26] Sanchez LA. Midterm experience with the endovascular treatment of isolated iliac aneurysms. J Vasc Surg 1999;30:907–13.
[27] Casana R. Midterm experience with the endovascular treatment of isolated iliac aneurysms. Int Angiol 2003;22:32–5.

[28] Patel NV. Open vs. endovascular repair of isolated iliac artery aneurysms: A 12-year experience. J Vasc Surg 2009;49: 1147-53.
[29] Pitoulias GA. Isolated iliac artery aneurysms: Endovascular versus open elective repair. J Vasc Surg 2007; 46: 648-54.
[30] Dorigo W. The treatment of isolated iliac artery aneurysm in patients withnon-aneurysmal aorta. Eur J Vasc Endovasc Surg 2008; 35: 585-89.
[31] Boules TN. Endovascular management of isolated iliac artery aneurysms. J Vasc Surg 2006;44:29-37.
[32] Char RA. Isolated iliac artery aneurysms: A contemporary comparison of endovascular and openrepair. J Vasc Surg 2008; 47: 708-13.
[33] Ferreira J. Isolated iliac artery aneurysms: six-year experience. InteractCardio Vasc Thorac Surg 2010; 10: 245-48.
[34] Hiromatsu S. Strategy for isolated iliac artery aneurysms. Asian Cardiovasc Thorac Ann 2007; 15:280-4.

18

Concomitant Abdominal Aortic Aneurysm and Malignancy: Simultaneous Minimally Invasive Repair

Gabriele Piffaretti[1], Luigi Boni[2], Matteo Tozzi[1], Nicola Rivolta[1], Giovanni Mariscalco[3] and Patrizio Castelli[1]

[1]*Vascular Surgery – Department of Surgical Sciences, University of Insubria School of Medicine, Varese*

[2]*General Surgery 1 – Department of Surgical Sciences, University of Insubria School of Medicine, Varese*

[3]*Cardiac Surgery – Department of Surgical Sciences, University of Insubria School of Medicine, Varese, Italy*

1. Introduction

Concomitant diseases were defined as those detected during the preoperative diagnostic evaluation for symptomatic abdominal aortic aneurysm (AAA) or occasional finding during oncological staging and/or follow-up, or as an intraoperative unsuspected findings at laparotomy. Malignancies presenting synchronously with AAA more frequently include primary or metastatic cancer of the gastrointestinal or genitor-urinary systems; more anecdotally, lung or endocrine cancers have been reported to be treated with AAA repair.

The association of AAA and malignancies is rare. In fact, although the true incidence of concomitant malignancy and AAA is difficult to establish, most centers report a low incidence of co-existence: discrepancy in incidence between the various studies probably depends on whether all aneurysms are included or just those operated on, and also whether only simultaneously diagnosed malignancies are included or all malignancies associated with a patient with an AAA (Jibawi et al., 2011). Malignancies were found in 4% of AAA cases in an extensive experience that covered 22 years (Szilagyi et al.). In the UK in 1995 there were approximately 7000 elective and emergency operations for AAA, giving an estimated annual incidence of concomitant colorectal malignancy of between 35 and 105 (Morris et al. 1998).

Since the milestone report of Szilagyi's four decades ago (Szilagyi et al.), surgical procedures for synchronous AAA and tumors have been constantly performed but reports have been mainly represented by single case series with small numbers. More recently, the advent of mini-invasive technology have (potentially) widened the indication to treat both lesions more extensively. A simultaneous minimally invasive treatment should be intended as the single-stage operation that couples an endovascular treatment to exclude the AAA and an additional minimally invasive technique to treat or excise the concomitant malignant lesion.

2. Radiologic work-up and patient selection

Regardless of the type of tumor, a multidisciplinary team help to direct the work-up and choose the type of imaging studies to determine AAA repair as well as the resectability of the cancer.

The goals of the radiologic work-up are the following items:

- to confirm the diagnosis and specify the morphology and sizing of the AAA
- define the local extent of the malignancy and the presence of metastases

When possible, preoperative evaluation should be carried out following a specific protocol, performing routine preoperative blood test, chest X-rays, ECG transthoracic echocardiography, plethymsography, and thoraco-abdominal CT-angiography (Fig. 1).

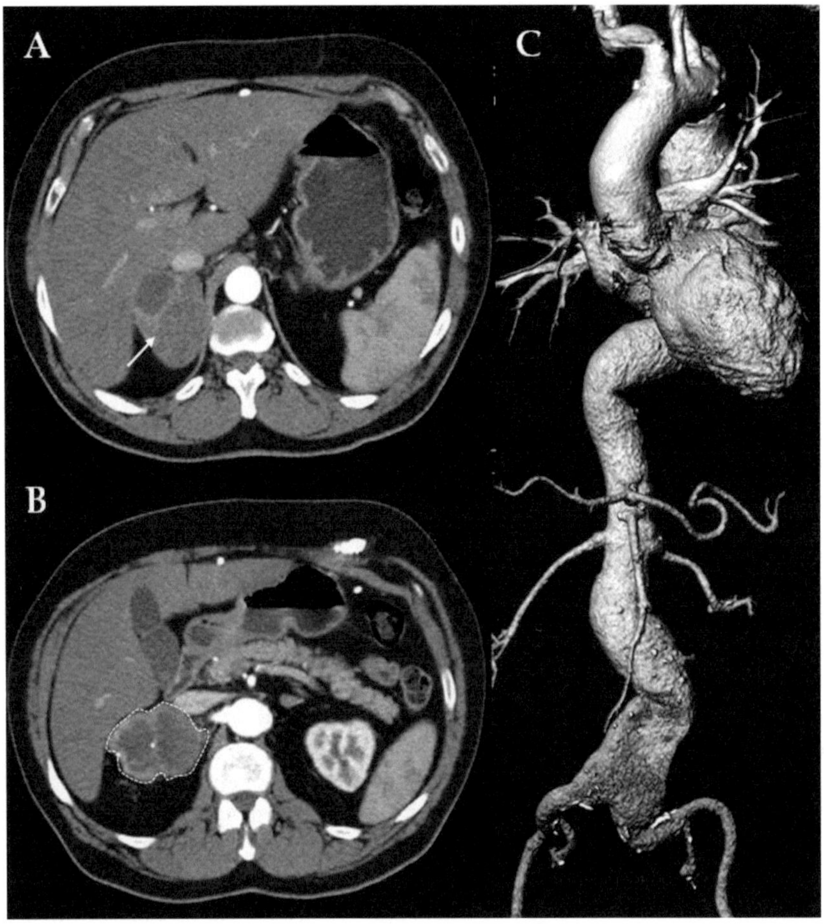

Fig. 1. Preliminary CT-angiography showing the presence of a mass (A, *arrow*) protrusing from the upper portion of the right kidney (B, *dotted line*) and a huge 6.5cm fusiform infrarenal AAA (C)

Esofagogastroscopy and/or flexible colonoscopy, liver ultrasound and other staging examinations were performed depending on the location of the tumor. The combination of these studies is needed to determine surgical resectability and to plan the type of

reconstruction, and therefore to guide the type of surgical approach and to assess the feasibility of the mini-invasive approaches.
Pathologic tumor staging should be classified according to the most recent TNM system.
Post-operative follow-up should be scheduled at periodic intervals (generally, 1, 6 and 12 months) coupling clinical visit, serological tests using oncologic markers, and CT-angiography to confirm the technical success or detect any type of complications (Fig. 2).

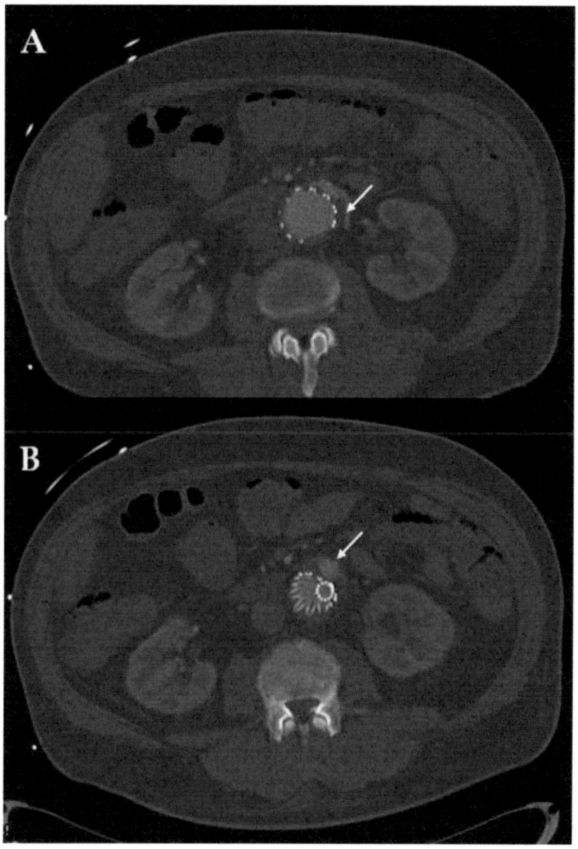

Fig. 2. Follow-up CT-angiography detecting an early type 2 endoleak (B, *arrows*) because of the inverted flow into the inferior mesenteric artery (A)

For decades, surgical intervention were rarely performed for several reasons: many cancers presented in advanced stage and carried poor prognosis, extent of the procedure especially for debilitated patients who had associated co-morbidities that placed them at high operative risk, many patients had undergone previous attempts of surgical resection or received adjuvant chemotherapy or radiation therapy that increased technical difficulties. More recently, improvements in preoperative imaging studies, surgical techniques, intraoperative anesthetic management, postoperative care, and the success of prosthetic grafts have burdened the impetus for a more aggressive surgical approach in selected patients. Nowadays, those patients with localized tumor, few co-morbidities (e.g. renal, liver, cardiopulmonary), and a good performance status could be considered candidates for operation. Careful patient evaluation is critical to outcome; a multidisciplinary approach to the evaluation and treatment of these patients is an integral component for patient selection involving both the medical evaluation of the candidate along with a precise assessment of both AAA and tumor extension. Dealing with a similar clinical challenge, such as the combination of liver resection with caval vascular reconstruction, a patient's performance status could be determined using general criteria which provides an assessment of the patient's physical conditioning and has been a useful measure of functional quality of life for patients with malignant disease in that situation (Bower et al, 2000).

3. Indication

All agree that definitive treatment of both processes confers the best overall prognosis; nevertheless, concerns still remain toward decision-making strategy, whether it is better to treat both diseases simultaneously or as staged procedures. Clinical consensus is to treat the most life-threatening process first: prioritization is determined by the urgency of addressing each of the identified conditions (Kiskinis et al., 2004). In the past, surgical strategy was determined by the patient's general condition, the patient's symptoms, the surgeon's preference, the AAA size, and cancer stage.

Up to date, we have paucity of experiences with small number of cases treated, with wide heterogeneities of the oncologic lesions: hence, because of all these uncertainties, there is no consensus on the best therapeutic approach for patients with simultaneous AAA and malignancy. In addition, detailed management strategies vary however, among different authors with some choosing simultaneous over sequential operations on the basis of cancer type and stage (Oshodi et al., 2000).

The main goal of the single-stage is either to prevent cancer progression or to prevent AAA rupture; the advantages of the simultaneous intervention are clear:

- treating two lethal diseases with a single laparotomy reduces technical difficulties due to scarred or post-attinic tissues;
- the specific risk related to general anaesthesia, particularly high in these patients often affected by significant co-morbidities (vascular, respiratory and metabolic) and the advanced age, it is reduced by treating both condition at one time;
- the risk of cancer progression is kept at minimum since there is no delay between tumour diagnosis and surgical treatment

The main disadvantage of the combined intervention is that single-stage operation carries potential risk of graft infection; in addition, it lengthens the operation time and decreases the bowel perfusion.

The advantages of the delayed intervention are:

- lower risk of graft infection due to the reduced risk of septic disease
- it reduces splanchnic ischemia (reduces potential leakages of the gastrointestinal or genitor-urinary anastomosis)
- it allows a definitive and specific staging of the oncologic disease

The main disadvantage of the two-stage intervention is that when AAA repair is performed first, the physiological immunosuppression effect can lead to cancer progression, whereas it has been demonstrated that, when the malignant tumour is resected first, there is a systemic release of protheolytic enzymes that could lead to the growth and rupture of the aneurysmatic sac (Lin et al., 2008). In addition, it is unquestionable that the two stage approach is definitively technically more complex due to the presence of peritoneal adhesions that, in some patients, could be extremely hard to dissect.

4. Intervention techniques

Generally, in conventional AAA repair a standard transperitoneal approach using a midline laparotomy has been performed; few Authors suggested a retroperitoneal approach to avoid contamination (Grego et al., 2003). Surgical reconstruction of the AAA have been preferentially performed using Dacron graft: silver or antibiotic-bonded prostheses should be supported in order to reduce the risk of infection in a potentially contaminated fields. Cancer resection was carried out following the main oncological principles (no touch techniques and vessels legation at their origins).

With the availability of laparoscopic surgery, as well as other minimally invasive therapies such as cryoablation for conditions including renal lesions, endovascular aortic repair (EVAR) nowadays represents an attractive alternative treatment modality with a less traumatic strategy (Porcellini et al., 2007). In addition to the management of primary AAAs, late sequelae of traditional repair such as anastomotic aneurysm, can also be addressed. Endografting confers the benefit of eliminating the need for a second laparotomy and creates flexibility in managing concomitant malignancy in rapid succession or simultaneously (Lee et. al, 2002). The devices can be placed prior to transabdominal resection and thus post-laparotomy rupture can be avoided. Hence, more recently, the single stage approach has been proposed using EVAR: the availability of this minimally invasive treatment strategy has created an alternative therapeutic paradigm, particularly in patients with synchronous challenging settings (Rivolta et. al, 2007). Results are still preliminary, and paucity of documentation exists concerning the application of EVAR to these patients as well as data pertaining to perioperative events.

Very few data have been published on the outcomes of synchronous treatment of AAA and tumors: we should take into account that the different etiology of cancers and the small number of patients preclude definitive conclusions regarding survival for such extensive interventions performed with open surgery. The advent of minimally invasive techniques with their encouraging results have been recently confirmed from different teams; in particular, EVAR intuitively should offer clinical and postoperative survival benefits in those patients at higher risk for conventional open repair. However, concerns remain about the definition of high-risk patient. Is the patient with concomitant diseases at higher risk for mini-invasive operations? In previous clinical experiences, ASA score have been used to identify high-risk patients; this is a variable objectively assessed by an independent auditor (anesthesiologist); it has been reported a 7.8% hospital mortality for ASA class 4, a 15-times higher than the rate for low-risk patients in that center (Verzini et al., 2002). If we consider the results of a large pivotal trial, attempt to identify the predictors of survival we could observe that malignancy was the cause of death in 30% of the patients, overall especially in the second year of that experience (Matsumura et al., 2009). More recently, our results have been in consonance with these data: in the long-term analysis, ASA was an independent factors of mortality but we did not consider the stage of malignant disease in the concept of high-risk patient despite tumors cancer was the second leading cause of death (11%) in our personal series (Lomazzi et al., 2011).

5. Literature review

The first ever report of minimally invasive treatment of synchronous malignancy and AAA was reported in 1998 by Herald et al. who performed full rectal wall thickness endoanal local excision of the rectal tumor but delayed the EVAR of the aneurysm three weeks later (herald et al., 1998). Similarly, Hafez et al. reported 3 cases of combined treatment for kidney tumors and AAA, but again the Authors did go 97 days between the two procedures (hafez et al., 2000). The most extensive clinical experience in the surgical management of patients with synchronous AAA and colo-rectal cancer have been reported by Lin et al. over 108 cases (lin et al., 2008). In their data, a total of 92 patients formed the basis of the study: twelve patients underwent EVAR but they were primarily treated for the AAA and then the colo-rectal cancer followed. They had no aortic graft infections, regardless of whether surgical treatment was performed in a staged or simultaneous fashion; however, they stated that despite the reported safety by several researchers about combined surgical repair of these synchronous lesions, we believe such a simultaneous surgical approach should be avoided whenever possible. It reflected the relatively small sample size in each group, rather than the safety of various treatment modalities. They concluded suggesting that: 1) staged open AAA repair followed by colo-rectal excision should be performed with caution because of the higher operative morbidity and mortality rates; 2) although combining rectal resection with EVAR during a single operation may seem to be an attractive option, concerns still remain about the potential endograft infection because of the seeding from the perioperative bacteremia related to the colon resection.

The attractive alternative to repair in a single-stage operation both lesions was brought to the fore by Lee et al. in 5 patients with different malignancies including renal, urinary bladder, esophageal, lung, and prostate (Lee et al., 2002). Endovascular exclusion was successfully accomplished in all cases, and surgical conversions were never needed; the postoperative course was uneventful with mean length of stay was 3.4 days. The Authors concluded that EVAR of either an aneurysm or other aortic pathology in patients with an associated malignancy can be performed safely, but remains an individualized option with a multidisciplinary team necessary to explore this type of approach.

The advantage of EVAR repair in patients with different (colon-rectum, bladder, pancreas, esophagous, prostate, kidney) concomitant abdominal malignancy was finally highlighted in a recent report by Porcellini et al. who compared 14 patients undergoing conventional open AAA repair vs. 11 patients who received endografting (Porcellini et al., 2007). Among those who received conventional open repair, 7 patients had simultaneous operations, with operative mortality and aortic graft infection rates of 14% and 14%, respectively. The overall operative morbidity and mortality rates of those treated with conventional open aneurysm repair were 34% and 21%, respectively. This was in contrast to the EVAR patient cohorts, who suffered no operative mortality and a relatively low operative morbidity rate of 8%. These short-term benefits are extremely important in patients who require further treatment for the concomitant oncologic lesion; even an advantage that was maintained after a mean follow-up of approximately 3 years. Furthermore, it is also likely that improvement of endovascular devices, refined technique, and enhanced operator experience will have an impact on the long-term outcome of EVAR.

6. Personal experience

Between august 1989 and December 2010, our overall experience consisted of 31 cases of synchronous repair of AAA and malignancy using the single-stage approach. The single stage minimally invasive approach was performed in 10 cases: we operated 9 males and 1 female, with a median age of 72 years (range 52-79). Most of the patients had co-morbidities: hypertension (n = 9), ischemic heart disease with prior cardiac revascularization (n = 4), chronic obstructive pulmonary (FEV_1 < 1lt, n = 4), and mild (creatinine >2mg/dL) chronic renal insufficiency (n = 1). Oncologic lesions included colo-rectal cancer (n = 5), kidney (n = 2), adrenal gland (n = 1), liver metastasis (n = 1), and lung cancer (n =1). Aortic disease included atherosclerotic fusiform AAA (n = 9), and saccular aneurysm complicating an ulcerated plaque (n = 1). All AAAs were infra-renal with a mean diameter of 58 mm (range, 44-92). Aneurysms were treated using bifurcated (n = 9) or tube (n = 1) endograft (infrarenal n = 8, transrenal n = 2). Oncologic operations included laparoscopic colectomy (left n = 4, right n = 1) for colo-rectal cancers, thermoablation with radiofrequency (n = 3), laparoscopic right nephrectomy (n = 1), and thoracoscopic wedge resection (n = 1). The mean blood loss was 312 ± 54 ml (range 154-400). Intensive care unit was never needed. Two patients had a major postoperative complication: acute on chronic renal insufficiency (n = 1) but hemofiltration or dialysis were not required, and acute pulmonary oedema (n = 1). Hospital mortality was not observed; there was no evidence of perioperative endograft infection. Mean hospitalization was 7 days (range 4-12). All patients were discharged alive and well; no patient was lost to follow-up. Median follow-up was 14 months: endograft infection was never observed, 2 patients died because of disseminated cancer disease (liver) and pulmonary thromboembolism without clinical or radiological signs of recurrency (kidney).

7. Comment

While co-existing AAA and malignancy is not a common problem, it presents a challenging dilemma in terms of operative management. Most physicians agree that treatment priority should be focused on the symptomatic or more life threatening lesion (Baxter et al., 2002). But because the majority of these concomitant lesions are asymptomatic at the time of diagnosis, physicians frequently are confronted with a therapeutic dilemma when dealing with this potentially challenging surgical problem. When the vascular surgeon discovers intra-abdominal malignancy before or during laparotomy the main considerations are to treat both lesions effectively, and to minimize the risks of graft infection and of postoperative rupture of the aneurysm.

The simultaneous combined treatment has not been used extensively; Literature lacks of experiences, especially those with long-term follow-up (Table 1).

Less often minimally invasive techniques have been used to treat concomitant lesions in a single-stage intervention. This because it has been considered inappropriate to resects aneurysms less than 50 mm or less in diameter, synchronously with a major gastrointestinal lesion if they are asymptomatic (Matsumoto et al., 1999). However, we should also pointed out that literature reported worse outcomes for patients with larger aneurysms, because they are often associated with a less favorable anatomy for EVAR (Zarins et al., 2006). In contrast, given the excellent results of EVAR in the short-term period in terms of morbidity and mortality, coupled with the most recent endograft improvement, as well as the shorter life-expectancy of these patients and the need to receive adjuvant therapies for the malignant lesion, a more aggressive management for the AAA could be supported legitimately.

Author	Cases (*number*)	Aortic disease	K location	K operation	Delay (*weeks*)	L.O.S. (*days*)	Follow-up (*mean, months*)	Complication
Herald et al.	1	aneurysm	colo-rectal	endoanal	3		12	no
Hafez et al.	3	aneurysm	kidney	open	13		57	no
Sheen et al.	1	aneurysm	pancreas	open	1		1	no
Lee et al.	5	aneurysm (4)	mainly genitourinary	open	simultaneous	3.4	10.1	no
Chai et al.	2	aneurysm	colo-rectal	open	1		12	endograft thrombosis
Kiskinis et al.	2	aneurysm	colo-rectal	open	simultaneous (1)	8	9	no
Lin et al.	12	aneurysm	colo-rectal	open	1		n.r.	no
Porcellini et al.	11	aneurysm	mainly gastrointestinal	open (9)	<1	n.s.	37.7	limb occlusion (2)
*Personal**	10	aneurysm	mainly gastrointestinal	video-assisted (7)	simultaneous	7	14	no

The main critic against a synchronous repair has been believed to be the increased risk of graft infection; to tell the truth, several previous papers focused on the outcome of a simultaneous intervention for AAA and cancer finally did not highlighted an increased risk for this type of complication. The risk of direct graft contamination by gut or urinary tract bacterial agents may be reduced by a combination of preoperative and bowel preparation, meticulous surgical technique and antimicrobial therapy with long-term antibiotic prophylaxis. Moreover, endograft placement should theoretically prevent exposure of the graft to an infected or potentially contaminated operative field: in fact, laparotomy is avoided and the aneurysmatic sac potentially protects the endograft from bowel contamination because of contiguity. In addition, septic complications following EVAR has been reported in only 0.43%, still lower than the 0.5-3% of the conventional open repair (Ducasse et al., 2004).

It is unquestionable whether the single-stage intervention using minimally invasive techniques has technically decreased complexity and less traumaticity. Intuitively, it remains desirable but even doubtful that a prospective randomized controlled study with sufficient statistical power will ever take place to definitively formulate a standardized treatment strategy in patients with these concomitant diseases.

8. Conclusion

Lacks of extensive series as well as long-term follow-up do not allow to drawn definitive conclusions. Simultaneous AAA repair and malignancy excision using minimally invasive techniques has been rarely reported in a single-stage operation. Nevertheless, the few papers actually available reported encouraging technical and clinical results especially in the short-term period, provided that aortic anatomy is suitable. If this is the case, it may be considered an attractive alternative to standard open repair.

9. References

Baxter NN, Noel AA, Cherry K, & Wolff BG. Management of patients with colorectal cancer and concomitant abdominal aortic aneurysm. *Dis Colon Rectum* 2002;45:165-170

Bower TC, Nagorney DM, Cherry KJ Jr, Toomey BJ, Hallett JW, Panneton JM, & Gloviczki P. Replacement of the inferior vena cava for malignancy: an update. *J Vasc Surg* 2000;31:270-278

Chai CY, Lin PH, Bush RL, & Lumsden AB. Aortic endograft thrombosis after colorectal surgery in lithotomy position. *J Vasc Surg* 2004;39:1112-1114

Ducasse E, Calisti A, Speziale F, Rizzo L, Misuraca M,& FioraniP. Aortoiliac stent graft infection: current problems and management. *Ann Vasc Surg* 2004;18:521-526

Grego F, Lepidi S, Bassi P, Tavolini IM, Noventa F, Pagano F, & Deriu GP. Simultaneous surgical treatment of abdominal aortic aneurysm and carcinoma of the bladder. *J Vasc Surg* 2003;37:607-614

Hafez KS, El Fettouh HA, Novick AC, & Ouriel K. Management of synchronous renal neoplasm and abdominal aortic aneurysm. *J Vasc Surg* 2000;32:1102-1110

Herald JA, Young CJ, White GH, & Solomon MJ. Endosurgical treatment of synchronous rectal cancer and abdominal aortic aneurysm, without laparotomy. *Surgery* 1998;124:932-933

Jibawi A, Ahmed I, El-Sakka K, & Yusuf SW. Management of concomitant cancer and abdominal aortic aneurysm. *Cardiol Res Pract* 2011;19;2011:516146

Kiskinis D, Spanos C, Melas N, Efthimiopoulos G, Saratzis N, Lazaridis I, & Gkinis G. Priority of resection in concomitant abdominal aortic aneurysm (AAA) and colorectal cancer (CRC): review of the literature and experience of our clinic. *Tech Coloproctol* 2004;8:S19-21

Lee JT, Donayre CE, Walot I, Kopchok GE, & White RA. Endovascular exclusion of abdominal aortic pathology in patients with concomitant malignancy. *Ann Vasc Surg* 2002;16:150-156

Lin PH, Barshes NR, Albo D, Kougias P, Berger DH, Huynh TT, LeMaire SA, Dardik A, Lee WA, & Coselli JS. Concomitant colorectal cancer and abdominal aortic aneurysm: evolution of treatment paradigm in the endovascular era. *J Am Coll Surg* 2008;206:1065-1073

Lomazzi C, Mariscalco G, Piffaretti G, Bacuzzi A, Tozzi M, Carrafiello G, & Castelli P. Endovascular treatment of elective abdominal aortic aneurysms: independent predictors of early and late mortality. *Ann Vasc Surg* 2011;25:299-305

Matsumoto K, Nakamaru M, Obara H, Hayashi S, Harada H, Kitajima M, Shirasugi N, & Nouga K. Surgical strategy for abdominal aortic aneurysm with concurrent symptomatic malignancy. *World J Surg* 1999;23:248-251

Matsumura JS, Katzen BT, Sullivan TM, Dake MD, & Naftel DC. Excluder Bifurcated Endoprosthesis Investigators. Predictors of survival following open and endovascular repair of abdominal aortic aneurysms. Ann Vasc Surg *2009*;23:153-158

Oshodi TO, Abraham JS, Brigg JK, & Kelly JF. Management of co-existing intra-abdominal disease in aortic surgery. *Eur J Vasc Endovasc Surg* 2000;19:43-46

Piffaretti G, Rivolta N, Mariscalco G, Tozzi M, Maida S, & Castelli P. Aortic endograft infection: A report of 2 cases. *Int J Surg* 2010;8:216-220

Porcellini M, Nastro P, Bracale U, Brearley S, & Giordano P. Endovascular versus open surgical repair of abdominal aortic aneurysm with concomitant malignancy. *J Vasc Surg* 2007;46:16-23

Rivolta N, Piffaretti G, Tozzi M, Lomazzi C, Riva F, Alunno A, Boni L, & Castelli P. Management of simultaneous abdominal aortic aneurysm and colorectal cancer: the rationale of mini-invasive approach. *Surg Oncol* 2007;16 Suppl 1:S165-167

Sheen AJ, Baguneid M, Ellenbogen S, Walker MG, & Siriwardena AK. Sequential endovascular repair and pancreaticoduodenectomy for abdominal aortic aneurysm copresenting with periampullary cancer. *Ann Vasc Surg* 2006;20:114-116

Szilagyi DE, Elliott JP, & Berguer R. Coincidental malignancy and abdominal aortic aneurysm. Problems of management. *Arch Surg* 1967;95:402–412

Verzini F, Cao P, Zannetti S, Parlani G, De Rango P, Maselli A, Lupattelli L, & Parente B. Outcome of abdominal aortic endografting in high-risk patients: a 4-year single-center study. J Endovasc Ther *2002*;9:736-742

Zarins CK, Crabtree T, Bloch DA, Arko FR, Ouriel K, & White RA. Endovascular aneurysm repair at 5 years: Does aneurysm diameter predict outcome? *J Vasc Surg* 2006;44:920-929

19

Aortic Aneurysms in Takayasu Arteritis

Guido Regina, Domenico Angiletta, Alessandro Bortone, Martinella Fullone, Davide Marinazzo and Raffaele Pulli
University of Bari
Italy

1. Introduction

Takayasu arteritis is a non-atherosclerotic chronic inflammatory vascular disease of unknown etiology that affects the aorta, proximal parts of its major branches and the pulmonary arteries. The disease may cause stenosis, occlusions and sometimes aneurysm formation in the aorta and/or the affected arteries. As the use of arteriography gradually became a more widespread and the procedure was more generally available, more details of the disease and its manifestation began to be described.

From the historical perspective, Mikito Takayasu is credited with having been the first to describe the disease in 1908, when he presented a case of a 21-year old woman with a peculiar optic fundus abnormality, characterized by arteriovenous anastomosis around the papilla (fig. 1). He made no mention of whether or not radial pulses were absent or diminished. Two other ophthalmologists, Onishi and Kagoshima, also described patients very similar to the one described by Takayasu, adding that their patients had no radial pulses. This is why nowadays, the disease is called Takayasu-Onishi aorto-arteritis. Probably the first description of the disease we now call Takayasu arteritis was actually done by Giovan Battista Morgagni in 1771. Patients with pulseless disease or aortic syndrome were also described by Adams in 1827, Devy in 1839 and William Broadbent in 1875. In 1856, the English surgeon William Savory described pathological and clinical examination findings in a patient who died of pulseless disease and aortic arch syndrome. In this 22-year old woman, autopsy revealed obliteration of left internal carotid artery, together with bilateral subclavian artery occlusion.

Histological descriptions of Takayasu arteritis were reported by Beneke in 1925 and Harbitz in 1926.

2. Epidemiology

Although Takayasu arteritis was first described in the Orient and is undoubtedly more prevalently among patients in India, Africa and South America, the disease has a worldwide distribution, with an increasing incidence in western countries. Retrospective reviews conclude that Takayasu arteritis is more frequent than was previously believed. Although most series collected in the United States include some Asians, these patients are mostly white. The disease affects women in the reproductive age group 5 to 8 times more commonly than men (Lupi-Herrera et al., 1977; Hall et al., 1985; Sato et al., 1998). In India and Japan is responsible for about

5% of all vascular cases. It has a worldwide incidence of 2.6 cases per million inhabitants, but the frequency appears to be increasing, as testified by Mayo Clinic data, in which 22% of patients with diseases of supra-aortic trunks requiring surgery have Takayasu arteritis. In Europe, aortoarteritis has been described in Russia, Scandinavia, France and Italy.
Takayasu arteritis can occur at any age, but it seems more frequent between ages of ten and twenty. However, aorto-arteritis is also present in younger children, who are often misdiagnosed as having rheumatic fever, coartation of the aorta and acute glomerulonephritis. Involvement of the descending thoracic and abdominal aorta occurs more commonly in young adults.
Numerous single case reports and some studies show a strict correlation between pregnancy and Takayasu arteritis.

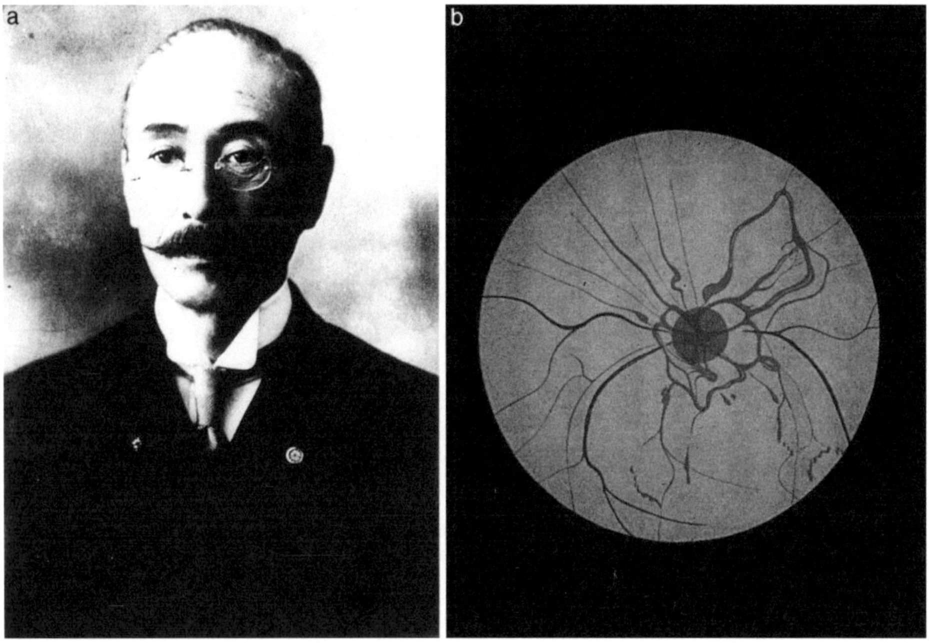

Fig. 1. In 1908, for the first time the Japanese ophthalmologist Mikito Takayasu (a) reported the case of a 21-year old woman with a peculiar optic fundus abnormality, characterised by arteriovenous anastomosis around the papilla (b).

3. Etiology and pathogenesis

Despite the fact that there are no specific immunologic markers of aortoarteritis, autoimmune mechanisms are undoubtedly involved in the pathogenesis. There have been reports of coincidence of Takayasu arteritis and other autoimmune diseases such as rheumatoid arthritis, juvenile rheumatoid arthritis, Still's syndrome, ankylosing spondylitis, Reiter's syndrome, inflammatory bowel disease, systemic sclerosis, systemic lupus erythematosus, glomerulonephritis and renal amyloidosis.
Moreover, rheumatoid factor and antinucleal antibodies have been identified. The erythrocyte sedimentation rate (ESR) is elevated during the inflammatory phase. The pathophysiology of Takayasu arteritis is multifactorial. Nevertheless, aorto-arteritis may be

classified as an autoimmune disease, in which cellular immunity is predominant while the role of humoral immunity has still to be fully defined.

The pathologic sequence imcludes stimulation by an antigen of an unknown nature that triggers heat shock protein (HSP)-65 expression in aortic tissue, which induces the expression of MHC class I chain-related gene A (MICA). Gamma-delta T cells and natural killer (NK) cells expressing NKG2D receptors then infiltrate the arterial wall, recognize MICA on vascular smooth muscle cells and trigger a cytotoxic response, provoking an acute inflammation. These inflammatory cells release perforin, a membrane disrupting protein as well as proinflammatory cytokines. These molecules amplify the inflammatory response, recruiting more infiltrating cells and inducing matrix metalloproteinases (MMP) that degrade elastin and collagen in the arterial wall.

Alpha-beta T cells will then start to infiltrate and specifically recognize one or several autoantigens presented by a shared epitope associated with specific MHC on the dendritic cells. The dendritic cells, together with the B cells, could give rise to a humoral immune reaction mainly featuring anti-endothelial cell autoantibodies, that could trigger complement-dipendent cytotoxicity against endothelial cells (Arnaud et al., 2006; Seko et al., 2000).

4. Pathology

Takayasu arteritis is a non-specific inflammatory disease that primarily affects large arteries such as the aorta and its branches. The term includes both occlusive and aneurismal disease. Thickening of the aorta with an intima exhibiting focal and raised plaques is demonstrated in Takayasu arteritis. Stenosis or occlusions of the aortic branches are also frequent. Ecstasias or aneurysms are more frequently found in the distal thoracic and abdominal aorta. Aortic intramural haematoma, dissection with rupture as well as a combination of ascending, arch, descending and abdominal aortic aneurysms are also described (O'Connor et al., 2008; Gupta et al., 2007).

In the absence of pathognomonic clinical findings and laboratory tests, a biopsy could be very helpful but it must be borne in mind that the histopathologic results may depend by the clinical phase of the disease and that a negative histology cannot rule out the possibility of an aorto-arteritis.

Results of laboratory tests, clinical and radiological findings, together with hystopathologic observations, are all pieces of the same puzzle, that need to be fitted together to obtain a correct diagnosis.

Histologically, the "early phase" is characterized by edema, patchy necrosis of the media and elastin and diffuse chronic inflammation with infiltration of the media, adventitia and vasa vasorum by lymphocytes, plasma cells, a variable number of eosinophils, histiocytes and rare giant cells, leading to thickening of the intima and perivascular inflammation determining arterial wall thickening (Fig. 2).

The early patchy destruction of the medial muscolo-elastic lamellae is replaced by progressive fibrosis. Heggtueit et al. (1963) described a band of infarct-like necrosis in several cases. These histopathological findings can be present even in patients receiving immunodepressive drug treatment and even in clinically successful conditions obtained by long-term corticosteroid therapy.

In the "late" or "pulseless phase", transmural sclerosis with a scanty infiltrate or no inflammatory cells is characteristic of aorto-arteritis. The proliferation and adventitia fibrosis are proportional to the duration and severity of the disease. A secondary thrombosis can occur, with partial or complete occlusion of the arteries.

In the subacute phase and burned-out stage, Takayasu arteritis may escape recognition and be mistaken for arteriosclerosis by a pathologist who is unfamiliar with this systemic arteritis. A disorganization or absence of the elastic lamina of the media, with inadequate supportive fibrous tissue, and focal intimal weakness in this phase, could be responsible for arterial dilatation and aneurysm formation.

Although other causes of aortic aneurysms include extensive degeneration of the media elastic fibres (e.g. Marfan syndrome, Ehlers-Danlos syndrome), the dense adventitial fibrosis and perivasculitis characteristic of Takayasu arteritis will be absent. The lack of atherosclerotic plaques, giant cells, gummas, helps to rule out inflammatory aneurysms, giant cell arteritis and syphilitic aortitis.

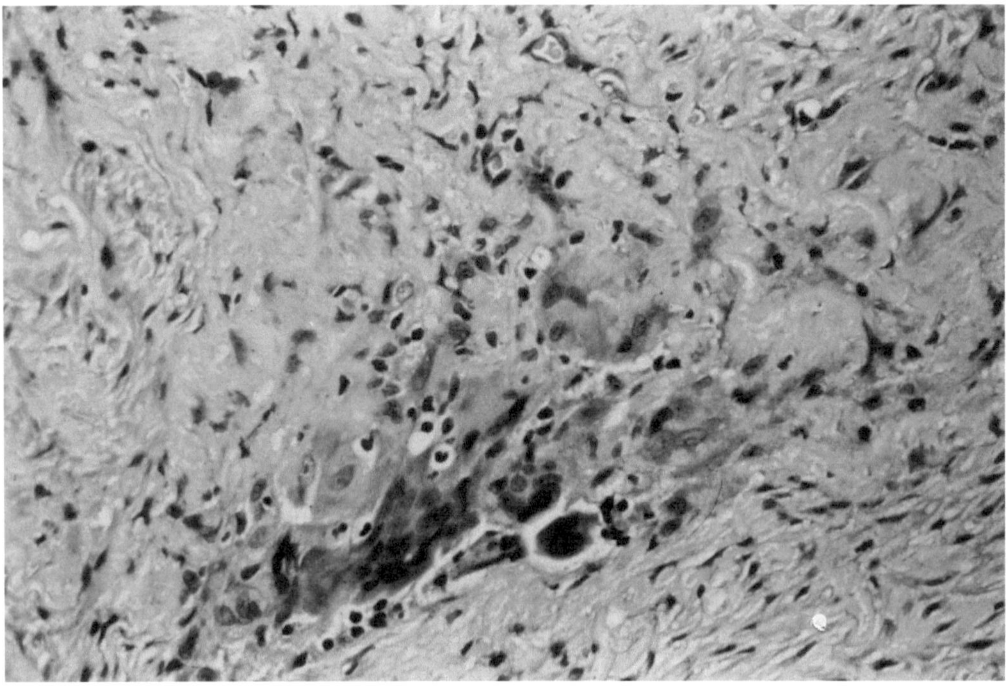

Fig. 2. Histopathologic findings characteristic of Takayasu arteritis: mononuclear inflammatory infiltrate in the media and adventitia with multinucleated giant cells-rich granulomas (hematoxylin-eosin, 100x).

Even if the arteritic process of Takayasu arteritis was originally thought to be confined to the aortic arch and brachiocephalic branches, subsequent clinical and pathological studies resulted in the classification of four topographic types of arterial lesions: type one, originally described by Shimizu and Sano, in which the involvement is limited to the aortic arch and its branches; this affects 8.4% of patients and includes an aneurismal subtype; type two corresponds to the middle aortic syndrome (Kymoto type) with lesions localized in the descending and abdominal aorta and affects 11.2% of cases; type three (Inada type), shares features of types one and two and affects 65.4% of patients. Type four (Lupi-Herrera type) denotes involvement of the pulmonary arteries and is observed in 15% of patients (fig. 3).

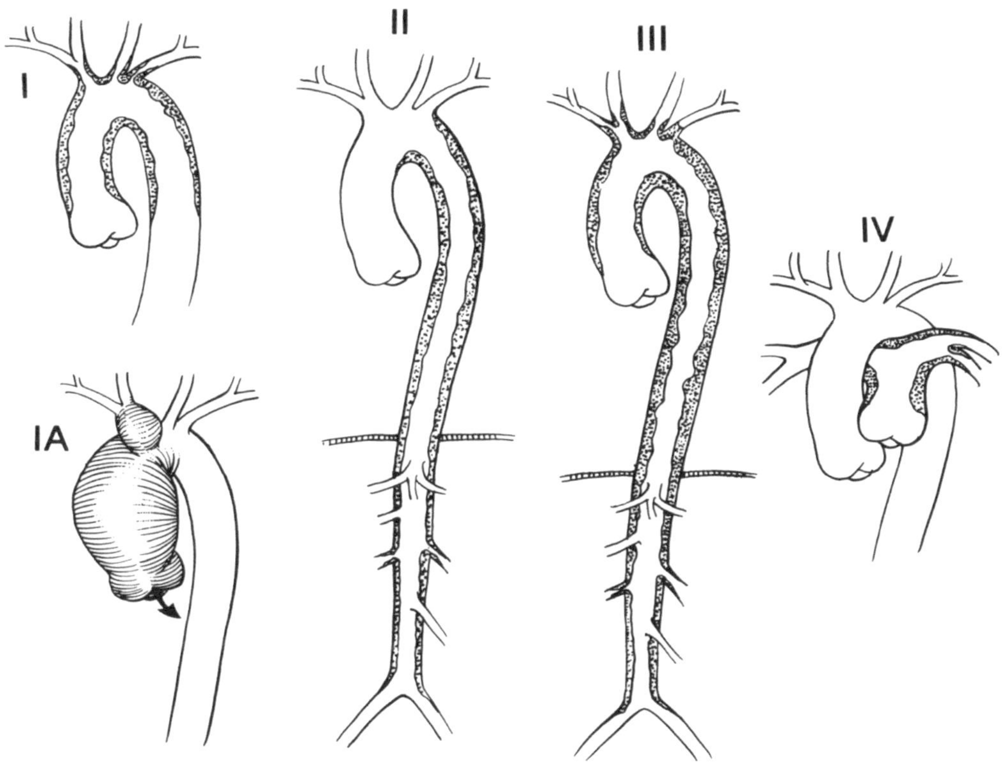

Fig. 3. Topographic classification of Takayasu arteritis (Ueno et al., 1967; Lupi-Herrera et al., 1975).

5. Clinical presentation and natural history

The symptoms of Takayasu arteritis reflect both the systemic inflammatory process and the alterations caused by arteritis. In the early phase of the illness non-specific symptoms are present; they include fatigue, malaise, fever, night sweats, cough, pleurisy with pleural effusion, weight loss, arthralgia, myalgia, skin rush, abdominal pain, vomiting, an elevated erythrocyte sedimentation rate and abnormal plasma protein count (Strachan RW, 1964; Johnston et al., 2002; Nastri et al., 2004).

The incidence of these symptoms is variable. Nakao et al. (1967) reported a history of systemic illness in 53 (63%) of 84 patients, while Lande found systemic symptoms only in 5 (14%) of 35 patients. The age of onset of the aorto-arteritis was between 10-20 years of age in 77% of the cases reported by Lupi-Herrera et al. (1977), between 10 and 29 years of age in 67% of the cases described by Nakao et al. (1967), while the 96 cases reported by Ishikawa (1998) were all under 40 years of age. In all these series, 85 to 90% of the patients were women.

In the pre-pulseless phase, Takayasu arteritis often goes unrecognized, leading to a misdiagnosis. A report by the Mayo Clinic cited a mean delay of 18 months before the true nature of the process is recognized, often not untill the appearance of manifestation of the late phase. These are characterized by arterial stenosis or occlusion after an interval of some months or even years.

The late phase is marked by diminished pulses, vascular bruits, extremitiy claudication, cerebral, ocular or facial ischemia, aortic insufficiency, pulmonary hypertension, cardiomyopathy, angina and myocardial infarction as a result of ostial coronary artery stenosis. Systemic hypertension is frequent in patients with Takayasu arteritis and indicates renal artery stenosis or a baroreceptors disfunction or alterated vascular compliance. Gastroenteric symptoms are extremely rare, because of the rich collateral flow at that level. Ocular symptoms are mainly due to common carotid and/or vertebral artery involvement, and can sometimes depend on systemic hypertension.

Isolated aneurysms are described in only 2% of the patients reported by Sheikhzadeh series (Sheikhzadeh et al., 2002). An association of stenotic and aneurismal lesions is present in nearly all patients with Takayasu arteritis. This observation, together with the high prevalence of systemic hypertension, has led to speculation that elevated blood pressure is an important contributor to aneurysm formation.

The aneurysmal symptoms include a pulsatile mass, embolism from mural thrombus and rupture leading to hemotorax or death. Rupture of aneurysms is uncommon perhaps because their wall tents to be rather thick (Matsumura et al., 1991). The natural history of Takayasu arteritis has not been well elucidated because of the paucity of reported series and numbers of patients.

Most patients with Takayasu arteritis have a favorable prognosis because the disease progresses slowly and the progress of the disease can be arrested if adequate treatment is provided.

During a follow-up study (ranging from 3 months to 15 years) by Morooka et al. (1972), an aortitis syndrome was observed in 64 patients: 4 died of heart failure, 3 of cerebral haemorrhage, 2 of cerebral infarction, 2 perioperatively, 1 of respiratory failure and 1 by suicide. In the review of experiences and studies of pulseless disease reported by Sano and Saito (1972), 77 patients were followed up from 1 to 21 years: 5 died of heart failure, 3 of cerebral embolism, 2 following corrective surgery, 1 of renal failure and 6 of unspecified cause.

In the series of 197 patients (24 men and 173 women) reported by the Japanese National Committee on the Study of Aortitis, death occurred in 25 (12%) cases. In the series of 54 patients reported by Ishikawa (1978) 8 deaths (15%) occurred during an 18-year follow-up period: 3 patients of stroke, 3 of congestive heart failure, 1 during aortic reconstruction and 1 of steroid withdrawal shock.

As regard non-Japanese patients, of the 107 cases (90 women, aged 4 to 45 years) from Mexico reported by Lupi-Herrera et al. (1977), 16 (15%) died during the 19 year follow up: 10 of heart failure, 3 of renal failure, 1 of cerebral haemorrhage, 1 of a ruptured subclavian aneurysm and 1 of perforation of a gastric ulcer.

Of 88 patients (34 men and 54 women, aged 6 to 48 years) from India reported by Subramanyan et al. (1989), 10 (11.4%) deaths occurred during follow-up (83.6+/-74.4 months): 4 of hearth failure, 2 of stroke, 1 of hemoptysis, 1 of ischemic myocardial arrest and 2 of unknown causes.

In a study on 32 North American patients (6 men and 26 women, aged 15 to 48 years) reported by Hall et al. (1985), 2 died during the 13-year follow-up, 1 of a ruptured aortic aneurysm and 1 of pneumonia.

In a small series of 20 cases (all women, aged 7 to 57 years) reported by Shelhamer et al. (1985), only 1 died during the follow-up period lasting a mean of 4.67 years (range 2 to 113 months).

In a series of 73 patients (61 women) reported by Sato et al. (1998), 5 deaths occurred during mean 5-year follow-up, 2 due to heart failure, 2 due to active disease and sepsis and 1 during abdominal aorta surgery.
The overall survival rate in patients with Takayasu disease after the onset of symptoms is reported to be 83% to 94% at 5 years and 83% at 15 years (Ishikawa & Metani, 1994; Sato et al., 1998; Subramanyan et al., 1989; Hall et al., 1985; Ishikawa, 1981).
Usually, aneurismal dilatation develops in patients over the age of 40, although cases of a descending thoracic aorta aneurysm have been reported in a 23-year-old woman (Chieh et al., 2003) and in a 25-year-old man (Regina et al., 2007). The annual risk of rupture is relatively low, ranging from 1% to 7% (Matsumura et al., 1991; Sunramanyan et al., 1989). In a series of 120 patients (111 women, 9 men), Ishikawa & Maetani (1994) reported 16 deaths related to Takayasu disease during a median follow-up of 13 years (range 1 month to 34 years), 5 of congestive heart failure, 4 of cerebrovasclar incidents, 3 after postoperative complications, 2 of acute myocardial infarction and 2 of other causes.
However, these Authors warned that a progressive disease course as well as complications arising from the disease, including aneurysm formation, have a poor long-term prognosis. Indeed, they reported that the 15-year survival rate for patients with both a progressive disease course and major complications, such as aneurysmal changes, was 43% compared with a survival rate of 96.4% in patients with no complications.
The rate of growth and risk of rupture of Takayasu aneurysms are thought to be lower than those of atherosclerotic aneurysms (Robbs et al., 1994). Sueyoshi and colleagues (2000) followed 17 aneurysms in 14 patients with Takayasu arteritis by CT scans for a mean follow-up period of 52.9 months. Eight of these aneurysms did not increase in size, while six grew slowly (at a mean growth rate of 0.03 cm/year). Only three aneurysms increased rapidly in size and ruptured (the mean growth rate was 1.16 cm/year for these aneurysms). They also showed that calcium deposits in the scarred media and intima seems to limit further enlargement of aortic aneurysms. Aortic wall scars are more severe in patients with Takayasu arteritis than in those with atherosclerosis. Therefore, aneurysms associated with this disease increase in size more slowly than atherosclerotic aortic aneurysms.

5.1 Diagnostic criteria

In 1990, the American College of Rheumatology (Arend WP et al., 1990) defined specific criteria for clinical diagnosis of Takayasu arteritis (Tab. 1).
For the purposes of classification, a patient is deemed to have Takayasu arteritis if at least three of the following six criteria are present: age at disease onset less than or equal to 40 years; claudication of the extremities; a diminished brachial artery pulse; a blood pressure difference between the arms more than 10 mmHg; an audible bruit over the subclavian arteries or abdominal aorta; angiographic abnormalities.
The presence of any three or more criteria yields a sensitivity of 90.5% and a specificity of 97.8%.

5.2 Laboratory findings

Although there are no specific diagnostic laboratory tests, the non-specific Erythrocytes sedimentation rate (ESR) is elevated in 68 to 83% of the patients tested. C-Reactive-Protein, gamma-globulin, antistreptolysin-O titers are also abnormal. A mild anemia and a mild to moderate leukocytosis may be present. The Mantoux test is positive in a high percentage of cases. Less than 10% of patients show rheumatoid factor, antinuclear antibodies or LE cells. Albuminuria and hematuria can be found, but are rare.

Criteria	*Definition*
Age of disease onset ≤ 40 years	Development of symptoms or findings related to Takayasu arteritis at age of ≤ 40 years
Claudication of extremities	Development and worsening of fatigue and discomfort in muscles of one or more extremity while in use, especially the upper extremities
Decreased brachial artery pulse	Decreased pulsation of one or both brachial arteries
Blood pressure difference >10 mmHg	Difference of >10 mmHg in sistolic blood pressure between arms
Bruit over subclavian arteries or aorta	Bruit audible on auscultation over one or both subclavian arteries or abdominal aorta
Arteriogram abnormality	Arteriographic narrowing or occlusion of the entire aorta, its primary branches, or large arteries in the proximal upper or lower extremities, not caused by arteriosclerosis, fibromuscolar dysplasia, or similar causes; changes usually focal or segmental

Table 1. American College of Rheumatology criteria for clinical diagnosis of Takayasu arteritis (1990).

6. Imaging techniques

6.1 Angiography

Angiography is still considered to be the gold standard technique. Thoracic and abdominal aortic angiography must be performed in order to visualize the entire aorta and all its branches (Kissin et al., 2004; Johnston et al., 2002; Nastri et al., 2004). Three basic arteriographic patterns are observed: (1) varying degrees of aortic and/or arterial narrowing; (2) saccular and/or fusiform aneurysm; (3) a combination of both (Fig. 4 a-b).

Angiography can also demonstrate dissections, pulmonary artery involvement and the subclavian steal phenomenon and is useful as a basis for selecting endovascular procedures such as angioplasty and stenting. The disadvantages of angiography include the substantial radiation dose and the frequent need to use a large amount of iodinated contrast medium. Moreover, angiography can evaluate only the intraluminal effects of the pathologies but cannot distinguish between acute and chronic disease.

In case of aneurysms, the dilatation may involve long segments of the aorta or the entire aorta. In some patient a saccular aneurysm is superimposed on diffuse aortic dilatation.

"Skipped" areas of aortic involvement, in which aneurysm and narrowing lesions are alternated with normal segments, are the most characteristic aortographic findings in Takayasu arteritis.

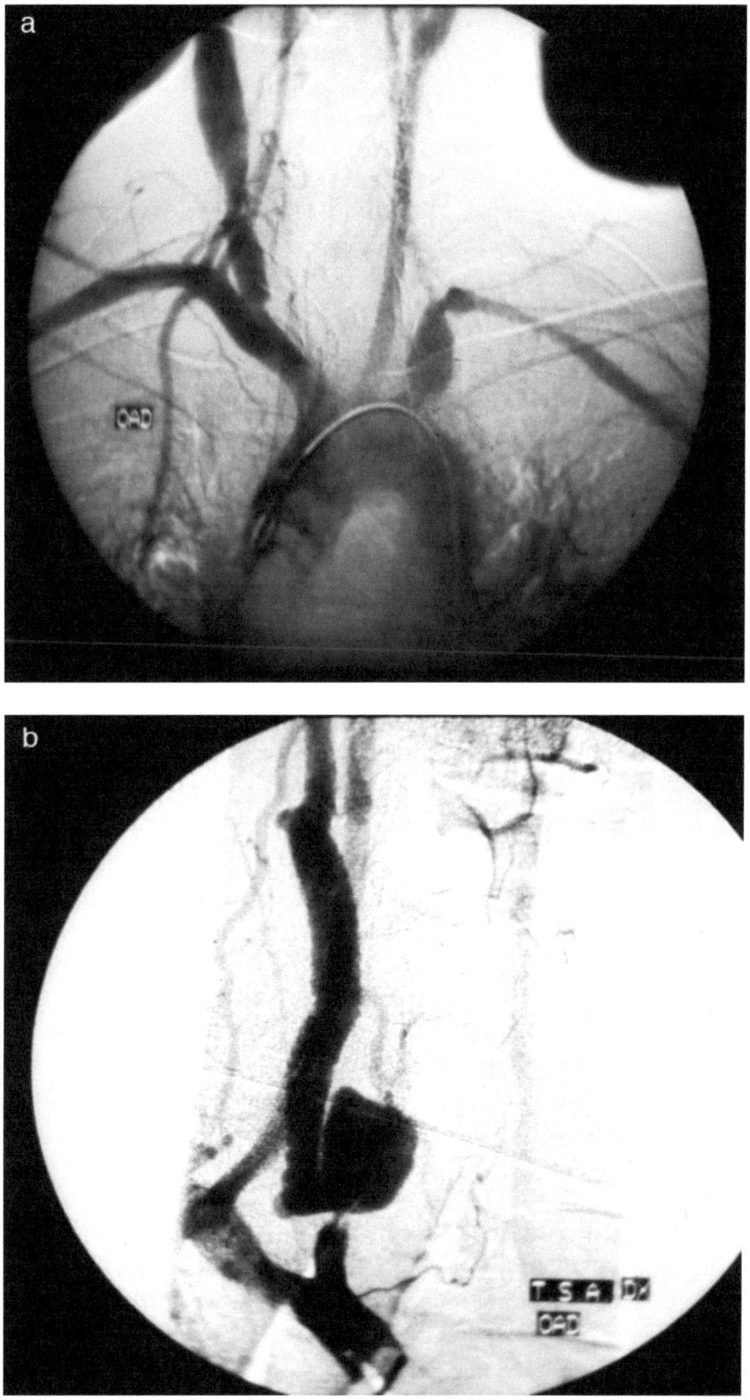

Fig. 4. Angiographic imaging: (a) aneurysmal dilatations of the right common carotid artery and the left intrathoracic sublcavian artery; (b) Pseudoaneurysm after common carotid artery replacement by Dacron graft for Takayasu arteritis aneurysm.

6.2 Ultrasonography (US)

Assessment of the disease activity in patients with Takayasu arteritis is challenging; the advantage of ultrasonography is that it can measure the wall thickness of the superficial vessels (e.g. carotid intima-medial thickness, a marker of the activity). US provides a higher axial resolution than other cross-sectional modalities (Taylor, 1992). If calcification is absent and there is concentric thickening of the artery, a differential diagnosis of the disease from atherosclerotic changes is easily made.

Color-Doppler visualization of the arterial lumen also allows a better estimation of the hemodynamic changes in both deep seated and fairly visible arteries (Canyigit et al., 2007). The freedom from radiation and contrast media, cost effectiveness and availability are all advantages of this technique. However, it is highly operator-dependent and has limited reproducibility. The examination can be technically difficult in the case of obese patients or when overlying bowel gas obscures the abdominal vasculature.

By using intravascular ultrasound (IVUS), a thickening and altered echogenicity of the media, adventitia and perivascular tissue, even in some portions of the aorta that looked normal at angiography, can be observed (Sharma et al., 1998).

Trans-esophageal-echocardiography has also proven efficacious in evaluating the stage of Takayasu arteritis in patients with aortic aneurysms.

In aorto-arteritis two patterns have been described: (1) intima-media thickening and dense echogenic layers outside the intima-medial thickeness, corresponding to the acute stage, or (2) a single thickened echogenic homogeneous layer corresponding to the scar stage. These results indicate that the ultrasound imaging can accurately determining the phase of Takayasu arteritis.

6.3 Computerized Tomography (CT) angiography

CT angiography has been suggested to be very useful in the evaluation of disease activity of Takayasu arteritis, as it allows evaluation of wall thickness. Moreover, it can provide information about wall enhancement during the active phase of the disease. It is also an excellent method for demonstrating stenosis, dissections, occlusions, calcifications, thrombus formation, concentric wall thickening of the aorta and its branches, pulmonary arteries and coronary arteries and aneurysms. In addition, it allows volumetric data acquisition thanks to high quality two or three-dimensional reconstruction.

CT imaging is quick, but less detailed than conventional angiography in the evaluation of stenotic lesions. Moreover, it carries the disadvantages of exposing the patients to high doses of radiation and iodinated contrast medium.

6.4 Magnetic Resonance Imaging (MRI)

Due to its excellent sensitivity MRI is an established screening modalities for central nervous system vasculitis, although it has limited specificity.

Contrast-enhanced MRI and three-dimensional contrast MR angiography can easily demonstrate stenotic lesions in branches of vessels and detect subtle morphologic and pathologic changes in the arterial wall.

A significant enhancement within and around the aorta is observed on post-contrast MR images in the acute phase of Takayasu arteritis. Enhancement of the vessel walls is also present in the chronic stage, indicating the activity of the disease at the tissue level (Matsunanga et al., 2003; Halefoglu et al., 2005; Nastri et al., 2004).

MRI is very useful in the serial evaluation of patients with aorto-arteritis because it does not involve the use of radiation and iodinated contrast material. Fusiform vascular dilatations, vascular occlusions, mural thrombi and multifocal stenosis have been described at MRI. The major disadvantages of this modality are the longer imaging times, as well as contraindications associated with electronic devices and artifacts from surgical clips.

7. Treatment

7.1 Medical treatment

Anti-inflammatory and immunosuppressive agents are the cornerstone of medical therapy for Takayasu arteritis. Corticosteroids are still used in the active phase of Takayasu arteritis. Disease activity is indicated by the onset or worsening of systemic features (fever and arthralgias with no identified cause), by an elevated erythrocyte sedimentation rate, vascular ischemia or inflammation (claudication, diminished or absent pulses, bruits, asymmetric blood pressure in upper or lower limbs or both, carotidynia).

Several reports have claimed that long term prednisolone therapy contributes to an angiographic improvement (Kulkarni et al., 1974; Ishikawa & Yonekawa, 1987). Some patients, in whom withdrawal from corticosteroids is difficult, may require additional cytotoxic immunosuppressive drugs such as cyclophosphamide or azathioprine. The use of other drugs, such as mycophenolate mofetil and infliximab, has been reported in literature. These agents are usually continued for at least one year after remission and are then tapered until discontinuation. Sometimes, long term low-dose corticosteroid therapy may be required. Osteoporosis preventive measures when patients are started on corticosteroids should be seriously considered.

The management of traditional cardiovascular risk factors such as dyslipidemia, hypertension and lifestyle factors is also important. Thrombosis in the affected vessels with stenotic or occlusive lesions or embolism from aneurysms is usually a complication of the disease. This is the reason why long term aspirin therapy is mandatory to prevent thrombus formation in vessels with endothelial damage. Hypertension related to atypical coartation or stenotic disease of the renal arteries should also be controlled with calcium antagonists, beta-blockers, hypotensive diuretics, cardiac glycoside and coronary vasodilator agents.

7.2 Surgical treatment

Numerous reports have shown that surgery on patients with Takayasu arteritis can safely be performed (Tab. 2). There are very low morbidity and mortality rates except in cases of surgery of an aortic aneurysm, especially of a ruptured aneurysm. There is always a concern about the development of anastomotic aneurysms in arteries that have been used for either inflow or outflow bypasses.

The durability of the reconstructions varies in different reports. However, a high incidence of restenosis or pseudoaneurysm has been described (Robbs et al., 1994). Constant surveillance of patients who have undergone these procedures is necessary. It is not clear whether anastomotic stenoses are due to the recurrence of Takayasu arteritis at the level of the anastomosis or to other reasons (Giordano et al., 1991). Nevertheless, they can be treated with either another surgical procedure or possibly even by percutaneous transluminal angioplasty (PTA).

Less than 20% of adult patients require surgical treatment (Ishikawa & Maetani, 1994). In the pediatric field Kalangos et al. (2006) instead found that 80% of the patients required surgery for stenotic or occlusive lesions; 70% were in the active phase of the arteritis, thus necessitating steroid therapy before and after surgery to prevent disease progression.

As reported by Giordano and coll. (1991) there are general principles that all surgeons should take into account in the evaluation and treatment of these patients. Takayasu arteritis is not the same as atherosclerosis. Patients with atherosclerosis are usually elderly, while patients with Takayasu disease are young. It should not be assumed that because the patient is young, he or she may not suffer significant medical complications.

The multi-arterial involvement could mean that the individual has significant renal disease, cardiac disease and other problems that could affect the overall surgical outcome. This is the reason why a complete preoperative evaluation is essential. It is important to maintain a conservative attitude to the management of patients with Takayasu disease.

Surgery should only be resorted to if there is a very significant problem that could affect a patient's prognosis or seriously interfere with the patient's lifestyle. Emergency surgery is not usually necessary since the lesions tend to be chronic, allowing time for collateral circulation to form. It is preferable to avoid surgery during the acute phase of the disease.

PTA has become an effective alternative to surgery for occlusive disease. Initially, there was considerable concern about the long term overall results of this procedure. Dilating a chronic lesion might initially be successful, but long term follow-up might show a restenosis. Restenosis does occur, but since the development of stents, the long term incidence of restenosis seems to be considerably less, although more cases are needed to confirm the effectiveness of this therapy (Takahashi et al., 2002). Therefore it is important, in the initial management of patients who are candidates for operation, to conduct an appropriate pre-surgical work-up to determine the feasibility of PTA.

Surgery always consists in occlusive or stenotic lesion bypassing from proximal to distal vessels, provided that they appear normal on angiography. It must be noted, however, that biopsies of arterial anastomotic sites, even if normal at arteriography, have still shown a 44% incidence of microscopic involvement by Takayasu disease (Kerr et al. 1994).

In case of multiple location of the disease, multistage surgery will need to be selected to reduce the surgical invasiveness. Single-stage surgery is generally preferable, especially for extensive thoracic aortic aneurysms (e.g. aortic arch and descending aorta aneurysm), but because of the excessive invasiveness of this approach, staged surgery must sometimes be performed.

The surgical priority of multiple aneurysms must be decided upon based on the diameter, morphology and propensity for dilatation of the lesion. When staged surgery is selected, rupture of the residual lesion during the interval period is always a concern, so the second stage of surgery must be scheduled as soon as possible after the first. Safi et al. (2001) reported a mortality rate of 5.1% for the first stage and 6.2% for the second stage. The mortality rate during the interval between operations was 3.6%, 75% of these deaths being caused by aneurysm rupture.

Occlusive disease is more prevalent in the United States and Europe, whereas aneurysmal disease is more common in Japan, India, Thailand, Mexico and Africa (Desiron et al., 2000; Matsumura et al., 1991; Kumar et al., 1990). It is not quite clear why there is such a difference.

Study, year	Patient no.	Type of lesions	Treatment	Morbidity	Mortality	Follow-up
Sasaki, 1998	14	Aortic aneurysms (6 type I; 2 type II, 2 type III)	6 graft; 1 aneurysmorraphy; 1 patch angioplasty; 1 Hardy op.; 2 AVR; 3 AVR + wrapping / aneurysmorraphy	4 redo surgery	3 (21.4%) hospital; 5 (35.7%) late	2-252 months
Ando, 2000	87	43 aortic aneurysms (31 type I; 6 type II; 6 type III); 44 aortic regurgitation	38 graft; 5 wrapping; 42 AVR; 2 valved conduit	3 valve detachment; 3 valve failure; 5 subsequent aneurysm op.	5 (5.7%) hospital; 15 (13%) late	1-246 months
Sasaki, 2000	10	Aortic aneurysms (2 type I; 5 type II; 3 type III)	6 graft; 1 patch angioplasty; 1 aneurysmorraphy; 1 Hardy op.; 1 modified Bentall op.	3 redo surgery	1 (10%) hospital; 3 (30%) late	88.8 +/- 46.8 months
Miyata, 2003	106 (155 lesions)	120 occlusive disease; 29 aortic aneurysms	137 graft; 6 patch angioplasty; 4 wrapping; 2 ligation; 2 TEA; 4 other	18 early graft fail 7 late graft fail 31 anastomotic aneurysm	12 (11.3%) hospital; 31 (32.8%) late	8-501.6 months
Kieffer, 2004	33	Aortic aneurysms (27 type II; 6 type III)	32 graft; 1 TEVAR	3 paraplegia; 4 artificial ventilation > 48h; 5 redo surgery	3 (9%) hospital; 2 (6%) late	3-240 months
Fields, 2006	42	39 occlusive disease; 3 aortic aneurysms (1 type I; 2 type II)	Graft	4 early graft thrombosis; 2 minor stroke; 2 cerebral hyperperfusion syndrome; 6 late graft thrombosis	0 hospital; 1 (2.3%) late	1-231.6 months
Lee, 2009	24 (35 lesions)	Occlusive disease	PTA +/- stenting	11 restenosis	0	46.8 months
Yukun, 2010	48 (101 lesions)	Occlusive disease	PTA +/- stenting	8 restenosis	0	3-6 months

AVR: aortic valve replacement; TEA: tromboendoarterectomy; TEVAR: thoracic endovascular aneurysm repair

Table 2. Outcomes following surgical treatment of Taykayasu disease.

Matsumura et al. (Matsumura et al., 1991) described aneurysms in 31.9% of patients with Takayasu arteritis, with a higher frequency in patients over the age of 40, and mostly within the ascending aorta. Aneurysms are a marker of extreme disease activity and are usually found in older patients with a longer history of the disease.

Aneurysm formation is considered one of the major complications related to the prognosis in Takayasu arteritis.

The real incidence of rupture of either the abdominal or thoracic aortic aneurysms is not known, but seems to be low (Matsumura et al., 1991). However, it should be remembered that young patients may have 40 to 50 more years of life expectancy and therefore the risks of aneurysm rupture over that period of time might be quite significant. Repair of abdominal and thoracic aortic aneurysms is indicated if they reach sizes greater than 5 cm.

The new endovascular approach may provide an interesting alternative to patients with thoracic or abdominal aortic aneurysms. Aneurysms also occur in the subclavian, innominate and carotid arteries (Regina et al., 1998). This presents technical problems, since resection and replacement of these arteries can be difficult with a relatively high incidence of stroke. Decision making in these cases must be tailored to the individual, depending upon the extent of involvement and the symptoms and also evaluating the possibility of hybrid intervention with the use of endovascular stent graft (Angiletta et al., 2004).

Operative mortality can certainly be affected by whether the problem treated is occlusive or aneurismal disease. Kieffer et al. (2004) reported a satisfactory surgical outcome of descending thoracic and thoracoabdominal aortic aneurysm in 33 patients with Takayasu arteritis operated between 1974 and 2001, despite the extent of the aneurysmal lesions and high frequency of association with visceral and supra-aortic vessel lesions. Robbs et al. (1994), from South Africa, reported an operative mortality of 3% to 4% in their patients with Takayasu arteritis, most of whom had aneurysms. The mortality was related to ruptured aneurysms.

After surgery for Takayasu arteritis, anastomotic false aneurysms (anastomotic detachment) can occur at any time in the long term, although the incidence seems to be low even in the active phase of the disesase. In Western countries, the development of an anastomotic false aneurysm is reportedly rare. To prevent this complication, reinforcement of the sutures with the use of a Teflon felt strip and/or suppression of active or persisting inflammation with corticosteroids, are recommended. In addition, if possible, sites of normal tissue without inflammatory changes should be chosen as anastomotic sites (Miyata et al., 1998).

In surgical repair of aortic aneurysm due to Takayasu arteritis, the outcome has been improved thanks to technical advances. Successful endovascular aneurysmal repair (stent-grafting) for dilated lesions due to aorto-arteritis has been reported (Baril et al., 2006). However, reintervention for a ruptured stent graft and new aneurysm formation after endovascular treatment was also described (Regina et al., 2007) (Fig. 6). The long term efficacy of endovascular aneurysmal repair remains uncertain even for atherosclerotic disease. In inflammatory lesions due to Takayasu arteritis, a positive but cautious approach may be best.

8. Conclusion

Takayasu arteritis can present in wide variety of forms and should be considered in differential diagnosis of a calcified aorta in young women, even in absence of occlusive or stenotic lesions. The presence of a thoracic aortic aneurysm is regarded as a major complication of this disease. Treatment of aneurysms related to Takayasu arteritis may require a different therapeutic strategy from that generally adopted for atherosclerotic aneurysms, because of the diffuse, progressive and relapsing nature of the disease and, moreover, the patients' greater life expectancy.

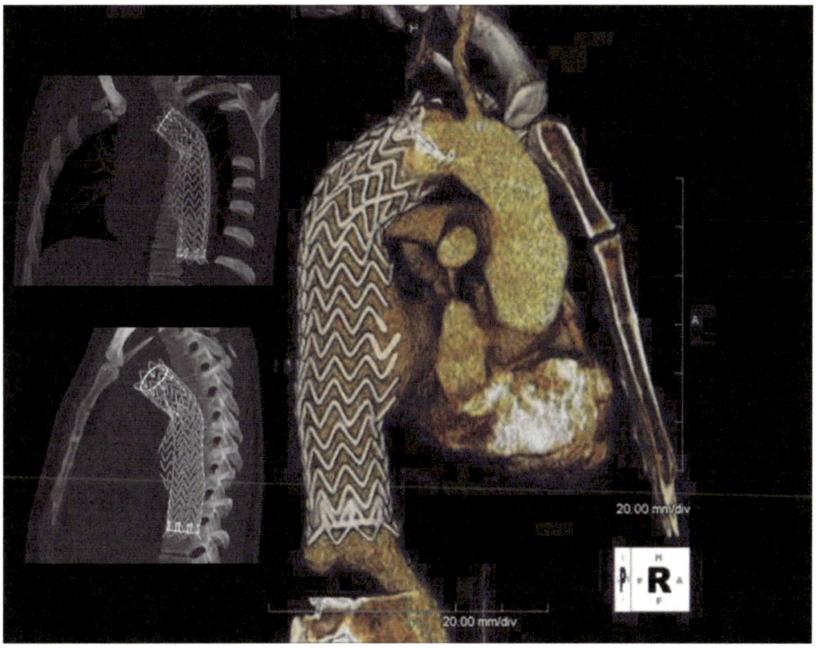

Fig. 6. Thoracic stent-graft bulging rupture after descending aortic aneurysm endovascular repair in a patient with Takayasu arteritis.

Therefore, it is important for physicians to coordinate medical and surgical therapy carefully. An effective control of traditional atherosclerotic risk factors, in addition to achieving suppression of the disease activity, is essential in the management of Takayasu arteritis. Radical surgical treatment of aortic aneurysms is highly recommended if technically feasible.

Long term monitoring of vascular reconstructions in patients with Takayasu arteritis, especially in patients with active disease at the time of initial operation, is mandatory.

9. References

Ando M, Okita Y, Sasako Y, Kitamura S & Matsuo H (2000). Evaluation of the results of surgical treatment for dilatative lesions associated with Takayasu's arteritis. *International Journal of Angiology,* 9:194-7

Angiletta D, Impedovo G, Pestrichella F, Martiradonna F, Fullone M & Regina G (2004). Endovascular treatment of two rare cases of aneurysms of the supra aortic trunks. *Italian journal of vascular and endovascular surgery,* 11:139-42

Arend WP, Michel BA, Bloch DA, Hunder GC, Calabrese LH, Edworthy SM, Fauci AS, Leavitt RY, Lie JT & Lightfoot RW Jr (1990). The American College of

Rheumatology 1990 criteria for the classification of Takayasu arteritis. *Arthritis Rheum,* 33:1129-34

Arnaud L, Kahn JE, Girszyn N, Piette AM & Bletry O (2006). Takayasu's arteritis: An update on physiopathology. *Eur J Intern Med,* 17(4): 241-6

Baril DT, Carroccio A, Palchik E, Ellozy SH, Jacobs TS, Teodorescu V & Marin ML (2006). Endovascular treatment of complicated aortic aneurysms in patients with underlying arteriopathies. *Ann Vasc Surg,* 20: 464–471

Canyigit M, Peynircioglu B, Haziloran T, Dagoglu MG, Cil BE, Haliloglu M, Balkanci F & Besim A (2007). Imaging Characteristics of Takayasu Arteritis. *Cardiovasc Intrvent Radiol.* 30:711-718

Chieh JJ, Brevetti LS, Scholz LS, Graham AM & Ciocca RG (2003). Multiple isolated aneurysms in a case of "burned out" Takayasu aortitis. *J Vasc Surg.* 37(5):1094-7

Desiron Q & Zeaiter R (2000). Takayasu's arteritis. *Acta Chir Belg.* 100:1-6

Fields CE, Bower TC, Cooper LT, Hoskin T, Noel AA, Panneton JM, Sullivan TM, Gloviczki P & Cherry KJ (2006). Takayasu's arteritis: operative results and influence of disease activity. *J Vasc Surg,* 43:64-71

Gupta M, Bhan A, Khanzode S, Das S & Ray R (2007). Total aorta replacement in Takayasu arteritis. *Heart, Lung and Circulation,* 16:382–384

Giordano J, Leavitt RY, Hoffman G & Fauci AS (1991). Experience with surgical treatment of Takayasu's disease. *Surgery,* 109:252

Halefoglu AM & Yakut S (2005). Role of magnetic resonance imaging in the early diagnosis of Takayasu arteritis. *Australas Radiol.* 49:377–381

Hall S, Barr W, Lie JT, Stanson AW, Kazmier FJ & Hunder GC (1985). Takayasu arteritis. A study of 32 North American patients. *Medicine (Baltimore),* 64:89–99

Heggtueit HA, Hannigar GR & Morrione TG (1963). Panaortitis. *Am J Pathol.* 42:151-172

Ishikawa K (1978). Natural history and classification of occlusive thromboaortopathy (Takayasu's disease). *Circulation.* 57: 27-35

Ishikawa K (1981). Survival and morbidity after diagnosis of occlusive thromboaortopathy (Takayasu's disease). *Am J Cardiol.* 47:1026-32

Ishikawa K. (1988). Diagnostic approach and proposed criteria for the clinical diagnosis of Takayasu's arteriopathy. *J Am Coll Cardiol.* 12:964-972

Ishikawa K & Maetani S (1994). Long-term outcome for 120 Japanese patients with Takayasu's disease. Clinical and statistical analyses of related prognostic factors. *Circulation.* 90:1855–60

Ishikawa K & Yonekawa Y (1987). Regression of carotid stenoses after corticosteroid therapy in occlusive thromboaortopathy (Takayasu's disease). *Stroke.* 18:677–679

Johnston SL, Lock RJ & Gompels MM (2002). Takayasu arteritis: A review. *J Clin Pathol.* 55:481–486

Kalangos A, Christenson JT, Cikirikcioglu M, Vala D, Buerge A, Simonet F, Didier D, Beghetti M & Jaeggi E (2006). Long-term outcome after surgical intervention and interventional procedures for the management of Takayasu's arteritis in children. *J Thorac Cardiovasc Surg.* 132:656–664

Kerr GS, Hallahan CW, Giordano J, Leavitt RY, Fauci AS, Rottem M & Hoffman GS (1994). Takayasu's arteritis. *Ann Intern Med,* 120:919

Kieffer E, Chiche L, Bertal A, Koskas F, Bahnini A, Bla Try O, Cacoub P, Piette JC & Thomas D (2004). Descending thoracic and thoracoabdominal aortic aneurysm in patients with Takayasu's disease. *Ann Vasc Surg.* 18: 505–513

Kissin EY & Merkel PA (2004). Diagnostic imaging in Takayasu arteritis. *Curr Opin Rheumatol.* 16:31–37

Kulkarni TP, D'Cruz IA, Gandhi MJ & Dadhich DS (1974). Reversal of renovascular hypertension caused by nonspecific aortitis after corticosteroid therapy. *Br Heart J.* 36:114 -116

Kumar S, Subramanyan R, Mandalam KR, Roa VR, Gupta AK, Joseph S, Unni NM & Rao AS (1990). Aneurysmal form of aortoarteritis (Takayasu's disease): analysis of thirty cases. *Clin Radiol,* 42:342

Lande A, Bard R, Rossi P, Passariello R & Castrucci A (1976). Takayasu's arteritis. A worldwide entity. *N Y State J Med.* 76(9):1477-82

Lee BB, Laredo J, Neville R & Villavicencio JL (2009). Endovascular management of Takayasu arteritis: is it a durable option? *Vascular,* 17:138-46

Lupi-Herrera E, Sanchez-Torres G, Horwitz S & Gutierrez FE (1975). Pulmonary artery involvement in Takayasu's arteritis. *Chest.* 67: 69-74

Lupi-Herrera E, Sanchez-Torres G, Marcushamer J, Mispireta J, Horwitz S & Vela JE (1977). Takayasu's arteritis. Clinical study of 107 cases. *Am Heart J.* 93:94–103

Matsumura K, Hirano T, Takeda K, Matsuda A, Nakagawa T, Yamaguchi N, Yuasa H, Kusakawa M & Nakano T (1991). Incidence of aneurysms in Takayasu's arteritis. *Angiology.* 42:308–15

Matsunaga N, Hayashi K, Okada M, & Sakamoto I (2003). Magnetic resonance imaging features of aortic diseases. *Top Magn Reson Imaging.* 14:253–266

Miyata T, Sato O, Deguchi J, Kimura H, Namba T, Kondo K, Makuuchi M, Hamada C, Takagi A & Tada Y (1998). Anastomotic aneurysms after surgical treatment of Takayasu arteritis: a 40-year experience. *J Vasc Surg.* 27:438–445

Miyata T, Sato O, Koyama H, Shigematsu H & Tada Y (2003). Long-term survival after surgical treatment of patients with Takayasu's arteritis. *Circulation,* 108:1474-80

Morooka S, Ito I, Yamaguchi H, Takeda T & Saito Y (1972) Follow-up observation of aortitis syndrome. *Jpn Heart J.* 13:201-213

Nakao K, Ikeda M, Kimata S & Niyahara M (1967). Takayasu's arteritis. Clinical report of eighty-four cases and immunological studies of seven cases. *Circulation.* 35(6):1141-55

Nastri MV, Baptista LP, Baroni RH, Blasbalg R, de Avila LF,Leite CC, de Castro CC & Cerri GG (2004). Gadolinium-enhanced three-dimensional MR angiography of Takayasu arteritis. *Radiographics,* 24:773–786

O'Connor MB, Murphy E, O'Donovan N, Murphy M, Phelan MJ & Regan MJ (2008). Takayasu's Arteritis presenting as a dissecting aortic aneurysm history: a case report. *Cases Journal.* 21:52

Regina G, Bortone A, Impedovo G, De Cillis E, Angiletta D & Marotta V (2007). Endovascular repair of thoracic stent-graft bulging rupture in a patient with multiple thoracic aneurysms due to Takayasu disease *J Vasc Surg,* 45:391-4

Regina G, Fullone M, Testini M, Todisco C, Greco L, Rizzi R, Caruso G & Ettorre GC (1998). Aneurysms of the supra-aotic trunks in Takayasu's disease. Report of two cases. *J Cardiovasc Surg (Torino),* 39(6):757-60

Robbs JV, Abdool-Carrim AT & Kadwa AM (1994). Arterial reconstruction for non-specific arteritis (Takayasu's disease): medium to long term results. *Eur J Vasc Surg.* 8:401–7

Safi HJ, Miller CC, Estrera AL, Huynh TT, Rubenstein FS, Subramaniam MH & Buja LM (2001). Staged repair of extensive aortic aneurysms: morbidity and mortality in the elephant trunk technique. *Circulation.* 104:2938-2942

Sano K & Saito I (1972). Pulseless disease: summary of our experiences and studies. *Schweiz Arch Neurol Neurochir Psychiatry,* 111:417-43

Sasaki S, Yasuda K, Takigami K, Shiiya & Sakuma M (1998). Surgical experiences with inflammatory arterial aneurysms due to Takayasu's arteritis. *International Journal of Angiology,* 7:92-6

Sasaki S, Kubota S, Kunihara T, Shiiya N & Yasuda K (2000). Surgical experience of the thoracic aneurysm due to Takayasu's arteritis. *International Journal of Cardiology,* 75:129-34

Sato EI, Hatta FS, Levy-Neto M & Fernandes S (1998). Demographic, clinical, and angiographic data of patients with Takayasu arteritis in Brazil. *Int J Cardiol.* 66 Suppl 1:S67–70; discussion S71

Seko Y, Takahashi N, Tada Y, Yagita H, Okumura K & Nagai R (2000). Restricted usage of T-cell receptor Vg-Vd genes and expression of co-stimulatory molecules in Takayasu'sarteritis. *Int J Cardiol,* 75:S77–83

Sharma S, Sharma S, Taneja K, Bahl VK & Rajani M (1998). Morphological mural changes in the aorta in nonspecific aortoarteritis (Takayasu's arteritis): assessment by intravascular ultrasound imaging. *Clin Radiol.* 53:37 - 43

Sheikhzadeh A, Tettenborn I, Noohi F, Eftekharzedeh M & Schnabel A (2002). Occlusive thromboaortopathy (Takayasu disease): Clinical and angiographic features and a brief review of literature. *Angiology.* 53:29-40

Shelhamer JH, Volkman DJ, Parrillo JE, Lawley TJ, Johnston MR & Fauci AS. (1985). Takayasu's arteritis and its therapy. *Ann Intern Med.* 103(1):121-6

Strachan RW (1964) The natural history of Takayasu's arteriophaty. *Q J Med.* 33:57-69

Subramanyan R, Joy J & Balakrishnan KG (1989). Natural history of aortoarteritis (Takayasu's disease). *Circulation.* 80:429–37

Sueyoshi E, Sakamoto I & Hayashi K (2000). Aortic aneurysms in patients with Takayasu's arteritis: CT evaluation. *Am J Roentgenol.* 175:1727–33

Taylor KJW (1992). Arterial vascular ultrasonography. *Radiol Clin North Am.* 30:865–878

Takahashi JC, Sakai N, Manaka H, Iihara K, Sakai H, Sakaida H, Higashi T, Ishibashi T & Nagata I (2002). Multiple Supra-aortic Stenting for Takayasu Arteritis: Extensive Revascularization and Two-Year Follow-up *AJNR Am J Neuroradiol.* 23:790–793

Ueno A, Awane Y, Wakabayaschi A & Shimizu K (1967). Successfully operated obliterative brachiocephalic arteritis (Takayasu) associated with the elongated coarctation. *Jpn Heart J.* 8: 538-44

Yukun H, Luxiang C, Zhiyuan S, Guoxiang H, Maoqin S, Jianping L, Shifei T, Tao J & Li Z (2010). Curative effects of endovascular therapy on Takayasu arteritis: report of 48 cases. *Acta Academiae Medicinae Militaris Tertiae,* 32(23).

20

Conventional Surgery in Type IV Thoracoabdominal Aortic Aneurysm

Arash Mohammadi Tofigh
*Imam Hossein Medical Center, Shahid Beheshti University of Medical Sciences
Iran*

1. Introduction

Type IV thoracoabdominal aortic aneurysms (TAAAs) affect the aorta between the diaphragm and aortic bifurcation (Fig. 1). For technical reasons, the aneurysms affecting only the part of aorta from which visceral arteries arise are also categorized as type IV. The level of difficulty of surgical treatment for type IV TAAAs lies between that of type II, which involve descending thoracic and abdominal aorta, and that of the most frequent aneurysm of the aorta: infra renal aortic aneurysm. Like all other TAAAs, the most frequent complication of surgical repair of type IV aneurysms is renal and visceral ischemia. However the risks of pulmonary, spinal and hemorrhagic complications are also important. Except for a few specific cases, surgical repair is carried out in a conventional way according to the technical method explained by Crawford in 1974. Endovascular techniques require specialized teams and will not be addressed in this chapter.

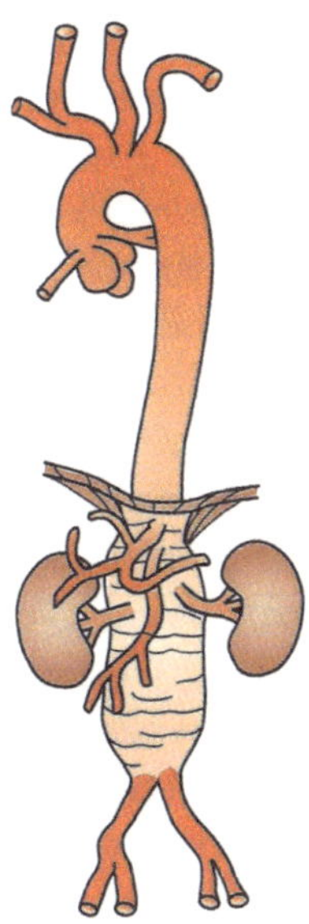

Fig. 1. Type IV thoracoabdominal aortic aneurysm

2. Epidemiology and etiology

Type IV TAAAs represent nearly 20% of all TAAAs (De Latour et al., 2005). They mostly have atheromatous etiology and develop by a degenerative process identical to infra renal aortic aneurysms. Many of these aneurysms happen in a diseased aorta that has undergone surgery to treat an infrarenal aneurysm, and the degenerative process has reached the upper parts of the aorta. This is mostly seen after an emergency repair of a ruptured infrarenal aortic aneurysm where the technical difficulties of the surgery (or even absence of preoperative imaging) can force the surgeon to suture the prosthesis on a diseased aortic neck. Type IV aneurysms may also develop in previously operated type I and type III aortic dissections and in dissections treated by stent grafts. These types require more complicated treatment than atherosclerotic aneurysms. Rarely, infectious aneurysms, saccular aneurysms secondary to focal weakness in the suprarenal aorta and inflammatory aneurysms associated with Takayasu's disease, are observed.

3. Indications for surgery

In contrast to abdominal or thoracic aortic aneurysms, no study has been undertaken on the natural history of type IV TAAAs. This is explained by their relative rarity and the fact that they are generally classified as type II or type III in the literature. Existing data are not sufficient for clinical decision making. Hence, surgeons rely on general data from abdominal aortic aneurysms or other thoracoabdominal types. Except for the symptomatic aneurysms, surgical intervention is usually recommended if the aneurysm diameter reaches 55-60 mm (Wahlgren & Wahlberg, 2005). However, several parameters should be considered other than aneurysm diameter: age, general condition, renal and cardiac comorbidities. The ratio of aneurism diameter to the diameter of the normal aorta in each patient must also be considered. For example, a 55 mm diameter aneurysm developed on an aorta diameter of 20 mm is considered to be at a higher risk of rupture than one that develops on an aorta diameter of 28 mm (De Latour et al. 2005). The aortic aneurysm is at risk of rupture if it doubles in diameter compared with the original aorta. The speed of development and the quality of hypertension control should also to be considered, particularly if Marfan's syndrome is present or if the patient has a family history of aortic rupture. Infectious and saccular aneurysms often show a faster and more dangerous pattern of evolution than atherosclerotic aneurysms. Type IV TAAAs are usually seen in subjects over the age of sixty. They impose a clamping of the aorta at the diaphragmatic level which induces visceral and renal ischemia. The surgeon must rely on a clear body of evidence to advise surgery. This reflects the great importance of preoperative assessment in this patient cohort.

4. Anatomic assessment

The entire thoracic and abdominal aorta, its visceral and renal branches, iliac arteries and preferably the lower limb arteries, should be evaluated. It is important to study the descending thoracic aorta to verify the presence of ectasia or dual aneurysms that could change the surgical procedure. It also helps in assessing the lower limit of the mural thrombus in the descending thoracic aorta which, if present, might become destabilized by clamping and embolizing the branches. However, small crescents of a few millimeters of mural thrombus located on the descending thoracic aorta are not a contraindication to aortic clamping above the celiac trunk. Another important parameter to consider is the distance between the celiac trunk and the neck of the aneurysm, where it will be clamped. Based on the data collected, the surgeon will decide whether to carry out a proximal aortic anastomosis followed by separate reimplantation of the visceral patch, or a single aortic anastomosis encompassing the proximal aorta and the visceral arteries. It is therefore possible, before surgery, to have an idea of the likely duration of clamping of the renal arteries and to predict if protection of the renal parenchyma is needed. The anatomic assessment should include an accurate analysis of visceral and renal arteries (topography and distribution) and the existence of associated stenotic, occlusive or aneurismal lesions that might change the approach or the strategy of surgery. Multi-detector computerized tomography angiography (CTA) can be used to obtain a dynamic analysis of the lesions. It also allows three-dimensional reconstructions and provides all data necessary for the procedure (Fig. 2&3).

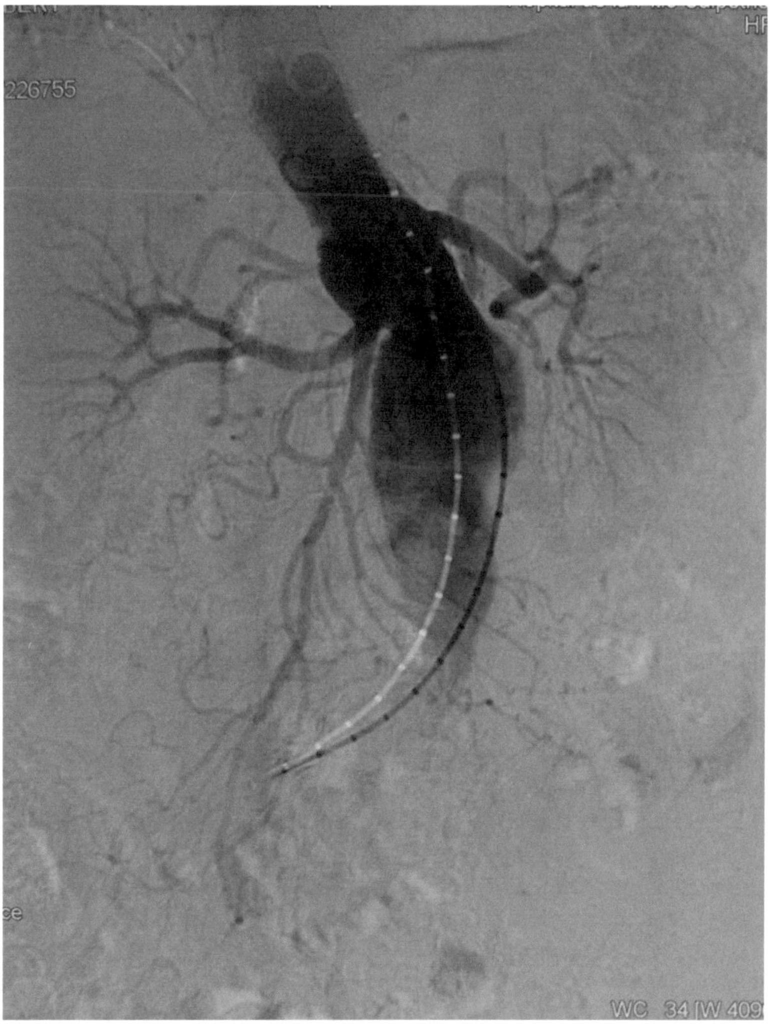

Fig. 2. Angiography of a Type IV thoracoabdominal aortic aneurysm

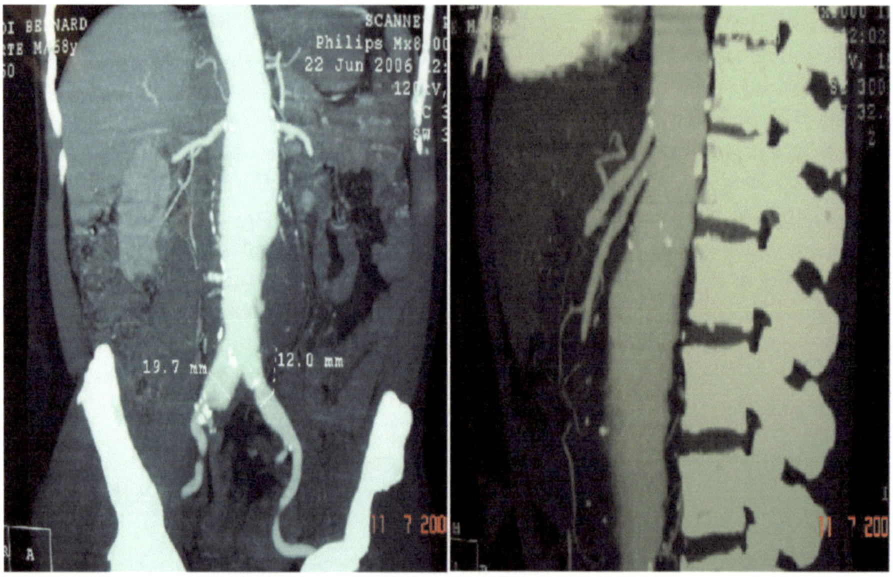

Fig. 3. CT angiography of a type IV thoracoabdominal aneurysm

5. Preoperative evaluation

Preoperative evaluation determines the patient's ability to cope with aggressive surgery and allows the team to anticipate possible postoperative decompensation. Four essential systems are checked for these reasons as outlined below.

5.1 Cardiac

Surgery for type IV TAAAs requires aortic clamping at the diaphragm level. This causes a sudden increase in cardiac afterload. Conversely, at declamping, there is a sudden collapse in peripheral resistance. In both circumstances, there is a significant increase in cardiac work. Furthermore, many of the patients undergoing this type of surgery are hypertensive and aged>60 years. Associated coronary artery disease is also common. The risk of intraoperative acute heart failure is high, so exact preoperative study of myocardial, coronary and valvular status is important (Suzuki et al., 2003).

Undertaking coronary angiography (which is questionable before the surgery of infra renal aortic lesions) is indispensable here, even in the absence of a positive history or clinical signs. An exception may be made in young adults suffering from Marfan's syndrome. Transthoracic echocardiography in search of associated valve diseases is necessary to eliminate severe aortic insufficiency, which would lead to clamping intolerance. An ejection fraction < 30% or severe coronary lesions should mean temporarily postponement or even canceling the intervention. Transesophageal echocardiography is helpful to evaluate the ascending and descending thoracic aorta, particularly in patients with renal insufficiency. Coronary artery revascularization may be indicated. If coronary stenting is undertaken to achieve this, aneurismal repair should be delayed for 6 weeks, while Clopidogrel should be used. Drug eluting stents might not be used preoperatively. If coronary artery bypass graft (CABG) is selected, use of the left internal mammary artery is not suitable because it is the most important collateral artery to the spinal cord.

5.2 Pulmonary

The surgical approach used for treatment of type IV TAAAs can be a left retroperitoneal or thoracoretroperitoneal approach via a left flank incision, or a thoracoabdominal incision in the tenth left intercostal space. These incisions result in reduction of pulmonary capacity with the possibility of postoperative atelectasis and pleural effusion. Chronic obstructive pulmonary disease (COPD) is common among these patients, and is associated with increased mortality after aneurysm repair. Preoperative assessment of respiratory function can be used to detect patients at risk and help to better prepare them. Pulmonary function tests and arterial blood gas analysis are undertaken routinely. Smoking cessation, appropriate medications and an adequate exercise program improve pulmonary capacity and lower the risk of complications (Knapp et al. 2007).

5.3 Renal

Kidneys are frequently associated with postoperative morbidity. Acute renal failure increases mortality and predicts increased non-renal complications. It has been suggested that preoperative renal insufficiency can be a relative contraindication to proceed with repair. Preoperative measurement of blood urea nitrogen (BUN), creatinine clearance, or glomerular filtration is needed. These serve as a benchmark for judging the postoperative functional outcome of the kidneys. This allows explaining to the patient the possibility of temporary or permanent postoperative dialysis if creatinine clearance is < 30 mL / min. In case of a significant reduction in preoperative creatinine clearance, it is important to have Doppler ultrasound images of the renal arteries and renal parenchyma. A significant functional difference between the kidneys may lead to changes in the surgical strategy to minimize the time of renal ischemia on the best kidney (Biknell et al., 2003). In all cases, detection of renal failure should lead to strengthening the level of renal protection pre- and intraoperatively. Preoperative hydration and avoidance of nephrotoxic agents is also important. Severe renal artery stenosis might be treated pre- or intraoperatively.

5.4 Carotids

Assessment of the carotid arteries by Doppler ultrasound is routinely requested to identify a possible cerebral circulatory insufficiency. Even if there is no strong evidence in the literature, it is likely that the hemodynamic changes often encountered during this type of surgery can predispose the patient to stroke. Hence, most surgeons prefer a correction of carotid artery stenosis before considering the repair of type IV aneurysms.

6. Anesthesia

During surgery for juxta-diaphragmatic aneurysms, the anesthesiologist will be faced with multiple problems. The right lateral decubitus position, the possible opening of the pleural space and incision of the diaphragm are the most important obstacles for good ventilation. Moreover, COPD is frequently associated with this type of disease. This explains the need for good preoperative chest physiotherapy and the use of bronchodilators. Double lumen endobronchial intubation is not necessary for this type of surgery. During closure of the chest wall, introduction of catheters in the intercostal spaces allows for repeated injections of local analgesics, which is more important just after extubation. The cardiac index should be maintained at >3 to ensure good perfusion of tissue. Systolic blood pressure should be maintained ~ 100 -- 120 mm-Hg to reduce the negative effects of a high afterload on cardiac function. This double constraint (low pressure and high flow condition) is usually provided during the clamping time, through the use of a short acting vasodilator such as sodium nitroprusside. Dobutamine can be added for better cardiac performance. Infusion of nitroprusside should be started a few minutes before clamping of the aorta and stopped minutes before declamping to avoid the risk of cardiovascular collapse due to reperfusion. Blood pressure is then rebalanced by increasing the intravascular volume. A cardiac index >3 and a mean arterial pressure >70 mm-Hg are maintained during the first 48 hours after surgery. These measures increase the visceral, renal and spinal perfusion and decrease the prevalence of complication after a low-flow state (Acher et al., 1997).Simultaneous use of different drugs can be difficult, particularly if there is significant bleeding and hypothermia. A short clamping time and cooling of the kidneys cannot guarantee renal protection. To optimize renal perfusion, flow and perfusion pressure are equally important and can be measured intraoperatively. The use of diuretics with osmotic effect (e.g. mannitol) remains controversial. They are used, however, to maintain renal diuresis if postoperative renal failure occurs (De Latour et al., 2005). Bleeding disorders due to clamping of the hepatic circulation can be prevalent. Although minimal doses of heparin are used during surgery, the coagulation profile is often disturbed postoperatively, with a rising prothrombin time and reduced serum fibrinogen level. We can undertake re-transfusion of autologous red packed cells without plasma or clotting factors through cell saver machines. It is therefore important to provide fresh frozen plasma, platelet and fibrinogen just after declamping the aorta. The complementary use of aprotinin provides much more rapid control of postoperative bleeding due to oozing. Oozing is a consequence of hypothermia that is commonly seen in this type of surgery because of the very large incision and opening of the abdominal and thoracic cavities. Hypothermia may promote further arrhythmia that the anesthesiologist must take into account during the procedure (Knapp et al., 2009).

7. Surgical procedure

7.1 Approaches

Two approaches have been described for surgical treatment of type IV TAAAs. The retroperitoneal approach is by far the most commonly practiced. Left flank incision with resection of the eleventh rib or thoracoabdominal incision in the tenth left intercostal space provide excellent exposure throughout the abdominal aorta, left renal artery and the first centimeters of the superior mesenteric artery (SMA). However, the right renal artery beyond the inferior vena cava, SMA in its distal parts and the hepatic artery remain inaccessible. If these arteries need to be accessed, the transperitoneal approach via a laparatomy is preferred.

7.1.1 Retroperitoneal approach

After introduction of a urinary catheter, a central venous catheter, a Swan- Ganz catheter, a radial arterial catheter (and possibly an intrathecal catheter for drainage of cerebrospinal fluid (CSF)), the patient is positioned in the partial right lateral decubitus with shoulders at 60° to the operating table and the left hip at 45°. This position allows access to the right femoral artery if necessary. It also facilitates access to the left crus of the diaphragm. The juxta-diaphragmatic aorta can be approached by the thoraco-retroperitoneal route, with resection of the eleventh rib, with or without division of the diaphragm. The two approaches are quite similar and differ only by the aortic exposure achieved in the cephalic direction. The incision is made in the left flank in the tenth intercostal space, and the eleventh rib is resected. If the diaphragm is not divided, the exposure of the higher portion of the aorta is less, as well as the diaphragmatic related postoperative complications. Only the left crus of the diaphragm is sectioned and the pleura is often opened in the corner of the incision. However, the gap does not exceed a few centimeters and can be sutured directly at the end of surgery without thoracic drainage. Conversely, if the diaphragm is divided, the aorta can be achieved much higher and control of the descending thoracic aorta is possible. However, the diaphragmatic incision and the significant opening in the pleura which mandate drainage of the thoracic cavity, have negative effects on postoperative pulmonary function.

Two criteria determine the choice between these two surgical approaches, as shown below.

- The exact point where the aneurysm starts and the length of the upper neck of the aneurysm. If the starting point appears on the crus of the diaphragm or slightly below it under CTA, the thoraco-retroperitoneal approach in the tenth intercostal space with resection of the eleventh rib, and isolated dissection of the left crus of the diaphragm without diaphragm incision might be suitable. However, if the aneurismal neck is shorter, the clamp should be placed above the diaphragm and the latter is divided.
- The patient morphotype. If the patient is tall, the costal margin covers broadly the hypochondriac fossa. The diaphragmatic dome is higher, the intercostal spaces are narrower, and exposure of the juxta-diaphragmatic aorta more difficult. Hence, it is better to use a thoraco-retroperitoneal approach in the tenth intercostal space with resection of the eleventh rib and diaphragm incision because it provides better exposure. In short patients with a wide chest, the exposure difficulties are less problematic and the diaphragmatic incision can often be avoided (unless obesity makes it difficult to mobilize the viscera). A flank incision in the tenth intercostal space starting 3- 4 cm from the spine is made (Fig 4). Its caudal extension is dependent upon the extent of the aneurysm. If there is no involvement of the iliac arteries and reconstruction stops at the aortic bifurcation, the incision goes down near to the umbilicus. If the iliac axes are involved in the aneurysm, the incision stops halfway between the pubic tubercle and the umbilicus. After division of the intercostal muscles and external oblique muscles, the eleventh rib is resected. Blunt dissection of the peritoneum begins when retroperitoneal fat appears and, by mobilizing the peritoneum and its contents medially, the retroperitoneum and aorta are exposed.

This incision allows for the introduction of a self-retaining retractor or a Finochietto retractor between the costal margin and the anterior superior iliac spine. After the retroperitoneal space is entered, the inferior surface of the diaphragm is mobilized medially until the left crus of the diaphragm is fully visualized. The left kidney can be mobilized superiorly and medially to expose the retroperitoneum up to the level of the diaphragm. The ureter should also be identified and mobilized superiorly. The left crus of the diaphragm is divided for exposure of the aorta above the celiac axis. Now the aorta can be readily palpated (especially in its diaphragmatic orifice). If the aorta has a normal size at the orifice, it is not necessary to continue the dissection upward: it will be clamped at this point. If the aneurismal neck is too short or the aneurysm continues cephalically, the diaphragm is divided parallel to its costal attachment. A 2 cm diaphragmatic fringe is left along the chest wall to ease the final repair. The diaphragmatic incision extends along its attachments to the costal margin, to the left crus that was previously cut. This approach allows finding a safe area for clamping the distal descending thoracic aorta. By cutting only the periphery of the diaphragm, injury to the branches of the phrenic nerve is avoided which offers better postoperative pulmonary function. Before clamping and incising the aorta, all para-aortic tissue is transected along the line of the intended aortotomy. Veins lateral to the aorta (e.g. renal lumbar vein) must be tied and transected. The time spent for preparation, reduces bleeding during aortic reconstruction, and helps the anesthesiologist to adjust the hemodynamic.

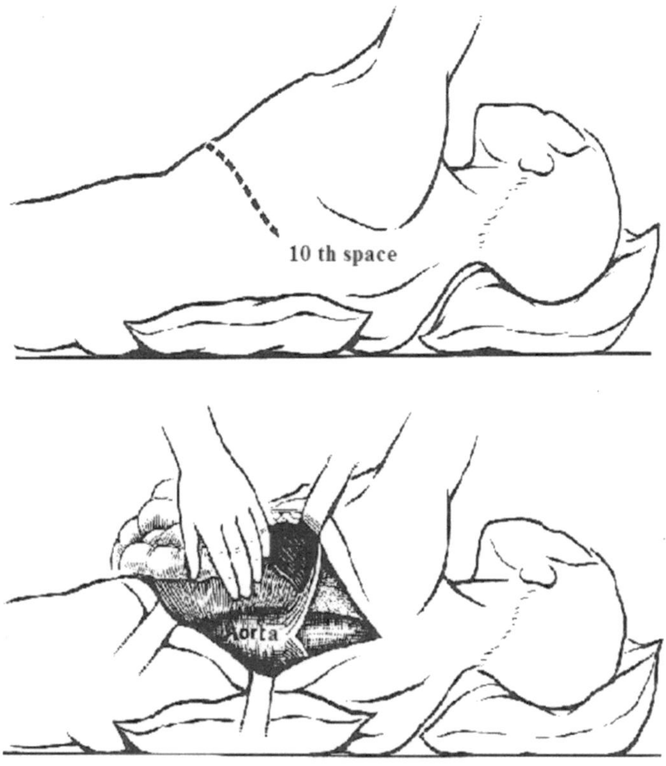

Fig. 4. Flank incision in the 10th intercostals space and exposure of the aorta

7.1.2 Transperitoneal approach

The transperitoneal approach via a laparotomy is intended for patients in whom surgical intervention on the right renal artery, common hepatic artery, or distal part of SMA is expected. A midline incision is most frequently used. It should extend from the xiphoid to the symphysis pubis to provide maximal exposure. Once the intra-abdominal contents have been inspected, a left medial visceral rotation is made by releasing the splenic flexure of the colon and mobilizing the spleen and pancreas medially until the suprarenal aorta is exposed. Division of the left crus of the diaphragm provides additional proximal exposure of the suprarenal aorta. The left kidney can be kept in the renal fossa or mobilized medially, which increases the risk of a postoperative pancreatic reaction. By mobilizing the right colon in continuity with the duodenum and shifting the orientation of the SMA and the root of the mesentery, the right renal artery beyond its retrocaval portion is exposed. Finally, the common hepatic artery and its branches, and the SMA beyond its original segment are exposed in this approach.

7.2 Aortic reconstruction

In most cases of type IV TAAAs, reconstruction of the aorta is by the inclusion technique described by Crawford. Once proximal and distal control is achieved and systemic heparinization initiated, the aneurysm is entered by incising the aorta from its bifurcation distally to the aneurismal neck proximally. Attention should be paid to the ostium of the left renal artery, which is normally situated in the posterior but might be moved upward if the kidney is mobilized superiorly. Hence, the incision should be situated in the left border of the aorta near the spine. If the incision passes near the ostium of the left renal artery, the ostium should be detached with a wide aortic patch (as Carrell patch) that will help reimplantation of the left kidney on the graft. Then the thrombus is evacuated and sent for laboratory analysis. Occlusive catheters are placed in the renal artery, celiac artery and SMA. Backbleeding lumbar arteries, as well as the inferior mesenteric artery are oversewn from within the sac. In this step, the quality of the aortic wall and degree of separation of origins of the renal and visceral arteries should be rapidly assessed. The surgical strategy will be decided based on these data. Two situations are most often encountered as shown below.

1. In most cases, the distance between the celiac trunk and SMA is short. The anastomosis is created at the level of the renal arteries with an oblique technique incorporating the visceral arteries and right renal artery (Fig.5). If the inter-renal distance is not too large, there is no need for separate button reimplantation of the renal arteries. In this situation, the clamping time of the visceral and renal arteries is short (normally <30 min) with minimal postoperative ischemic complications. The twelfth pair of intercostal arteries is usually included in the patch. However, in most cases, this distance is remarkable and cutting a large patch including the four ostia will leave diseased aortic tissue - the source of secondary dilation. Hence, the left renal artery is treated separately by amputating its origin as a Carrell patch and reimplating it in the graft. (Fig.6)
2. In the case of substantial separation of the origin of the celiac artery and SMA, a convenient technique is to amputate the celiac origin as a Carrell patch, defer its reconstruction, and use a single inclusion button for the SMA and the right renal artery. The left renal artery is treated as described above. The distance between these anastomoses is just a few millimeters and has two drawbacks as shown below.

- If bleeding occurs from the suture line after declamping, repair would be difficult. The proximity of the two suture points between the prosthesis and the aorta does not allow mobilization and exposure of the posterior suture line. To reduce this risk, it seems preferable to completely sever the aorta circumferentially and to not carry out the in-lay suture technique. This allows for better visualization of the passage of sutures and safer anastomosis.
- Commonly there is a pair of large intercostal arteries between the celiac trunk and the upper limit of the aneurysm. The narrow spaces in this area do not allow for another anastomosis for the intercostal arteries, hence, they should be included in one of the visceral patches. Ligation or thrombosis of the intercostal arteries is probably one of the causes of postoperative paraplegia encountered in this type of surgery.

Once the aorto-prosthetic anastomosis is realized, the celiac axis, SMA and right renal artery are reimplanted as an inclusion button in the graft. Then the left renal artery is reimplanted or bypassed separately in the tube graft. (Fig.7) This anastomosis should be placed on the left postero-lateral side of the graft to avoid kinking of the artery after repositioning the left kidney. The inferior mesenteric artery is in general ligated and finally the distal anastomosis done. This anastomosis can be created between a tube graft and the distal portion of the aorta, or between a bifurcated graft and both iliac arteries (including hypogastric arteries) depending on the extent of the aneurysm. Colonic perfusion can be examined by opening the peritoneum and, if sigmoidal ischemia is present, the inferior mesenteric artery should be reimplanted. Protamine is then administered and extensive hemostasis undertaken. The aneurismal layer is closed over the graft, and the muscular layers of the crus firmly closed. The diaphragm is repaired with heavy absorbable sutures and attached to the parietal flap, left *in situ* during the initial section. A chest tube is inserted and the retro peritoneum drained. Two catheters can be positioned on either side of the tenth intercostal space to infuse analgesic in the postoperative phase.

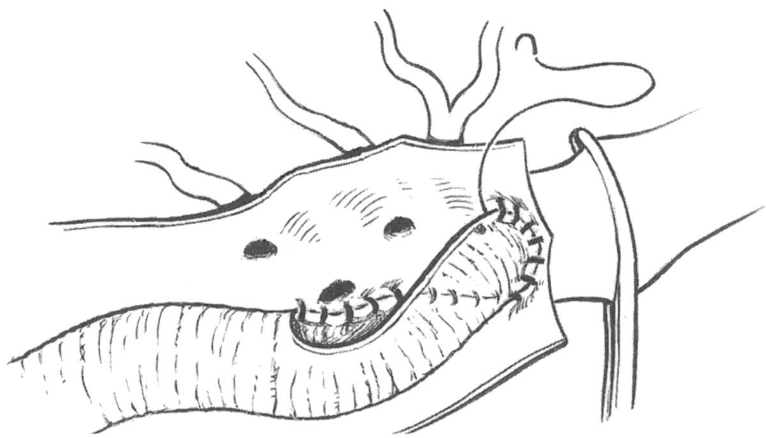

Fig. 5. Anastomosis between the aorta and graft including visceral and renal arteries

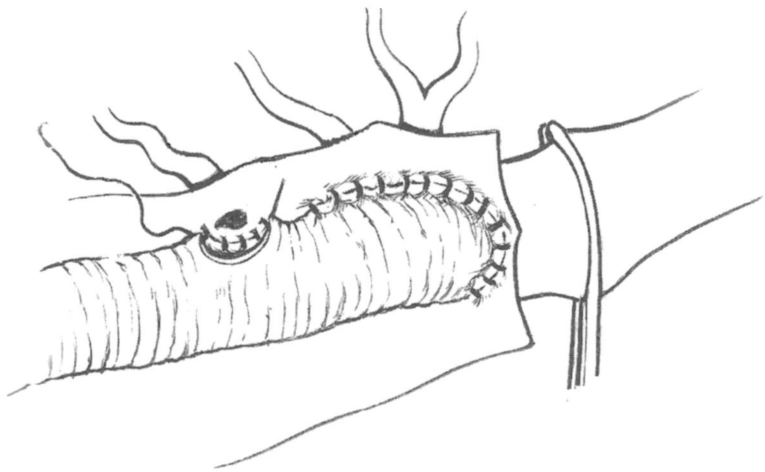

Fig. 6. Separate anastomosis of the left renal artery in the graft

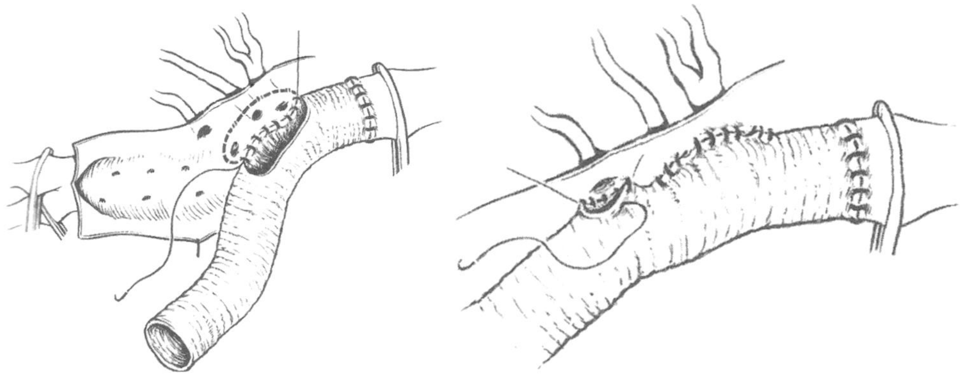

Fig. 7. Separate anastomosis between the graft and the aorta and the visceral patch

7.3 Spinal protection

As mentioned above maintaining good hemodynamic is the main protective method for perfusion of the spinal cord. The other protective method for the spinal cord in this type of surgery is to include the ostia of the lowermost pair of intercostal arteries in the aortic anastomosis or in the visceral patch. If the upper anastomotic line lies above the diaphragm, cerebrospinal fluid (CSF) drainage is carried out (Safi et al., 2003). There is no need for extracorporeal circulatory support.

7.4 Renal protection

The prevalence of postoperative renal failure varies between 0% and 21% (table 1). It is mainly dependent upon the initial renal function, clamping time, and quality of the surgical procedure (postoperative occlusion of a renal or polar artery). In our surgical unit, the best results are obtained if preoperative renal function is in the normal range, the upper anastomotic patch includes both renal arteries and the duration of renal clamping is <30 min. Under these conditions intraoperative renal protection is not needed. If the patient has preoperative renal failure, then each kidney is perfused with 300 mL of cold (+4 ° C) Ringer's lactate solution after opening the aneurysm. The infusion is undertaken for 4 - 5 min at 150 mm-Hg through a coronary cannula. Such high pressure is important to eliminate micro-thromboses in the capillary bed (as has been demonstrated in kidney transplantation). Proximal anastomosis is then carried out. If the repair is more complex, with separate reimplantation of both renal arteries, the clamping time might be much longer. It is preferable to carry out renal cold perfusion with the same technique but it is repeated for the left renal artery, after declamping the right renal artery. Finally, maintaining a high cardiac output and mean arterial pressure > 70 mm-Hg during and after surgery are two major elements to ensure satisfactory diuresis. This maintenance of good hemodynamic is also necessary for protecting the spinal cord (Coselli, 2010).

8. Special conditions

8.1 Dissecting aneurysms

A descending thoracic aortic dissection can be transformed to a type IV TAAA several months or even years after the acute episode (Conrad et al., 2010). The external diameter of the descending thoracic aorta may be conserved near the normal range as it expands slightly, whereas immediately after crossing the diaphragm a significant expansion occurs, (especially if an intimal tear is present between the diaphragm and renal arteries). Technically the aortic wall is thick and sclerotic and does not pose a problem for suturing. There are, however, two other practical challenges:

- The proximal anastomosis will be carried out on a dissected area. Hence, the inner membrane should be resected to create a wider stoma. The suture should be placed on the outer layer. If a parietal thrombus is present, it should be evacuated to avoid embolization upon declamping.
- The existence of a false channel strongly modifies the endoaortic appearance. Unlike atherosclerotic aneurysms, ostia of the renal and visceral arteries are not always easily distinguished (especially if the false lumen ends on an ostium or it continues along the branched artery). Simple resection of the inner membrane leaves a fibrous bead in the origin of the artery which can induce postoperative thrombosis. This bead should not be included in the prosthetic suture line. It is better to bury it in the aortic wall with a few sutures to eliminate local turbulence. If the false lumen extends to the right renal artery it is recommended to detach it from the aorta. It will be later reimplanted on the aortic graft with a short prosthetic graft.

8.2 Simultaneous occlusive lesions

Preoperative evaluation may reveal significant stenosis of renal and visceral arteries. If located on the left renal artery (or if purely ostial), they can be treated by the Crawford technique described above. However, in cases of extensive lesions on the right renal artery, SMA or hepatic artery, this technique is no longer possible due to the incision not exposing the distal parts of the arteries. There are several options to solve this condition:

- Balloon expandable angioplasty of the diseased arteries before surgery can be a convenient technical expedient.
- Using a laparotomy approach in which the spleen and pancreas are mobilized medially until the suprarenal aorta is exposed (as described in transperitoneal approach section). This approach allows extensive dissection of diseased arteries and carrying out reconstruction by a bypass from the prosthesis.
- If a long segment of the SMA is involved or if a prolonged ischemia on the left dominant kidney should be avoided, revascularization can be achieved first on the visceral arteries. The left diaphragm and its crus are completely divided and the distal 5-6 cm of the thoracic aorta exposed. The aorta is then partially clamped by a side biting clamp and a graft anastomosed at this level to the aorta. It is then used for antegrade revascularization of the visceral or renal arteries. Once visceral revascularization has been completed, the aorta is clamped and the procedure continues as described above (Ballard et al., 2002).
- It is possible to carry out this surgery in two stages. Extra-anatomic revascularization of occluded arteries (hepato-renal or right ilio-mesenteric bypass) or kidney auto-transplantation can be done in the first surgery. The patient is then operated a few days or weeks later for treatment of the aneurysm. The disadvantage of this approach is the multiplication of surgical approaches and surgical risks. However, in some cases, this two-step approach, can minimize the risk of visceral or renal ischemia during the clamping of the aorta, and thus should be considered (Etz et al., 2010).

8.3 Retro-aortic left renal veins

As an anatomic variation the left renal vein can be retro-aortic. In this case, by mobilizing the kidney anteriorly during retroperitoneal exposure, the renal vein completely ties around the aneurysm and hinders incision and opening of the aorta. Hence, there is no choice apart from renal auto-transplantation. The left kidney should be completely released and its ureter dissected down to the iliac vessels. The renal artery is cut near its ostium and the renal vein cut close to the spine. The kidney is then washed and cooled continuously in a sterile tray positioned above the pubis while the ureter is still contiguous. Once the aortic reconstruction is completed, the kidney is auto-transplanted to the iliac vessels.

8.4 Isolated aneurysm of the visceral part of the aorta

Aneurysms affecting only the visceral part of the aorta where the SMA and celiac arteries branch, are mostly saccular with infectious etiology (Fig.8) or are secondary to rupture of a calcified plaque. In these cases, it is recommended to excise the aneurismal sac and to repair the aortic wall with a Dacron patch or cryopreserved arterial homograft. The latter material is preferred if infectious or mycotic etiologies are suspected (Vogt et al., 1998). This repair is not always readily undertaken due to the poor quality of the aortic wall and a resection that is wider than expected. Also, the ostium of the aneurysm may be near the origin of the renal or visceral arteries, which makes simple repair unachievable. In these cases, it is recommended to do the reconstruction by the Crawford's inclusion technique described above.

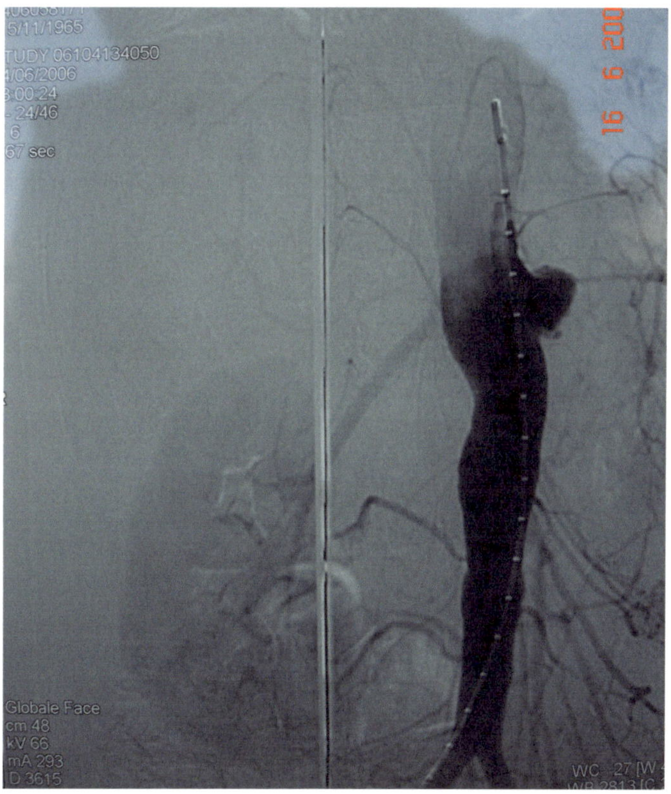

Fig. 8. A saccular aneurysm of the suprarenal part of the aorta with infectious origin

8.5 Reoperations

Surgical treatment of type IV TAAAs (like any prosthetic reconstruction) is subject to possible secondary degradation (Dardick et al., 2001). The occurrence of an anastomotic pseudoaneurysm or dilatation of the aortic patch may require further surgery if the lesion diameter becomes unacceptably large. Reoperation and a direct approach to the lesion are not easy and, since the advent of aortic stent grafts, a hybrid technique is preferred (Patel et al., 2009). In this technique, retrograde revascularization of the visceral arteries is followed by covering the aneurysm by a stent graft.

After laparotomy, visceral arteries are dissected a few centimeters from the aorta and an 8-mm Dacron graft is anastomosed to a common iliac artery or to the infrarenal aorta. The SMA is then ligated at its origin and an end to side anastomosis made between it and the right side of the Dacron graft. The graft is then carefully tunneled beneath the pancreas and an end to side anastomosis made between it and the common hepatic artery. The celiac trunk is then ligated at its origin. A bifurcated Dacron graft is then anastomosed on the same iliac artery, the contralateral iliac artery or on the infrarenal aorta to revascularize the renal arteries. Once renal and visceral revascularization is confirmed, an aortic stent graft is placed to cover the aneurysm (Fig.9).

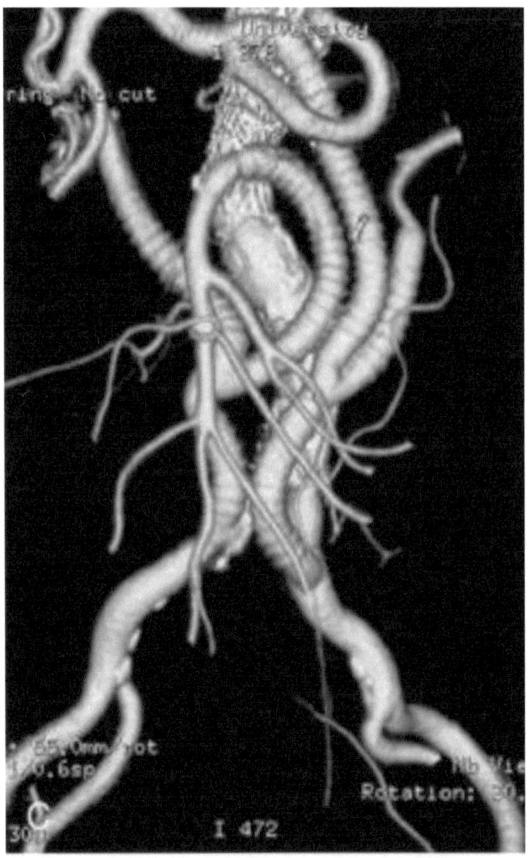

Fig. 9. Postoperative CTA of a hybrid reconstruction of a type IV thoracoabdominal aneurysm

9. Results

Results of the studies conducted on type IV TAAAs which are published in the literature are summarized in Table 1. Some results correspond to series with only type IV aneurysms; others have been extracted from series covering all TAAAs. The overall postoperative mortality is higher than that for infrarenal aneurysms, and is 3.6% -- 17 %(mean 8.8%). Most deaths are due to multi-organ failure secondary to low-cardiac output and renal failure. Postoperative bleeding is also a significant cause of death, immediately after multi-organ failure. The differences found among these studies might be caused by "The center effect". The prevalence of postoperative renal failure is difficult to analyze because the criteria are highly variable from one series to another. The risk of postoperative dialysis is much more dependent upon preoperative renal function than on clamping time. Overall, in the contemporary series, the prevalence of dialysis after surgery varies from 0% to 21 %(mean 9%). The occurrence of postoperative renal failure requiring dialysis significantly increases postoperative mortality. In surgery for type IV TAAAs, spinal cord ischemia due to aortic clamping is less common than for surgery for type II or III. The prevalence of paraplegia varies from 0% to 4% in elective surgery and from 0 %to 20% in urgent and emergency surgery. There is no evidence supporting that further protective measures (CSF drainage, extracorporeal circulatory support, visceral perfusion) reduce the risk of this complication. When the anastomoses of the upper neck of the aorta and the visceral patch are separated, CSF drainage appears to be the logical approach. Also, in these patients clipping or ligating the lower intercostal arteries which may arise between the two anastomoses should be avoided (Safi et al., 2003).

Author	Period of study	n (patients)	Paraplegia n (%)	Renal insufficiency n(%)	Mortality n(%)
Richards et al.	2000-2010	53	1(2)	-	3(6)
Ockert et al.	1997-2004	30	1(1.6)	1(1.6)	2(6)
Lombardi et al	1993-2003	56	0(0)	2(4)	7(13)
Schepens et al.	1981-2003	42	2(5)	4(6)	3(7)
Coselli et al.	1986-2001	329	6(2)	22(7)	12(4)
Cina et al.	1990-2001	42	0(0)	9(21)	2(5)
Cambria et al	1987-2001	66	1(1.5)	-	5(8)
Bicknell et al.	1993-2001	130	6(5)	20(15)	22(17)
Ballard et al.	1996-2001	20	2(6)	0(0)	2(6)

Table 1. Results of conventional surgery of type IV thoracoabdominal aortic aneurysm.

10. Conclusion

Open repair of type IV TAAA may be undertaken using different approaches with acceptable levels of morbidity and mortality. The surgery is not as difficult as that for type II or III TAAAs. Compared with the surgical procedure described by Crawford for TAAAs, (which requires wide opening of the thorax and abdomen, spinal cord protection, reimplantation of the intercostal arteries and usually extracorporeal circulatory support) this intervention is simpler and could be described as "modified Crawford procedure". Despite this relative simplicity, surgical risks should not be underestimated. A specialized team is required in all cases, especially for the management of hemodynamic complications.

11. Acknowledgments

I would like to thank Dr. K. Sheibani for his help in preparing this chapter and the staff of the Clinical Research Center of Imam Hossein Medical Center for their support.

12. References

Acher , CW; Wynn, MM; Hoch, JR & Kranner, PW.(1998). Cardiac function is a risk factor for paralysis in thoracoabdominal aortic replacement. *Journal of Vascular Surgery*, Vol. 27, No. 5,(May 1998), pp. 821-828

Ballard, JL; Abou Zam-Zam, AM & Teruya,TH. (2002). Type III and IV thoracoabdominal aortic aneurysm repair: result of a trifurcated two graft technique. *Journal of Vascular Surgery*, Vol. 3, No. 2, (August 2002), pp. 211-216

Biknell, CD; Cowan, AR & Kerle MI. (2003). Renal dysfunction and prolonged visceral ischemia increase mortality rate after suprarenal aneurysm repair. *British Journal of Surgery*, Vol. 90, No. 9, (September 2003), pp. 1142-1146

Cambria, RP; Clouse, WD; Davidson, JK; Dunn, PF & Corey, M.(2002). Thoracoabdominal aneurysm repair: results with 337 operations performed over a 15 year interval. *Annals of Surgery*, Vol.236, No.4, (October 2002), pp. 471- 479

Cina, CS; Lagana, A & Bruin, G. (2002). Traitement chirurgical des anévrysmes de l'aorte thoraco-abdominale : étude prospective d'une cohorte de 121 malades. *Annales de Chirurgie Vasculaire*, Vol. 16, (2002), pp. 631-638

Coselli, JS. (2010). Strategies for renal and visceral protection in thoracoabdominal aortic surgery. *Journal of Thoracic and Cardiovascular Surgery*, Vol. 140, No. 6 Suppl, (December 2010), pp. S147-149

Coselli, JS; Conklin, LD& Lemair, SA. (2002). Thoracoabdominal aortic aneurysm repair: review and update of current strategy. *Annals of thoracic surgery*, Vol. 74, No. 5, (November 2002), pp. S1881-S1884

Conrad, MF; Chung, TK; Cambria, MR; Paruchuri, V; Brady, TJ & Cambria RP. (2010). Effect of chronic dissection on early and late outcomes after descending thoracic and thoracoabdominal aneurysm repair. *Journal of Vascular Surgery*, Vol. 53, No. 3, (March 2010), pp. 600-607

Crawford,ES. (1974). Thoraco-abdominal and abdominal aortic aneurysms involving renal, superior mesenteric and coeliac arteries. *Annals of Surgery*, Vol. 179, No. 5, (May 1974), pp. 763-772

Dardick, A; Perler,BA; Rose Borough, GS &Williams, GA.(2001) Aneurismal expansion of The visceral patch after thoracoabdominal aortic replacement, an argument for limiting patch size. *Journal of Vascular Surgery*, Vol. 36, No.3, (September 2001), pp.405-409

De Latour, B ; Camilleri, JP ; Nourissat, G ; Favre, JP & Barral, X. (2005). Traitement chirurgical conventionnel des anévrysmes thoraco-abdominaux de type IV, In : *Traitement des anévrysmes de l'aorte abdominale,* Kieffer & Koskas, pp. 83-95, Editions AERCV, ISBN: 2-907232-19-3, Paris

Etz ,CD; Zoli, S; Mueller, CS; Bodian, CA; Di Luozzo, G; Lazala, R; Plestis, KA & Griepp, RB. (2010). Staged repair significantly reduces paraplegia rate after extensive thoracoabdominal aortic aneurysm repair *Journal of thoracic and cardiovascular surgery,* Vol.139, No. 6, (June 2010), pp. 1464-1472

Knapp, J; Bernhard, M; Rauch, H; Hyhlik-Dürr, A; Böckler, D & Walther A.(2009). Anesthesiologic procedures for elective aortic surgery, *Anaesthesist*, Vol. 58, No. 11, (November 2009), pp. 1161-1182

Lombardi, JV; Carpenter, JP; Pochetino,A ; Sonnad, SS & Bavaria, JE. (2003). Thoracoabdominal aortic aneurysm surgery repair after prior aortic surgery. *Journal of Vascular Surgery*, Vol. 38, No.6, (December 2003), pp. 1185-1190

Ockert, S; Riemensperger, M; Von Tengg-Kobligk, H; Schumacher, H; Eckstein, HH & Böckler, D.(2009). Complex abdominal aortic pathologies: operative and midterm results after pararenal aortic aneurysm and typeIV thoracoabdominal aneurysm repair. *Vascular,* Vol.17, No.3, (May- June 2009), pp. 121-128

Patel, R; Conrad, MF; Paruchuri, V; Kwolek, CJ; Chung, TK & Cambria, RP.(2009). Thoracoabdominal aneurysm repair: hybrid versus open repair. *Journal of Vascular Surgery,* Vol. 50, No. 1, (July 2009), pp. 15-22

Richards, JM; Nimmo, AF; Moores, CR; Hansen, PA; Murie, JA & Chalmers, RT. (2010). Contemporary results for open repair of suprarenal and type IV thoracoabdominal aortic aneurysms. *British Journal of Surgery*, Vol. 97, No. 1, (January 2010), pp. 45-49

Safi, Hj; Miller, CC 3rd & Huynh, TT. (2003). Distal aortic perfusion and cerebrospinal fluid drainage for thoraco abdominal and descending thoracic aortic repair: ten years of organ protection. *Annals of surgery*, Vol. 238, No.3, (September 2003), pp. 372-381

Schepens, M; Dossche, K & Morshuis, W.(2004). Introduction of adjuncts and their influence on changing results in 402 consecutive thoracoabdominal aortic aneurysm repair. *European Journal of Cardiothoracic Surgery*, Vol. 25, No. 5, (May 2004), pp. 701-707

Suzuki, S; Davis 3rd, CA; Miller 3rd, CC; Huynh, TT; Estrera, AL; Porat, EE; Vinnerkvist, A & Safi, HJ. (2003). Cardiac function predicts mortality following thoracoabdominal and descending thoracic aortic aneurysm repair. *European Journal of Cardiothoracic Surgery*, Vol. 24, No. 1, (July 2003), pp. 119-124

Vogt, PR; Brunner-La Rocca, HP; Carrel, T; von Segesser, LK; Ruef, C; Debatin, J; Seifert, B; Kiowski, W & Turina ,MI.(1998). Cryopreserved arterial allografts in the treatment of major vascular infection: a comparison with conventional surgical techniques. *Journal of Thoracic and Cardiovascular Surgery*, Vol. 116, No. 6, (December 1998), pp. 965-972

Wahlgren, CM & Wahlberg, A. (2005). Prise en charge des anévrysmes thoraco-abdominaux de type IV, In: *EMC Techniques chirurgicales, chirurgie vasculaire,* pp. 43-152, Elsevier Sas, Paris

21

Spinal Cord Protection for Descending or Thoracoabdominal Aortic Aneurysm Repair

Nobuyoshi Kawaharada, Toshiro Ito and Tetsuya Higami
Department of Thoracic and Cardiovascular Surgery
Sapporo Medical University School of Medicine
Japan

1. Introduction

The mortality and morbidity of extensive thoracoabdominal aorta replacement has improved markedly in recent years [1]. However, postoperative paraplegia from spinal cord infarction remains the most devastating complication that faces patients undergoing surgery on the thoracoabdominal aorta because loss of lowerlimb function imposes severe constraints on the quality of life. Additionally, paraplegia is associated with higher postoperative mortality and morbidity. Despite advances in spinal cord protection, the risk of spinal cord ischemia or infarction as a consequence of open surgical repair of thoracoabdominal aortic aneurysms (TAAAs) remains within the range of 8-28%[2,3]. The registry of the Japanese Association for Thoracic Surgery reported that the hospital mortality for surgery on the thoracoabdominal aorta was 14.2% in 561 patients during 2008 [4]. The U.S. multicenter registry in 2001 disclosed that early mortality after thoracoabdominal aortic surgery was 20% [5].

There are two major events during which injury to the spinal cord can occur. Firstly, spinal cord injury happens depending on the duration and degree of ischemia during cross-clamping. The surgeon must temporarily interrupt aortic blood flow to the lower body, which renders the distal organs (including the spinal cord) ischemic, in order to resect the aneurysm. Secondly, damage may occur from the loss of blood flow to the spinal cord after the period of aortic cross-clamping because of failure to reattach the intercostal and lumbar arteries that are critical to the spinal cord blood supply.

Essentially, being a neural tissue, the spinal cord tolerates ischemia poorly and if infarction ensues, paraplegia results. A number of adjunctive measures have been used successfully to counteract the consequences brought about by spinal cord ischemia during surgical intervention and a precarious spinal cord blood supply postoperatively. The incidence of paraplegia and paraparesis at centers for aneurysm repair has been decreasing then. Occasionally, a case of spinal cord injury still occurs, and the most important factors for the prevention of either immediate or delayed paraplegia remain to be elucidated [6-10].

In this chapter, we review the contemporary anatomical and pathophysiological understanding of spinal cord blood supply and present the scientific basis for clinical interventions used during descending and thoracoabdominal aortic surgery in order to reduce the incidence of paraplegia.

2. Blood supply of the spinal cord

2.1 Arterial supply of the spinal cord

The vessels that supply the spinal cord are derived from the branches of the vertebral, deep cervical, intercostal, and lumbar arteries. The spinal cord is supplied by three longitudinal arteries, which include an anterior spinal artery and two posterior spinal arteries. These vessels are reinforced by blood from segmental vessels called radicular arteries. The anterior artery is larger than the two posterior arteries and provides 75% of spinal blood flow. The posterior spinal arteries arise as small branches of either the vertebral or posterior inferior cerebellar arteries. Between the anterior and posterior arteries, collateral blood flow is minimal.

2.2 Spinal arteries

The anterior spinal artery is formed by the union of two small branches from the vertebral arteries. It runs the length of the spinal cord in the anterior median fissure and supplies the anterior two-thirds of the spinal cord. The caliber of this artery varies according to its proximity to a major radicular artery. It is usually smallest in the T4 to T8 region of the cord.

2.3 Radicular arteries

The radicular arteries arise from the spinal branches of the vertebral, deep cervical, ascending cervical, posterior intercostal, lumbar, and lateral sacral arteries. They enter the vertebral canal through the intervertebral foramina and divide into anterior and posterior radicular arteries. The anterior radicular arteries supply the anterior spinal artery and the posterior radicular arteries contribute blood to the posterior spinal arteries. The radicular arteries supply the vertebrae, meninges, and spinal arteries. They pass along the dorsal and ventral roots of the spinal nerves to reach the spinal cord.

2.4 Anatomy of the arteria radicularis magna (artery of Adamkiewicz)

One segmental artery has assumed particular importance in the pathogenesis of spinal cord ischemia. The arteria radicularis magna (ARM), also known as the artery of Adamkiewicz, is an exceptionally large radicular artery that anastomoses into the mid-segment of the anterior spinal artery. The segmental reinforcements of blood supply from the radicular arteries are very important in supplying the anterior and posterior spinal arteries. The spinal cord may also suffer circulatory impairment if the radicular arteries, particularly the great anterior radicular artery, are narrowed by obstructive arterial disease or by ligation during surgery of the intercostal or lumbar arteries from which they arise.

Through the anterior spinal artery , the ARM supplies the major flow to the lower thoracic and lumbar cord segments. The ARM can arise from any segmental artery between T7 and L4 on either side, or directly from the aorta, but frequently originates from one of the left segmental arteries between T8 and L1. In a study of 102 cadavers, Koshino et al. found that approximately 70% of Adamkiewicz arteries originated from the intercostal and/or lumber arteries on the left side, frequently at the T8-L1 vertebral level [11]. The study reported that there was no significant correlation between the diameter of the ARM and the diameters of the intercostal and lumbar arteries, from which the ARM originated.

Furthermore, within the Th8 to L1 vertebral level, the diameters of the intercostal and lumbar arteries varied considerably and did not correlate with the diameter of the ARM.

Morishita et al. reported that the anterior spinal artery was continuous in adult cadavers and that its diameters above and below the ARM were inconsistent. Furthermore, distal spinal blood supply becomes progressively dependent on the ARM at the narrowest point of the anterior spinal artery. Although larger compared with other radicular arteries, the ARM is of variable diameter ranging from 0.25 to 1.07 mm in cadaveric examinations [12].

3. Strategies to prevent spinal cord ischemia

3.1 Preoperative examination and monitoring of spinal cord function

3.1.1 Preoperative detection of the artery of Adamkiewicz

Kieffer et al.[13] performed preoperative spinal cord arteriography in patients with thoracic and thoracoabdominal aneurysms and identified the arteria radicularis magna (ARM) in 85%. They reported that the risk of paraplegia was 5% if the ARM was identified preoperatively and reimplanted; whereas, it was 50% if the ARM was not reattached back in the 1980s. The complexity and invasiveness of the method, however, prevented its widespread diffusion. There is growing evidence that the Adamkiewicz artery may, nowadays, be visualized through noninvasive methods, such as magnetic resonance angiography (MRA) or computed tomographic angiography (CTA)[14-16]. In a review of literature, Melissano et al.[17] revealed the identification of the artery of Adamkiewicz in 84% of patients by using MRA or CTA. Through examination of the angiographic location of the spinal cord blood supply and its relationship to postoperative paraplegia, they concluded that selective intercostal angiography was safe and the procedure provided information to help understand the mechanisms and risks of spinal cord complications after thoracoabdominal aneurysm repair.

3.1.2 Somatosensory-evoked potentials and motor-evoked potentials

Popularized by Cunningham and associates in the early 1980s [18], somatosensory-evoked potentials (SSEPs) record cortical stimulations through the scalp after peripheral electrical stimulation of the posterior tibial or peroneal nerves. SSEPs are designed to monitor spinal cord perfusion [19]. Schepens et al.[20] demonstrated the usefulness of SSEPs in lowering the incidence of spinal cord injury in patients undergoing thoracic and thoracoabdominal aneurysm repair; however, the tracing of SSEPs has several limitations. First, the tracings are altered by some anesthesic agents, hypothermia, and neuromuscular blockade. Second, SSEPs only evaluate the function of the posterior and lateral columns of the spinal cord. Third, there are reports of false-positive and false-negative responses during the intraoperative monitoring of SSEPs [21].

These limitations of SSEPs can be explained anatomically. Since SSEPs are transmitted through the posterolateral tracts, they primarily reflect ischemia in the region of the posterior spinal arteries. The SSEPs are neither sensitive nor specific monitors of the corticospinal tracts in the anterior spinal cord (supplied by the anterior spinal artery); but, the anterior spinal cord is usually the first region affected during spinal ischemia which causes paraplegia. Therefore, while SSEPs detect extensive spinal ischemia affecting global cord function, smaller degrees of ischemia limited to the anterior spinal motor territories may not be detected.

However, due to a great variance of sensitivity and specificity to the spinal ischemia in many clinical studies [22,23], the use of motor evoked potentials (MEPs) has been proposed. The MEP is a more logical way to detect impending paraplegia as it directly monitors nerve conduction in the corticospinal tract. MEPs can evaluate the function of the anterior columns of the spinal cord. Use of MEPs greatly increases the sensitivity and specificity of evoked potentials in detecting spinal ischemia compared with monitoring of SSEPs alone [24]. To detect MEPs, the motor cortex or spinal cord proximal to the aortic clamp level is stimulated, and potentials are recorded in the lower spinal cord, peripheral nerves, or muscles. Unlike the SSEPs, which may have a slow response time, inadequate cord perfusion can result in loss of MEPs within as little as 1 min[25]. Laschinger et al.[26] evaluated the usefulness of MEPs to monitor spinal cord perfusion; while van Dongen et al.[27] reported that MEPs monitoring was feasible during low-dose propofol, fentanyl/50% N2O in O2 anesthesia, and partial neuromuscular blockade.

3.2 Strategy to reduce the severity of spinal cord ischemia

When prolonged spinal cord ischemia is anticipated, it is important to minimize the severity of the ischemia. Various methods have been proposed to increase the tolerance of the cord to ischemic insult [28].

3.2.1 Distal perfusion techniques

Deterioration of blood flow to the spinal cord and abdominal viscera contributes significantly to the development of ischemic complications. Distal perfusion techniques perfuse the abdominal aorta during the period of aortic cross-clamping, which permit blood supply to the spinal cord via the intercostal, lumbar, and hypogastric vessels. Although distal perfusion techniques were used by some surgeons in the 1960s， they were not widely adopted because the results were variable, such that some surgeons suggested the inefficacy of the technique due to the greater rate of incidence of paraplegia [29]. Although the clamp-and-sew technique is used successfully in most cases [30,31], several studies confirm the need for an additional protective measure if the aortic cross-clamp time is longer than 30min [31,32]. Katz et al.[33] reported a 71% incidence of spinal cord injury in patients with disease of the descending thoracic aorta and cross-clamp times longer than 30 min. To date, abundant experimental and clinical evidences reveal that these techniques do reduce the incidence of paraplegia compared with the simple clamp-and-sew approach. Notably, data from studies that concurrently employed distal perfusion and clamp-and-sew procedures have demonstrated that the exponential rise in paraplegia rates when clamp times exceeds 30 min with clamp-and-sew technique alone does not occur [34]. Several techniques have been advocated for the perfusion of the distal aorta, such as femoro-femoral bypass, passive shunts, and left heart bypass.

3.2.1.1 Passive shunts

Historically, the use of the passive shunt was the method of choice for distal perfusion. During the 1960's, the Gott shunt tube was used as a passive shunt [35]; however, according to two published reports of traumatic tear of the thoracic aorta, the Gott shunt did not decrease the incidence of paraplegia from that associated with the clamp-and-sew technique [36,37]. Moreover, the distal aortic perfusion pressure necessitated to be greater than or equal to 60mmHg in order to minimize spinal cord injury, which made the Gott shunt less desirable than techniques that allowed the flow to be actively maintained. The shunt was too small with an internal diameter of 5-6 mm; thus the blood flow was not adequate for distal aortic perfusion, and the proximal aorta could not be adequately decompressed. These problems led to the development of left heart bypass or partial cardiopulmonary bypass.

3.2.1.2 Left heart bypass

The centrifugal pump is used for left heart bypass [38], and provides the best means of maintaining distal aortic perfusion. The left heart bypass is set up with cannulation of the left atrium or left pulmonary vein. Blood is returned to one of the femoral arteries for distal perfusion. Minimal heparinization is needed, but it is recommended especially for patients with femoral occlusive disease. With the use of the pump, the distal aortic perfusion can be maintained at 60–70 mmHg. According to Kaplan et al.,[39] active distal bypass perfusion achieved significantly greater distal aortic pressure than either the clamp and sew technique or passive shunting.

3.2.1.3 Partial cardiopulmonary bypass

To overcome the limitation of poor oxygenation of the left heart bypass, partial cardiopulmonary bypass including the artificial lung and blood reservoir in the circuit has been utilized mainly in Japan. With the aid of heart-lung bypass and full heparinization, intraoperative shift from normothermic bypass to deep hypothermia was easily achieved, and unrestricted blood aspiration was possible. Detrimental effects of prolonged cardiopulmonary bypass (CPB), including heparin-related bleeding, cannot be ignored though [40].

3.2.2 Cerebrospinal fluid drainage

Blaisdell and Cooley[41] and Miyamoto et al.[42] reported that CSF drainage was beneficial for reducing the incidence of spinal cord injury in a dog model. It was shown that the relative spinal cord perfusion pressure increased with the CSF drainage, which led to reduction of spinal cord injury. McCullough et al.[43] also reported the protective effect of CSF drainage in reducing the incidence of paraplegia in a canine model. The combined effects of decreased arterial pressure and increased CSF pressure during aortic cross-clamping resulted in decreased spinal cord perfusion pressure. The perfusion pressure can be maintained by decreasing CSF pressure through CSF drainage. Based on the results of these experiments, the concept of CSF drainage has been applied clinically. Crawford et al.[44] performed a prospective randomized study on the effectiveness of CSF drainage for preventing paraplegia and reported that it was not beneficial in this regard. Conversely, a more recent prospective randomized study of CSF drainage by Coselli et al.,[45] and a report by Safi et al.,[46] showed that CSF drainage did help to prevent spinal cord injury. Many reports regarding reversal of paraplegia by commencing CSF drainage after surgery or endovascular stent-grafting also substantiated the importance of lowering the CSF pressure.

The use of CSF drainage as a therapeutic measure for delayed-onset paraparesis or paraplegia after open or endovascular repair is more accepted because there are several published case reports and anecdotal accounts of successful reversal of paraplegia by employing CSF drainage [47,48]. Wada et al.[49] manipulated the mean arterial and CSF pressures intraoperatively and found that ischemic SSEPs normalized when a combination of CSF drainage and arterial pressure manipulation was used to obtain a spinal perfusion pressure above 40mmHg. On the basis of their data, spinal perfusion pressure should always be maintained above 40mmHg, which confirmed previous similar observations from animal studies. Manipulation of spinal perfusion pressure assumes greater importance in patients with respiratory compromise, as autoregulation of spinal blood flow is lost with hypoxia and hypercarbia, thereby, making spinal blood flow more sensitive to changes in perfusion pressure [50].

In view of these encouraging clinical results, CSF drainage has been incorporated as one of the most important components in the modern multimodality approach to spinal cord protection. Since not all cases of spinal cord ischemia are accompanied by increased CSF pressure; however, CSF drainage alone cannot be relied upon to prevent or reverse paraplegia and should be regarded as part of a multimodality approach to the prevention of spinal cord injury. Most importantly, this procedure is not immune to serious complications, such as intracranial bleeding, perispinal hematoma, and meningitis.

3.2.3 Systemic hypothermia

Systemic hypothermia is the most reliable protective adjunct for the prevention of spinal cord injury and is used by many surgeons [51,52]. Hypothermia is one of the most promising methods for protecting neural tissue during ischemia with the advantage that even longer periods of ischemia are tolerated compared with normothermic techniques. Because ventricular fibrillation or severe bradycardia is invariable with profound hypothermia, total body circulatory arrest is necessarily a component of this technique. Experimental work has shown that during the periods of aortic cross-clamping, hypothermia confers a protective effect on spinal cord function [53]. Hypothermia increases the tolerance of neural tissue to ischemia [54,55] by decreasing oxygen demand and metabolic rate, and mild hypothermia confers a marked protective effect on the spinal cord [56]. Kouchoukos and Rokkas reported an 8% 30-day mortality with a paraplegia or paraparesis rate of 2.8%. They concluded that the use of hypothermic CPB and circulatory arrest provided substantial protection against paraplegia and allowed complex operations on the descending thoracic and thoracoabdominal aorta to be performed safely [57]. Depending upon the extent of aortic replacement and vessel reimplantation, the whole procedure may be undertaken during circulatory arrest, or, for more extensive thoracoabdominal procedures, circulation is resumed after completion of the proximal and intercostal anastomoses. The advantages of this approach, in terms of spinal protection, are more uniform cooling of the cord, avoidance of the need for selective intercostal or visceral perfusion, and ability to perform open aortic and intercostal anastomoses; thus, potential steal phenomenon can be avoided. Okita et al. reported the clinical advantages of using deep hypothermia in patients for thoracoabdominal repair [58]. The main candidate for deep systemic hypothermia is a good-risk patient with less blood reserve in the spinal cord, such as one with a prior aortic replacement, severe atherosclerosis, or chronic aortic dissection.

On the other hand, the employment of CPB necessitates full heparinization; wherein, hypothermia itself may cause coagulopathy. The resultant intrabronchial bleeding in the left lung is then problematic. Furthermore, the requirement for full CPB and profound hypothermia introduces additional new problems and potential complications, including cardiac dysfunction (due to ventricular distension during cooling), brain injury, and possibly higher infection risk. Various results in the literature are demonstrated, and there are several small series reporting the high morbidity and mortality associated with this technique [59]. For this reason, most surgeons reserve deep hypothermic circulatory arrest techniques for only the most complex cases.

3.2.4 Regional cooling

Apart from systemic hypothermia, regional hypothermia has been used for spinal cord protection. Experiments have shown that regional hypothermic perfusion applied to the epidural or intrathecal space may protect the spinal cord during cross-clamping of the aorta [60]. Direct cooling of the spinal cord has been applied in both the laboratory and clinical settings, and has the theoretical advantage of deep cooling of the spinal cord whilst avoiding the drawbacks of profound systemic hypothermia.

In 1961, Albin et al. demonstrated the effect and safety of regional spinal cord cooling [61]. In 1993, Tabayashi et al.[62] and Marsala et al.[63] evaluated the effect of spinal cord cooling during spinal cord ischemia and reported its usefulness in preventing ischemic spinal cord injury. Davison et al.[64] devised and applied this method in eight patients undergoing thoracic or thoracoabdominal aneurysm repair in 1994 and reported that epidural cooling was a safe and effective technique of increasing the ischemic tolerance of the spinal cord.

The most systematically applied in the clinical setting has been the technique of Cambria et al.[65]; in which, normal saline at 4°C is continuously infused into the epidural space through a catheter. Using epidural cooling with CSF drainage, segmental artery reimplantation, and almost exclusive use of a clamp-and-sew technique without distal bypass (98% of patients), Cambria et al.[66] reported a paraplegia rate of 2% in 170 cases. The major risk associated with this approach is a potential for an increase in CSF pressure; hence, the necessity for CSF pressure monitoring and drainage is described. Their data show that epidural cooling is an effective method of spinal protection and may offer an alternative to distal bypass. Whilst regional cooling has been shown to be a safe alternative to distal perfusion in the majority of cases, it is not known whether it adds further protection if used in addition to distal perfusion.

3.2.5 Segmental artery perfusion

Some studies further attempt to reduce spinal cord ischemia by continuously perfusing the lower intercostal arteries. Experimentally, it has been demonstrated in pigs that segmental artery perfusion can protect the spinal cord for up to 60 min of ischemia [67]. In this study, the control group has simple aortic cross-clamping without distal perfusion, which is not reflective of the clinical scenario where adjuncts are frequently used. Selective spinal cord perfusion has been applied clinically utilizing a special cannulae [68] or through a Dacron graft [69].

Kawaharada et al. reported that trials to perfuse the critical intercostal arteries have been tried based on preoperative identification of the ARM [70]. Perfusion of the intercostal arteries from the study on the measurement of blood flow of the intercostal artery or lumbar artery with the use of transthoracic Doppler sonography was conducted [71]. They attempted to perfuse the intercostal arteries mainly through the Adamkiewicz artery for the purpose of maintaining spinal cord perfusion pressure during the cross-clamping of the aorta. By this technique, total blood flow quantity in the spinal cord becomes equal to or more than a certain constant level. Selective spinal perfusion maintains the quantity of total blood flow in the spinal cord and is very useful for reducing the incidence of ischemic injury of the spinal cord during operation.

3.2.6 Spinal cord steal syndromes

Steal is one concept that unifies most of the various successful strategies for reduction of paraplegia rates. When the aneurysm is opened, free back-flow of blood from the patent intercostal arteries is usually observed with retrograde flow into the operating field through the opened intercostal and lumbar vessels, instead of going through the ASA due to a steal mechanism [72].

The various collaterals of the spinal cord arterial supply mean that blood can be diverted toward or away from the spinal cord and toward or away from other competing vascular beds in the cervical, thoracic, and lumbar/hypogastric regions. The importance of steal syndromes in the context of aortic surgery has been less appreciated. Although the possibility of steal as a cause of paraplegia after aortic resection was suggested by Cole and Gutelius [73] in 1969, it was largely unacknowledged until only recently. In the early 1990s, Wadouh et al.[74] revisited the concept of steal and suggested that spinal cord injury during aortic clamping resulted from a steal phenomenon. Using a pig model, they concluded that after aortic cross-clamping, blood had the tendency to drain away from the spinal cord than to supply it longitudinally. These experiments suggest that simple clamp techniques, especially where a proximal clamp only is applied, may result in more steal away from the cord compared with other approaches. Kawanishi et al. had experimentally demonstrated that control of the intercostal back-flow in the rabbit's opened aorta could reduce the incidence of spinal cord ischemia [75]. Using aortic injection and spinal artery perfusion in cadavers, Biglioli et al. [76] demonstrated the anatomical existence of a functional steal pathway; wherein, the blood was diverted from the spinal cord to the ARM during aortic clamping.

Another potential steal pathway is into the open thoracic cavity. If the aneurysm is opened prior to ligation of segmental arteries, back-bleeding is evident from the intercostal and lumbar orifices into the aorta. As there is no resistance to blood flow from these segmental vessels, blood from the anterior spinal artery will preferentially bleed out into the thorax through the ARM; thus, the spinal ischemia that has already resulted from the loss of intercostal supply from the excluded aortic segment is compounded [77]. The clinical existence of spinal steal as a possible cause of neurological injury is supported by the relatively low incidence of paraplegia in endovascular stent graft procedures, which entirely avoid steal phenomenon. Thus, external clamping of the intercostal arteries before opening the aneurysm or intraluminal insertion of a balloon-tipped catheter into the intercostal arteries after opening the aneurysm is a routine procedure to minimize blood reflux from the intercostal arteries. It seems prudent therefore to include measures for prevention of steal in spinal protection strategies.

3.2.7 Management of segmental arteries

3.2.7.1 Reattachment of the intercostal and lumbar arteries

Reattachment of segmental arteries after reconstructive surgery of the aorta is a controversial subject. A markedly lower incidence of spinal cord ischemia after endovascular stent-grafting stimulated the controversy, as well as a search for insights regarding the etiologies of spinal cord ischemia [78]. Some surgeons avoid intercostal reattachment. In fact, Acher et al.[79] demonstrated excellent operative results without reattachment of intercostal arteries. They reported that quick oversewing of the intercostal arteries with CSF drainage and naloxone administration could help reduce the incidence of spinal cord injury. Griepp et al.[80] also showed that reattachment could be avoided by ligating the intercostal arteries before aortic cross-clamping while monitoring somatosensory evoked potential. These reports suggest that existing collateral vessels might improve the perfusion pressure. However, in 2008, Acher et al. [81] reported their clinical experience with thoracoabdominal aorta repair and the impact of intercostal artery implantation, in which the incidence of paraplegia decreased from 4.83% to 0.88% for neuroprotective strategies. The concept of oversewing segmental vessels with appropriate monitoring of the spinal cord is based on the fact that many clinical studies demonstrate the increasing rate of postoperative paraplegia with the increase in cross-clamping time. Time might be saved by not reattaching the noncritical segmental arteries. However, when a large number of intercostal and lumbar arteries are oversewn, the risk of neurological complications may be increased. Some surgeons attempt to identify the critical segmental vessels and selectively reimplant them. Traditionally, which vessels are important is decided intraoperatively by observing the intercostal arteries and reimplanting the larger vessels and those with greatest back-bleeding. Other surgeons base their decisions on the extent of resection; in which, vessels are reimplanted only during extensive thoracoabdominal resections. Anatomical studies have, however, shown no correlation between the size of the intercostal arteries and their likelihood of feeding the ARM [11]. The assumption that the arteries with greatest back-bleeding should be implanted is also flawed, since the presence of bleeding after aortic transection implies that a vessel is well collateralized and is effectively stealing blood retrograde from the spinal cord; hence, such vessels can be ligated without consequence. In contrast, vessels that do not back-bleed suggest a lack of collateralization and their reimplantation may improve spinal circulation.

Most surgeons who advocate selective reimplantation do not rely on intraoperative assessment but undertake preoperative angiography to localize the ARM. Preoperative localization helps target intercostal reimplantation, such that only a few intercostal arteries are reimplanted. Preoperative detection of an intercostal artery that may be related to the ARM is useful for establishing the best operational strategy for thoracoabdominal aortic aneurysm repair because surgical repair can be performed while taking care to revascularize the intercostal and lumbar arteries at or near the level of the ARM. Consequently, the occurrence of spinal cord injury can be reduced.

With this reconstruction method, the operation time, distal perfusion time, and clamp time needed for thoracoabdominal aortic aneurysm repair may be reduced. However, there is still no prospective randomized study that shows a significant reduction in the risk of postoperative paraplegia through reattachment of the segmental arteries. With the refinement of techniques in identifying the critical intercostal arteries and monitoring of evoked potentials, selective reattachment of the critical segmental arteries may be achieved.

3.2.7.2 Sacrificing of the intercostal and lumbar arteries

Systematic sacrifice of the intercostal vessels has been employed by Griepp et al.[80] and Gala et al.[82]. Intercostal reimplantation is not an integral part of their technique and is only undertaken if evoked potentials suggest spinal ischemia when intercostal arteries are occluded. Vessels are occluded thrice every 10 min, after which motor and sensory potentials are recorded. If the evoked potentials remain normal after 5 min of occlusion, then these vessels are sacrificed. The advantages of the Griepp approach include reduction of aortic cross-clamp time (and hence decrease in the overall duration of spinal ischemia), diminution of steal (as all intercostals are ligated prior to aortic transection), and prevention of unnecessary reimplantation of intercostals (with its attendant risks). The postoperative spinal circulation is more predictable and is not subject to abrupt changes resulting from problems with intercostal reimplantation (such as acute occlusion from thrombosis, which

has been postulated as one mechanism for delayed-onset paraplegia). Other potential advantages are the avoidance of technical problems associated with performing anastomoses or oversewing intercostals in a severely atherosclerotic aneurysm and the absence of residual aortic tissue in the replaced segment of the aorta.
Sacrificing of the intercostal inflow to the spinal circulation, however, means that the part of the thoracic cord is totally dependent upon extrasegmental supply and inflow from the cervical and hypogastric/lumbar arteries postoperatively. The spinal perfusion pressure, therefore assumes greater importance as the principal determinant of spinal blood flow to critical regions. For this reason, evoked potentials are monitored until the patient is awake and can be evaluated neurologically. Mean arterial pressures are kept in a supranormal range (80-90 mmHg mean) and, with concomitant CSF drainage, cerebrospinal pressures are kept below 10 mmHg. Sustained hypotension in the absence of the intercostal inflow will almost certainly result in paraparesis, which, if untreated, could develop into paraplegia.

4. Conclusions

Reconstructive surgery of the thoracoabdominal aorta remains a challenging surgical procedure with a recognized incidence of postoperative neurological complications. The complications pose not only the physical disability described but also a higher mortality rate among patients. The etiology of the aforementioned postoperative neurological problems has now been well described, and attempts have been made to reduce the incidence based on our knowledge of the pathophysiology of spinal cord ischemia. In open repair, recognized important strategies that reduce the risk of paraplegia include maintenance of the total amount of blood flow of the spinal cord during the cross-clamping of the aorta, provision of maximum collateral blood flow, reduction of nervous tissue oxygen demand, prolongation of ischemic tolerance of the spinal cord, and reduction of reperfusion injury. However, understanding the development and prevention of spinal cord complications is a prerequisite for a successful surgery on the thoracoabdominal aorta.

5. References

[1] Svensson LG. Paralysisafteraorticsurgery:insearchoflostcordfunction. Surgeon 2005; 3:396-405.
[2] Greenberg RK, Lu Q, Roselli EE, Svensson LG, Moon MC, Hernandez AV, Dowdall J, Cury M, Francis C, Pfaff K, Clair DG, Ouriel K, Lytle BW.Contemporary analysis of descending thoracic and thoracoabdominal aneurysm repair: a comparison of endovascular and open techniques.Circulation. 2008 Aug 19;118(8):808-17. Epub 2008 Aug 4.
[3] Messé SR, Bavaria JE, Mullen M, Cheung AT, Davis R, Augoustides JG, Gutsche J, Woo EY, Szeto WY, Pochettino A, Woo YJ, Kasner SE, McGarvey M. Neurologic outcomes from high risk descending thoracic and thoracoabdominal aortic operations in the era of endovascular repair. Neurocrit Care. 2008;9(3):344-51.
[4] Sakata R, Fujii Y, Kuwano H. Thoracic and cardiovascular surgery in Japan during 2008: annual report by the Japanese Association for Thoracic Surgery. Gen Thorac Cardiovasc Surg 2010;58:356–83.

[5] Derrow AE, Seeger JM, Dame DA, Carter RL, Ozaki K, Flynn TC, et al. The outcome in the United States after thoracoabdominal aortic aneurysm repair, renal artery bypass, and mesenteric revascularization. J Vasc Surg 2001; 34:54–61.

[6] Safi HJ, Estrera AL, Miller CC, Huynh TT, Porat EE, Aziz- zadeh A, et al. Evolution of risk for neurologic deficit after descending and thoracoabdominal aortic repair. Ann Thorac Surg 2005;80:2173–9; discussion 2179.

[7] Coselli JS, LeMaire SA. Descending and thoracoabdominal aortic aneurysms. In: Cohn LH, editor. Cardiac surgery in the adult. New York: McGraw-Hill; 2008. p. 1277–98.

[8] Cambria RP, Clouse WD, Davison JK, Dunn PF, Corey M, Dorer D. Thoracoabdominal aneurysm repair: results with 337 operations performed over a 15-year interval. Ann Surg 2002;236:471–9.

[9] Etz CD, Luehr M, Kari FA, Bodian CA, Smego D, Plestis KA, et al. Paraplegia after extensive thoracic and thoracoab- dominal aortic aneurysm repair: does critical spinal cord ischemia occur postoperatively? J Thorac Cardiovasc Surg 2008;135:324–30.

[10] Maniar HS, Sundt TH III, Prasad SM, Chu CM, Camillo CJ, Moon MR, et al. Delayed paraplegia after thoracic and thoracoabdominal aneurysm repair: a continuing risk Ann Thorac Surg 2003;75:113–20.

[11] Koshino T, Murakami G, Morishita K, Mawatari T, Abe T. Does the Adarnkiewicz artery originate from the larger segmental arteries? J Thorac Cardiovasc Surg 1999;117(5):898-905

[12] Morishita K, Murakami G , Fujisawa Y, Kawaharada N, Fukada J, Saito T et al. Anatomical study of blood supply to the spinal cord. Ann Thorac Surg 2003;76(6):1967-1971.

[13] Kieffer E, Ricard T, Chiras J, Godet G, Cormier E. Preoperative spinal cord arteriography in aneurysmal disease of the descending thoracic and thoracoabdominal aorta: preliminary results in 45 patients. Ann Vasc Surg 1989;3:34–46.

[14] Yamada N, Okita Y, Minatoya K, Tagusari O, Ando M, Takamiya M, Kitamura S.Preoperative demonstration of the Adamkiewicz artery by magnetic resonance angiography in patients with descending or thoracoabdominal aortic aneurysms. Eur J Cardiothorac Surg. 2000 Jul;18(1):104-11.

[15] Kawaharada N, Morishita K, Hyodoh H, Fujisawa Y, Fukada J, Hachiro Y, Kurimoto Y, Abe T. Magnetic resonance angiographic localization of the artery of Adamkiewicz for spinal cord blood supply. Ann Thorac Surg. 2004 Sep;78(3):846-51; discussion 851-2.

[16] Yoshioka K, Niinuma H, Ehara S, Nakajima T, Nakamura M, Kawazoe K. MR angiography and CT angiography of the artery of Adamkiewicz: state of the art. Radiographics. 2006 Oct;26 Suppl 1:S63-73. Review.

[17] Melissano G, Bertoglio L, Civelli V, Amato AC, Coppi G, Civilini E, Calori G, De Cobelli F, Del Maschio A, Chiesa R.Demonstration of the Adamkiewicz artery by multidetector computed tomography angiography analysed with the open-source software OsiriX. Eur J Vasc Endovasc Surg. 2009 Apr;37(4):395-400. Epub 2009 Feb 20.

[18] Cunningham JN Jr, Laschinger JC, Merkin HA, Nathan IM, Colvin S, Ransohoff J, et al. Measurement of spinal cord ischemia during operations upon the thoracic aorta: initial clinical experience. Ann Surg 1982;196(3):285-296.

[19] Shiiya N, Yasuda K, Matsui Y, Sakuma M, Sasaki S. Spinal cord protection during thoracoabdominal aortic aneurysm repair: re- sults of selective reconstruction of the critical segmental arteries guided by evoked spinal cord potential monitoring. J Vasc Surg 1995;21:970–5.

[20] Schepens MA, Boezeman EH, Hamerlijnck RP, ter Beek H, Vermeulen FE. Somatosensory evoked potentials during exclu- sion and reperfusion critical aortic segments in thoracoabdominal aortic aneurysm surgery. J Card Surg 1994;9:692–702.

[21] Takai O, Okumura F. Application and limitation of somatosen- sory evoked potential monitoring during surgical procedures on the thoracoabdominal aorta. J Thorac Cardiovasc Surg 1987;94: 266–70.

[22] Guerit JM, Witdoeckt C, Verhelst R, Matta AJ, Jacquet LM, Dion RA. Sensitivity, specificity, and surgical impact of somatosensory evoked potentials in descending aorta surgery. Ann Thorac Surg 1999;67(suppl):1943–6.

[23] De Haan P, Kalkmann CJ, Ubags LH. A comparison of sensitivity of epidural and myogenic transcranial motor- evoked responses in the detection of acute spinal cord isch- emia in the rabbit. Anesth Analg 1996;83:1022–7.

[24] Meylaerts SA, Jacobs MJ, van Iterson V, De Haan P, Kalkman CJ. Comparison of transcranial motor evoked potentials and somatosensory evoked potentials during thoracoabdominal aortic aneurysm repair. Ann Surg. 1999 Dec;230(6):742-9.

[25] Reuter DG, Tacker WA Jr, Badylak SF, Voorhees WD 3rd, Konrad PE. Correlation of motor-evoked potential response to ischemic spinal cord damage. J Thorac Cardiovasc Surg. 1992 Aug;104(2):262-72.

[26] Laschinger JC, Owen J, Rosenbloom M, Cox JL, Kouchoukos NT. Direct noninvasive monitoring of spinal cord motor function during thoracic aortic occlusion: use of motor evoked potentials. J Vasc Surg 1988;7:161–71.

[27] van Dongen EP, ter Beek HT, Schepens MA, Morshuis WJ, Langem HJ, Kalkman CJ, et al. The influence of nitrous oxide to supplement fentanyl/low-dose propofol anesthesia on transcranial myogenic motor-evoked potential during thoracic aortic surgery. J Cardiothorac Vasc Anesth 1999;13:30–4.

[28] Svensson LG, Crawford ES. Aortic dissection and aortic aneurysm surgery: clinical observation and experimental investigations, and statistical analysis. Part II. Curr Probl Surg 1992;29:915–1057.

[29] Crawford ES, Rubio PA. Reappraisal of adjuncts to avoid ischemia in the treatment of aneurysms of descending thoracic aorta. J Thorac Cardiovasc Surg. 1973 Nov;66(5):693-704.

[30] Crawford ES, Snyder DM, Cho GC, Foehm JO. Progress in treat- ment of thoracoabdominal and abdominal aortic aneurysms in- volving celiac, superior mesenteric and renal arteries. Ann Surg 1978;188:404–22.

[31] Schepens MA, Defauw JJ, Hamerlijnck RP, Geest RD, Vermeulen FE. Surgical treatment of thoracoabdominal aortic aneurysms by simple crossclamping, risk factors and late results. J Thorac Cardiovasc Surg 1994;107:134–42.

[32] Grabits K, Sandmann W, Stuhmeier K, Mainzer B, Godehardt E, Ohke B, et al. The risk of ischemic spinal cord injury in patients undergoing graft replacement for thoracoabdominal aortic aneu- rysms. J Vasc Surg 1996;23:230–40.
[33] Katz NM, Blackstone EH, Kirklin JN, Karp RB. Incremental risk factors for spinal cord injury following operation for acute trau- matic aortic transection. J Thorac Cardiovasc Surg 1981;81:669– 74.
[34] Schepens MA, Vermeulen FE, Morshuis WJ, Dossche KM, van Dongen EP, Ter Beek HT, Boezeman EH. Impact of left heart bypass on the results of thoracoabdominal aortic aneurysm repair. Ann Thorac Surg. 1999 Jun;67(6):1963-7; discussion 1979-80.
[35] Gott VF, Whiffen JD, Dutton RC. Heparin bonding on colloidal graphite surface. Science 1963;142:1297.
[36] Duhaylongsod FG, Glower DD, Wolfe WG. Acute traumatic aortic aneurysm: the Duke experience from 1970 to 1990. J Vasc Surg 1992;15:331–43.
[37] Hilgenberg AD, Logan DL, Akins CW. Blunt injuries of the thoracic aorta. Ann Thorac Surg 1992;53:233–9.
[38] Svensson LG, Hess KR, Coselli JS, Safi HJ. Influence of segmen- tal arteries, extent, and atriofemoral bypass on postoperative paraplegia after thoracoabdominal aortic operations. J Vasc Surg 1994;20:255–62.
[39] Kaplan DK, Atsumi N, D'Ambra MN, Vlahakes GJ. Distal circu- latory support for thoracic aortic operations: effects on intra- cranial pressure. Ann Thorac Surg 1995;59:448–52.
[40] Kazui T, Komatsu S, Yokoyama H. Surgical treatment of aneurysms of the thoracic aorta with the aid of partial car- diopulmonary bypass: an analysis of 95 patients. Ann Thorac Surg 1987;43:622–7.
[41] Blaisdell FW, Cooley DA. The mechanism of paraplegia after temporary thoracic aortic occlusion and its relationship to spinal fluid pressure. Surgery 1962;51:351–5.
[42] Miyamoto K, Ueno A, Wada T, Kimoto S. A new and simple method of preventing spinal cord damage following temporary occlusion of the thoracic aorta by draining the cerebrospinal fluid. J Cardiovasc Surg 1960;1:188–97.
[43] McCullough JL, Hollier LH, Nugen M. Paraplegia after thoracic aortic occlusion: influence of cerebrospinal fluid drainage; experi- mental and early clinical results. J Vasc Surg 1988;7:153–60.
[44] Crawford ES, Svensson LG, Hess KR, Shenaq SS, Coselli JS, Safi HJ, et al. A prospective randomized study of cere- brospinal fluid drainage to prevent paraplegia after high-risk surgery on the thoracoabdominal aorta. J Vasc Surg 1991;13:36–45.
[45] Coselli JS, LeMaire SA, Koksoy C, Schmitting ZC, Curling PE. Cerebrospinal fluid drainage reduces paraplegia following thoracoabdominal aortic aneurysm repair: results of a prospective randomized trial. J Vasc Surg 2002;35:631–9.
[46] Safi HJ, Miller CC III, Huynh TTT, Estera AL, Porat EE, Winnerkvist AN, et al. Distal aortic perfusion and cerebrospinal fluid drainage for thoracoabdominal and descending thoracic aor- tic repair: ten years of organ protection. Ann Surg 2003;238:372– 81.
[47] Estrera AL, Miller CC 3rd, Huynh TT, Azizzadeh A, Porat EE, Vinnerkvist A, Ignacio C, Sheinbaum R, Safi HJ. Preoperative and operative predictors of delayed neurologic deficit following repair of thoracoabdominal aortic aneurysm. J Thorac Cardiovasc Surg. 2003 Nov;126(5):1288-94.

[48] Oberwalder PJ, Tiesenhausen K, Hausegger K, Rigler B. Successful reversal of delayed paraplegia after endovascular stent grafting. J Thorac Cardiovasc Surg. 2002 Dec;124(6):1259-60

[49] Wada T, Yao H, Miyamoto T, Mukai S, Yamamura M. Prevention and detection of spinal cord injury during thoracic and thoracoabdominal aortic repairs. Ann Thorac Surg. 2001 Jul;72(1):80-4; discussion 85.

[50] Afifi S. Pro: cerebrospinal fluid drainage protects the spinal cord during thoracoabdominal aortic reconstruction surgery. J Cardiothorac Vasc Anesth. 2002 Oct;16(5):643-9.

[51] Borst HG, Schaudig SA, Rudolph W. Arteriovenous fistula of the aortic arch: repair during deep hypothermia and cir- culatory arrest. J Thorac Cardiovasc Surg 1964;48:443–7.

[52] Crawford ES, Coselli JS, Safi HJ. Partial cardiopulmonary bypass, hypothermic circulatory arrest, posterolateral expo- sure for thoracic aortic aneurysm operation. J Thorac Car- diovasc Surg 1987;94:824.

[53] Beattie EJ, Adovasio D, Keshishian JM. Refrigeration in experimental surgery of the aorta. Surg Gynecol Obstet 1953;96:711–3.

[54] Fox SL, Blackstone E, Kirklin JW. Relationship of brain blood flow and oxygen consumption to perfusion flow rate during profoundly hypothermic cardiopulmonary bypass: an experi- mental study. J Thorac Cardiovasc Surg 1984;87:658–64.

[55] Colon R, Frazier DH, Cooley DA. Hypothermic regional perfusion for protection of the spinal cord during periods of ischemia. Ann Thorac Surg 1987;43:643–93.

[56] Ginsberg MD, Globus MYT, Dietrich R. Temperature mod- ulation in ischemic brain injury: a synthesis of recent advances. Prog Brain Res 1993;96:13–22.

[57] Kouchoukos NT, Rokkas CK. Hypothermic cardiopulmonary bypass for spinal cord protection: rationale and clinical results. Ann Thorac Surg 1999;67s:1940–2.

[58] Okita Y, Takamoto S, Ando M, Morota T, Yamaki F, Mat- sukawa R, et al. Repair of aneurysm of the entire descending thoracic aorta or thoracoabdominal aorta using a deep hypo- thermia. Eur J Cardiothorac Surg 1997;125:120.

[59] Juvonen T, Biancari F, Rimpiläinen J, Satta J, Rainio P, Kiviluoma K. Strategies for spinal cord protection during descending thoracic and thoracoabdominal aortic surgery: Up-to-date experimental and clinical results -- a review. Scand Cardiovasc J. 2002 May;36(3):136-60.

[60] Salzano RP Jr, Ellison LH, Altonji PF, Richter J, Deckers PJ. Regional deep hypothermia of the spinal cord protects against ischemic injury during thoracic aortic cross-clamping. Ann Thorac Surg. 1994 Jan;57(1):65-70; discussion 71.

[61] Albin MS, White RJ, Donald DE, Maccarty CS, Faulconer A Jr. Hypothermia of the spinal cord by perfusion cooling of the subarachnoid space. Surg Forum. 1961;12:188-9.

[62] Tabayashi K, Niibori K, Konno H, Mohri H. Protection from postischemic spinal cord injury by perfusion cooling of the epidu- ral space. Ann Thorac Surg 1993;56:494–8.

[63] Marsala M, Vanicky I, Galik J, Radonak J, Kundrat I, Marsala J. Panmyelic epidural cooling protects against ischemic spinal cord damage. J Surg Res 1993;55:21–31.

[64] Davison JK, Cambria RR, Vierra DJ, Columbia MA, Koustas G. Epidural cooling for regional spinal cord hypothermia during thoracoabdominal aneurysm repair. J Vasc Surg 1994;20:304–10.
[65] Cambria RP, Davison JK, Zannetti S, L'Italien G, Brewster DC, Gertler JP, Moncure AC, LaMuraglia GM, Abbott WM. Clinical experience with epidural cooling for spinal cord protection during thoracic and thoracoabdominal aneurysm repair. J Vasc Surg. 1997 Feb;25(2):234-41; discussion 241-3
[66] Cambria RP, Davison JK, Carter C, Brewster DC, Chang Y, Clark KA, Atamian S. Epidural cooling for spinal cord protection during thoracoabdominal aneurysm repair: A five-year experience. J Vasc Surg. 2000 Jun;31(6):1093-102.
[67] Meylaerts SA, De Haan P, Kalkman CJ, Jaspers J, Vanicky I, Jacobs MJ.Prevention of paraplegia in pigs by selective segmental artery perfusion during aortic cross-clamping. J Vasc Surg. 2000 Jul;32(1):160-70
[68] Sueda T, Morita S, Okada K, Orihashi K, Shikata H, Matsuura Y.Selective intercostal arterial perfusion during thoracoabdominal aortic aneurysm surgery. Ann Thorac Surg. 2000 Jul;70(1):44-7
[69] Ueda T, Shimizu H, Mori A, Kashima I, Moro K, Kawada S. Selective perfusion of segmental arteries in patients undergoing thoracoabdominal aortic surgery. Ann Thorac Surg. 2000 Jul;70(1):38-43.
[70] Kawaharada N, Ito T, Koyanagi T, Harada R, Hyodoh H, Kurimoto Y, Watanabe A, Higami T. Spinal cord protection with selective spinal perfusion during descending thoracic and thoracoabdominal aortic surgery. Interact Cardiovasc Thorac Surg. 2010 Jun;10(6):986-90; discussion 990-1.
[71] Koyanagi T, Kawaharada N, Kurimoto Y, Ito T, Baba T, Nakamura M, Watanebe A, Higami T. Examination of intercostal arteries with transthoracic Doppler sonography. Echocardiography. 2010 Jan;27(1):17-20
[72] Griepp RB, Ergin AM, Galla JD, Klein IT, Spielvogel C, Griepp E. Minimizing spinal cord injury during repair of descending thoracic and thoracoabdominal aneurysms: the Mount Sinai approach. Semin Thorac Cardiovasc Surg 1988;10:25–8.
[73] Cole PT, Gutelius JR. Neurologic complications of operations on the descending thoracic aorta. Can J Surg. 1969 Oct;12(4):435-43.
[74] Wadouh F, Wadouh R, Hartmann M, Crisp-Lindgren N. Prevention of paraplegia during aortic operations. Ann Thorac Surg. 1990 Oct;50(4):543-52.
[75] Kawanishi Y, Okada K, Tanaka H, Yamashita T, Nakagiri K, Okita Y. The adverse effect of back-bleeding from lumbar arteries on spinal cord pathophysiology in a rabbit model. J Thorac Cardiovasc Surg 2007;133:1553–8.
[76] Biglioli P J Thorac Cardiovasc Surg 2004;127(4):1188-1192.
[77] Griepp RB, Semin Thorac Cardiovasc Surg 1998; 10(1):25-28.
[78] Bavaria JE, Appoo JJ, Makaroun MS, Verter J, Yu ZF, Mitchell RS. Endovascular stent grafting versus open surgi- cal repair of descending thoracic aortic aneurysms in low-risk patients: a multicenter comparative trial. J Thorac Cardio- vasc Surg 2007;133:369–77.
[79] Acher CW, Wynn MM, Hoch JR, Popic P, Archibald J, Archibald J, et al. Combined use of cerebral spinal fluid drainage and nalox- one reduces the risk of paraplegia in thoracoabdominal aortic aneurysm repair. J Vasc Surg 1994;19:236–48.

[80] Griepp RB, Ergin MA, Galla JD, Lansman S, Khan N, Quintana C, et al. Looking for the artery of Adamkiewicz: a quest to minimize paraplegia after operations for aneurysms of the descending thoracic and thoracoabdominal aorta. J Thorac Cardiovasc Surg 1996;112:1202–15.

[81] Acher CW, Wynn MM, Mell MW, Tefera G, Hoch JR. A quantitative assessment of the impact of intercostal artery reimplantation on paralysis risk in thoracoabdominal aortic aneurysm repair. Ann Surg. 2008 Oct;248(4):529-40.

[82] Galla JD, Ergin MA, Lansman SL, McCullough JN, Nguyen KH, Spielvogel D, Klein JJ, Griepp RB. Use of somatosensory evoked potentials for thoracic and thoracoabdominal aortic resections. Ann Thorac Surg. 1999 Jun;67(6):1947-52; discussion 1953-

22

Rehabilitation for Spinal Cord Injury Caused by Thoracic Aortic Aneurysm

Ohsawa, Suguru and Hirabayashi, Shinji
Sumitomo Hospital & Osaka Rosai Hospital
Japan

1. Introduction

Aortic aneurysm (AA) is a life threatening condition. Large AA carries a substantial risk of rupture. Observational studies have reported a 14.1% annual incidence rate of aortic rupture. Once the aorta has reached a diameter of 6 cm the risk of rupture increases in proportion to the aortic diameter (Elefteriades, 2002). The 5-year cumulative risk of rupture has been estimated to be 31 % among aneurysms wider than 6 cm (Clouse et al., 1998). A ruptured thoracic aortic aneurysm (TAA) is a medical catastrophe, and the survival rate is extremely low (Johansson et al., 1995).
The incidence of thoracoabdominal aortic aneurysm (TAAA) was estimated to be 16.3 per 100,000 males and 9.1 per 100,000 females in a recent review of the Swedish National Healthcare Register, which reported increasing incidences over a 15-year period (Olsson et al., 2006). The incidence of thoracic aortic aneurysms in Rochester, Minnesota, was 5.9 per 100,000 (Bickerstaff et al., 1982).
The Swedish register study also found that the frequency of thoracoabdominal aortic surgery had increased from 7 to 15 fold during the study period. A series of 1004 patients who underwent thoracoabdominal aortic operations were reported to have a 5-year mortality of 39% compared with a matched population of untreated patients with a 5-year mortality of 87% (Miller III et al., 2004).
However, aneurysm surgery also carries a risk of death (Rectenwald et al., 2002): mortality at 30 days ranges from 4.8%-8.3% (Coselli et al., 2000; Etz et al., 2006; Greenberg et al., 2008; Svensson et al., 1993). Moreover, the complications associated with this type of surgery are devastating and unpredictable, e.g., thoracic spinal cord infarction (Crawford et al., 1970; Grace & Mattox, 1977; Sliwa & Maclean, 1992) and renal failure caused by renal artery occlusion (Coselli & Le Maire, 1999; Svensson et al., 1991; 1993), which can induce a sedentary state. Aortic aneurysm is a degenerative condition, which means that the patients with this condition are usually elderly, except for those with Marfan syndrome (Etz et al., 2006). Elderly patients are susceptible to respiratory system complications. In long operations, such as open thoracotomy, paraplegia and recurrent laryngeal nerve (RLN) palsy can also occur (discussed later), leading to respiratory system failure. Spinal cord injury (SCI) rehabilitation is hard and requires a long period of exercise. Severely impaired patients with SCI and/or respiratory failure and/or renal failure are often elderly; therefore, it is very hard for them to undergo rehabilitation. These above issues are discussed in this chapter together with our experiences.

2. Incidence of spinal cord injury after thoracoabdominal aortic aneurysm repair

The incidence of SCI as a complication of TAAA repair ranges from 8% to 28% (Greenberg et al., 2008; Messe et al., 2008). Aneurysmal expansion influences the incidence of SCI. Crawford classified aortic aneurysms into several types (Fig. 1): Type I involves most of the descending thoracic aorta and the celiac and superior mesenteric arteries but not the renal arteries. Type II involves most of the descending thoracic aorta and the abdominal aorta including all of the renal and visceral arteries. Type III involves less than half of the descending thoracic aorta and all of the abdominal aorta. Type IV involves all of the abdominal aorta including the renal and mesenteric arteries (Fig 1, Acher et al., 2008).

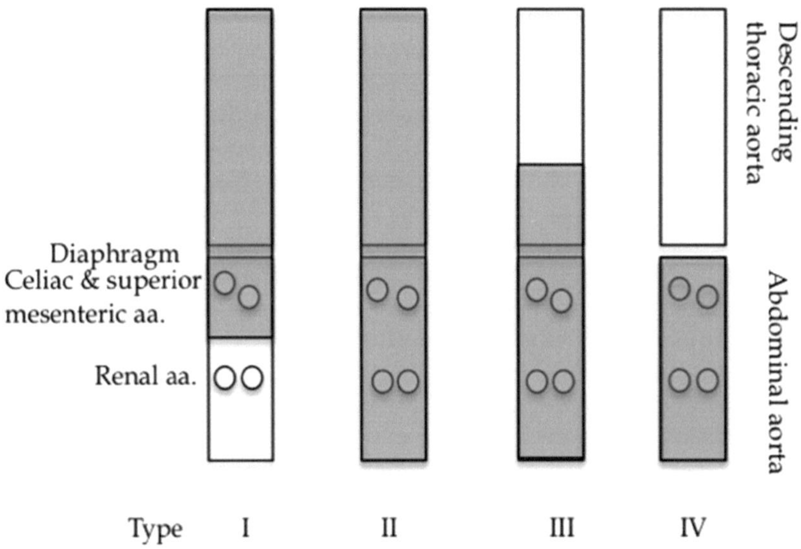

Fig. 1. Crawford classification of descending thoracic and abdominal aortic aneurysm (aneurysm: shadow)

The advent of thoracic endovascular aortic repair (TEVAR) was expected to decrease the rate of complications; however, the incidence of spinal cord infarction did not change much (3-7 %) (Table 1, Dake et al., 1998; Greenberg et al., 2008; Matsuda et al., 2010; Sinha & Cheung, 2010).

	Crawford classification	C-I	C-II	C-III	C-IV
Incidence of SCI (%)	Endovascular	10	19	5	3
Incidence of SCI (%)	Open surgery	14	22	10	2

Table 1. Incidence of spinal cord injury and TAAA Crawford classification (Greenberg et al., 2008; Sinha & Cheung, 2010)

Neurologic complications are strongly associated with mortality. Messe et al. reported that 64% of stroke patients died compared with 17% of those who did not suffer a stroke and that 39% of patients with spinal cord ischemia died compared to 14% of those without spinal cord ischemia (Table 2).

Neurologic complication	Yes	No
Mortality of AA repair (Stroke)	64%	17%
Mortality of AA repair (SCI)	39%	14%

Table 2. Mortality of aortic aneurysm repair complicated with central nervous system (Messe et al., 2008)

3. Anatomy of the spinal cord circulation

The spinal cord depends on a single longitudinal anterior spinal artery and two posterior spinal arteries for blood flow, all of which originate from the vertebral arteries. The anterior and posterior spinal arteries receive segmental circulation from segmental arteries for their blood supply; the largest of these is the artery of Adamkiewicz, which originates from the lower thoracic aorta in the majority of people (Fig 2).

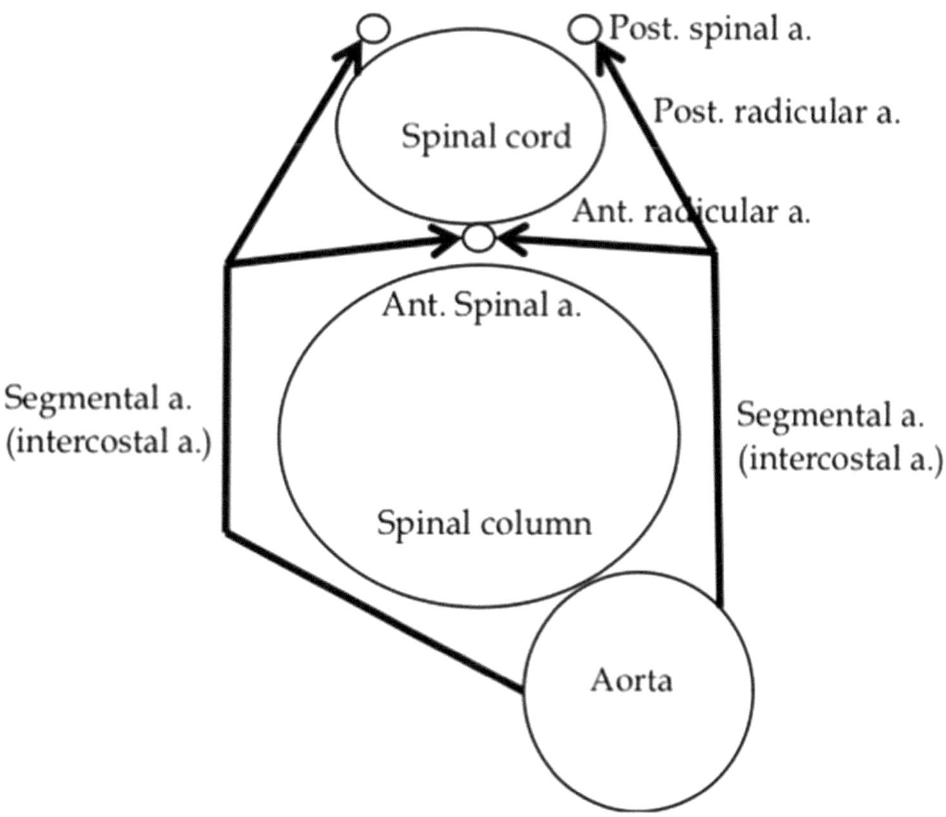

Fig. 2. The arterial supply to the spinal cord (Sliwa & Maclean, 1992)

This large intercostal (segmental) artery has various origins, but originates from T8-L1 in most patients.

Intraoperative ischemia in the spinal cord is thought to be, at least in part, related to the interruption of blood flow through these intercostal arteries due to cross-clamping of the aorta and surgical ligation during aneurysmal resection. In patients with significant thoracic aortic aneurysms, spinal cord integrity may also be maintained by an extensive network of collateral arteries, including supplies from the lumbar and pelvic circulation (Fedorow et al., 2010). Spinal cord ischemia is caused by aortic cross-clamping and interruption of the blood supply to the spinal cord via critical intercostal arteries. The cause of SCI during TAA repair is thought to depend on various factors, including clamping time, reperfusion injury, and hemodynamics. As for the arterial blood supply to the spinal cord, the mid-thoracic area is poorly vascularized with one (or occasionally no) anterior medullary artery that originates from the intercostal arteries. The distance between medullary arteries is greatest and the watershed effect is most striking in the thoracic area. Embolic processes induced by reversed flow might be responsible for reduced flow to the anterior spinal artery.

Fedorow et al. summarized the risk factors for paraplegia after open TAAA repair; emergency presentation (aortic dissection or rupture), postoperative hypotension, more extensive aneurysms (Crawford Type I or II), ligation of spinal collateral vessels, prolonged aortic cross-clamp time, previous abdominal aortic aneurysm repair, diabetes, advanced age(Fedorow et al., 2010). Similar risk factors for spinal cord ischemia after TEVAR were also listed by Sinha & Cheung; longer extent of aneurysm, hypotension, emergency operation, open operative repair, acute aortic rupture, aortic dissection, longer duration of aortic cross-clamp, failure to re-implant segmental arteries, prior distal aortic surgery, severe peripheral vascular disease, anemia (Sinha & Cheung, 2010).

In addition, periarterial edema around the very small radicular arteries as a result of ischemia- reperfusion induced inflammatory responses could play an etiologic role (Jacobs et al., 2006).

4. Prevention of paralysis during surgery

Various methods have been devised to protect against spinal cord ischemia during surgery for TAA (Bicknell et al., 2009; Tabayashi, 2005), such as cerebrospinal fluid drainage (Acher et al., 1994; Coselli, et al., 2002; Fedorow et al., 2010; Griepp et al., 1996; Griepp & Griepp, 2007), hypothermia (Griepp et al., 1996), epidural cooling (Cambria et al., 1997), monitoring of somatosensory (SSEP) (Crawford et al., 1988) and motor evoked potentials (MEP) (de Haan et al., 1997; Jacobs et al. 2006), intercostal artery reattachment (Acher et al., 2008), distal aortic perfusion (Crawford et al., 1988; Safi et al., 2003), and direct spinal cord cooling (Davison et al., 1994).

Spinal cord perfusion is regulated according to the following formula,

$$[\text{Tissue perfusion}]=[\text{Input blood pressure}]-[\text{Tissue back pressure}].$$

Maximizing systolic blood pressure increases the input pressure to the tissue, and removing spinal cord fluid reduces tissue back pressure, which reduces the need for significant input pressure (Acher & Wynn, 2009). This technique can be performed safely with excellent technical results (Estrera et al., 2009).

Reducing the risk further may be dependent on identifying radicular perforators that are critical to the spinal cord blood supply between the cephalad and caudal supply. Spinal cord angiography was used to identify the main supply to the spinal cord (Kieffer et al., 2002). In another study, MRI was used for the detection of the Adamkiewicz artery (Kawaharada et al., 2004), and multidirectional row CT has also been used for the same purpose (Shiiya et al., 2009). The Adamkiewicz artery is the major blood supply to the lumbar spinal cord, and its reimplantation after TAA surgery reduced the risk of paralysis to 5-6%. However, other radicular perforators may also be critical in some patients (Acher et al., 2008). A group from Mount Sinai Hospital discussed avoiding back-bleeding through the intercostal and lumber arteries, in order to prevent loss from the collateral circulation to the spinal cord, by sacrificing the segmental arteries before opening the aneurysm. As a result, the postoperative paraplegia rate in their series was 2% (Etz et al., 2006). However, when more than 10 arteries were sacrificed, the risk of paraplegia increased 29 fold (Gripp et al., 1996).

Monitoring nerve potentials (especially MEP) has been used to identify important vessels, and their reimplantation reduced the risk of paralysis even further (to below 5%) (Sloan, 2008). However, in a prospective study, SSEP monitoring and temporary distal aortic perfusion did not reduce the prevalence of early or delayed neurologic complications after surgery for thoracic aortic aneurysm (Crawford et al., 1988). One reason for the failure of SSEP to identify patients at risk is that the response of the dorsal columns to spinal cord ischemia is slow and does not reflect motor function (de Haan et al., 1997). However, MEP monitoring is an effective technique for detecting spinal cord ischemia within minutes, as a guide for the distal aortic perfusion technique, and for identifying segmental arteries that need to be preserved (de Haan et al., 1997).

Safi et al. reported that distal aortic perfusion and cerebrospinal fluid drainage (DAP+CFD) were safe and effective; immediate neurologic deficits occurred in 36 (3.6%) of 1004 patients overall, including 18 (2.4%) of 741 who received DAP+CFD and 18 (6.8%) of 263 who did not ($p<0.0009$). Among patients with high-risk Crawford type II aneurysms, 11 (6.6%) of 167 who received the DAP+CFD and 11 of those who did not (29%) suffered immediate neurologic deficits (Table 3, Safi et al., 2003).

DAP+CFD	Overall	Yes	No
Rate of neurologic deficit	36/1004 (3.6%)	18/741 (2.4%)	18/263 (6.8%)

Table 3. The effects of distal aortic perfusion (DAP) and cerebrospinal fluid drainage (CFD) (Safi et al., 2003)

After the release of the cross-clamp, the spinal cord is at further risk of ischemia secondary to hypercapnia and hypotension, which can result in decreased tissue perfusion. Metabolic acidosis after the release of the cross-clamp causes an increase in cerebral blood flow, resulting in increases in intracranial pressure and cerebrospinal fluid pressure (Fedorow et al., 2010), which increase tissue back pressure, leading to decreased spinal cord perfusion due to ischemia.

Epidural morphine for postoperative pain relief also carries a risk of paraplegia. Kakinohana et al. reported morphine-induced motor dysfunction after spinal ischemia and relief of the paralysis via the injection of naloxone and investigated the mechanisms responsible for these effects using an animal model (Kakinohana et al., 2003; Nakamura et al., 2004). Acher et al. reported good clinical results for naloxone treatment and cerebral spinal fluid drainage (Acher et al., 1994). The strategies to prevent and treat spinal cord ischemia are summalized in Table 4.

- Minimize spinal cord ischemia time:
    1. Segmental reconstruction of the descending aorta
    2. Distal aortic perfusion with a passive shunt
    3. Partial left heart bypass
- Increase tolerance of ischemia:
    1. Deliberate mild systemic hypothermia
    2. Deep hypothermic circulatory arrest
    3. Selective spinal cord hypothermia by epidural cooling
    4. Pharmacologic neuroprotection
- Augmentation of spinal cord perfusion:
    1. Deliberate hypertension
    2. Lumber cerebrospinal fluid (CSF) drainage
    3. Preservation of subclavian artery flow
- Early detection of spinal cord ischemia:
    1. Intraoperative MEP
    2. Intraoperative SSEP monitoring
    3. Serial postoperative neurologic examination

Table 4. Strategies to prevent and treat spinal cord ischemia (Sinha & Cheung, 2010)

5. Elderly patients: Dysphagia and aspiration pneumonia

In the general population, studies have shown a number of changes that result in the gradual loss of respiratory system function with advancing age (Robbins et al., 1992). Langmore et al. reported that predictors of aspiration pneumonia in elderly people were being dependent for feeding, dependent for oral care, the number of decayed teeth, tube feeding, more than one medical diagnosis, the number of medications being taken, and smoking (Table 5, Langmore et al., 1998).

- Dependent for feeding
- Dependent for oral care
- Decayed teeth
- Tube feeding
- Complications
- Medications
- Smoking

Table 5. Predictors of aspiration pneumonia (Langmore et al.)

Older age at the time of injury is also associated with a higher risk of respiratory complications. The combined effects of SCI and older age are likely to pose a significant risk of respiratory tract complications, such as pneumonia and atelectasis (Charlifue et al., 2010). The most commonly considered mechanism is pulmonary aspiration of the gastric contents, resulting in acid-induced injury. Beta agonists might contribute to gastroesophageal reflux (GER) by decreasing lower esophageal pressure (Yamaya et al., 2001). GER probably occurs more often when the patient is bedridden, and vomiting may be more frequent in patients with GER, adding to the risk of aspiration pneumonia (Feinberg et al., 1990). Aspiration pneumonia contributes to infection of the lung due to the aspiration of bacteria contained in oropharyngeal or gastric secretions. Normal hosts are less likely to develop pneumonia (Barish et al., 1985) because they either aspirate smaller volumes or are able to clear bacteria rapidly. But, an extremely small volume (0.01 ml) of saliva can contain pathogenic numbers of bacteria, and elderly patients with a predisposition to aspiration frequently aspirate oropharyngeal or gastric secretions containing high numbers of bacteria (Bartlett et al., 1974; Johanson & Harris, 1980; Toews et al., 1990). The progressive loss of protective swallowing and cough reflexes with age is thought to be one of the major risk factors for aspiration pneumonia in older people (Pontoppidan & Beecher, 1960). Impaired swallowing and cough reflexes have been demonstrated in elderly patients who develop aspiration pneumonia (Nakazawa et al., 1993; Sekisawa et al., 1990; Yamaya et al., 2001), as has a high incidence of silent aspiration in elderly patients with community-acquired pneumonia (Kikuchi et al., 1994); nevertheless, normal elderly people display no deterioration in their coughing reflex (Katsumata et al., 1995) (Table 6).

- Loss of respiratory system function
- GER
- Impaired swallowing
- Silent aspiration
- Impaired cough reflex

Table 6. Characteristics of elderly patients

Leder & Ross reported that 29% of the total referral population in an tertiary-care teaching hospital exhibited aspiration while 44% of patients with vocal fold immobility aspirated, indicating that vocal fold immobility was associated with a 15% increased incidence of aspiration in patients already suspected of dysphagia. Left vocal fold immobility most frequently occurred due to surgical trauma (60%). A liquid bolus was aspirated more often than a puree bolus (Leder & Ross, 2005). Aspiration caused by RLN palsy has also been reported (Heitmiller et al., 2000; Perie et al., 1998). As a consequence, the nerve is particularly vulnerable to pathological conditions involving these structures (Ortner, 1897; Thirlwall, 1997; Woodson & Kendrick, 1989). In cases of thoracic aortic aneurysm, the incidence of left RLN (LRLN) palsy has been reported to range from 5% to 12% (Stoob et al., 2004). The incidence of LRLN palsy was 8.6% in a study of 500 patients (de Bakey et al., 1978) and 5% in another study of 168 cases (Teixido & Leonetti, 1990). Ishimoto et al. reported an incidence of vocal cord immobility of 32% (20/62), which was confirmed by laryngoscopy after surgery for TAA, and 16 out of 19 patients (84 %) who were followed for more than 6 months did not fully recover (Ishimoto et al., 2002)

As shown in Table 7, postoperative paraplegia closely related to respiratory failure. Crawford Type II aneurysms occurred in 32% of patients with respiratory failure and in 28% of the patients that developed postoperative pneumonia (Money et al., 1994). Five out of seven patients with total paraplegia developed respiratory failure (86%) and that 7 of the 14 patients (50%) with muscle weakness developed respiratory failure, whereas respiratory failure developed in 29 (38%) patients with normal muscle function (p=0.041) (Svensson et al., 1991).

Muscle function	Paraplegia	Paraparesis	Normal
Respiratory failure	5/7 (86%)	7/14 (50%)	29/77 (38%)

Table 7. Paraplegia and respiratory failure (Svensson et al., 1991)

6. Rehabilitation of spinal cord injury in elderly patients

For patients who suffer spinal cord injuries during surgery for AA, the mortality rate is high: Kiwerski et al. reported that 18 out of 74 (24%) patients with traumatic paraplegia died during rehabilitation (Kiwerski et al., 1992). Life-threatening complications are more frequent following spinal cord injuries in elderly patients. This dangerous situation is caused by several factors including a diminished inspiratory reserve volume, circulatory system disease, and poor tolerance to prolonged immobilization (Kiwerski et al., 1992).
Searching the SCI databases in Japan (Sumida et al., 2001a; 2001b) and the USA (Chen et al., 1999; DeVivo et al., 1999; Eastwood et al., 1999; Graves et al., 1999; Hall et al., 1999; Marino et al., 1999) revealed that the complication rates of pneumonia and aspiration were higher in our cases (Ohsawa et al., 2008).

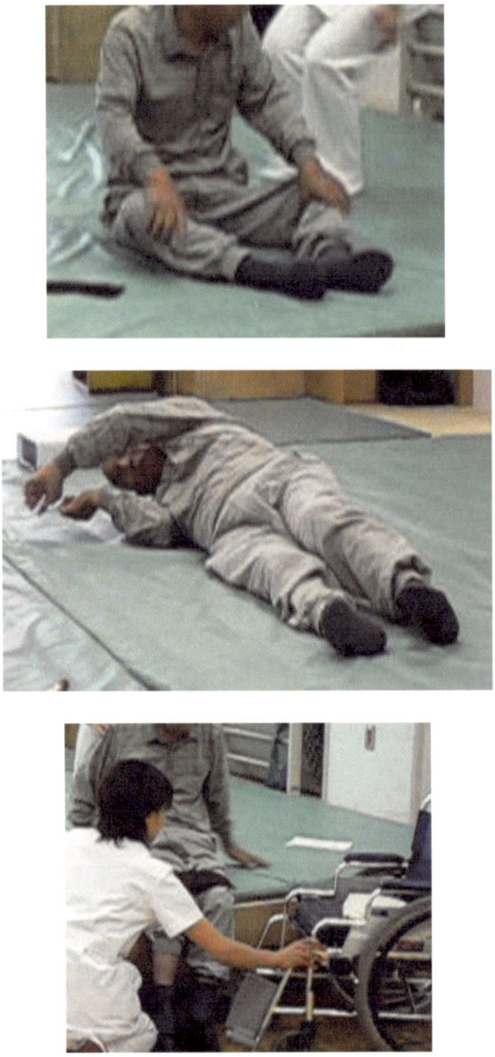

Fig. 3. Basic exercises for patients with SCI (long sitting, roll over, transfer to wheel chair)

Elderly patients with thoracic SCI receive rehabilitation as following exercises; a shot-legged sitting on the edge of the bed, transfer to wheelchair in a ward, then, roll over, long leg sitting, wheelchair drive in rehabilitation center. However, upper limb muscle weakness, excess body weight, renal failure which causes restricted exercise times, respiratory failure, decubitus, all these factors drive them deconditioned and sedentary state. Motor scores of functional independence measure of our patients (FIM, Table 8; Granger et al., 1986; Ottenbacher et al., 1996) before rehabilitation and at discharge were also lower than those in the databases, as were the gain in FIM and the rate of FIM gain during hospitalization.

Finally, SCI associated with thoracic aortic aneurysm surgery was especially marked in the elderly patients requiring airway assistance such as intubation, tracheostomy, or mini-tracheostomy. Due to the long operation time, tracheal secretion is increased, resulting in longer stays in intensive care units and a worse state (Fig 4).

The abovementioned problems can easily worsen a patient's general condition, and such the resultant vicious cycle leads to a poor prognosis. DeVivo et al. reported a high mortality rate for traumatic spinal cord injury older patients (61-86 years-old), who tend to be complicated with pneumonia, ($p=0.031$); moreover, for survivors in the oldest age group (61-86), there was a high likelihood of having to live in a nursing home (DeVivo et al., 1990).

The incidence of pressure sores was very high in our series. In the Japanese database, the incidence is 45.4% for the complete paraplegic SCI patients aged 30 years or higher and 17.3% for those aged less than 30 years. However, the United State database showed no difference in age (23.7%). These results can be attributed to the smaller nursing facilities in Japan (Table 9).

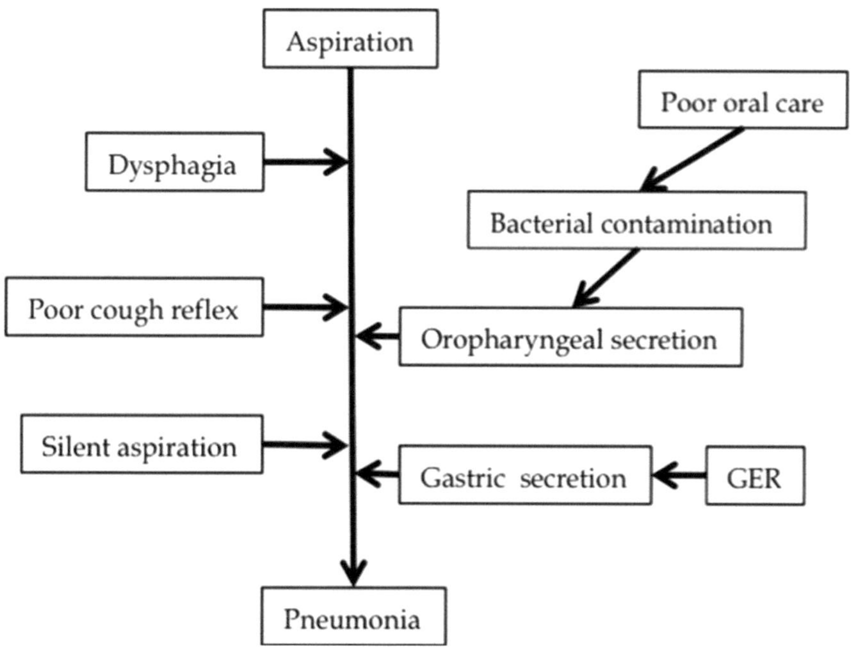

Fig. 4. Aspiration pneumonia in elderly patients

FIM (motor)

- Self care
  1. Eating
  2. Grooming
  3. Bathing
  4. Dressing upper body
  5. Dressing lower body
  6. Toileting
- Sphincter control
  1. Bladder management
  2. Bowel management
- Transfer
  1. Bed, chair, wheelchair
  2. Toilet
  3. Tub
  4. Shower
- Locomotion
  1. Walk/wheelchair
  2. Stairs

FIM (cognitive)

- Communication
  1. Comprehensive
  2. Expression
- Social cognition
  1. Social interaction
  2. Problem solving
  3. Memory

Table 8. FIM domain (Ottenbacher et al., 1996)

	Our cases	Japanese database> 30 years old	Japanese database < 30 years old	USA database
Incidence	11/19 (58%)	45.4%	17.5%	23.4%

Table 9. Incidence of pressure sore

Special consideration to swallowing and deglutitive rehabilitation is needed (Table 10, Honda & Mizojiri, 2000).

- Auscultation: swallowing sound, respiratory sound (Fig 5)
- Water drinking test (1ml, 30ml)
- RSST (repetitive saliva swallowing test)
- Videofluoroscopic swallowing study (VFSS)
- Fiberoptic endoscopic examination of swallowing (FEES)

Table 10. Assessment of swallowing

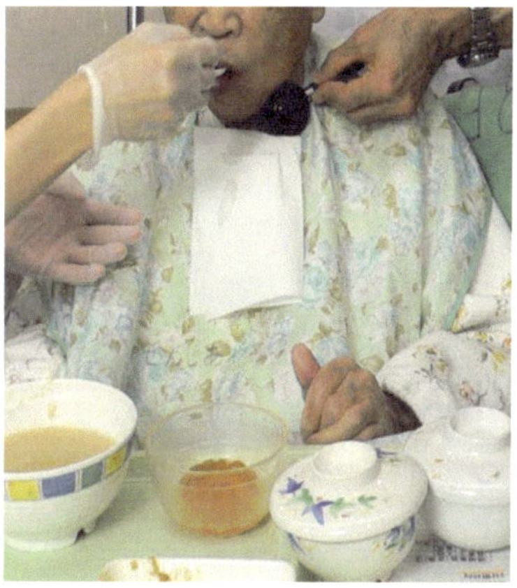

Fig. 5. Auscultation

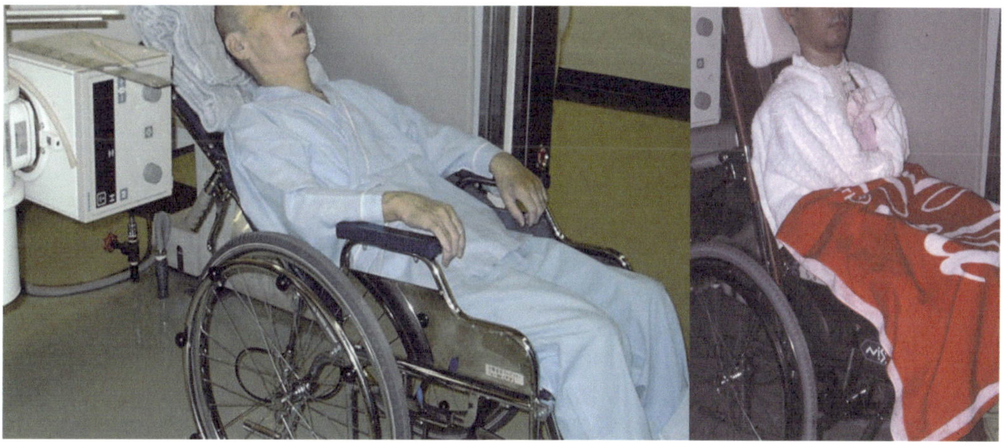

Fig. 6. Positions of VFSS, keeping neck flexion to avoid aspiration during eating

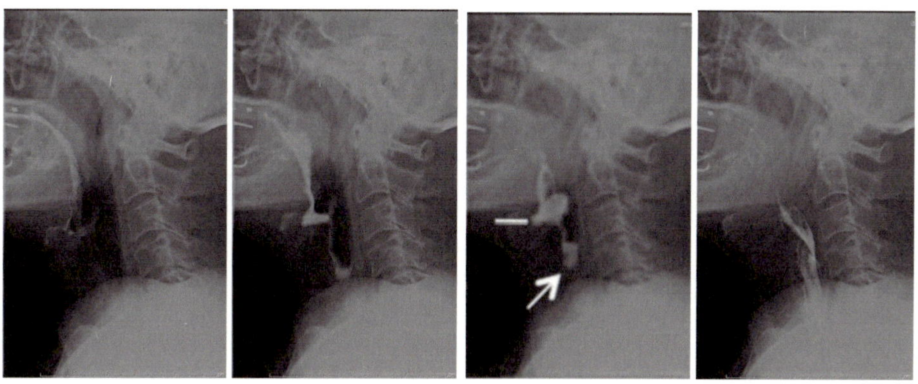

Fig. 7. VFSS (74 year-old man), series of a swallow, no aspiration, delayed swallowing, pooling bolus in the vallecular pouch (line) and the piriformis sinus (arrow) with thick iopamidol liquid

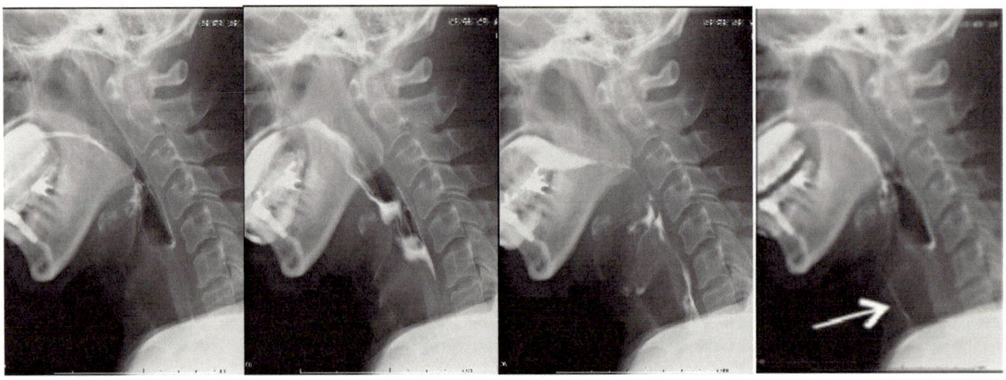

Fig. 8. VFSS (57 year-old man), series of a swallow, thin iopamidol liquid, aspiration (arrow)

This could involve the use of diagnostic tools such as videofluoroscopic study (Fig 6,7,8,) and endoscopy (Langmore, 2003); oral care to prevent pneumonia (Fig 9, Yoneyama et al., 1999);

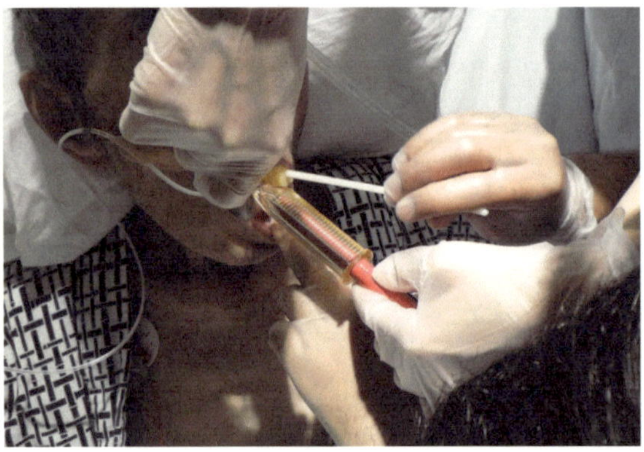

Fig. 9. Oral care by dental hygienists

neck muscle exercises to improve swallowing activity (Shaker et al., 1997); and the monitoring of food temperature, which affects the swallowing reflex; i.e., temperatures above and below body temperature accelerate the triggering of the swallowing reflex (Watando et al., 2004).

The final outcome in our series was poor. Only one third of the patients were able to live independently in their homes. One of the reasons for this was that their main caregiver was often also old. This dearth of care potential led to long-term care in hospitals (Ohsawa et al., 2008).

7. Factors influencing outcomes

In our series, two elderly women (78 and 80 years old) died during hospitalization. Both of them had TAA complicated with aspiration pneumonia. One of them experienced intubation, and the other underwent mini-tracheostomy. One of them had LRLN palsy, which was diagnosed postoperatively with a laryngoscope. Both of them had a long smoking history. They also had renal failure, and one of them was receiving haemodialysis, which meant that

they became sedentary and it was difficult for them to undergo rehabilitation therapy every day. Their poor general condition led to a delay in the start of rehabilitation. Only pulmonary rehabilitation and range of motion exercises were performed in the intensive care unit. They also suffered sacral decubitus due to deterioration of their general condition and long bed rest. In general, among elderly patients with vascular ischemic spinal cord injury, males were more independently mobile than females (Kay et al., 2010).
In our series, our previously reported cases and seven recently rehabilitated patients; i.e., a total of 19 patients, were analyzed. Two died in hospital, and another patient died 13 months after the operation. The American Spinal Injury Association (ASIA) (Table 11, Ditunno et al., 1994, Maynard et al., 1997) motor score at the beginning of the rehabilitation was 55.8 points, and the mean improvement was 7.9 points, giving a mean score of 64.0 points at discharge. The motor FIM at the beginning of rehabilitation was 31.4, and the mean improvement was 26.1 points, giving a mean score of 59.4 points at discharge (Table 12).

Key muscles

- C5: elbow flexors
- C6: wrist extensors
- C7 elbow extensors
- C8: Finger flexors to the middle finger
- T1: small finger abductors
- L2: Hip flexors
- L3: knee extensors
- L4: Ankle dorsiflexors
- L5: Long toe extensors
- S1: Ankle plantar flexors

Table 11. ASIA motor score (Marino et al., 1999; Maynard et al., 1997), numerical sum of motor grades of all key muscles as determined by motor testing

Six patients were referred to another hospital. The other three were transferred to a long-term care hospital such as a nursing home. Renal failure and LRLN palsy occurred in four and nine cases, respectively, before rehabilitation. In eight of the nine cases, LRLN palsy probably developed perioperatively. Postoperatively, seven patients suffered respiratory failure that was managed with intubation, tracheostomy, or mini-tracheostomy. Sacral decubitus developed in nine patients and in other regions in three. Most of them had slightly reddish skin on the sacral region without ulcer formation. As shown in Table 12, we compared the gain in motor FIM during hospitalization and the rate of this gain with those in the reported databases. The independent patients at home had a mean gain in motor FIM of 37 points, and their rate of improvement was also very high ((gain of mFIM/LOS); 0.30 (0.17)) compared with those of the other patients, who had comparatively good outcomes for non-traumatic SCI patients (Kay et al., 2010; New & Epi, 2005; Yokoyama et al., 2006). Our series were obtained from an acute care hospital, and selected patients were transferred to tertiary rehabilitation centers. Most traumatic SCI patients will be in a similar situation. Hagen & Kennedy reported that elderly patients with traumatic SCI also displayed significant improvement during rehabilitation (Hagen et al., 2005; Kennedy et al., 2003).

	Our case, mean (SD)	Japanese database	USA database
Pneumonia	5/19	3.7%	15.2%
Aspiration	5/19	n	1.5%
mASIA at start	55.8 (17.1)	48.5 (28.6)*	50-74**
mASIA at discharge	64.0 (19.3)	61.4 (29.5)*	51-81**
Gain of mASIA	7.9 (9.3)	12.9 (14.5)*	2.6-21.0**
mFIM at start	31.4 (16.7)	37.6	33.3
mFIM at discharge	59.4 (26.7)	71	72.7
Gain of mFIM	26.1 (14.5)	34.1	39.4
Gain/LOS	0.19 (0.14)	0.21	0.72

* paraplegia+tetraplegia, ** reported according to each Frankel grade (A-D)

Table 12. Comparison between the databases of thoraco-lumbar SCI (Ohsawa et al, 2008 with further cases added) mASIA: ASIA motor score, mFIM: motor FIM, LOS: length of stay, n: not mentioned,

8. Conclusions

In conclusion, thoracic aortic aneurysm surgery has improved in recent years, and better outcomes are now being achieved. However, when thoracic aortic aneurysm surgery is complicated with SCI, respiratory complications, or renal failure, it is life threatening. Such complications produce a vicious cycle, which worsens outcomes. This vicious cycle can be broken by intensive and comprehensive rehabilitation. Smoking ban before operation and pulmonary rehabilitation in perioperative period improve patients' cardiopulmonary conditions. Checking hoarseness and aspiration by auscultation before food intake under safe position (maintaining 30-degree head of the bed elevation with neck flexion) are mandatory. After suture removal, muscle exercise of the upper limb and reducing body weight are encouraged. Then, comprehensive spinal cord injury rehabilitation started. Above precautious rehabilitation plan drives them better condition than that of reported (Fig 10).

9. Abbreviations

AA: aortic aneurysm, ASIA: American spinal injury association, CFD: cerebrospinal fluid drainage, DAP: distal aortic perfusion, FEES: fiberoptic endoscopic examination of swallowing, FIM: functional independence measure, GER: gastroesophageal reflux, LOS: length of stay, LRLN: left recurrent laryngeal nerve, MEP: motor evoked potential, mFIM: motor FIM , RLN: recurrent laryngeal nerve, SC: spinal cord, SCI: spinal cord injury, SSEP: somatosensory evoked potential, TAA: thoracic aortic aneurysm,
TAAA: thoracoabdominal aortic aneurysm, TEVAR: thoracic endovascular aortic repair,
VFSS: videofluoroscopic swallowing study

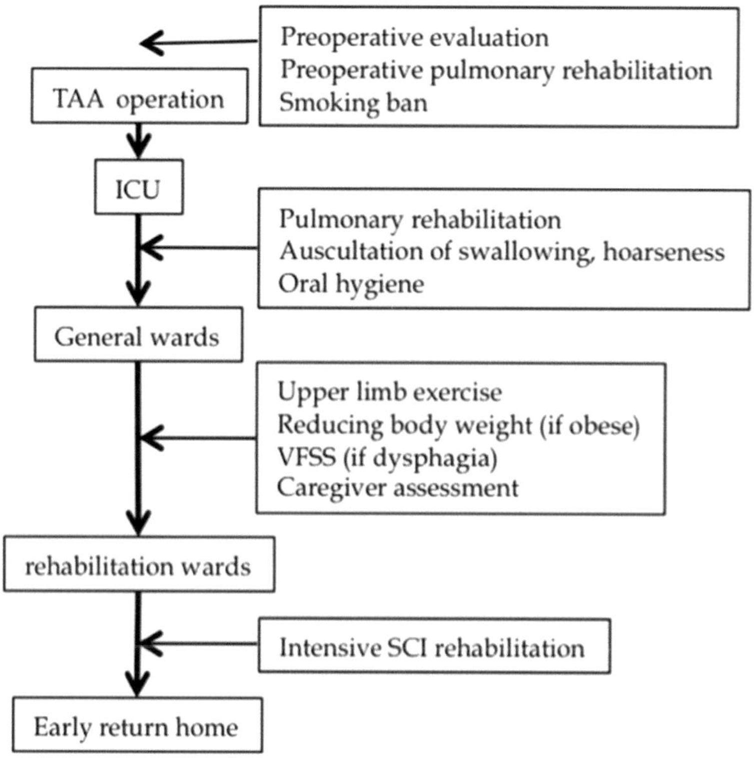

Fig. 10. Comprehensive rehabilitation for thoracic aortic aneurysm repair

10. References

Acher, CW. & Wynn, M. (2009). A modern theory of paraplegia in the treatment of aneurysms of the thoracoabdominal aorta: An analysis of technique specific observed/expected ratios for paralysis. *J Vasc Surg*, Vol. 49, No.5, (May 2009), pp. 1117-1124, ISSN 0741-5214

Acher, CW., Wynn, MM., Hoch, JR., Popic P., Archibald, J., & Turnipseed, WD. (1994). Combined use of cerebral spinal fluid drainage and naloxone reduces the risk of paraplegia in thoracoabdominal aneurysm repair. *J Vasc Surg*, Vol. 19, No. 2, (February 1994), pp. 236-248, ISSN 0741-5214

Acher, CW., Wynn, MM., Mell, MW., Tefera, G., & Hoch, JR. (2008). A quantitative assessment of the impact of intercostal artery reimplantation on paralysis risk in thoracoabdominal aortic aneurysm repair. *Ann Surg*, Vol. 248, No. 4, (October 2008), pp. 529-540, ISSN 0003-4932

Barish, CF. Wu, WC., & Castell DO. (1985). Respiratory complications of gastroesophageal reflux. *Arch Intern Med*, Vol. 145, (October 1985), pp. 1882-1888, ISSN 0003-9926

Bartlett, JG., Gorbach, SL., & Finegold, SM. (1974). The bacteriology of aspiration pneumonia. *Am J Med*, Vol. 56, (February 1974), pp. 202-207, ISSN 0002-9343

Bickerstaff, LK., Pairolero, PC., Hollier, LH., Melton, LJ., Van Peenen, HJ., Cherry, KJ., Joyce, JW., & Lie, JT (1982). Thoracic aortic aneurysms: A population-based study. *Surgery*, Vol. 92, No. 6, (December 1982), pp. 1103-1108, ISSN 0039-6060

Bicknell, CD., Riga, CV., & Wolfe, JHN. (2009). Prevention of paraplegia during thoracoabdominal aortic aneurysm repair. *Eur J Vasc Endovasc Surg*, Vol. 37, pp. 654-660, ISSN 1078-5884

Cambria, RP., Davison, JK., Zannetti, S., L'Italien, G., Brewster, DC., Gertler, JP., Moncure, AC., LaMuraglia, GM., & Abbott, WM. (1997). Clinical experience with epidural cooling for spinal cord protection during thoracic and thoracoabdominal aneurysm repair. *J Vasc Surg*, Vol. 25, No.2, (February 1997), pp. 234-243, ISSN 0741-5214

Charlifue, S., Jha, A., & Lammertse, D. (2010). Aging with spinal cord injury. *Phys Med Rehabil Clin N Am*, Vol. 21, pp. 383-402, ISSN 1047-9651

Chen, D., Apple Jr., DF., Hudson, LM., & Bode, R. (1999). Medical complications during acute rehabilitation following spinal cord injury- Current experience of the model systems. *Arch Phys Med Rehabil*, Vol. 80, (November 1999), pp. 1397-1401, ISSN 0003-9993

Clouse, WD., Hallett Jr., JW., Schaff, HV., Gayari, MM., Ilstrup, DM., & Melton III, LJ. (1998). Improved prognosis of thoracic aortic aneurysms. A population-based study. *J Am Med Assoc*, Vol. 280, No. 22, (December 1998), pp. 1926-1929, ISSN 0002-9955

Coselli, JS., & LeMaire, SA. (1999). Surgical techniques. Thoracoabdominal aorta. *Cardol Clin N Am*, Vol. 17, No. 4, (November 1999), pp. 751-765, ISSN 0733-8651

Coselli, JS., LeMaire, SA., Koeksoy, C., Schmittling, ZC., & Curling, PE. (2002). Cerebrospinal fluid drainage reduces paraplegia after thoracoabdominal aortic aneurysm repair: Results of a randomized clinical trial. *J Vasc Surg*, Vol. 35, No.4, (April 2002), pp. 631-639, ISSN 0741-5214

Coselli, JS., LeMaire, SA., Miller III, CC., Schmittling, ZC., Koeksoy, C., Pagan, J., & Curling, PE. (2000). Mortality and paraplegia after thoracoabdominal aortic aneurysm repair: A risk factor analysis. Ann Thorac Surg, Vol. 69, pp. 409-414, ISSN 0003-4975

Crawford, ES., Fenstermacher, JM., Richardson, W., & Sandiford, F. (1970). Reappraisal of adjuncts to avoid ischemia in the treatment of thoracic aortic aneurysms. *Surgery*, Vol.67, No. 1, (January 1970), pp182-196, ISSN 0039-6060

Crawford, ES., Mizrahi, EM., Hess, KR., Coselli, JS., Safi, HJ., & Patel, VM. (1988). The impact of distal aortic perfusion and somatosensory evoked potential monitoring on prevention of paraplegia after aortic aneurysm operation. J Thorac Cardiovasc Surg, Vol. 95, No. 3, (March 1988), pp. 357-367, ISSN 0025-5223

Dake, MD., Miller, DC., Mitchell, RS., Semba, CP., Moore, KA., & Sakai, T. (1998). The "first generation" of endovascular stent-grafts for patients with aneurysms of the descending thoracic aorta. *J Thorac Cardiovasc Surg*, Vol. 116, No. 5, (November 1998), pp. 689-704, ISSN 0022-5223

Davison, JK., Cambria, RP., Vierra, DJ., Columbia, MA., & Koustas, G. (1994). Epidural cooling for regional spinal cord hypothermia during thoracoabdominal aneurysm repair. *J Vasc Surg*, Vol. 20, No. 2, (August 1994), pp. 304-310, ISSN 0741-5214

De Bakey, ME., McCollum, CH., & Graham, JM. (1978). Surgical treatment of aneurysms of the descending thoracic aorta. Long- term results in 500 patients. *J Cardiovas Surg*, Vol. 19, pp. 571-576, ISSN 0021-9509

De Haan, P., Kalkman, CJ., De Mol, BA., Ubags, LH., Veldman, DJ., & Jacobs, MJHM. (1997). Efficacy of transcraninal motor-evoked myogenic potentials to detect spinal cord ischemia during operations for thoracoabdominal aneurysms. *J Thorac Cardiovasc Surg*, Vol. 113, No.1, (January 1997), pp. 87-101, ISSN 0022-5223

DeVivo, MJ., Krause, JS., & Lammertse, DP. (1999). Recent trends in mortality and causes of death among persons with spinal cord injury. *Arch Phys Med Rehabil*, Vol. 80, (November 1999), pp. 1411-1419, ISSN 0003-9993

DeVivo, MJ., Kartus, PL., Rutt, RD., Stover, SL., & Fine, PR. (1990). The influence of age at time of spinal cord injury on rehabilitation outcome. *Arch Neurol*, Vol. 47, (June 1990), pp. 687-691, ISSN 0003-9942

Ditunno, Jr., JF., Young, W., Donovan, WH., & Creasey, G. (1994). The international standards booklet for neurological and functional classification of spinal cord injury. *Paraplegia*, Vol. 32, pp. 70-80, ISSN 0031-1758

Eastwood, EA., Hagglund, KJ., Ragnarsson, KT., Gordon, WA., & Marino, RJ. (1999). Medical rehabilitation length of stay and outcomes for persons with traumatic spinal cord injury - 1990-1997. *Arch Phys Med Rehabil*, Vol. 80, (November 1999), pp. 1457-1463, ISSN 0003-9993

Elefteriades, JA. (2002). Natural history of thoracic aortic aneurysms: Indications for surgery, and surgical versus nonsurgical risks. *Ann Thoracic Surg*, Vol. 74, pp. S1877-S1880, ISSN 0003-4975

Estrera, AL., Sheinbaum, R., Miller, CC., Azizzadeh, Ali., Walkes, J-C., Lee, T-Y., Kaiser, L., & Safi, HJ. (2009). Cerebrospinal fluid drainage during thoracic aortic repair: Safety and current management. *Ann Thorac Surg*, Vol. 88, pp. 9-15, ISSN 0003-4975

Etz, CD., Halstead, JC., Spielvogel, D., Shahani, R., Lazala, R., Homann, TM., Weisz, DJ., Plestis, K., & Griepp, RB. (2006). Thoracic and thoracoabdominal aneurysm repair: Is reimplantation of spinal cord arteries a waste of time? *Ann Thorac Surg*, Vol. 82, pp. 1670-1678, ISSN 0003-4975

Fedorow, CA., Moon, MC., Mutch, WAC., & Grocott, HP. (2010). Lumber cerebrospinal fluid drainage for thoracoabdominal aortic surgery: Rationale and practical considerations for management. *Anesth Analg*, Vol. 111, No.1, (July 2010), pp. 46-58, ISSN 0003-2999

Feinberg, MJ., Knebl, J., Tully, J., & Segall, L. (1990). Aspiration and the elderly. *Dysphagia*, Vol. 5, pp. 61-71, ISSN 0179-051X

Grace, RR., & Mattox, KL. (1977). Anterior spinal artery syndrome following abdominal aortic aneurysmectomy. Case report and review of the literature. *Arch Surg*, Vol. 112, (July 1977), pp. 813-815, ISSN 0004-0010

Granger, CV., Hamilton, BB,, Keith, RA., Zielezny, M., & Sherwin, FS. (1986). Advances in functional assessment for medical rehabilitation. *Top Geriatr Rehabil*, Vol. 1, No.3, (April 1986), pp. 59-74, ISSN 0882-7524

Graves, DE., Frankiewicz, RG., & Carter, RE. (1999). Gain in functional ability during medical rehabilitation as related to rehabilitation process indices and neurologic measures. *Arch Phys Med Rehabil*, Vol. 80, (November 1999), pp. 1464-1470, ISSN 0003-9993

Greenberg, RK., Lu, Q., Roselli, EE., Svensson, LG., Moon, MC., Hernandez, AV., Dowdall, J., Cury M., Francis, C., Pfaff, K., Clair, DG., Quriel, K., & Lytle, BW. (2008). Contemporary analysis of descending thoracic and thoracoabdominal aneurysm repair. A comparison of endovascular and open techniques. *Circulation*, Vol. 118, (August 2008), pp. 808-817, ISSN 0009-7322

Griepp, RB., Ergin, MA., Galla, JD., Lansman, S., Khan N., Quintana, C., McCollough, J., & Bodian, C. (1996). Looking for the artery of Adamkiewicz: A quest to minimize paraplegia after operations for aneurysms of the descending thoracic and thoracoabdominal aorta. *J Thorac Cardiovasc Surg*, Vol. 112, No. 5, (November 1996), pp. 1202-1215, ISSN 0022-5223

Griepp, RB., & Griepp EB. (2007). Spinal cord perfusion and protection during descending thoracic and thoracoabdominal aortic surgery: The collateral network concept. *Ann Thorac Surg*, Vol. 83, No. 3, (March 2007), pp. S865-S869, ISSN 0003-4975

Hagen, EM., Aarli, JA., & Gronning, M. (2005). The clinical significance of spinal cord injuries in patients older than 60 years of age. *Acta Neurol Scand*, Vol. 112, pp. 42-47, ISSN 1600-0404

Hall, KM., Cohen, ME., Wright, J., Call, M., & Werner, P. (1999). Characteristics of the functional independence measure in traumatic spinal cord injury. *Arch Phys Med Rehabil*, Vol.80, (November 1999), pp. 1471-1476, ISSN 0003-9993

Heitmiller, RF., Tseng, E., & Jones, B. (2000). Prevalence of aspiration and laryngeal penetration in patients with unilateral vocal fold motion impairment. *Dysphagia*, Vol. 15, pp. 181-187, ISSN 0179-051

Honda, T & Mizojiri, G. (May 25, 2000). *Handbook of eating and swallowing disorder for physicians and dentists*. Ishiyakusyuppan, ISBN 4-263-21516-8, Tokyo

Ishimoto, S-I., Ito, K., Toyama, M., Kawase, I., Kondo, K., Oshima, K., & Niimi, S. (2002). Vocal cord paralysis after surgery for thoracic aortic aneurysm. *Chest*, Vol. 121, No. 6, (June 2002), pp. 1911-1915, ISSN 0012-3692

Jacobs, MJ., Mess, W., Mochtar, B., Nijenhuis, RJ., Van Eps, RGS., & Schurink, GWH. (2006). The value of motor evoked potentials in reducing paraplegia during thoracoabdominal aneurysm repair. *J Vasc Surg*, Vol. 43, No.2, (February 2006), pp. 239-246, ISSN 0741-5214

Johanson, WG., & Harris, GD. (1980). Aspiration pneumonia, anaerobic infections, and lung abscess. *Med Clin North Am*, Vol. 64, No.3, (May 1980), pp. 385-394, ISSN 0025-7125

Johansson, G., Markstroem, U., & Swedenborg, J. (1995). Ruptured thoracic aortic aneurysms: A study of incidence and mortality rates. *J Vasc Surg*, Vol. 21, No.6, (June 1995), pp. 985-988, ISSN 0741-5214

Kakinohana, M., Marsala, M., Carter, C., & Davison, JK. (2003). Neuraxial morphine may trigger transient motor dysfunction after a noninjurious interval of spinal cord ischemia. A clinical and experimental study. *Anesthesiology*, Vol. 98, No. 4, (April 2003), pp. 862-870, ISSN 0003-3022

Katsumata, U., Sekizawa, K., Ebihara, T., & Sasaki, H. (1995). Aging effects on cough reflex. *Chest* , Vol. 107, No. 1, (January 1995), pp.290-291, ISSN 0012-3692

Kay, E., Deutsch, A., Chen, D., Semik, P., & Rowles, D. (2010). Effects of gender on inpatient rehabilitation outcomes in the elderly with incomplete paraplegia from nontraumatic spinal cord injury. *J Spinal Cord Med*, Vol. 33, No. 4, (October 2010), pp. 379-386, ISSN 1079-0268

Kawaharada, N., Morishita, K., Hyodoh, H., Fujisawa, Y., Fukada, J., Hachiro, Y., Kurimoto, Y., & Abe, T. (2004). Magnetic resonance angiographic localization of the artery of Adamkiewicz for spinal cord blood supply. *Ann Thorac Surg*, Vol. 78, pp. 846-851, ISSN 0003-4975

Kennedy, P., Evans, MJ., Berry, C., & Mullin, J. (2003) Comparative analysis of goal achievement during rehabilitation for older and younger adults with spinal cord injury. *Spinal Cord*, Vol. 41, No. 1, pp. 44-52, ISSN 1362-4393

Kieffer, E., Fukui, S., Chiras, J., Koskas, F., Bahnini, A., & Cormier, E. (2002). Spinal cord arteriography: A safe adjunct before descending thoracic or thoracoabdominal aortic aneurysmectomy. *J Vasc Surg*, Vol. 35, No.2, (Feburary 2002) pp. 262-268, ISSN 0741-5214

Kikuchi, R., Watabe, N., Konno T., Mishina, N., Sekizawa, K., & Sasaki, H. (1994). High incidence of silent aspiration in elderly patients with community-acquired pneumonia. *Am J Respir Crit Care Med*, Vol. 150, pp. 251-253, ISSN 1073-449X

Kiwerski, JE. (1992). Injuries to the spinal cord in elderly patients. *Injury*, Vol. 23, No. 6, pp. 397-400, ISSN 0020-1383

Langmore, SE. (2003). Evaluation of oropharyngeal dysphagia: which diagnostic tool is superior? *Curr Opin Otolaryngol Head Neck Surg*, Vol. 11, pp. 485-489, ISSN 1068-9508

Langmore, SE., Terpenning, MS., Schork, A., Chen, Y., Murry JT., Lopatin, D., & Loesche, WJ. (1998). Predictors of aspiration pneumonia: How important is dysphagia? *Dysphagia*, Vol. 13, pp. 69-81, ISSN 0179-051X

Leder, SB., & Ross, DA. (2005). Incidence of vocal fold immobility in patients with dysphagia. *Dysphagia*, Vol. 20, pp. 163-167, ISSN 0179-051X

Marino, RJ., Ditunno Jr., JF., Donovan, WH., & Maynard Jr., F. (1999). Neurologic recovery after traumatic spinal cord injury: Data from the model spinal cord injury systems. *Arch Phys Med Rehabil*, Vol. 80, (November 1999), pp. 1391-1396, ISSN 0003-9993

Matsuda, H., Fukuda, T., Iritani, O., Nakazawa, T., Tanaka, H., Sasaki, H., Minatoya, K., & Ogino, H. (2010). Spinal cord injury is not negligible after TEVAR for lower descending aorta. Eur J Vasc Endovasc Surg, Vol. 39, pp. 179-186, ISSN 1078-5884

Maynard, FM., Bracken, MB., Creasey, G., Ditunno, Jr., JF., Donovan, WH., Ducker, TB., Garber, SL., Marino, RJ., Stover, SL., Tator, CH., Waters, RL., Wilberger, JE., & Young W. (1997). International standards for neurological and functional classification of spinal cord injury. *Spinal Cord*, Vol. 35, pp. 266-274, ISSN 1362-4393

Messe, SR., Bavaria JE., Mullen, M., Cheung, AT., Davis, R., Augoustides, JG., Gutsche, J., Woo, EY., Szeto, WY., Pochettino, A., Woo, YJ., Kasner, SE., & McGarvey, M. (2008). Neurologic outcomes from high risk descending thoracic and thoracoabdominal aortic operations in the era of endovascular repair. *Neurocrit Care*, Vol. 9, pp. 344-351, ISSN 1541-6933

Miller III, CC., Porat, EE., Estrera, AL., Vinnerkvist, AN., Huynh, TTT., & Safi, HJ. (2004). Number needed to treat: Analyzing of the effectiveness of thoracoabdominal aortic repair. *Eur J Vasc Endvasc Surg*, Vol. 28, (August 2004), pp. 154-157, ISSN 1078-5884

Money, SR., Rice, K., Crockett, D., Becker, M., Abdoh, A., Wisselink, W., Kazmier, F., & Hollier, L. (1994). Risk of respiratory failure after repair of thoracoabdominal aortic aneurysms. *Am J Surg*, Vol 168, (August 1994), pp. 152-155, ISSN 0002-9610

Nakamura, S., Kakinohana, M., Sugahara, K., Kinjo, S., & Miyata, Y. (2004). Intrathecal morphine, but not buprenorphine or pentazocine, can induce spastic paraparesis after a noninjurious interval of spinal cord ischemia in the rat. *Anesth Analg*, Vol. 99, pp.1528-1531, ISSN 0003-2999

Nakazawa, H., Sekizawa, K., Ujiie, Y., Sasaki, H., & Takishima, T. (1993). Risk of aspiration pneumonia in the elderly. *Chest*, Vo. 103, No. 5, (May 1993), pp. 1636-1637, ISSN 0012-3692

New, PW., & Epi, MC. (2005). Functional outcomes and disability after nontraumatic spinal cord injury rehabilitation: Results from a retrospective study. *Arch Phys Med Rehabil*, Vol. 86, (February 2005), pp. 250-261, ISSN 0003-9993

Ohsawa, S., Tamaki, M., & Hirabayashi, S. (2008). Medical rehabilitation of the patients with spinal cord injury caused by aortic aneurysm and its operation. *Spinal Cord*, Vol. 46, pp. 150-153, ISSN1362-4393

Olsson, C., Thelin S., Stahle, E., Ekbom, A., & Granath, F. (2006). Thoracic aortic aneurysm and dissection. Increasing prevalence and improved outcomes reported in a nationwide population-based study of more than 14000 cases from 1987 to 2002. *Circulation*, Vol. 114, (December 2006), pp. 2611-2618, ISSN 0009-7322

Ortner, N. (1897). Recurrenslaehmung bei Mitralstenose. *Wien Klin Wochenschr*, Vol. 33, pp. 753-755, ISSN 0043-5325

Ottenbacher, KJ., Hsu, Y., Granger, CV., & Fiedler, RC. (1996). The reliability of the functional independence measure: A quantitative review. *Arch Phys Med Rehabil*, Vol. 77, (December 1996), pp. 1226-1232, ISSN 0003-9993

Perie, S., Laccourreye, O., Bou-Malhab, F., & Brasnu, D. (1998). Aspiration in unilateral recurrent laryngeal nerve paralysis after surgery. *Am J Otolaryngol*, Vol. 19, No.1, (January-February 1998), pp. 18-23, ISSN 0196-0709

Pontoppidan, H. & Beecher, HK. (1960). Progressive loss of protective reflexes in the airway with the advance of age. *J Am Med Assoc*, Vol. 174, No. 18, (December 1960), pp. 2209-2213, ISSN 0002-9955

Rectenwald, JE., Huber, TS., Martin, TD., Ozaki, K., Devidas, M., Welborn, MB., & Seeger, JM. (2002). Functional outcome after thoracoabdominal aortic aneurysm repair. *J Vasc Surg*, Vol.35, No. 4, (April 2002), pp. 640-647, ISSN 0741-5214

Robbins, J., Hamilton, JW., Lof, GL., & Kempster, GB. (1992). Oropharyngeal swallowing in normal adults of different ages. *Gastroenterology*, Vol. 103, No. 3, (September 1992), pp. 823-829, ISSN 0016-5085

Safi, HJ., Miller III, CC., Huynh, TTT., Estrera, AL., Porat, EE,, Winnerkvist, AN., Allen, BS., Hassoun, HT., & Moore, FA. (2003). Distal aortic perfusion and cerebrospinal fluid drainage for thoracoabdominal and descending thoracic aortic repair. Ten years of organ protection. *Ann Surg*, Vol. 238, No. 3, (September 2003), pp. 372-381, ISSN 0003-4932

Sekizawa, K., Ujiie, Y., Itabashi, S., Sasaki, H., & Takishima, T. (1990). Lack of cough reflex in aspiration pneumonia. *Lancet*, Vol. 335, (May 1990), pp. 1228-1229, ISSN 0140-6736

Shaker, R., Kern, M., Bardan, E., Taylor, A., Stewart, ET., Hoffmann, RG., Arndorfer, RC., Hofmann, C., & Bonnevier, J. (1997). Augmentation of deglutitive upper esophageal sphincter opening in the elderly by exercise. *Am J Phsiol*, Vol. 272, pp. G1518-G1522, ISSN 0002-9513

Shiiya, N., Wakasa, S., Matsui, K., Sugiki, T., Shingu, Y., Yamakawa, T., & Matsui, Y. (2009). Anatomical pattern of feeding artery and mechanism of intraoperative spinal cord ischemia. *Ann Thorac Surg*, Vol. 88, pp768-772, ISSN 0003-4975

Sinha ,AC., & Cheung, AT. (2010). Spinal cord protection and thoracic aortic surgery. *Curr Opin Anaesthesiol*, Vol. 23, pp. 95-102, ISSN 0952-7907

Sliwa, JA., & Maclean, IC. (1992). Ischemic myelopathy: A review of spinal vasculature and related clinical syndromes. *Arch Phys Med Rehabil*, Vol. 73, No.4, (April 1992), pp. 365-372, ISSN 0003-9993

Sloan, TB. (2008). Advancing the multidisciplinary approach to spinal cord injury risk reduction in thoracoabdominal aortic aneurysm repair. *Anesthesiology*, Vol.108, No.4, (April 2008), pp. 555-556, ISSN 0003-3022

Stoob, K., Alkadhi, H., Lachat, M., Wildermuth, S., & Pfammatter, T. (2004). Resolution of hoarseness after endovascular repair of thoracic aortic aneurysm: a case of Ortner's syndrome. *Ann Otol Rhinol Laryngol*, Vol. 113, pp. 43-45, ISSN 0003-4894

Sumida, M., Fujimoto, M., Tokuhiro, A., Tominaga, T., Magara, A., & Uchida, R. (2001a). Early rehabilitation effect for traumatic spinal cord injury. *Arch Phys Med Rehabil*, Vol. 82, (March 2001), pp. 391-395, ISSN 0003-9993

Sumida, M., Tokuhiro, A., Magara, A., Toyonaga, T., & Uchida, R. (Eds.) (November 1, 2001b). Clinical Outcome of Spinal Cord Injury. Ishiyaku Publishers, ISBN 4-263-21125-1, Tokyo

Svensson, LG., Crawford, ES., Hess, KR., Coselli, JS., & Safi, HJ. (1993). Experience with 1509 patients undergoing thoracoabdominal aortic operations. *J Vasc Surg*, Vol. 17, No. 2, (February 1993), pp. 357-370, ISSN 0741-5214

Svensson, LG., Hess, KR., Coselli, JS., Safi, HJ., & Crawford, ES. (1991). A prospective study of respiratory failure after high-risk surgery on the thoracoabdominal aorta. *J Vasc Surg*, Vol.14, No. 3, (September 1991), pp. 271-282, ISSN 0741-5214

Tabayashi, K. (2005). Spinal cord protection during thoracoabdominal aneurysm repair. *Surg Today*, Vol. 35, pp. 1-6, ISSN 0941-1291

Teixido, MT., & Leonetti, JP. (1990). Recurrent laryngeal nerve paralysis associated with thoracic aortic aneurysm. *Otolaryngol Head Neck Surg*, Vol. 102, No. 2, (February 1990), pp. 140-144, ISSN 0161-6439

Thirlwall, AS. (1997). Ortner's syndrome: A centenary review of unilateral recurrent laryngeal nerve palsy secondary to cardiothoracic disease. *J Laryngol Otol*, Vol. 111, (September 1997), pp. 869-871, ISSN 0022-2151

Toews, GB., Hansen, EJ., & Strieter, RM. (1990). Pulmonary host defenses and oropharyngeal pathogens. *Am J Med* , Vol. 88, No. Suppl 5A, (May 1990) pp. 20S-24S, ISSN 0002-9343

Watando, A., Ebihara, S., Ebihara, T., Okazaki, T., Takahashi, H., Asada, M., & Sasaki, H. (2004). Effect of temperature on swallowing reflex in elderly patients with aspiration pneumonia. *J Am Geriatr Soc*, Vol. 54, No. 12, (December 2004), pp. 2143-2144, ISSN 0002-8614

Woodson, GE., & Kendrick, B. (1989). Laryngeal paralysis as the presenting sign of aortic trauma. *Arch Otolaryngol Head Neck Surg*, Vol. 115, (September 1989), pp. 1100-1102, ISSN 0886-4470

Yamaya, M., Yanai, M., Ohrui, T., Arai, H., & Sakai, H. (2001). Interventions to prevent pneumonia among older adults. *J Am Geriatr Soc*, Vol. 49, No. 1, (January 2001), pp. 85-90, ISSN 0002-8614

Yokoyama, O., Sakuma, F., Itoh, R., & Sashika, H. (2006). Paraplegia after aortic aneurysm repair versus traumatic spinal cord injury: Functional outcome, complications, and therapy intensity of inpatient rehabilitation. *Arch Phys Med Rehabil*, Vol. 87, (September 2006), pp. 1189-1194, ISSN 0003-9993

Yoneyama, T., Yoshida, M., Matsui, T., Sasaki, H., & the Oral Care Working Group (1999). Oral care and pneumonia. *Lancet*, Vol.354, (August 1999), p. 515, ISSN 0140-6736

23

Relationships Between AAA and Cauda Equina Syndrome

Masood Rehman Moghul and Bassel El-Osta
North-West London Hospitals NHS Trust, UK

1. Introduction

Lower back pain is one of the most common clinical presentations in general practice, with a lifetime prevalence of around 70-80% [1,2]. A small proportion of these patients will be recommended for immediate further investigation, those that demonstrate: loss of sphincter control, progressive lower limb motor weakness, saddle anaesthesia or signs of bilateral nerve root involvement; all symptoms and signs of the surgical emergency Cauda Equina syndrome (CES) [3].

2. Vertebral column

The vertebral column consists of 33 [4] individual vertebrae: 7 cervical, 12 thoracic, 5 lumbar, 5 sacral and 4 (this can vary between 3 and 5 [5]) coccygeal bony vertebrae [4,5]; protecting the spinal cord (and nerves) that traverse between them [4,6]. The sacral and coccygeal vertebrae are normally fused in adults leaving 24 articulating vertebrae [4,5]. This is demonstrated in figure 1.

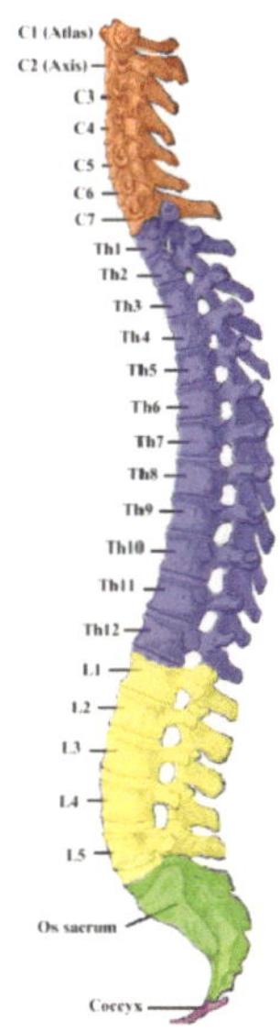

Fig. 1. Showing the vertebral column.

2.1 Vertebrae

The vertebrae are bound together via several ligaments and between each vertebrae, resting on the body of each, lie the strong intervertebral discs. Anteriorly and posteriorly are the anterior longitudinal and posterior longitudinal ligaments respectively [4,5,7]. In addition the posterior aspects of the vertebrae are attached to one other by the supraspinous and intraspinous ligaments, posterior facet joints and the ligamentum flavum. [5,7]. Figure 2 illustrates these.

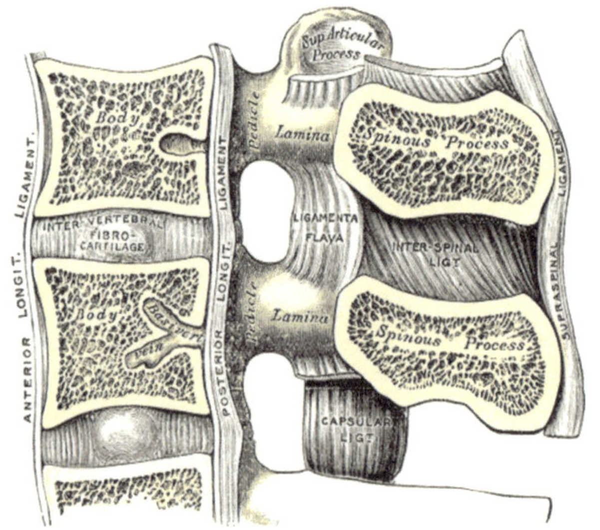

Fig. 2. Showing the ligaments of the vertebral column.

2.2 Spinal cord

The spinal cord is the extension of the medulla oblongata of the brainstem [4,6]. Measuring between 42cm and 45cm (from the foramen magnum to L2) it is the structure responsible for relaying information to the brain, and passing commands down [4,6,8]. It passes through the vertebral canal, which is made by the vertebral foraminae of consecutive vertebrae using the body, pedicles and vertebral arch [4], as well as the iv discs [5]. The canal continues in the fused sacrum through the sacral canal [5]. It has two enlargements due to innervations for upper and lower limbs, cervical and lumbar (upper and lower limbs respectively) [4,6]. Caudal to the lumbar enlargement the cord suddenly narrows to form a cone shaped termination: conus medullaris [6] at L1-L2 (although this may be as high as T12 or as low L3 [4]). Hence the spinal cord only occupies the superior two-thirds of the vertebral canal [4]. This is due to a slower growth rate of the cord compared with the vertebral column [4,6].

The cord itself is a cylindrical structure [6]. It is split into an 'H' shaped darker grey matter surrounded by the peripheral white matter [6,8]. The four projections of the grey matter (two dorsal and two ventral horns) are sites of attachment for peripheral nerves [6]. The dorsal horn contains sensory afferent fibres whilst the ventral horn contains efferent motor (skeletal muscle) fibres [6]. A lateral horn is also present at thoracic and upper lumbar levels, containing autonomic neurones [6]. The white matter is organised into a series of longitudinally running ascending and descending neuronal tracts [6]. This is demonstrated in figure 3.

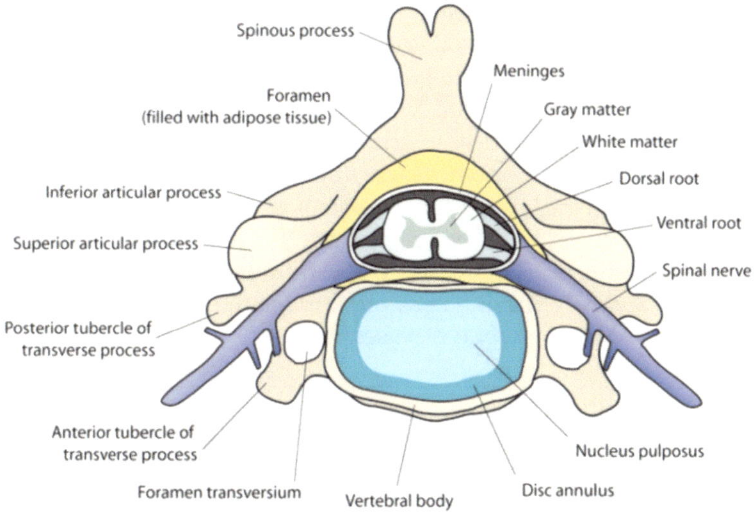

Fig. 3. Showing a cross-sectional view of a typical cervical vertebrae with the spinal cord.

2.3 Spinal nerves

The spinal cord connects to the periphery via 31 pairs of spinal nerves: 8 cervical, 12 thoracic, 5 lumbar, 5 sacral and a solitary coccygeal nerve [4,6]. Each nerve is formed by the uniting of ventral and dorsal nerve roots close to the cord [4,5]. The mixed spinal nerves pass within the intervertebral foraminae (formed by the joining of subsequent superior and inferior vertebral notches [4]) and immediately divide into dorsal and ventral rami [4,5,6]. The dorsal ramus (thinner and posterior) supplies the true muscles and skin of the back region [4,6]. The ventral (larger and anterior) ramus supplies skin and muscles of front of body and limbs [4,6], giving rise to the myotome and dermatome distribution patterns [6].

Due to the differing lengths of the cord and canal, below the cervical region successive spinal nerve roots follow a progressively longer course to reach their respective intervertebral foraminae, through which they must exit. This is most notable in the Cauda Equina [6]. The Cauda Equina contains the dorsal and ventral nerve roots of lumbar, sacral and coccygeal nerves [4,6]. Each level of the spinal cord is numbered according to the IV foraminae through which the dorsal and ventral roots exit the vertebral canal [4,8].

2.4 Meninges

As with the brain the spinal cord has 3 meningeal coverings. The innermost is the pia mater; a thin, delicate, vascular membrane, covering the cord, nerve roots and cauda equina [4,6]. The arachnoid mater is a loose-fitting layer separated from the pia mater by the subarachnoid space containing cerebrospinal fluid [6]. The outermost covering, the dura mater, is tougher, fibrous sheath, continuous with its cranial counterpart [4,6]. The dura is kept away from the walls of the vertebral canal by adipose tissue and internal vertebral venous plexuses [4,6]. Even though the spinal cord terminates at L1-L2 the arachnoid and dural sheaths continue to S2, even forming meningeal sleeves that cover the nerve roots, which later become continuous with the epineurium sheathing the spinal nerve [4,6]. The filum terminale is a remnant of the embryological spinal cord made out of connective tissue [4,6]. It exits the dural sac at S2 and attaches to the coccyx, securing the cord [4,6].

2.5 Vasculature of the vertebral column

Most vertebrae are supplied by segmental vessels and spinal arteries, which distribute to the vertebrae, are branches of the (descending order): cervical, posterior intercostal, subcostal, lumbar, iliolumbar and sacral arteries [4]. These spinal arteries enter the IV foraminae and divide into terminal radicular arteries, which supply dorsal and ventral roots and their coverings (and also some of the superficial grey matter), although some radicular arteries continue as medullary segmental arteries that anastamose with spinal arteries [4].

As previously mentioned internal venous plexuses lie within the vertebral canal, and external plexuses lie outside [4]. They receive blood from large tortuous basivertebral veins lying within vertebral and IV veins (both passing through the IV foraminae), which receives veins from the spinal cord and vertebral plexuses [4].

2.6 Spinal cord vasculature

Arterial supply to the spinal cord is through three main longitudinal spinal arteries: one anterior and two posteriors [4,6]. The anterior spinal artery, formed by the joining of the vertebral arteries (at the level of the medulla), runs in the anteromedian fissure of the cord itself [4,6,9-12]. Sulcul (central) arteries from it enter the cord through the fissure [9], supplying two-thirds of the cross-sectional area of the spinal cord [4,10,11]. Blood flow through the anterior spinal artery is predominantly caudal (away from the head) [9]. The posterior arteries are branches of either the vertebral artery or posterior-inferior cerebellar arteries [4,6,11], with blood flow towards the head (rostral) [9]. They supply the posterior one thirds of the cord and receive collaterals from around 12 unpaired radicular arteries, whilst the anterior cerebral arteries have a less effective collateral circulation with 6-10 unpaired radicular brances [11,12].

The anterior longitudinal artery only supplies the superior cord, with the remainder being supplied by the segmental medullary and radicular arteries previously mentioned (4,6). These run along spinal nerve roots and in the case of segmental medullary arteries are located where the need for blood is greatest: at the cervical and lumbosacral cord enlargements (4,6). Deficiencies in the number of segmental arteries increase susceptibility to ischemia [10].

The great anterior segmental medullary artery of Adamkiewicz (GRA) forms from the inferior intercostal or upper lumbar arteries and enters the vertebral canal via one of their IV foraminae [4,6,9]. It arises around T9-L2 and is larger than other segmental arteries and has significance as it reinforces circulation to the inferior cord including the lumbosacral enlargements [4,11,12)].

Spinal veins follow similar paths as arteries but with 3 anterior and 3 posterior spinal veins [4,6]. They communicate with each other freely and are drained by up to 12 anterior and posterior radicular and medullary veins [4,6]. They also join internal venous plexuses in the extradural space, which communicate with the external plexuses and then the ascending lumbar, azygous and hemiazygous veins [4,6].

3. Spinal injury – Cauda equina

There are various types of spinal injury, however most remain out of the scope of this chapter. This chapter focuses particularly on two types: Cauda Equina syndrome and spinal cord ischaemia, also known as spinal stroke and in particular how they may share characteristics. Cord damage and compression can cause similar symptoms in any area of the cord however; CES is a particular syndrome when this happens in the inferior cord.

Cauda Equina syndrome is caused by injury to the lumbosacral nerve roots, contained within the Cauda Equina (figure 4) grossly causing pain, bladder and bowel disturbances as well as focal neurology in the lower limb [4,8]. Essentially any mechanism which can cause compression of the spinal nerve roots, thereby causing shear stresses as well as obstructing blood flow in the vasculature of the nerve roots can cause CES [13]. The most common is cause herniation of the nucleus pulposus, 2% of which cause CES [14,15]. This is especially common in the lumbar spine where the lumbosacral enlargement means the spinal nerves are increasing in size caudally, but the IV foraminae size decrease [4]. The 5th lumbar disc is the most common "slipped disc" causing trauma to the roots of the first sacral nerve [6].

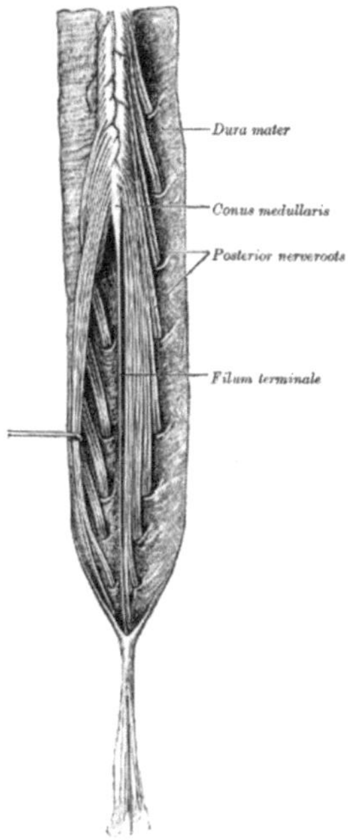

Fig. 4. Showing the cauda equina.

Other causes are: spinal cord stenosis, blunt or direct injury through the cauda equina, sacral fractures [16], hematomas, abscesses, lymphomas, solid tumors and other space-occupying lesions [11,14,15]. Rare causes include: ankylosing spondylitis, inferior vena cava thrombosis, sarcoid, and demyelinating lesions [14,15]. CES can occur as a complication of spinal anaesthesia but is rather rare [17]. The cauda equina is supplied by blood from the sacral arteries, which arise from the hypogastric artery [11].

Symptoms can vary depending on the size and location of the lesion. Above the vertebrae L1 (conus medullaris) damage can affect the cord itself or the roots, or both simultaneously however, below this level only the roots can be damaged [11]. Root damage causes lower motor neurone effects and sensory impairment in the affected root only, whilst segmental damage to the cord causes similar effects in the same segmental level but will also cause upper motor neurone effects and a sensory deficit below the level of the lesion [11]. This is due to interruption of the cord fibres. Root damage causes severe sharp, shooting, even burning pain radiating in the specific myotome and dermatome distribution of the root, exacerbated with movement [11]. Segmental damage causes continuous deep, aching pain,

which radiates into either one lower limb or one half of the body, and that is not affected by movement [11]. Hence upper cauda equina may cause root or segmental effects with late bladder involvement, whilst a lower cauda equina lesion causes root damage, with early bladder incontinence and saddle anaesthesia (S2-S5) [11].
History and examination can frequently yield key clues to the diagnosis. Spinal imaging is usually required to confirm diagnoses with MRI being the gold standard, CT scanning can illustrate protrusions, X-rays are of little benefit but can show loss of disc space or collapse [11].

4. Spinal cord infarction ("spinal stroke")

Spinal cord infarction is a stroke that occurs within the spinal cord or the arteries that supply it, usually caused by atherosclerosis of the major arteries to the spinal cord [18-20]. It is rare compared to cerebral stroke [10,14,21], accounting for approximately 1-2% of all strokes [22,23]. Spinal stroke can be categorised into two types: local interference with the blood supply (trauma, embolism, aortic surgery, aortic dissection etc.), and generalised hypoxia/hypoperfusion (e.g. cardiac arrest) where often the brain is impacted as well but careful examination can show the spinal cord is also affected [10,14,19]. Spinal cord ischaemia is a serious neurological condition and causes neuronal death, functional neurological loss and paraplegia in up to 33% of patients affected [19]. Thus prompt diagnosis and treatment may significantly alter outcomes. Often there is no relevant past medical history, or signs of inflammation [14], although vascular risk factors are usually present, less than 50% of spinal strokes have a definite cause [24].
The mid-thoracic cord around T4-T8 is known as the ischaemic "watershed region" and because of fewer radicular arteries and narrowing of the anterior spinal artery in this area, was thought to be particularly sensitive to hypoperfusion [11,22]. However in terms of spinal stroke, this traditional view has recently come under scrutiny [12,25] and as seen in post-mortem studies conducted by Duggal et al. 66 patients which had ischaemic myelopathy (secondary to cardiac arrest or severe systemic hypotension) showed 95.5% had involvement of the lumbosacral cord, whilst the thoracic cord was only affected in 7.6% of cases [26)]. Hence the lumbosacral cord which, is mainly supplied by the singular artery of Adamkiewicz, is the most sensitive to hypoperfusion; possibly due to its greater metabolic demands (lumbosacral enlargement) [22,26]. A saddle embolus can cause occlusion of the GRA causing distal cord ischaemia [27]. The cauda equina is mainly supplied by lateral and medial sacral arteries, which arise from the internal iliac artery [27].
Spinal cord infarction presents with sudden onset of severe pain, radiating down the legs (radicular) [24] and progressive sensori-motor deficits in the initial stages. In lumbosacral involvement there may be a rapidly progressive bilateral flaccid paresis initially, with loss of tendon reflexes, possibly an absent plantar response and urinary retention [10,11,14,22,24]. Bowel dysfunction can also develop [19]. The pain may be throbbing or burning in nature and disappear after 2 to 3 days [24]. A sensory level below the infarction is usually present however passive movement may be retained if the posterior circulation is preserved [10,11], with gross rather than fine sensation more affected [14]. As it happens the anterior circulation is more often affected [14], with 88% of infarcts in the central territory of the anterior spinal artery [24]. If the infarction is established it is irreversible and spastic paraplegia, spastic bladder and hyper-reflexia may develop [10,11]. Cervical infarction can cause bilateral paresis in the upper limb [14]. Saddle anaesthesia may also be present [24].

Investigations involve excluding other causes, and later confirmation of the ischaemia with T2 weighted MRI imaging [11,14]. In the initial stages diffusion weighted MRI can detect spinal cord oedema, which is a precursor to infarction [14]. CSF protein can also be raised in some cases [9,11,24]. Treatment is usually symptomatic with a variable outcome [11].

5. Abdominal aortic aneurysms, spinal stroke and CES

As we can see, the symptoms and even aetiology of spinal stroke and CES may well overlap. Although history and examination can indicate other causes of CES, spinal stroke is moreover a diagnosis of exclusion, confirmed only by MRI[**] (fig 5,6) of the cord [11]. In the literature, there are not many cases to report relationship between the abdominal aortic aneurysm, spinal stroke and cauda equina syndrome.

P. Jauslin et al[32] in 1991 describe a case report of cauda equina syndrome associated with an Aorto-caval Fistula. In this particular case history and clinical examination demonstrated symptoms of: pain, tachycardia, peri-umbilical tenderness and a systolo-diastolic murmur. The patient was apyrexial and normotensive with femoral pulses present but cyanosis in both legs. Neurologically, there was perineal anaesthesia *("anesthesie en selle")* with markedly reduced anal sphincter tone, paresis and anaesthesia of the left leg in the L1 territory. Lumbar percussion was painless and deep sensitivity was intact.

Verneuil A et Al[33] in 1997 reported a case of persistent cauda equina syndrome following bilateral aortoiliac dissection as a complication of cardiac angiography. In this case report they describe the symptoms as follows: numbness in the gluteal region and the soles of the feet with urinary retention and faecal incontinence. In this case report, the MRI scan of the lumbar region was completely normal in the absence of anal tone in rectal manometry. Electromographic study (EMG) was consistent with cauda equine at level S1 & S2.

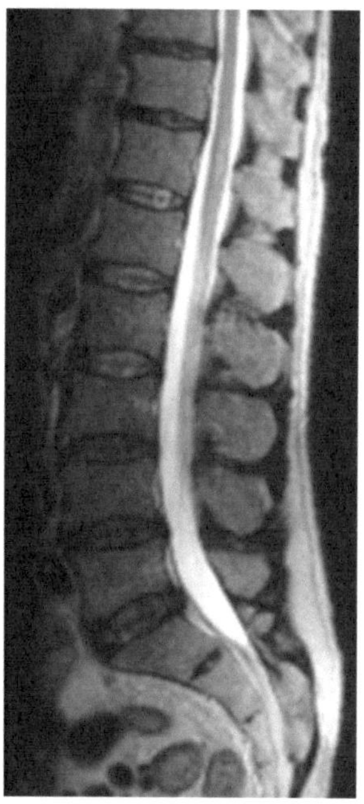

Fig. 5. Normal MRI scan

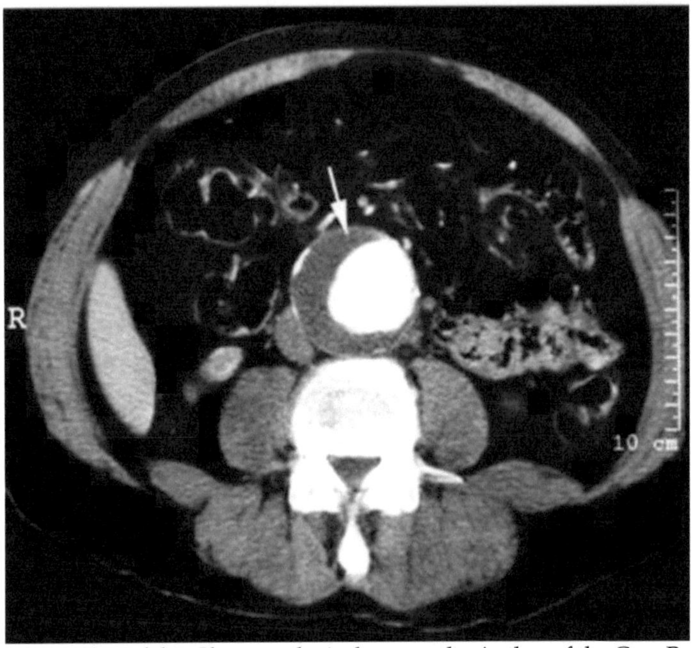

[**] Copyright for the Author of this Chapter who is the same the Author of the Case Report

Fig. 6. Abdominal Aortic Aneurysm

Patel NM et Al[34] published in 2002 a case report describing aortic dissection presenting as an acute cauda equina syndrome. In this case, the patient had acute, but transient, neck pain following a short coughing episode. The patient was able to walk to the restroom, but began to have severe low-back pain and lower extremity numbness and weakness that rapidly progressed to frank lower extremity paralysis. While en-route to the hospital, the patient became incontinent of both bowel and bladder. Upon admission to the emergency department, the patient complained of low-back pain, bilateral hip and thigh pain, and the inability to move or feel the lower extremities. The diagnosis of dissecting aortic aneurysm was made on the basis of a CT scan.

An unusual cause of spinal cord infarction, first documented in 2009 by EL-Osta et al. is from emboli thrown off an abdominal aortic aneurysm (AAA), with symptoms mimicking CES [28].

An aneurysm is a focal increase in diameter of the aorta of at least 50% in relation to the normal expected diameter [29]. Though by definition it can occur anywhere in the abdominal cavity the vast majority are infra-renal [30]. Thrombus frequently collects in the walls of an aneurysm and fragments can easily be thrown-off in the direction of a spinal artery, thus causing spinal cord ischaemia.

In this particular case the patient had sudden onset of lower back whilst heavy lifting. The pain radiated to his groins and there was a progressive bilateral weakness worse on one side. On examination profound neurological deficit was seen in both legs, with arreflexia, altered sensation and reduced bladder sensation and anal tone.

Although MRI showed lumbar disc protrusions there was no cord compression, hence spinal arteriography was performed. The final diagnosis was through a combination of clinical, diagnostic and radiological tests. CT had shown a 6.6 by 5.8cm infra-renal aneurysm[28].

As a result of reviewing the literature, it seems that patients who are admitted with query cauda equina syndrome and with unusual symptoms, should be investigated for other causes. It seems that the patient had more than simply weakness in the leg, paraesthesia and decreased anal tones. Some patients will present with abdominal discomfort and neck discomfort. Past medical history may be unremarkable with no trauma, but sudden onset cauda equina symptoms. In those particular cases, the responsible surgeon has to be extra cautious especially in orthopaedics.

In all four cases that have been reported in the literature, none of the patients recovered fully and in one case the patient deteriorated and died immediately. However, one patient did recover partially and the authors could not explain this. This implies that either way patients will have some gross disability and this may be as a result of delayed treatment.

6. Conclusion

Though spinal stroke is uncommon the high level of incidence and prevalence of AAAs may mean such cases may become more common, and hence should be an important thought in the surgeons mind when assessing CES. The key difference between atherosclerosis and thrombi in the spinal arteries will be the speed of onset of symptoms. With sudden CES-like symptoms affecting the patient with a significant spinal artery thrombus.

Initially after thorough history and examination (including abdominal examination for a pulsatile mass [31]) all other causes of CES must be ruled out, hence urgent CT/MRI of the spinal cord is appropriate.

On the other hand, when acute aortic dissection is suspected, an emergent diagnostic workup should be initiated with ultrasound techniques involving either a transthoracic or transesophageal approach or computerized tomography. Magnetic resonance imaging is also a diagnostic resource but may be difficult to obtain rapidly. Other vascular phenomena, such as aneurysms of the abdominal aorta or pelvic arteries, can also cause neurological symptoms, further pointing to the need for close attention to the vascular tree during orthopaedic examination[35].

Prompt diagnosis of such disorders may help in hastening treatment, which is particularly important in the context of neurological ischaemia, which can be irreversible. Thus this may help to improve outcomes for such patients in the future.

Figures

1. Gray H (1918). Lateral view of the vertebral column in: *Anatomy of the Human Body.* 20th U.S. edition. Philadelphia: Lea & Febiger. From www.wikipedia.com.
2. Gray H (1918). Median sagittal section of two lumbar vertebræ and their ligaments. *Anatomy of the Human Body.* 20th U.S. edition. Philadelphia: Lea & Febiger. From www.wikipedia.com.
3. Debivort user (2007). Annotated diagram of cervical vertebrae. From www.wikipedia.com.
4. Gray H (1918). Cauda equine in:*Anatomy of the Human Body.* 20th U.S. edition. Philadelphia: Lea & Febiger. From www.wikipedia.com.

5. El-Osta B, Ghoz A, Singh VK, Saed E, Abdunabi M (2009). Spontaneous spinal cord infarction secondary to embolism from an aortic aneurysm mimicking as cauda equina due to disc prolapse: a case report. *Cases J* **2**: 7460.

7. References

[1] Jensen MC, Brant-Zawadzki MN, Obuchowski N, Modic MT, Malkasian D, Ross JS (1994). Magnetic resonance imaging of the lumbar spine in people without back pain. *N Engl J Med* 14;331(2): 69-73.

[2] Deyo RA, Rainville J, Kent DL (1992). What can the history and physical examination tell us about low back pain? *JAMA* 12;268(6): 760-5.

[3] Referral Advice. A guide to appropriate referral from general to specialist services (2001). National Institute for Clinical Excellence.

[4] Moore KL & Dalley AF (1999). Clinically orientated anatomy. 4th edition. Lippincott Williams & Wilkins.

[5] Abrahams PH, Marks Jr SC, Hutchings RT (2003). McMinn's colour atlas of human anatomy. 5th edition. Mosby.

[6] Crossman AR & Neary D (2005). Neuroanatomy. An illustrated colour text. 3rd edition. Elselvier Churchill Livingstone.

[7] Holdsworth F (1970). Review article fractures, dislocations, and fracture-dislocations of the spine. *J Bone Joint Surg Am* 52: 1534-1551.

[8] Maynard FM Jr, Bracken MB, Creasey G, Ditunno JF Jr, Donovan WH, Ducker TB, Garber SL, Marino RJ, Stover SL, Tator CH, Waters RL, Wilberger JE, Young W (1997). International Standards for Neurological and Functional Classification of Spinal Cord Injury. American Spinal Injury Association. *Spinal Cord* 35(5): 266-74.

[9] Silver JR & Buxton PH (1974). Spinal stroke. *Brain* 97: 539-550.

[10] Editorial: spinal stroke (1974). *The Lancet* 30;2(7892): 1299-1300.

[11] Lindsay KW, Bone I (2004). Neurology and neurosurgery illustrated. Fourth edition. Churchill Livingstone.

[12] Cheshire WP, Santos CC, Massey EW, Howard JF Jr (1996). Spinal cord infarction: Etiology and outcome. *Neurology* 47:321-330.

[13] Olmarker K, Rydevik B, Holm S (1989). Edema formation in spinal nerve roots induced by experimental, graded compression. An experimental study on the pig cauda equina with special reference to differences in effects between rapid and slow onset of compression. *Spine* 14(6): 569-73.

[14] Küker W, Weller M, Klose U, Krapf H, Dichgans J, Nägele T (2004). Diffusion-weighted MRI of spinal cord infarction--High resolution imaging and time course of diffusion abnormality. *J Neurol* 251: 818-824

[15] Gitelman A, Hishmeh S, Morelli BN, Joseph SA Jr, Casden A, Kuflik P, Neuwirth M, Stephen M (2008). Cauda Equina Syndrome: A Comprehensive Review. *Am J Orthop* 37(11): 556-562.

[16] Bonnin JG (1945). Sacral fractures and injuries to the cauda equina. *J Bone Joint Surg Am* 27: 113-127.

[17] Auroy Y, Narchi P, Messiah A, Litt L, Rouvier B, Samii K (1997). Serious complications related to regional anesthesia: results of a prospective survey in France. *Anesthesiology* 87(3): 479-86.

[18] NINDS Spinal Cord Infarction Information Page. *National Institute of Neurological Disorders and Stroke.* http://www.ninds.nih.gov/disorders/spinal_infarction/spinal_infarction.htm#What_is

[19] Thurnher MM & Bammer R (2006). Diffusion-weighted MR imaging (DWI) in spinal cord ischemia. *Neuroradiology* 48: 795-801.

[20] Silver JR & Buxton PH (1974). Spinal stroke. *Brain* 97: 539-550.

[21] Börnke C, Schmid G, Szymanski S Schöls L (2002). Vertebral body infarction indicating midthoracic spinal stroke. *Spinal Cord* 40: 244-247.

[22] Rossi D, Goodwin D, Cruzzavala J (2008). Spinal cord infarction following coronary artery bypass grafting surgery. *W V Med J* 104(6): 24-25.

[23] Novy J, Carruzzo A, Maeder P, Bogousslavsky J (2006). Spinal cord ischemia. Clinical and Imaging Patterns, Pathogenesis, and Outcomes in 27 Patients. *Arch Neurol* 63:1113-1120.

[24] Masson C, Pruvo JP, Meder JF, Cordonnier C, Touzé E, de la Sayette V, Giroud M, Mas JL, Leys D (2004). Spinal cord infarction: clinical and magnetic resonance imaging findings and short term outcome. *J Neurol Neurosurg Psychiatry* 75: 1431-1435.

[25] Jellinger KA (1997) Spinal cord water- shed. *Neurology* 48:1474.

[26] Duggal N & Lach B (2002). Selective vulnerability of the lumbosacral spinal cord after cardiac arrest and hypotension. *Stroke* 33: 116-121.

[27] Chandrashekar G, Acharya PT, Rao J, Kumar RS, Nayak G (1994). Recovery from paraplegia following aortic saddle embolism. Case report. *Paraplegia* 32: 112-116.

[28] El-Osta B, Ghoz A, Singh VK, Saed E, Abdunabi M (2009). Spontaneous spinal cord infarction secondary to embolism from an aortic aneurysm mimicking as cauda equina due to disc prolapse: a case report. *Cases J* 2: 7460.

[29] Ernst CB (1993). Abdominal Aortic Aneurysm. *N Engl J Med* 328:1167-1172.

[30] Lederle FA, Johnson GR, Wilson SE, Chute EP, Littooy FN, Bandyk D, Krupski WC, Barone GW, Acher CW, Ballard DJ (1997). Prevalence and Associations of Abdominal Aortic Aneurysm Detected through Screening. *Ann Intern Med* 126: 441-449.

[31] Estes JE Jr (1950). Abdominal Aortic Aneurysm: A Study of One Hundred and Two Cases. *Circulation* 2: 258-264.

[32] Pierre A. Jauslin, Alex F. Müller, Peter Myers, Vladimir Velebit. Cauda equina syndrome associated with an Aorto-caval fistula. *Eur J Vasc Surg.* 1991 Aug;5(4):471-3.

[33] Verneuil A, Boeve BF, Fulgham JR, Johnson CM, Wright RS.Persistent cauda equina syndrome following bilateral aortoiliac dissection as a complication of cardiac angiography. Cathet Cardiovasc Diagn. 1997 Apr;40(4):377-9.

[34] Patel NM, Noel CR, Weiner BK. Aortic dissection presenting as an acute cauda equina syndrome : a case report. J Bone Joint Surg Am. 2002 Aug;84-A(8):1430-2

[35] Mignucci LA, Bell GR. Differential diagnosis of sciatica. *The spine*.4th ed; 1999. p 89-107.

24

Anesthetic Management of Aortic Aneurysm

Zsófia Verzár and Sándor Szabados
University of Pécs, Faculty of Medicine, Institute of Anesthesiology and Intensive Care and Heart Institute, Hungary

1. Introduction

Careful preoperative evaluation of patients undergoing vascular surgical intervention holds great significance since this group of patients has almost the highest percentage of accompanying diseases with poor outcome. It is well-known that vascular disease - irrespectively of its manifestation - is a generalized disorder, the majority of patients with vascular disease smoke and have chronic pulmonary disease, also suffers from diabetes and hypertension.

Hypertension and diabetes are often associated with coronary artery disease which determines the short and long-term survival of vascular procedures. Coronary artery disease is one of the most frequent cause of the perioperative mortality and morbidity (1-5%). Goldman et al. drew the attention to the frequency of cardiac complication of vascular operations as far back as 1977 and aimed to establish a multi-factorial score index. Based on detailed surveys which covered a large patient population the perioperative incidence of myocardial infarction among patient undergoing vascular surgical procedures is 2,1 - 8,0 %, whilst the mortality is 0,6 - 5,4 %. These examinations did not consider the type of operations - open or endovascular. Beside Goldman's classic risk index numerous task forces have established their own score system for the assessment of perioperative cardiac risk. All of these highlight the significance of the fact that after being aware of the clinical risk, consultation and mutual decision making of cardiologists, anesthetists and vascular surgeons in evaluation the long-term efficiency and risk ratio is essential. The most important weak point of all score system is the utilization of data derived from patients underwent elective operations. Kertai et al. developed a simplified risk index, which is suitable for the assessment of perioperative mortality of either acute or elective patients undergoing vascular surgical operations. The American College of Cardiologist and the American Heart Association has developed a guideline for the assessment of cardiovascular risk among patients with different diseases who are undergoing non-cardiac surgery. This guideline includes the risk assessment for the patient undergoing vascular surgery. Three categories of cardiac risk have been classified in the guideline, high, intermediate and low. High cardiac risk involves the history of acute coronary syndrome, congestive heart failure, significant arrhythmias and severe heart valve diseases. Among non-cardiac surgeries associated with higher cardiac risk, the acute operations, surgery on extremely old patient, operations of the aorta, prolonged operations, operations with excessive fluid or blood loss are considered to be high-risk while carotid endarterectomy should be considered within the intermediate-risk category. The most simple clinical determining factors of cardiac risk are the age, body weight, known diabetes, congestive heart failure, angina pectoris, history of myocardial infarction and previous coronary revascularization.

2. Preoperative evaluation

Preoperative examination should include the assessment of patient's functional capacity.

In the presence of lower extremity peripheral vascular disease performing exercise stress test may be difficult, thus pharmacological stress test or specific upper body exercise test should be carried out. Severely impaired functional capacity further increases the cardiac risk. Diseases of the aorta are frequently associated with severe coronary artery disease/ The incidence and severity of coronary artery disease are remarkably higher at the diseases of the aorta.

Preoperative examination should include the following:

Assessment of cardiac risk using different noninvasive examinations.Noninvasive stress testing are the following: dipyridamole myocardial perfusion scintigraphy, radionuclide ventriculography, Holter ECG monitoring, dobutamine stress echocardiography. Several authors (Eagle and collegues, Lee and coworkers) have examined the sensitivity and specificity of these methods, and have found the dobutamine stress echocardiography to be the most appropriate test to assess this group of patients. This examination not only assesses the left ventricular dysfunction but also provides other valuable information on the ground of echocardiography. However, choosing the most appropriate type of test is undoubtedly influenced by local availabilities and cost effectiveness, as well. After assessing the cardiac risk, what therapeutic options are available to decrease it? Beta-blocker therapy at high-risk vascular patient has been proven to improve not only the perioperative but also the long-term survival. Manago et al. carried out a study, which covered a large number of patients on the effect of bisoprolol and atenolol on mortality and cardiovascular morbidity after non-cardiac surgery. Treatment of hypertension: blood pressure fluctuation at high-risk vascular patients further increases the cardiac risk. Previous anti-hypertensive therapy should be broadened by administration of beta-blockers and the directly acting, alpha-2 agonist, clonidine. Perioperative ACE-inhibitors therapy may cause intraoperative hypotension, thus administration of them are not recommended.

What further medical therapy is available to decrease the perioperative risk?

Poldermans and colleagues evaluated the effectiveness of statin therapy, and they found that the perioperative statin therapy is associated with lower postoperative mortality.

Among the evaluated drug therapies, only the perioperative beta-blocker therapy has been found to significantly decrease the mortality. Increased risk of urgent surgery, especially in elderly patients, a longer surgery, excessive blood loss due to classify interventions in high-risk group.

Of smoking among patients with vascular risk factors are also important, so increased the perioperative complications between the role of pulmonary complications. Chronic obstructive pulmonary disease and chronic bronchitis, which often encounter. The kidney complications should be considered. First, the generalized vessel disease associated with hypertension, the renin-angiotensin system leads to damage, and the second associated with diabetes to nephropathy.

3. For each type of surgery

3.1 Aortic reconstruction – Lesions affecting the abdominal aorta

Growing the progressive aortic aneurysm rupture in the final output. In ruptured cases, the deaths of over 50% indicate a value and this value has not changed significantly over the past 40 years, developments in technology and the introduction of the endovascular technique does not like routine. If known and expanding aortic aneurysm is detected, and reconstruction is the surgical mortality rate is between 0.4 to 2.3%.
The technique of anesthesia during general anesthesia supplemented with epidural anesthesia benefits. We must work towards the introduction of anesthesia, the hemodynamic stability, to eliminate changes caused by intubation. Cross-clamping of the aorta, causes a sudden increse in the afterload. This growth, provoke arrhythmias and myocardial ischemia and left ventricular failure.

3.2 If a patient with acute surgery

Aortic aneurysm rupture due to a significant amount of blood in the abdomen, in any event be deemed hypovolemic. The abdominal muscle tone affects the capacity for intra-abdominal blood vessels, this relaxation is terminated and the formation of the blood pressure to fall, then a further decrease in blood pressure by opening the abdominal cavity should be expected. So close to the team's work comes to the fore the importance of continued vigilance isolation inhalating 100% oxygen, and then rapidly after induction opening the stomach , fast and high aortic cross clamp immediately save the patient's life. This type of surgery with surgical mortality of 50% is over, and over the past 4 decades has not changed.

3.3 Thoracic, thoraco-abdominal aneurysm

The anesthesia and surgical technique despite the development of the aorta during surgery thoraco-abdomial section of the complications and mortality has not changed significantly over the past 20 years. High-traffic, high number of sick institutions in 5-14% mortality rates reported.The paraplegia, paraparetikus complication rate of 50-40% of the shares are known. The percentage of complications depends on which section of the aorta, the exclusion should be carried out. The neurological complications after pulmonary complications to be expected. The monitoring of the thoracic aneurysm surgery should be extended. Close cooperation is required between the vascular surgeon and anesthesiologist, the surgical plan must be designed carefully crafted after, the every aspect of the monitoring and the distal aortic perfusion technique. Important aspects of the arteries of the spinal cord and the renal arteries perfusion ensure and the adequate oxygenation.
If the exclusion (cross clamping) is happening, a retrograde perfusion provides security for patients. In surgery for thoracic aortic aneurysm general anesthesia of suitable technology. The most important is protection of the spinal cord, 20-30 minute cross clamping time is safe for the patient . The hypothermia is one of the most suitable method for neuroprotection.

4. Perioperative management

The patient who has been diagnosed with significant coronary artery disease during preoperative examination and is a candidate for high-risk vascular surgery is the most

challenging. In case of acute operation beta-blockers remains the only therapeutic option, while in elective patients coronary revascularization should be carried out.
If the vascular procedure is not urgent, CABG operation is preferable over PCI. Elective non-cardiac surgery is not recommended within 6 weeks of coronary revascularization with PCI and stent implantation. In these cases careful risk assessment and effectiveness evaluation is necessary. Among patients with vascular disease tobacco smoking is a significant risk factor, thus perioperative pulmonary complications are frequent. Chronic obstructive pulmonary disease and chronic bronchitis are the most common ones. Perioperative blood gas analysis can be useful in assessing the risk. If the arterial carbon-dioxide partial pressure is higher than 45 mmHg, the risk for postoperative pulmonary complication is increased. If a tobacco smoking patient is presented at the preoperative evaluation meeting 2-4 weeks prior to the operation, it is reasonable to try to persuade the patient to cease the cigarette smoking, although, cessation will increase the amount of bronchial discharge. Smoking cessation 2-3 days prior to the surgery only results in decrease of the blood carboxi-hemoglobin level. In case of history of COPD and asthma preoperative glucocorticoid therapy (40 mg of prednisolon for two days) can decrease the risk of pulmonary complications. Treating the bronchial spasm, mobilizing the bronchial discharge and performing chest physiotheraphy would improve the patients' condition. One to two days prior to surgery preoperative pulmonary function test should be performed. Decreased FEV_1/FVC ratio suggests obstructive pulmonary disease. Performing regional anesthesia can lower the operative risk by eliminating the administration of the respiratory depressive opiates. On the other hand intraoperative blood CO_2 pressure monitoring is important, since the probability of developing hypercapnia is high, as well as the postoperative CO_2 level follow up, since the pain can lead to hypoventilation. Thus adequate pain management is strongly advisable.
Renal complications should also be taken into consideration, because of the pre-existing hypertension which is usually accompanied to generalized vascular disease and which can lead to impairment of the renin-angiotensin system. Preexisting diabetic nephropathy can also influence the development of postoperative renal complications.

5. Anaesthetic management

5.1 Infrarenal aortic aneurysm

The final outcome of aneurysms that present progressive growth is the rupture. In case of aneurysm rupture the mortality reaches the 50 %, this ratio has not changed over the last 40 years, despite the technical development and the introduction and routine application of endovascular techniques. Postoperative mortality rate of reconstruction of previously known and growing aortic aneurysm varies from 0,4 to 2,3 percents.
Preparation for the operation includes setting up the following:

1. two 14 G peripheral venous line
2. central venous line
3. arterial line
4. ECG monitoring from 5 different points
5. pulsoxymetry
6. urinary catheter
7. gastric tube
8. body temperature monitoring

9. noninvasive blood pressure measurement (from the opposite side than the direct arterial pressure line)
10. In case of impaired ejection fraction (less than 30 %) or suprarenal aortic cross-clamping, routine monitoring should be completed by the use of PICCO or Swan-Ganz catheter. In case of patients with significant diastolic dysfunction continuous intraoprative TEE (trans-esophageal echocardiography) monitoring can help to evaluate the need of fluid or catecholamine therapy.

The anticoagulation maintained with use of heparin 100 unit/kg, additional heparin necessary if the clamping time prolonged. Heparin can be reversed by protamine (4mg/kg over 15 minutes) it may lead to anaphylaxis, pulmonary hypertension and myocardial depression.

At aortic operations it is recommended to prepare 4 - 6 units of red blood cell transfusion, if possible, autologous transfusion should be performed. The use of cell saver (intraoperative cell salvage machine) improves the efficacy of transfusion therapy, if it is not available normovolaemic hemodilution is required. Hemodilution does not increase the oxygen deficit of the myocardium. During fluid therapy close monitoring the 24-hour diuresis and warming the fluid infusions increases patients' safety. (Myers G)

During anesthesia, general anesthesia can be completed by the benefits of application epidural anesthesia. The thoracic epidurals decrease the stress response to surgical procedure. During induction of anesthesia care must be taken to maintain the patient's hemodynamic stability and to eliminate the hyperdynamic response caused by the intubation. In case of aortic operation close attention must be paid to physiologic changes during aortic cross-clamping. In case of abdominal aortic operation the level of cross-clamping is infrarenal, i.e. aorta is fully cross-clamped under the origin of renal arteries. Changes in patient's condition appear rapidly, thus taking prompt actions are necessary. Aortic cross-clamping causes sudden increase in systemic vascular resistance, i.e. in afterload. This increase can provoke myocardial ischemia, arrhythmia and left ventricular failure. The more proximal the cross-clamping is, the more severe the myocardial adverse consequences are. Administration of vasodilators and activation the epidural anesthesia before the cross-clamping can stabilize the patient's condition and have beneficial effect. During aortic cross-clamping the lower extremities and certain parts of large intestines receive minimal blood flow through collateral circulation, but the renal circulation are also impaired. As a result of these circulatory changes inflammatory mediators are released by leukocytes, platelets and endothelial cells.

Cessation of aortic cross-clamping causes sudden decrease in afterload, which is on the one side caused by the discontinuation of mechanical obstruction but the accumulated vasodilator mediators by getting back into the systemic circulation plays also an important role in this. Beside vasodilation, metabolic acidosis and increased capillary permeability aggravates the condition. Providing adequate circulatory volume and maintaining stable blood pressure is necessary before releasing the aortic cross-clamp. Administering mannitol and pressor drugs can be helpful to fulfill this. Every efforts must be made in order to reach as short hypoperfusion time as possible.

In the postoperative period the close monitoring should be continued and care must be taken of the adequate pain management. If the infrarenal cross-clamp time exceeds 60 minutes, the subsequent pressure rise in the renal arteries may cause systemic hypertension in the early postoperative period, which is usually transient.

Patients require monitoring after abdominal aortic aneurysm operation. The postoperative pain management is important, the early extubation, and the enteral nutrition. Appropriate thrombotic profilaxis and postoperative gastrointestinal ulcus profilaxis, the use of antacids.

5.2 Emergency AAA surgery

In case of acute operation of ruptured aortic aneurysm, the patient should be considered hypovolaemic under all circumstances due to the excessive amount of extravascular blood found in the abdominal cavity. Increased abdominal muscle tone has a pressor effect on the intraabdominal capacity vessels, which is ceased if muscle relaxants are administered during the anesthesia and this causes subsequent blood pressure drop. Hypotension is further aggravated by the opening of abdominal cavity. This fact underlines the importance of team work. Isolation and draping of the operative field is carried out while the patient is awake, under simultaneous 100 % of oxygen inhalation, followed by rapid induction, quick opening the abdominal cavity and immediate high aortic cross-clamp which actions can only save the patient's life. Heparinization is not required until the aorta is not cross clamped. After the aorta is cross clamped the fluid resuscitation can be instituted with colloids and blood. The dilutional coagulopathy is precnse, FFP and platelets ordered for the patient, and heparin is omissioned. Mortality rate of these operations exceeds the 50 percents and has not changed over the past four decades. The predictors of the survival are the patients age, the total blood loss, and the time of hypotension.

Preparation for the operation includes setting up the following:

1. two 14 G peripheral venous line
2. blood count, electrolytes coagulation screen
3. arterial line
4. ECG monitoring from 5 different points
5. pulsoxymetry
6. urinary catheter
7. gastric tube
8. body temperature monitoring
9. noninvasive blood pressure measurement (from the opposite side than the direct arterial pressure line)

Drugs and fluids:

6-10 units of cross matched blood, fresh frozen plasma and platelets
Crystalloids and colloids
Inotropes (ephedrine 3 mg/ml, adrenaline 1:100 000) and vasopressor agents (phenylephrine 100 mcg/ml, metaraminol 0.5 mg/ ml)

5.3 Thoracic – Thoracoabdominal aneurysm

Operative complications and mortality rate of thoracoabdominal aneurysm surgeries has remained remarkably high despite the development of anesthetic and surgical techniques. High, 5-14 % of mortality rates have been reported by even specialized aneurysm centers which are dealing with a large number of patients. Paraplegia and paraparesis, as postoperative complications develop at 5 - 40 % of all cases. The incidence of complications is influenced by the site of the cross-clamp. The most commonly occurring neurological complications are followed by the pulmonary ones. At thoracic aneurysm operations more vital signs is required to be monitored. It also demands closer collaboration between the vascular surgeon and the anesthetist, because every step of the monitoring has to be set up after developing the operative plan. Particular attention must be paid to the perfusion technique of the distal aorta. Providing adequate perfusion of vertebral and renal arteries and application of satisfactory ventilation are also very important.

Preparation for the operation includes setting up the following:
1. High flow venous catheter, 2 peripheral venous line and 3-lumen central venous line
2. Radial arterial cannula , inserted in the right side if the cross-clamp is placed proximally to the left subclavian artery.
   Femoral arterial cannula, if the bypass is used to maintain the distal aortic flow.
   Radial + femoral , more information can be obtained about the circulation of the lower part of the body
3. Transesophageal echocardiography - intraoperative information: LVEDP, the myocardial function and the valves status
4. Preparation for unilateral ventilation
   Positioning the double-lumen tube can be helped by bronchofiberoscopic intubation.
5. Ten units of red blood cell transfusion, FFP and platelet transfusion.
6. Monitoring of SSEPs (somatosensory evoked potentials)
7. Body temperature monitoring: core and peripheral temperature.

The aneurysm of the ascending aorta is destroyed, need an urgent surgical procedure.
If cross-clamping is applied, significant pressure elevation proximally to the cross-clamping is common. Administration of nitrates and vasodilators is recommended, in case of patient with preserved myocardial systolic function administration of isofluran and desfluran is also suggested. Nitrates can optimize the preload and are able to decrease the left ventricular wall tension. If the operation is performed under the protection of cardiopulmonary bypass (CPB), patient safety is improved if retrograde aortic perfusion is used. In order to ensure appropriate therapy, direct arterial pressure monitoring is registered from two separate regions, above and under the cross-clamping.
In case of thoracic aortic aneurysm surgery balanced anesthesia is the appropriate technique of choice. Protection of the vertebral spine is the most important task, from 20 to 30 minutes of cross-clamping time is considered to be safety. Spinal blood pressure is equal to the difference of mean distal aortic pressure and the cerebrospinal fluid pressure. Cerebrospinal fluid pressure is approximately equal to the central venous pressure. The spinal perfusion autoregulation is similar to the cerebral, appropriate blood flow is maintained between 60-120 mmHg of perfusion pressure.
Applying hypothermia is one of the best solution to ensure adequate neuroprotection, 32 - 34 degrees of Celsius of body temperature is recommended during the operation.
Impairment of renal circulation can also lead to severe complications, administration of mannitol and loop-diuretics and applying hypothermia can prevent these adverse outcomes.
During anesthesia strict attention must be paid to maintain the patient's body fluid and electrolyte balance. If the procedure is done with the patient in the left lateral thoracotomy the CPB is constructed through the femoral artery with venous drainage through right atrial, bicaval, or femoral venous cannulation. Systemic hypothermia is used , with a circulatory arrest. Surface cooling is used along with core cooling and rewarming through the CPB heat exchanger. The cooling of the head with ice during core cooling and kept cold until the period of arrest is important. The core temperature is monitored in the esophagus or tympanic membrane. (Kumar N)

Drugs and fluids:

6-10 units of cross matched blood, fresh frozen plasma and platelets
Crystalloids and colloids

Inotropes (ephedrine 3 mg/ml, adrenaline 1:100 000) and vasopressor agents (phenylephrine 100 mcg/ml, metaraminol 0.5 mg/ ml).
It is very important during induction is to minimize the hypertensive response to laryngoscopy and intubation, which may lead to further spreading of the tear and result in rupture of an aneurysm or propagation of a dissection. Dispite the factthat we could make a long surgery, a large doses of pancuronium are generally avoided. This drug has a vagolytic and norepinephrine releasing effects, which produce hypertension and tachycardia. In patients with significant reduced myocardial function etomidate 0.2 to 0.3 mg/kg may provide the hemodynamic stability during induction. Anesthesia is maintained with inhalation agents, opiates and non-depolarizing muscle relaxants.
Airway management : lesions of the ascending and transverse aortic arch are managed with a single-lumen endotracheal tube. If the aortic lesions may cause tracheal or bronchial compression better to use a left-sided double-lumen tube (DLT). The tube should be placed with using fiberoptic bronchoscopy.
Bleeding and hematologic dysfunction: A thoracic aortic surgery involves using large amounts of blood. The amount of blood used for depends on the bypass time. The time of deep hypothermia has an effect on the clotting system.

Aneurysms of the descending thoracic and thoracoabdominal aorta

Aneurysm of descending thoracic aorta involves diffenert parts of the thoracic aorta and may extend to the abdominal aorta too. Several techniques can be used to control upper- and lower-body blood flow during the operation.

- **Aortic cross-clamping,** This is the method for resection in a short period of time. The problems are the organ ischemia because of arterial hypertension, and metabolic acidosis. The cross clamp duration and severity of complications is directly proportional. A cross-clamping time longer than 30 minutes increases the risk of spinal cord injury
- **Passive shunts,** the most commonly used shunt is the 9-mm heparin-coated conduit (Gott shunt), which does not require systemic anticoagulation.
- **Centrifugal pump bypass flow,** the left atriofemoral centrifugal pump bypass may be useful in patients with decreased left ventricular function, coronary artery disease, renal failere.. and anticipated longer then 30 minutes aortic cross-clamping time.
- **Partial Cardiopulmonary Bypass,** it is used from the femoral vein to the femoral artery, or from the right atria to the femoral artery. This techique adds the use of oxigenator.
- **Deep Hypothermic Circulatory Arrest** has been used to protect vital organs and the spinal cord. Despite the detailed research work has not found the perfect way to protect the spinal cord. Containing a high number of patients in studies based on the present position is that hypothermic protection with CPB and DHCA may be the useful methods.

6. Endovascular procedures

Endovascular stent graft implantation is one of the most suitable alternatives to open aortic aneurysm surgery today. Aortic operations have remarkably changed since the introduction of endovascular techniques. Extremities of implantation technique have been reported in the scientific literature, from the stent-grafts implanted in the X-ray lab percutaneously toward the open stent-graft implantation procedures. Stent-graft

implantation is less invasive, more tolerable for the patients, the length of surgery is shorter, less transfusion is required and the shorter ICU and hospital stay are also the advantages of this technique. Based on our experience stent-graft implantation is considered at those patients, who are referred to be high-risk due to the large number of severe accompanying diseases. In our institute we intend to perform epidural anesthesia at abdominal aortic aneurysm stent-graft repair operations and balanced anesthesia at thoracic cases. Standards of the monitoring technique are the same as that is described at the open procedures. Monitoring improves patient's safety.
Preparation for the procedure includes setting up the following:

1. two 14 G peripheral venous line
2. laboratory exams : blood count, electrolytes , coagulation screen
3. arterial line
4. ECG monitoring from 5 different points
5. pulseoxymetry
6. urinary catheter
7. body temperature monitoring - prolonged operations
8. noninvasive blood pressure measurement (from the opposite side than the direct arterial pressure line)

At the endovascular procedures hemodynamic changes caused by the cross-clamping are not presented. The postoperative period is better tolerated, the pain is milder and the cardiovascular status is more stable. Endovascular stent-graft repair of aortic aneurysms. At present, aortic stent-grafts are most frequently used to repair infrarenal aortic aneurysms. The hemodynamic consequences of infrarenal endovascular balloon inflation are minimal compared with those of suprarenal, supraceliac, or thoracic aortic occlusion. More significant hemodynamic changes are likely to be encountered during stent-graft repair of the descending thoracic aorta.
The high-risk patients undergoing endovascular stent-graft aortic repair appear to have greater hemodynamic stability compared with for the traditional open technique was . Despite this, hypotension and hemodynamic instability could detected, especially during manipulation with expended balloon. Causes of hypotension include hemorrhage and loss of blood into the aneurysm sac after graft implantation, release of endothelial vasoactive substances, and/or an autonomic reflex in response to endovascular balloon inflation.Along the course of the operation, theres is a significant advamtage with the change int he opersation technique, and that the clamping of the aorta is left out or restricted to only a few minutes. During the positioning of the graft , the measured systemic vascular resistence increases but the value (9,2 ±3%)compared to total aortic clamping (32,8 ± 7,6 %) is significantly lower. At this point , following clamping of the abdominal aorta, we experienced a decrease in stroke volume and cardiac output which reached 38% in the cross clamping patients. In patients with stent graft technique this value remained under 9% . The decrease in venous backflow is much lower and therefore the decrease in end diastolic pressure is also lower which influences the left ventricular filling pressure. In a series of 12 patients undergoing infrarenal aortic repair with an EVT endovascular graft under neuroaxial blockade (epidural or continuous spinal), 25% of patients had sudden severe bradycardia and hypotension necessitating immediate therapy. Accordingly, blood must be immediately available, and large-bore intravenous

access must be obtained before the procedure. Because of the high incidence of CAD, careful monitoring and aggressive treatment of myocardial ischemia is essential. Conversion to open repair may be required in 2% to 20% of patients (average, 9%) due to technical difficulty with graft deployment or acute surgical complications such as aneurysm rupture or arterial injury With increasing experience, the need for emergency conversion to open repair is decreasing to approximately 2% to 5% of cases but is still associated with increased morbidity and mortality in these high-risk surgical patients (Kumar N)

In patients with significant coexisting atherosclerotic vascular disease of major organs (heart, brain, kidneys), induced hypertension should be avoided altogether or its duration minimized. A stent-graft that does not require hemodynamic manipulations for its deployment would be more desirable in such patients. The anesthetic technique may consist of general anesthesia, regional anesthesia (epidural, spinal, or continuous spinal), or local anesthesia plus sedation . The choice of technique is influenced by multiple factors, including local customs and the experience of the surgical and anesthetic teams. Consideration should be given to the potential for intraoperative hemodynamic instability and the possible need to react rapidly to surgical complications. The anesthetic goals include analgesia, sedation, anxiolysis, patient immobility, and maintenance of hemodynamic stability. General anesthesia was the most commonly used method during the initial experience with endovascular infrarenal aortic repairs because it provided the ability to rapidly convert to open surgical repair. With evolving experience, regional anesthesia (epidural or spinal) and even local anesthesia with sedation and monitoring are being increasingly used for endovascular aortic repairs A variety of drugs have been used successfully for general anesthesia, including etomidate, , propofol, potent synthetic opioids, volatile anesthetics, and muscle relaxants In patients with severely impaired left ventricular function, etomidate together with a potent opioid such as fentanyl or sufentanil provides adequate hemodynamic stability. Advantages of regional anesthesia include minimization of systemic drug use, continuation of pain relief into the postoperative period, and the improved ability to detect symptoms of myocardial ischemia in patients who can report the occurrence of chest pain. Central neuroaxial blockade was shown to reduce the postoperative hypercoagulable state, which may result in a decreased incidence of deep vein thrombosis and vascular graft occlusion .

The infrarenal cross clamping acts on kidney function only bedside refle and hemodinamic changes. In our stent graft patients we did not experienced a decrease in the renal functions . The infrarenal aortic clamping convincingly increases renin release from the kidney. The increase in plasma renin and angiotensin levels causes a postoperative increase in blood pressure, compared to preoperative values. Because of the variable and unpredictable duration of these procedures, epidural anesthesia is the most commonly used technique because it has the flexibility of providing anesthesia of indefinite duration. Careful titration of the dermatomal level helps minimize the sympathectomy-related hypotension.

Continuation of epidural blockade beyond the operating room is an excellent method of providing postoperative analgesia. A normal coagulation profile must be assured before catheter placement and removal. Continuous spinal anesthesia using an intrathecally placed epidural catheter provides a more rapid onset of a more dense neuroaxial block than does epidural anesthesia. The stent graft technique not only makes the task of the surgeon easier but eases the work of the anesthesiologists. It is important to note that considering the high risk patients we cannot lax th tight monitoring end technical equipment which encure the patient's safety and well being.

6.1 Endovascular technique for ruptured aortic aneurysm: RAAA

The decision of using endograft configuration in the RAAA depends of several factors. For the anesthesia the most important is the hypotension. We are in the position to use intra-aortic occlusion balloons in hemodinamically unstable patients, after the unsuccesfull volumen resuscitaion. It seems to be the hemodinamical instability is the most important factor of the survival in the patients with RAAA undergoing endovascular aortic aneurysm repair.

7. Hybrid solutions in aortic surgery

Hybrid solutions are called for vascular interventions, which are the traditional methods of open vascular surgery and insertion of the endograft are combined in order to reduce the risk of interference. The anesthesiologist must be always ready for a planned change in surgical technique, and the situation has changed to provide the surgeon and the patient to the optimal situation.

8. Reperfusion injury and inflammatory responses following acute revascularization surgery

After revascularization of an acute arterial occlusion the development of a serious ischaemic-reperfusion injury is a menacing challenge and a hard task in vascular surgery. A whale of evidences point to oxidative stress, as an important trigger, in the complex chain of events leading to reperfusion injury.

Arató et al . made examinations, after reperfusion in the 2nd and 24th hours, and on 7th day. Superoxide-dismutase activity, reduced glutathion concentration and leukocytes free radical production were measured. The degree of lipidperoxidation was marked with the quantity of malondialdehyde. The expressions of adhesion molecules were measured with flowcytometry. The speed and rate of free radical production significantly increased in the early reperfusion ($p < 0.05$). The level of antioxidant enzymes decreased after revascularization. The CD11a and CD18 expression of the granulocytes significantly ($p < 0.05$) decreased right after the revascularization, but with a gradual elevation until the 7th day they exceed the ischaemic value. The results showed a time specific turnover of the sensitive antioxidant–prooxidant balance after revascularization operation.

Revascularization procedures performed on acutely ischaemized extremities are accompanied by metabolic and functional derangements which may be life threatening. Determination of selected biochemical, oxidative and inflammatory parameters which belong to the most objective criteria will alert physicians reducing the reperfusion injury cascade. Malondyaldehide plasma level has shown significant elevation after the operation and during reperfusion, it remained almost constant during first post operative week, this determines lipidperoxidation and membrane impairment (Fig. 1).

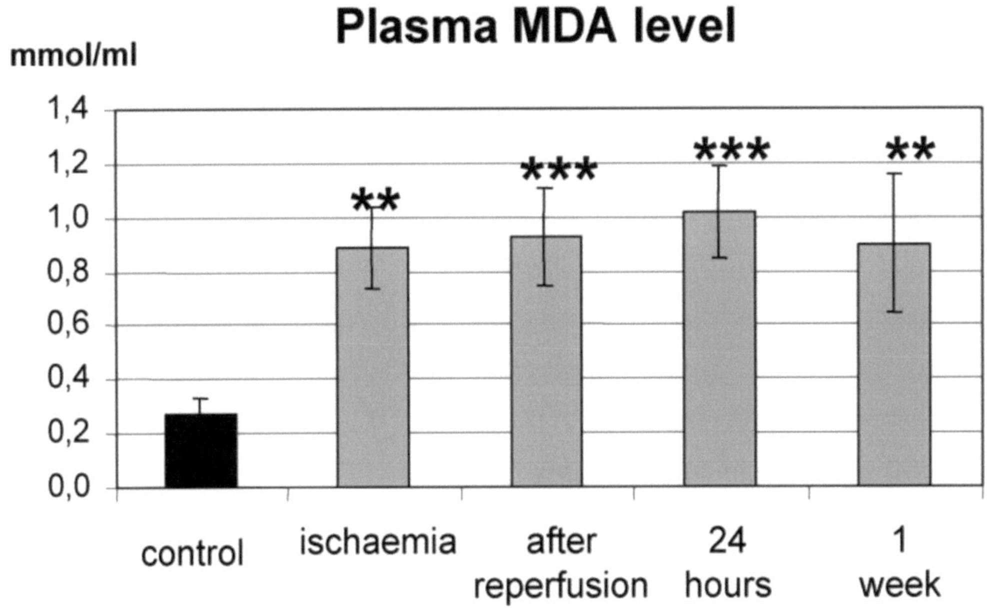

(**$p < 0.01$; *** $p < 0.001$ vs. control).

Fig. 1. The malondialdehyde plasma concentration elevated significantly in all of the operated groups

During early reperfusion period GSH level dramatically diminished ($p < 0.01$) at the sam e time -SH groups levels also decreased (Figs 2 and 3).

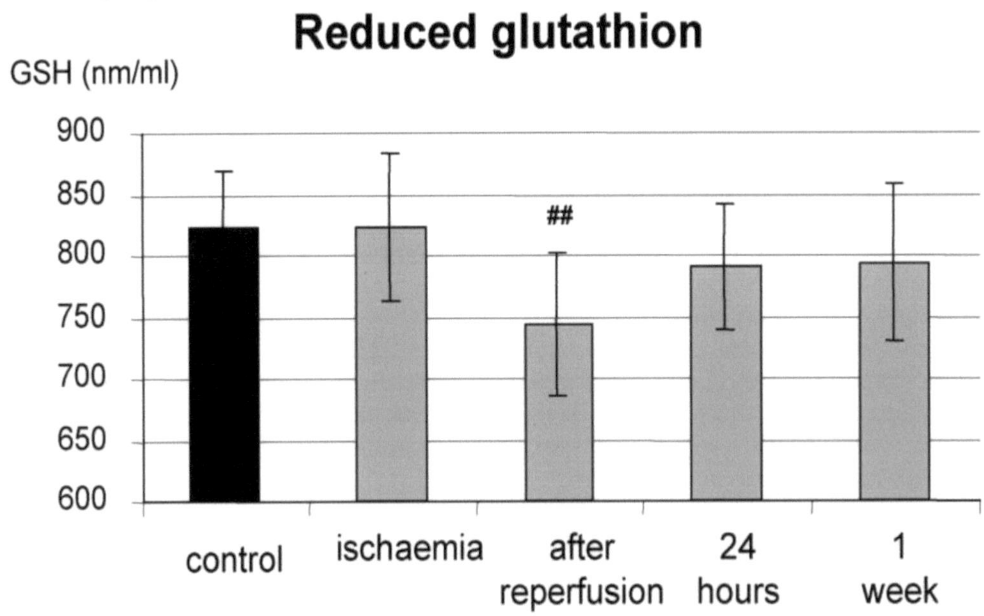

(##p < 0.01 vs. ischaemia).,

Fig. 2. The plasma concentration of reduced glutathion (GSH) decreased significantly in the early, acute phase of reperfusion

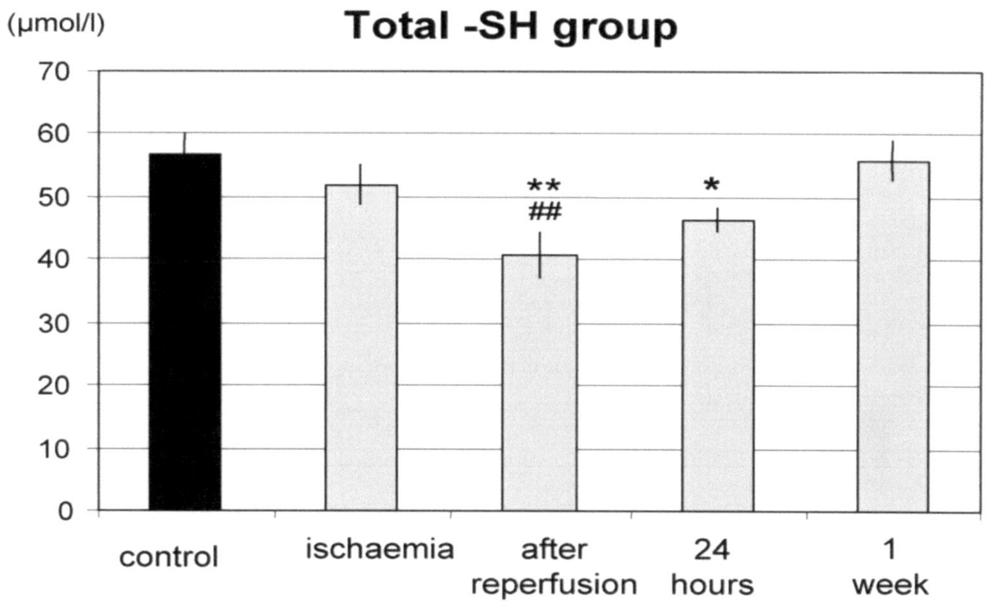

Fig. 3. Plasma concentration of -SH groups decreased significantly in the early reperfusion, then showed a slight elevation till the end of the week (##p < 0.01 vs. ischaemia, *p < 0.05 and **p < 0.01 vs. control).

Regarding SOD activation a notable difference has been noticed between the two groups (control: 894.34 ± 86.85 U/ml, study group: 415.43 ± 75.22 U/ml), and after 24 h a significant reduction has followed (*p* < 0.05) (Fig. 4).

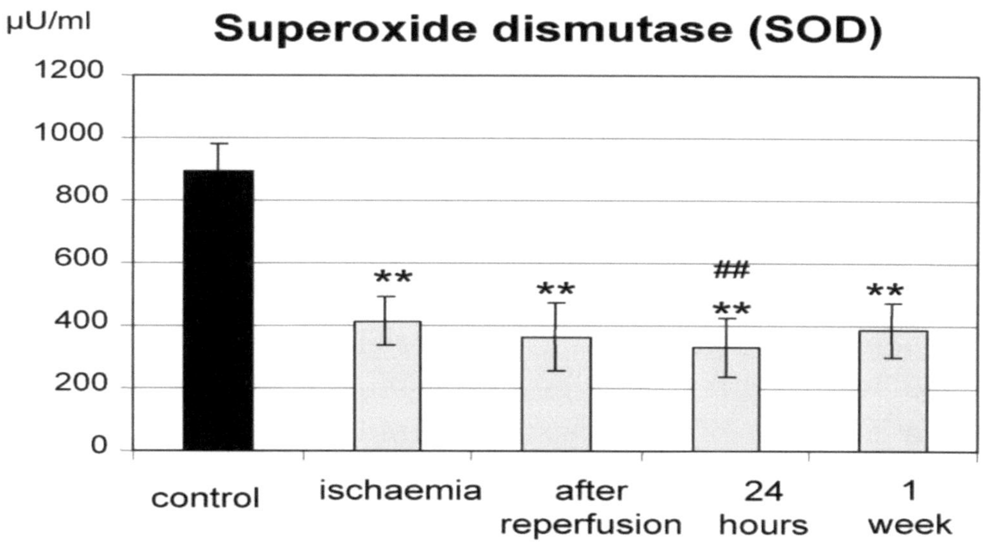

Fig. 4. Total superoxide dismutase activity was significantly lower during ischaemia versus control group, and decreased further in the 24th hour of reperfusion. Even, after a week could not reach the control value (**p < 0.01 vs. control; ##p < 0.01 vs.ischaemia).

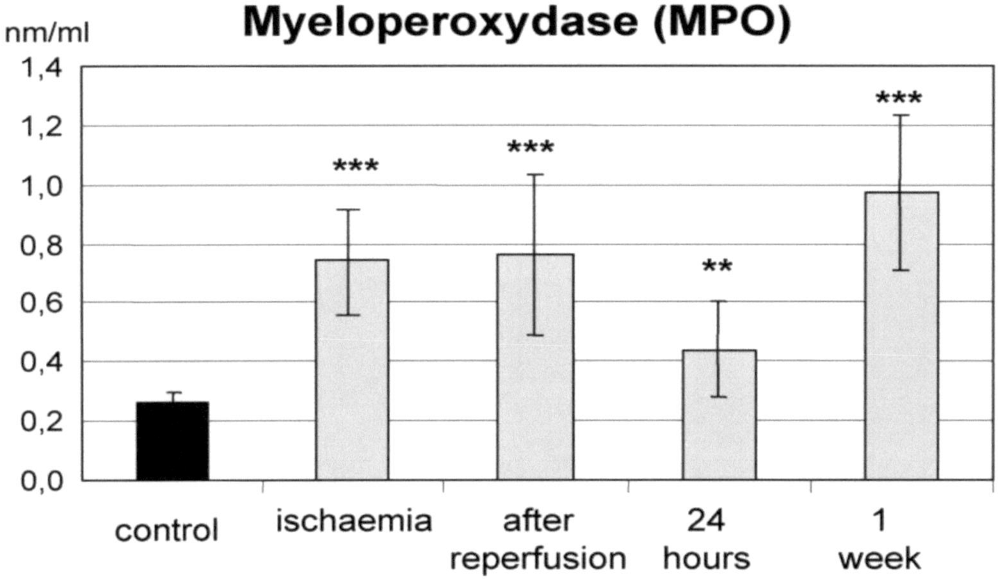

Fig. 5. Plasma myeloperoxidase (MPO) level elevated significantly after revascularization, shows a slight decrease in 24 hours,than increase further in the late reperfusion period (**p < 0.01; ***p < 0.001 vs. control)..

The results show that the reperfusion induced, prompt oxidative stress does not disappear after the early period, but persist until the examined one week postoperative period. The basic pathology in the early reperfusion injury is the oxidative burst with the generation of a mass of oxygen free radicals.

The postischaemic, immediately oxidative turnover induces a massive inflammatory response with the activation of the leukocytes after 24 hours and in the late period these tissue inflammatory responses will maintain the oxidative imbalance.

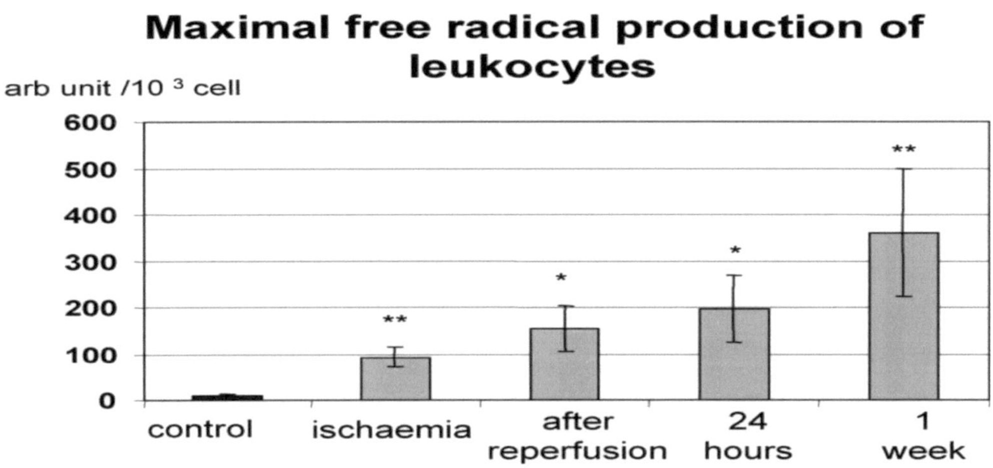

Fig. 6. Maximal free radical production of leukocytes was significantly higher during ischaemia (versus control), and continuously increased until the seventh day (*$p < 0.05$ and ** $p < 0.01$ vs. control).

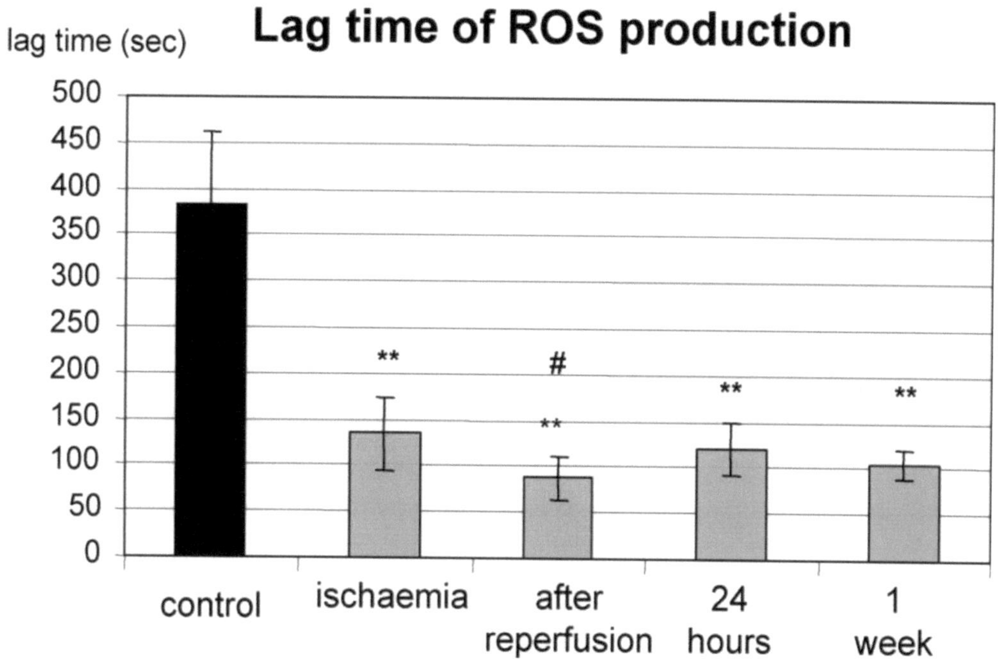

Fig. 7. The "lag time" (taking from induction until the superoxide production) decreased significantly during the reperfusion This showed the significant activation of the leukocytes (# $p < 0.05$ vs. ischaemia* $p < 0.05$ and ** $p < 0.01$ vs. control).

The long time monitoring of the oxidative and inflammatory changes in reperfusion helps to understand the pathology and to develop a more effective therapy.

During exclusion of blood from the circulation ischemia and acidosis appear in the surrounding tissues of the occluded vessels, which try to adapt to the absence of oxygen by switching their metabolism from aerobic to anaerobic, but finally these strategy will lead to tissue damage and loss. In the chronic or acute occlusive diseases the tissue injuries depend on the duration of hypoxia, the mass of tissues involved and the blood pressure of the patients. Reconstruction of the occluded vessels is not without risk, because it can cause volume, pressure and metabolic load, with further tissue damage resulting in the so-called reperfusion injury. Peripheral arterial diseases are a seriously under-diagnosed disorder affecting up to 20 % of the adult population worldwide. Atherosclerotic involvements frequently are in the background, thrombosis or embolization can occur within the narrowed or calcified vessels, or within the aneurismal sites, resulting in serious tissue ischemia.

It is very difficult to monitor the cellular processes, which influence the outcome of the surgical manoeuvres or serve as a marker of the following events. A huge amount of data emerged for the characterization of ischemia reperfusion injury, but function of thrombocytes has been hardly investigated by Kürthy M et al. In their study showed that the duration of hypoxia basically influenced the degree of reperfusion injury in revascularization surgery, resulting in a different outcome in ADP and collagen induced platelet aggregation in whole blood even one week after surgery. Platelet aggregation highly and significantly elevated , in spite of the intensive antiplatelet and antiaggregation therapy. Sinay et al. measured in an *in vivo* animal model the serum total peroxide concentration during infrarenal aortic cross clamping ischaemia and reperfusion. Reperfusion injury is an integrated response to the restoration of blood flow after ischaemia, and is initiated at the very early moments of reperfusion, lasting potentially for days. The extent of the oxidative stress and the consecutive generalized inflammatory response depends on the ischaemic-time, the ischaemic tissue volume, and the general state of the endothelium-leukocyte-tissue functional complex (diabetes, chronic ischaemia, drugs). The pathogenesis of reperfusion injury is a complex process involving numerous mechanisms exerted in the intracellular and extracellular environments. Hypoxia leads to intracellular ATP depletion with a consecutive hypoxanthine elevation. In the early seconds of reperfusion, when the molecular oxygen appears in the cell, the - xanthine oxidase catalised –hypoxanthine–xanthine conversion will produce a mass of superoxide radicals. Superoxide radical and the other reactive oxygen intermediates will damage the membrane-lipids (through lipidperoxidation), the proteins (causing enzyme defects and ion channel injury) and the DNA. These are the main pathways of the cellular oxidant injury. The endogenous antioxidant system defends against these radical injuries .Reactive oxygen species (ROS) will also induce local and systematic inflammatory responses through the inducing of cytokine expression and leukocyte activation. Inflammatory process leads to increased microvascular permeability, interstitial edema, and capillary perfusion depletion. The oxidative and inflammatory pathways will lead to a complex reperfusion injury (Jancsó G ,Fig.8).

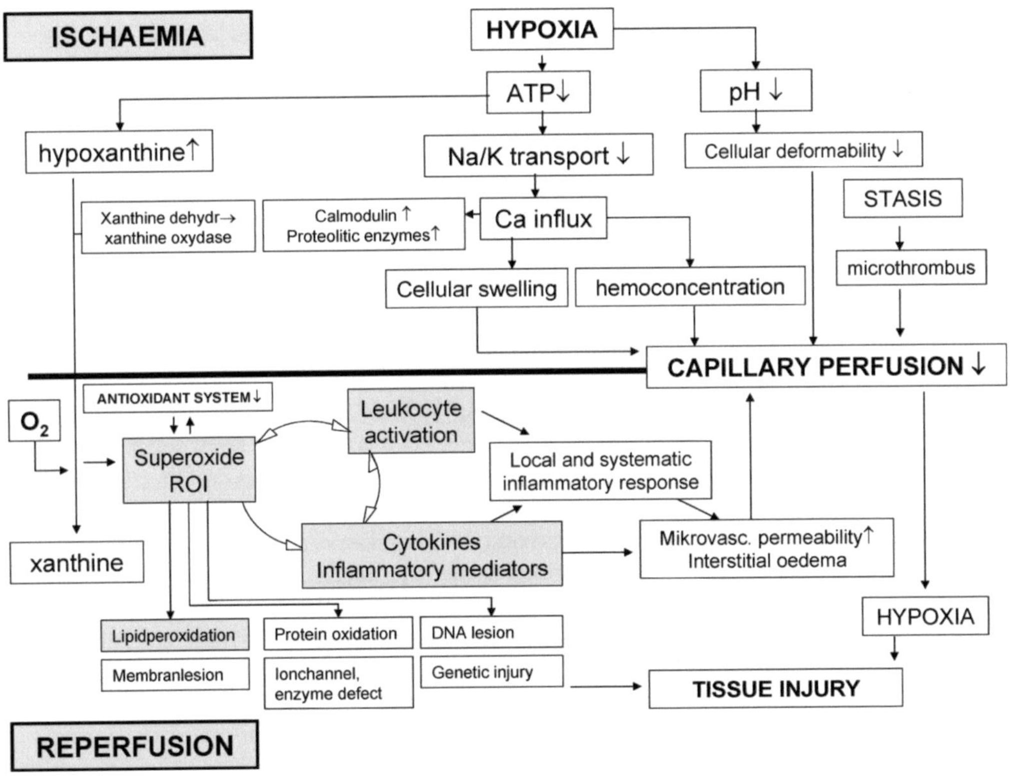

Fig. 8. Simplified presentation of the mechanism of ischaemic–reperfusion injury. Emphasizing, that the engine of reperfusion injury is the ROI–cytokine–leukocyte positive feedback circle (ROI: reactive oxygen intermediers; ATP: adenosine triphosphate; DNA: deoxyribonucleic acid).

9. Conclusions

The management of patients undergoing vascular surgery is one of the most challanging and contraversial area of anesthesiology. The high incidence of coexisting disease, the metabolic stress associated with cross-clamping and unclamping, the ischemic insults in the brain, the heart, the kidneys and the spinal cord resulting a relative high perioperative morbidity in these patients. While these pathways are well known in vascular surgery, there is no real effective tool in the hand of the operating team to treat or to prevent them. As we know how to limit ischemic damage (mostly by reducing the ischemia time via an early reperfusion, and improving O2 demand/supply balance), postconditioning might be the way to prevent or reduce reperfusion damage.

Postconditioning has the advantage of being a way to influence and modify ischaemia-reperfusion injury after it has occurred. This may open a therapeutic alternative in situations of unexpected and uncontrolled ischaemic injury, for instance in the situation where complications occur during surgery, making a simple procedure into a complicated one, and making aortic cross-clamping longer than anticipated.

10. References

Goldman L, Caldera DL, Nussbaum SR, et al.: Multifactorial index of cardiac risk in noncardiac surgical procedures N.Engl.J Med 297:845-850,1977

Manago DT: Perioperative cardiac morbidity. Anesthesiology 72:153-184,1990

Eagle K, Coley CM,Newell JB , et al: Combining clinical and thallium data optimizes preoperative assessment of cardiac risk before major vascular surgery . Ann Intern Med 110:859-866,1989

Lee TH, Marcantonio ER, Mangione CM, et al: Derivation and prospective validation of a simple index for prediction of cardiac risk of major non-cardiac surgery .Circulation 100:1043-1049, 1999.

Poldermans D, Boersma E, Bax JJ, et al: Bisoprolol reduced cardiac death and myocardial infarction in high risk patients as long as two years after succesful major vascualr surgery. Eur. Heart J 22: 1353-1358, 2001.

Myers G, Puskás F : Anesthesia for Vascular Procedures, UCH practice guide

Kumar N, Cowlishaw P, Telford R: Anesthesia for Abdominal Aortic Surgery www.frca.co.uk

Arató E, Jancsó G, Sinay L et al: Reperfusion injury and inflammatory responses following acute lower limb revascularization surgery Clin Hemorheology and Microcirculation 39 (2008) 79–85 79

Kürthy M, Arato E, Jancso G et al.: Duration of hypoxia influences platelet function due to free radical production in revascularization surgery of lower limb Perfusion 2007., 20:187-199

Sinay L, Kürthy M,. Horváth Sz, et al: Ischaemic postconditioning reduces peroxide formation, cytokine expression and leukocyte activation in reperfusion injury after abdominal aortic surgery in rat model Clinical Hemorheology and Microcirculation 40 (2008) 133–142 133

Jancsó G , Cserepes B, Gasz B et al: Expression and protective role of heme oxygenase-1 in delayed myocardial preconditioning Ann N Y 2007 Jan, 1095:251-61

Kertai MD:Preoperative coronary revascularization in high-risk patients undergoing vascular surgery: a core review Anesth Analg.2008.Mar;106(3):751-8.